Symposium on the neurologic aspects of plastic surgery

Volume seventeen

Symposium on the neurologic aspects of plastic surgery

Edited by

SIMON FREDRICKS, M.D., F.A.C.S.

Clinical Professor of Plastic Surgery, University of Texas Medical Branch;
Clinical Associate Professor of Plastic Surgery,
Baylor College of Medicine,
Houston, Texas

GARRY S. BRODY, M.D., F.A.C.S.

Clinical Assistant Professor of Surgery (Plastic),
University of Southern California;
Chief, Plastic and Reconstructive Surgery Service,
Rancho Los Amigos Hospital,
Downey, California

Proceedings of the Symposium of the Educational Foundation of the American Society of Plastic and Reconstructive Surgeons, Inc., held at Houston, Texas, January 27-30, 1977

with 385 illustrations

The C. V. Mosby Company

Saint Louis 1978

Volume seventeen

Printed in the United States of America

The C. V. Mosby Company
11830 Westline Industrial Drive, St. Louis, Missouri 63141

Library of Congress Cataloging in Publication Data

Symposium on the Neurologic Aspects of Plastic Surgery, Houston, Tex., 1977.
Symposium on the Neurologic Aspects of Plastic Surgery.

(Proceedings of the symposium of the Educational Foundation of the American Society of Plastic and Reconstructive Surgeons; v. 17)
Bibliography: p.
Includes index.
1. Neuromuscular diseases—Surgery—Congresses. 2. Nerves, Peripheral—Surgery—Congresses. 3. Surgery, Plastic—Congresses. I. Fredricks, Simon. II. Brody, Garry S. III. Series: American Society of Plastic and Reconstructive Surgeons. Educational Foundation. Proceedings of the symposium; v. 17. [DNLM: 1. Neurosurgery—Congresses. 2. Surgery, Plastic—Congresses. WL368 S992s 1977]
RD595.S95 1977 617'.483 78-7355
ISBN 0-8016-1679-4

TS/U/B 9 8 7 6 5 4 3 2 1

Contributors

Prof. Dr. Hans Anderl

University Professor, University Klinik fur Plastische- und Wiederherstellungschirurgie, Head: Prof. Dr. P. Wilflingreder, Innsbruck, Austria

Joseph Agris, M.D., D.D.S.

Assistant Professor of Surgery, Cora and Webb Mading Department of Surgery, Division of Plastic Surgery, Baylor College of Medicine; Chief of Surgery, Texas Institute for Rehabilitation and Research, Houston, Texas

Lois M. Barber, B.S., O.T.R.

Clinical Instructor, University of Southern California, School of Occupational Therapy; Chief Therapist, Downey Community Hospital, Hand Rehabilitation Center, Downey, California

Margaret E. Brand, M.B., B.S. (London)

Chief, Ophthalmology Department, Public Health Service Hospital, Carville, Louisiana; Associate Clinical Professor, Ophthalmology, Tulane University Medical School, New Orleans, Louisiana

Paul W. Brand, M.B., B.S. (London), F.R.C.S. (Eng.)

Chief, Rehabilitation Branch, Public Health Service Hospital; Clinical Professor of Surgery and Orthopedics, Louisiana State University Medical School, Carville, Louisiana

Garry S. Brody, M.D., F.A.C.S.

Clinical Assistant Professor of Surgery (Plastic), University of Southern California; Chief, Plastic and Reconstructive Surgery Service, Rancho Los Amigos Hospital, Downey, California

John Conley, M.D.

Professor Emeritus, Clinical Otolaryngology, Columbia Presbyterian Medical Center; Chief Head and Neck Service, St. Vincent Hospital, New York, New York

Raymond M. Curtis, M.D.

Chief, Division of Hand Surgery, Union Memorial Hospital; Associate Professor of Plastic Surgery, Associate Professor of Orthopaedic Surgery, Johns Hopkins University; Consultant (Hand Surgery) to the Surgeon General of the Army, Baltimore, Maryland

Jonathan J. Dora, M.D.

Cora and Webb Mading Department of Surgery, Division of Plastic Surgery, Baylor College of Medicine, Houston, Texas

Thomas B. Ducker, M.D.

Professor and Head of Neurosurgery, University of Maryland School of Medicine and University of Maryland Hospital; Attending Physician and Consultant, University Hospital, Maryland Institute of Emergency Medicine, and Mercy Hospital, Baltimore, Maryland

William W. Fish, M.D.

Assistant Professor, Orthopedic Surgery, McGill University; Assistant Professor, Department of Physical Medicine, Royal Victoria Hospital, Montreal, Quebec

Bromley S. Freeman, M.D., F.A.C.S.

Clinical Professor, Plastic Surgery, Baylor College of Medicine; Attending Plastic Surgeon, The Methodist Hospital, Houston, Texas

Frank J. Gerow, M.D., F.A.C.S.

Professor of Plastic Surgery, Cora and Webb Mading Department of Surgery, Division of Plastic Surgery, Baylor College of Medicine, Houston, Texas

Valerie Gonzales, O.T.R.

Occupational Therapist, Rancho Los Amigos Hospital, Downey, California

Patti Harder, R.P.T.

Staff Physical Therapist, Spinal Injury Service, Rancho Los Amigos Hospital, Downey, California

M. Mark Hoffer, M.D.

Chief, Department of Surgery, Rancho Los Amigos Hospital; Assistant Clinical Professor, University of Southern California, Department of Orthopaedics and Pediatrics, Downey, California

Melton J. Horwitz, M.D., F.A.C.S.

Clinical Assistant Professor, Division of Otolaryngology, University of Texas Medical School, Houston; Clinical Assistant Professor, Department of Otorhinolaryngology and Communicative Sciences, Baylor College of Medicine, Houston, Texas

John D. Hsu, M.D., F.A.C.S.

Attending Orthopaedic Surgeon; Chief, Muscle Disease Clinics, Rancho Los Amigos Hospital, Downey, California; Director, M.D.A.A. Clinic, Orthopaedic Hospital; Assistant Professor, Surgery (Orthopedics), University of Southern California, School of Medicine, Los Angeles, California

Michael E. Jabaley, M.D.

Professor and Chairman, Division of Plastic Surgery, University of Mississippi Medical Center, Jackson, Mississippi

Frederick C. Kauffman, Ph.D.

Associate Professor, Pharmacology and Experimental Therapeutics, University of Maryland, School of Medicine, Baltimore, Maryland

Thomas J. Krizek, M.D.

Professor of Surgery; Chief, Section of Plastic and Reconstructive Surgery, Yale University School of Medicine, New Haven, Connecticut

Timothy A. Miller, M.D.

Chief, Plastic Surgery, Wadsworth Veterans Hospital; Associate Professor of Surgery, Division of Plastic Surgery, UCLA School of Medicine, Los Angeles, California

Hanno Millesi, M.D.

Professor of Plastic Surgery; Head, Department of Plastic and Reconstructive Surgery at the First Surgical Clinic of the University of Vienna; Head, Ludwig Boltzmann Institute for Experimental Plastic Surgery, Vienna, Austria

Erik Moberg, M.D.

Professor Emeritus, Orthopedic and Hand Surgery, University of Göteborg, Göteborg, Sweden

Vert Mooney, M.D.

Professor and Chairman, Division of Orthopedics, University of Texas Health Science Center, Dallas, Texas

Dozent Dr. med. Wolfgang D. Mühlbauer

Department of Plastic Surgery, Technical University of Munich, Munich, Germany

George E. Omer, M.D., M.S. (Orthopaedic Surgery)

Professor and Chairman, Department of Orthopaedics and Rehabilitation; Professor and Chief, Division of Hand Surgery, Department of Surgery; School of Medicine, University of New Mexico, Albuquerque, New Mexico

James B. Reswick, Ph.D.

Director, Rehabilitation Engineering Center, Rancho Los Amigos Hospital, Downey, California

Walker L. Robinson, M.D.

Assistant Professor, Division of Neurosurgery, University of Maryland School of Medicine and University of Maryland Hospital; Consultant Neurosurgeon, Maryland Institute of Emergency Medicine, U.S. Public Health Hospital, Baltimore, Maryland

Martin C. Robson, M.D.

Professor of Surgery; Chief, Section of Plastic and Reconstructive Surgery, University of Chicago Pritzker School of Medicine, Chicago, Illinois

Bryan Roper, M.D.

Fellow in Orthopedic Surgery, Rancho Los Amigos Hospital, Downey, California

Leonard R. Rubin, M.D., F.A.C.S.

Diplomate, American Board of Plastic Surgery; Clinical Professor of Plastic Surgery, State University of New York at Stony Brook, Stony Brook, New York; Director, Plastic and Maxillofacial Surgery and the Burn Center, Nassau County Medical Center, East Meadow, New York

Michael Salcman, M.D.

Assistant Professor of Neurosurgery, University of Maryland School of Medicine and University of Maryland Hospital; Consultant Neurosurgeon, Maryland Institute of Emergency Medicine, Baltimore, Maryland

Melvin Spira, M.D.

Professor and Head, Division of Plastic Surgery, Baylor College of Medicine, Houston, Texas

E. Shannon Stauffer, M.D.

Professor and Chairman, Orthopaedics and Rehabilitation, Southern Illinois University School of Medicine, Springfield, Illinois; formerly Director of the Spinal Injury Center, Rancho Los Amigos Hospital, Downey, California

Susan Swank, M.D.

Fellow in Orthopedic Surgery, Rancho Los Amigos Hospital, Downey, California

David Taylor, M.D.

Resident in Orthopedic Surgery, University of California, Irvine, California

Julia K. Terzis, M.D., F.R.C.S. (C)

Assistant Professor of Surgery, McGill University; Assistant Surgeon, Royal Victoria Hospital, Montreal, Quebec

F. William Wagner, Jr., M.D.

Director, Amputee-Diabetic Service, Rancho Los Amigos Hospital, Downey, California

Robert L. Waters, M.D.

Chief, Stroke Service, Rancho Los Amigos Hospital, Downey, California

Ervin S. Wheeler, M.D.

Resident, Department of Surgery, UCLA School of Medicine, Los Angeles, California

Roger Wickenden, M.D.

Fellow in Orthopedic Surgery, Rancho Los Amigos Hospital, Downey, California

H. Bruce Williams, M.D.

Professor of Surgery; Chairman, Plastic Surgery, McGill University; Director, Plastic Surgery, Montreal General Hospital and Montreal Children's Hospital, Montreal, Quebec

Libby F. Wilson-Mackby, M.D.

Chief, Cleft Palate Service, Rancho Los Amigos Hospital; Assistant Clinical Professor, Department of Surgery, University of Southern California School of Medicine, Downey, California

The authors wish to dedicate this book
to their colleague

THEODORE F. WILKIE

whose efforts on behalf of cerebral palsy
children were unique.
His death at the height of his abilities
was precipitously premature.
His warmth and presence will be missed.

Symposium faculty

SIMON FREDRICKS, M.D., *Cochairman*
GARRY S. BRODY, M.D., *Cochairman*

Hans Anderl, M.D.
Lois M. Barber, O.T.R.
Margaret E. Brand, M.D.
Paul W. Brand, M.D.
John Conley, M.D.
Raymond M. Curtis, M.D.
Thomas B. Ducker, M.D.
Bromley S. Freeman, M.D.
Frank J. Gerow, M.D.
M. Mark Hoffer, M.D.
Melton J. Horwitz, M.D.
Michael E. Jabaley, M.D.
Timothy A. Miller, M.D.
Hanno Millesi, M.D.
Erik Moberg, M.D.
Vert Mooney, M.D.
Wolfgang D. Mühlbauer, M.D.
George E. Omer, M.D.
Martin C. Robson, M.D.
Leonard R. Rubin, M.D.
Morton Spinner, M.D.
Melvin Spira, M.D.
E. Shannon Stauffer, M.D.
Julia K. Terzis, M.D.
Robert L. Waters, M.D.
H. Bruce Williams, M.D.
Libby F. Wilson-Mackby, M.D.

Preface

We had a longing to perceive the possibilities still dim and in the distance.

The neuromusculo-receptor marriage is vital to a full-bodied and robust life. The nervous system serves as the coordinating communicator between the senses that reveal our environment and the muscular system, the motor-driven effector. Without one the other is nothing but wasted and lost potential.

To be afflicted by the conditions studied in this symposium is to endure and therefore to be miserable. They are conditions without the compassion of coma or an end point of death. These malfunctions are lifelong, agonizing, and frustrating. These patients truly suffer and deserve our attention.

To cure is elusive and for the foreseeable future perhaps impossible. But surely, to improve, to substitute for, or to mitigate is within our combined capabilities.

Problems of such complexity are best understood by a multidisciplinary approach. The interdigitation of all available knowledge by all concerned modalities was our intent and this volume the fruit of our combined deliberation.

Here we present in a portable, easily disseminated manner the current essence of understanding and therapeutics. The interface of such sincere and inventive workers was inspiring and appeared to produce a rededication of effort.

We wish to express our appreciation to the 125 participants of this symposium who made it possible.

We are humbled by the hopes and aspiration of the thousands whose lives we sincerely pray might be improved by the collection of offerings which is this text.

Simon Fredricks

Garry S. Brody

Contents

Color plate

Part I

Neurophysiology and sensation

Chapter 1

Metabolism of peripheral nerve injuries

Thomas B. Ducker
Michael Salcman
Frederick C. Kauffman

Injury to the whole or any part of an organism causes marked changes in the existing metabolic status. The peripheral nervous system of man is no exception. Knowledge about the metabolic alterations associated with peripheral nerve lesions aids in determining the timing of an operation and the chances of a successful nerve repair.

The central and peripheral nervous systems are a single functioning unit whose purpose is to process information. Impulses travel down the spinal cord and synapse on the anterior horn cell to initiate action throughout the body or the periphery. Peripheral nerves are simply bundles on axons, the long extensions of neuronal cell bodies located within the spinal cord and brain stem. If the central system is diseased, then inadequate or incorrect information will be passed to and from the periphery. If the peripheral system is diseased, the same principle applies. In addition, if a segment of the system dies, for example, as in poliomyelitis, there are not only central nervous system changes but also degenerative changes in peripheral nerves and muscle.

We will approach the metabolic factors in the surgery of peripheral nerves in a dual fashion. The normal metabolic state will be described first. Then the changes in metabolism that are seen with injury or disease will be outlined. These normal and abnormal metabolic states will be reviewed from central to peripheral along the nerves, starting with the central cell or the dorsal ganglion cell and ending with the muscle cell or the sensory end organ.

NERVE CELL BODY

Injury to a peripheral nerve or axon involves removal of a large portion of the nerve cell volume; however, the biochemical machinery required for repair remains largely intact because it is localized in the soma or cell body. Because of their unique geometry nerve cells must synthesize large amounts of structural material and transport these materials over relatively long distances. If the central cell body were the height of an average man, its axon would be 2 to 5 cm in diameter and would extend more than 3.2 km. The energy expenditure needed to synthesize structural materials, as well as factors associated with neurotransmission, and to transport these over long distances becomes very large and requires markedly enlarged and metabolically hyperactive cell bodies. The mature nerve cell is one of the most metabolically active cell types in our bodies.[67] With axonal injury or disease, even higher metabolic activity occurs, and profound changes take place in the structure as well as in the biochemical and physiologic properties of the cell body. Some of these changes may be viewed as particularly appropriate for the repair process. After axonal injury, chromatolysis, nuclear eccentricity, nucleolar enlargement, and cell swelling are the most conspicuous morphologic changes seen during the retrograde response.[47] For peripheral axons these changes have been associated with a reorganization and enhanced formation of cytoplasmic ribonucleic acid (RNA) to a more active state directed toward the reconstitution of lost axoplasm and recovery of peripheral connections.[6,55,69]

Increases in RNA synthesis, as expected, have been associated with enhanced cytoplasmic protein synthesis, demonstrated by the incorporation of radioactive amino acid precursors.[7,24,25,28,69] The changes in protein synthesis are complex and appear to involve a reordering of the various types of proteins synthesized by the injured neuron. Materials required for transmitter function are decreased, while materials required for regeneration of the axon are elevated. For example, in adrenergic neurons, decreases in dopamine-β-hydroxylase, dopa decarboxylase, monamine oxidase, and tyrosine hydroxylase activities occur after axonotomy.[15,45,60,61] Similar decreases in acetyl cholinesterase and choline acetyltransferase have been reported in axonotomized cholinergic neurons.[37,47] In contrast, the activity of glucose-6-phosphate dehydrogenase, a key enzyme by which glucose is converted to precursors required for the biosynthesis of nucleic acids and lipids, is significantly elevated in axonotomized neurons.[34,35,70]

A number of histochemical and biochemical studies have demonstrated that the activity of glucose-6-phosphate dehydrogenase is increased in axonotomized nerve cell bodies. Spinal anterior horn cells, facial nucleus, neurons, and sympathetic ganglion cells, all of which direct axons to peripheral structures, show such changes in the pentose phosphate pathway.[33,38,46,56,62] Increases in this activity are not observed in neuronal perikarya whose axons undergo wallerian degeneration.[50] In extended studies of metabolic changes in the rat superior cervical ganglion, strong evidencc has been obtained that increases in glucose-6-phosphate dehydrogenase occurring shortly after axonotomy are associated with increased metabolism of glucose via the anabolic pentose pathway.[34,35] This increase occurs in the absence of any gross alteration in the major energy-yielding reactions such as ATP utilization and oxygen consumption.

Enhanced metabolism via the pentose pathway may have special significance in injured peripheral neurons because two functions of this pathway are to generate NADPH for reductive biosynthetic reactions and to form ribose phosphate required for nucleic acid and ribonucleotide biosynthesis. Studies carried out on nonneuronal tissue provide strong evidence that the formation of NADPH by the pentose pathway is intimately related to the biosynthesis of fatty acids.[4] A similar relationship may exist in regenerating neural tissuse because significant increases in lipid synthesis begin within the first week after axonal injury.[34,35,52]

The regenerative process in nerve cell bodies is complicated by the simultaneous occurrence of extensive hydrolytic activity during the period of enhanced biosynthetic activity. A marked increase in acid phosphatase and a corresponding increase in the internal complexity and number of lysosome-like dense bodies has been frequently noted in axonotomized nerve cells.[49,65] Matthews and Raisman[49] have suggested that the increased hydrolytic activity is related to a digestion of transmitter storage granules in nerve cells. It is not known whether these changes are a necessary prerequisite for axonal sprouting and regeneration.

The regenerative capacity of neurons varies with age. Axonal outgrowth from proximal stumps of transected nerves appears to be more rapid, and reconnection with denervated end organs occurs more rapidly in younger animals than in older animals.[31,53] Pertinent histologic and temporal characteristics of the retrograde response of various classes of neurons in young animals have been recently reviewed by Brodal.[10] Data concerning biochemical differences between young and mature axonotomized nerve cells is minimal, and it is not clear what mechanisms account for the greater regenerative capacity of neural tissue from immature animals. Nerve cells from very young mammals tend to degenerate when axonal lesions are introduced at or during the first few days after birth.[29] These differences reflect but one aspect of the major biologic problem of the nature and control of cellular differentiation, which is itself poorly understood. Nevertheless, these findings have important practical implications for the physician. For example, the neuron's reparative demands may be readily met in a teenager who has a sharp cut of a digital nerve, indicating immediate repair. On the other end of the spectrum, a person in his 50s with a proximal blast injury to the ulnar nerve does not have significant regenerative powers until 2 to 3 weeks after injury, and even then the neuron may be so busy in an effort to survive that its regenerative efforts are, in essence, ineffective.

SUPPORTIVE GLIAL CELLS

The glial cells form the supportive structure of the central nervous system and are thought to help regulate metabolic events external to the neuronal membrane. They invest the neurons in such a way that sugars, amino acids, and other solutes freely circulating in the extracellular space are made available for the nerve cell's metabolism.[68] Neuroglia also have comparatively high resting membrane potentials and a high internal potassium level, which may serve to distribute potassium ions to aid or create surface potentials in active axons.[11,54]

Glial cells in close association with axonotomized neuronal perikarya undergo alterations that influence metabolic changes accompanying neuronal regeneration. A proliferation of microglia close to perikarya occurs shortly after axonotomy; in some cases this change is associated with displacement of synaptic boutons from the perikarya and dendrites of nerve cells. Activation of metabolism in glia surrounding injured neurons is suggested by hypertrophy of astrocytes in the vicinity of axonotomized nerve cell bodies.[48] Literature dealing with glial responses during antegrade and retrograde neuronal responses has been recently reviewed.[10] Relevant to defining those events that take place in glial elements and nerve cells, Watson[71] has shown that in contrast to neuronal responses the onset of metabolic changes in astrocytes surrounding nerve cells in the hypoglossal nucleus is independent of the level at which the hypoglossal nerve is injured.

PROXIMAL NERVE TRUNK

Regeneration of a damaged axon requires the restoration of large quantities of axonal lipids and proteins, which are synthesized in the nerve cell body and delivered to the growing axon by transport systems. There is more than one distinct transport process, and materials are transported at different rates. The slow component may be mediated by peristalsis in the nerve trunk plasms, and the fast component involves active participation of microtubules. Inconsistent results have been obtained in studies of the effect of axonotomy on fast axonal transport.[14,26,28,57] These inconsistencies may be explained by the recent findings that axonotomy produces different responses in different nerves of the same animal.[26] Griffin and associates[30] studied fast axoplasmic flow in regenerating rat sciatic nerves. They demonstrated that the rate of fast flow was not altered in the proximal nerve trunk and that the rapidly transported proteins were carried past the level of axonotomy into regenerating nerve sprouts. Materials moved down the sprouts at the normal rate of about 400 mm per day. Although rates of axoplasmic flow may not be altered in the regenerating axon, evidence has been obtained that the amount of protein transported is increased.[30] Functional adaptation of axoplasmic flow in regenerating axons may also involve a reordering of the types of proteins transported. As discussed above, the production of proteins associated with transmitter function seems impaired while formation of proteins associated with the repair process is enhanced in nerve cell bodies that have sustained axonal injury.

PROXIMAL NERVE STUMP

Within 1 hour of cutting a peripheral nerve, there is marked proximal swelling, as much as 1 cm, from the point of disruption. The amount of swelling is greater than previously realized, for the cross-sectional area of the nerve increases three times.[21] The swelling consists of both intracellular and extracellular edema, mostly a gellike amorphous substance that contains a large quantity of acid mucopolysaccharides.[13,59] It persists for a week or more and subsides slowly thereafter.

Within 2 to 3 days after transection of a nerve there are signs of demarcation of the nerve stump or healing over of the open end of the neuron. After a week there is vigorous sprouting of the axons. In traumatic blast wounds the axonal sprouting may be 1, 2, or even 3 cm proximal to the point of the actual severed end. In a clean operative sectioning this occurs for only a few millimeters retrograde. Between 1 and 3 weeks, axon buds begin to advance across the anastomosis of a primary neurorrhaphy.[43,44] The onset of this budding and regeneration occurs concomitantly with the anabolic hypertrophic phase of the cell body in the spinal cord or dorsal ganglion.

Thus all evidence indicates that there is a delay from a few days to a few weeks before the axon buds and crosses a repair site. Thus, operations for the repair of an injured nerve need to be planned when the regenerative efforts of the nerve are at their initial maximum performance.

Axon elongation and the transduction of chemical energy to sustain this process are central issues in the ongoing nerve regeneration. The process of axon elongation appears to originate at growth cones situated at the tip of axons.[74] Growth cones are characterized by a profuse elaboration of microspikes that explore the environment and establish direction for growth.[74] The direction as well as the amount of branching displayed by a growing axon is influenced by adhesion between the cell surface and the substratum upon which it grows.[64] Thus, initiation as well as maintenance of axon elongation may involve changes in the cell surface. Extension of a growing fiber seems to take place at the tip of the fiber.[9]

It is unlikely that sustained axonal growth could occur without the enhanced metabolic activity generated in the cell body during the retrograde reaction. This is supported by the finding that the rate of axonal outgrowth is faster after the second of two successive axonal injuries.[51] Presumably the necessary metabolic adaptation for optimal axonal regeneration has taken place prior to the second injury.[27]

Little information exists concerning the biologic signal that initiates nerve sprouting. Considerable evidence exists that trophic interactions occur between target tissues and nerves that somehow regulate innervation. One hypothesis that has gained support is that target tissues continually manufacture a substance that stimulates nerves to sprout; this substance is neutralized in a negative feedback manner by the release of neural factors that are carried to nerve endings by axoplasmic flow.[3] This hypothesis explains "denervation sprouting" and also explains the phenomenon of collateral sprouting. The recovery of function after sectioning of certain peripheral nerves may be best seen as the collateral sprouting of remaining fibers.[17]

SUPPORTIVE MESENCHYME AND NEUROECTODERM AT INJURY SITE

Within hours after transection of a nerve the metabolism of the Schwann cells, the perineural epithelial cells, and the epineurium increases. Two to three days after injury there is a cellular proliferation of nearly all elements in both proximal and distal stumps. After the first week the most active cell is the Schwann cell, which now has assumed a phagocytic function. The response of these cells is directly proportional to the severity of the wound. For example, battle injuries of peripheral nerves are characterized by a marked inflammatory response and retrograde demarcation of the nerve anatomy several centimeters from the actual point of severance of the nerve.[36] Conversely a clean operative injury or knife cut is not associated with a marked tissue reaction, and the response of the Schwann cell is minimal. As the debris is cleared from the injury area, a mesenchymal and neuroectodermal scar is left behind. This tissue is, for the most part, not longitudinally aligned, so that any early axonal regeneration becomes twisted and entangled. In time, a traumatic neuroma may form as the neuronal buds push into a reactive cellular conglomerate that has no anatomic planes.

At the site of injury, supportive cells from both stumps dominate the dynamic and metabolic action in the early posttraumatic period when there are only the earliest signs of axonal budding and regeneration. The orientation of the mesenchymal cells left behind after the debridement of Schwann cells is dependent on the state of the wound and local geometry rather than on chemotaxis and so on.[1,31] There is evidence that these cellular structures can be longitudinally aligned by mechanical devices such as wraps or tubes.*

*References 8, 12, 13, 20, 21, 32, 73.

With a repair, regardless of the timing, both proximal and distal stumps swell and become edematous. The swelling includes axons in the proximal stump, and the amount of the increase may be two to three times the normal cross-sectional area of the nerve in higher primates and in man.[21] Studies indicate that silicone rubber possesses physical properties that best delimit the mesenchymal proliferation and force longitudinal alignment, without constricting the nerve.[20] Larger tubes or cuffs allow for swelling in the immediate postrepair period and force longitudinal alignment of the rapidly proliferating supportive structures. Concurrently with the decrease in edema, the neuron bud advances and pushes into the intercellular spaces before the mesenchymal cellular and collagen proliferation becomes impermeable. With the more direct axonal spanning there should be improvement in functional return.[22,58] And with time and maturation the new nerve trunk returns to normal size, and the larger cuffs are not constrictive. Proper dimensions have been worked out and commercial nerve cuff kits are available.[22] If there is a longitudinal scar as opposed to a random scar at a repair site, there is more direct spanning of the regenerating axons. While the histologic picture of the repair site definitely improves with cuffing, there is only a little improvement in the final functional result. Sensory return is benefited the most by cuffing.[22,73]

It must be stressed that (1) the response to injury of the supportive structures is immediate, and thick collagen is laid down starting 3 weeks after injury, and (2) the response of the neuron at the site of injury is delayed until axonal budding and regeneration take place. Thus if nerve repairs are done immediately, the scar at the anastomosis may be too thick for effective axonal penetration. If the repair is delayed 3 weeks, the axonal sprouts from the now metabolically active central cell can push into the anastomotic site almost immediately before the supportive cells completely congest the repair site. Therefore a properly planned delayed operative repair, metabolically speaking, places the neurons and supportive elements on a more equal footing. The actual amount of delay depends on the level of the lesion, the severity of wounding, and the age and general condition of the patient.

DISTAL NERVE TRUNK

The distal nerve stump can react only with supportive structures. The axonal elements that are separated from their trophic centers die. A reactive schwannoma or peripheral glioma may form from the proliferating supportive elements and can inhibit regenerating axonal penetration. However, these metabolically active and dividing neurolemmal and mesenchymal cells can be cut away at the time of repair. They will react again, but in a sequence and with the timing outlined above.

Wallerian degeneration of the nerve is defined as the death of all neuronal elements distal to the site of injury. This term should be applied primarily to those changes in the distal stump or trunk. It can include deterioration of the proximal stump back to the next node of Ranvier. After injury, digestive enzymes are present in the axonal segments.[46,59] Parts of the axonal segments, often near the stump, may isolate themselves into small units that can survive up to 2 weeks, but most neuronal elements break down within a week. The surrounding myelin undergoes fragmentation and is digested by the Schwann cells. By 3 weeks most of this cellular debris is phagocytosed by the metabolically active Schwann cells. By 6 weeks the debridement is complete. Parts of the fascicular anatomy persist in the distal nerve, and the endoneural sheaths either shrink or become nonexistent.[39,40,41,63] The entire nerve shrinks, and in time the shrinkage becomes irreversible and downgrades the prognosis of unduly postponed nerve repair. The neuroectodermal and mesenchymal elements are in part dependent on the nerve fibers to maintain anatomic and metabolic existence.

With penetration of new axons the Schwann cell again increases its metabolic activity, but not for phagocytic function. Fresh myelin is layered around the nerves by the Schwann cells. The electron microscopic details of this process have been worked out, as well as certain metabolic features. To the surgeon who is repairing a peripheral nerve the axonal regrowth is the primary concern, and the myelin reconstitution will take place only if regeneration occurs. However, remyelinization is never as good as the premorbid state; and this fact, along with nerve size and endoneural tube size, accounts for the slower conduction times of the distal nerve trunk after repair.

Practically all the metabolites in the distal peripheral nerve trunk come from the central cell via axoplasmic flow. Enlargement of the central cell is not limited to the period soon after injury, but also occurs at the end of regeneration when the myoneural junctions are being formed. Engh and associates showed that there is a consistent increase in synthetic activity within the central cell that occurs with axonal maturation.[23,24] The combination of the building of new synaptic end-plates and the return of a trophic perikaryal stimulus to and from the reinnervated peripheral structure may cause a greater increase in metabolism in the central cell than occurs in the immediate posttraumatic period.

Regeneration down most peripheral distal nerve trunks averages about 1 mm per day or 2.5 cm per month. Initially however there is a delay until the neuron is clearly across the anastomosis. In some cases regeneration may occur as fast as 3 mm per day. There is a slowing of the regenerative process with the forming of new connections with the muscle or sensory organs or both.

MUSCLE CELL

The biochemical as well as electrophysiologic properties of skeletal muscles are influenced by peripheral nerves. After nerve injury the muscle cells shrink, the endomysium and perimysium thicken, and the muscle spindles atrophy. These changes may be ascribed, in part, to a loss of neurotrophic factors supplied to the muscles by the nerves. This long-term regulatory property of motor neurons is clearly distinct from the more commonly studied electrophysiologic properties.[2,18] The early alterations that occur after nerve section or injury include a decline in resting membrane potential, the appearance of extrajunctional acetylcholine sensitivity, and a decrease in muscle phosphocreatine.[2,42] The time course of these changes is dependent upon the distance from the muscle at which the nerve is transected as well as the type of muscle that has been denervated, but in general these changes take place over the first 3 days after nerve section in small mammals. Muscle atrophy begins at 2 to 16 weeks in animals and somewhat later in man; with time (2 years or more), muscle fibers may fragment and disintegrate.[3] Such changes take place despite good physical therapy or intermittent external electric stimulation or both. To date, denervation atrophy can be halted only by reinnervation, where constant stimuli from gamma and alpha fibers as well as delivery of neurotrophic substances result in sufficient drive of the metabolism of the muscle cell. Any denervation atrophy of the muscle is harmful because the thickening of the muscle sheath hinders end-plate formation, and formation of fibrous tissue in and around the muscle interferes with nerve regrowth and muscle contraction. Thus the sooner a nerve establishes connection with the muscle, the more likely the metabolism and anatomy of the muscle will be normal. If reinnervation is delayed to

1 year, function is very poor. A delay of 2 years allows irreversible changes to take place in the muscle cells, and any hope of motor return at that time is practically nil.

SENSORY END ORGANS

The sensory end organs are less dependent on nerve innervation for survival. In fact, the evidence from a World War II study yielded no evidence that the time from injury to nerve repair influenced sensory recovery in any way.[58] There are no metabolic studies of these cells to account for the clinical observations, but it is acceptable therapy to perform, for example, a markedly delayed sciatic nerve repair to gain protective sensation of the foot.

GENERAL SYSTEMIC METABOLIC STATUS

The age of the patient is the most important general factor influencing metabolic status. There are no statistical studies to validate the fact that the younger the patient, the better he regenerates a peripheral nerve; yet all experienced surgeons have made this observation. Children sometimes have close to 100% return after a distal nerve repair. Nerve growth factors found in the laboratory have not been tried in human patients. Clinically one suspects that growth hormone may be helpful, but it has not been used. There is evidence that thyroid hormone promotes peripheral nerve regeneration; however, the clinical usefulness of thyroid hormone in patients with injured or transected peripheral nerves has not been fully evaluated.[16]

The wound wherein the nerve was injured is important. Massive blast injuries result in thick scar formation and delayed healing. A regenerating nerve may become scarred and entrapped in such injuries, and motor and sensory recovery fails. Or, the blast injury can result in distal ischemia of the limb and irreversible changes in all structures, including the distal nerve trunk and distal muscles. Or, multiple war-inflicted injuries may result in a catabolic state of the patient for 2 or 3 months and adversely influence nerve regeneration.

When analyzing studies dealing with nerve regeneration in experimental animals it is important to consider phylogeny. Although regeneration of spinal cord is currently impossible in man, certain lizards regrow segments of spinal cord when the tail is cut off. Rats and dogs can have their nerves severed and not reanastomosed, yet their regenerative efforts are so strong that nerve continuity is restored and motor and sensory return will occur. Monkeys at times will do the same. The nerves of adult baboons and chimpanzees behave more like those of man.

SUMMARY

Respect for the metabolic changes within the neuron is critical in planning peripheral nerve surgery. Only by understanding the different metabolic responses of nerve tissue and supportive tissue can anastomosis be planned when the budding neuron stands its best chance of successfully regenerating across a repair site. Usually, a short delay in nerve repair is indicated. When all factors are ideal, good motor function can be counted on across one joint from the next group of muscles. Rarely is there good function across two. Protective sensory function can be achieved distally even under the most adverse metabolic conditions because of the independent metabolic state of these end organs.

REFERENCES

1. Abercrombie, M., Johnson, M. L., and Thomas, G. A.: Influence of nerve fibers on Schwann cell migration investigated in tissue culture, Proc. R. Soc. Med. **136:**460, 1949.
2. Albuquerque, E. X., and McIsaac, R. J.: Fast and slow mammalian muscles after denervation, Exp. Neurol. **26:**183-202, 1970.
3. Aquilar, C. E., Bisby, M. A., Cooper, E., and Diamond, J.: Evidence that axoplasmic transport is involved in the regulation of peripheral nerve fields in salamanders, J. Physiol. (Lond.) **234:**449-464, 1973.
4. Banquer, N. Z., Cascales, M., Teo, B. C., and McLean, P.: The activity of the pentose phosphate pathway in isolated liver cells, Biochem. Biophys. Res. Comm. **52:**263-269, 1973.
5. Bowden, R. E. M., and Gutmann, E.: Denervation and re-innervation of human voluntary muscle, Brain **67:**273-313, 1944.
6. Brattgard, S. O., Edstrom, J. E., and Hyden, H.: The chemical changes in regenerating neurons, J. Neurochem. **1:**316-325, 1957.
7. Brattgard, S. O., Edstrom, J. E., and Hyden, H.: The productive capacity of the neuron in retrograde, Exp. Cell Res. **5:**185-200, 1958.
8. Braun, R. M.: Comparative studies of neurorrhaphy and sutureless peripheral nerve repair, Surgery **122:**15-18, 1966.
9. Bray, D.: Model for membrane movement in the neural growth cone, Nature **244:**93-96, 1973.
10. Brodal, A.: Anterograde and retrograde degeneration of neurons in the central nervous system. In. Haymaker, W., and Adams, R. D., editors: Histology and histopathology of the nervous system, Springfield, Ill., 1973, Charles C Thomas, Publisher.
11. Bunge, R. P.: Structure and function of neuroglia: some recent observations. In Schmitt, I. O., editor: The neurosciences (second study program), New York, 1970, The Rockefeller Press.
12. Campbell, J. B., Bassett, C. A. L., and Bohler, J.:

Frozen-irradiated homografts shielded with microfilter sheaths in peripheral nerve surgery, J. Trauma **3:**303-311, 1963.

13. Campbell, J. B., and Luzio, J.: Symposium: facial nerve rehabilitation. Facial nerve repair: new surgical techniques, Trans. Am. Acad. Ophthalmol. Otolaryngol. **68:**1068-1075, 1964.
14. Carlsson, C. A., Bolando, P., and Sjostrand, J.: Changes in axonal transport during regeneration of feline ventral roots, J. Neurol. Sci. **14:**75-93, 1971.
15. Cheah, T. B., and Geffen, L. B.: Effects of axonal injury on norepinephrine, tyrosine hydroxylase and monoamine oxidase levels in sympathetic ganglia, J. Neurobiol. **4:**443-452, 1973.
16. Cockett, S. A., and Kiernan, J. A.: Acceleration of peripheral nervous regeneration in the rat by exogenous triiodothyronine, Exp. Neurol. **39:**389-394, 1973.
17. Coers, C., and Woolf, A. L.: The innervation of muscle; a biopsy study, Oxford, England, 1959, Blackwell Scientific Publications Ltd.
18. Deshpande, S. S., Albuquerque, E. X., and Guth, L.: Neurotrophic regulation of prejunctional and postjunctional membrane at the mammalian motor end plate, Exp. Neurol. 1978. In press.
19. Diamond, J., Cooper, E., Turner, C., and Macintyre, L.: Trophic regulation of nerve sprouting, Science **193**(4251):371-377, 1976.
20. Ducker, T. B., and Hayes, G. J.: Peripheral nerve injuries: a comparative study of the anatomic and functional results following primary nerve repair in chimpanzees, Milit. Med. **133:**298-302, 1968.
21. Ducker, T. B., and Hayes, G. J.: Experimental improvements in the use of silastic cuff for peripheral nerve repair, J. Neurosurg. **28:**582-587, 1968.
22. Ducker, T. B., Kempe, L. G., and Hayes, G. J.: The metabolic background for peripheral nerve surgery, J. Neurosurg. **30:**270-280, 1969.
23. Engh, C. A., and Schofield, B. H.: The review of the central response to peripheral nerve injury and its significance in nerve regeneration, J. Neurosurg. **37:**195-203, 1972.
24. Engh, C. A., Schofield, B. H., Doty, S. B., and Robinson, R. A.: Perikaryal synthetic function following reversible and irreversible peripheral axon injuries as shown by radioautography, J. Comp. Neurol. **142:**465-480, 1971.
25. Francoeur, J., and Olszewski, J.: Axonal reaction and axonplasmic flow as studied by radioautography, Neurology (Minneap.) **18:**178-179, 1968.
26. Frizell, M., and Sjostrand, J.: Transport of proteins, glyeoproteins and cholinergic enzymes in regenerating hypoglossal neurons, J. Neurochem. **22:**845-850, 1974.
27. Grafstein, B.: The nerve cell body response to axotomy, Exp. Neurol. **48**(3 pt. 2):32-51, 1975.
28. Grafstein, B., and Murray, M.: Transport of protein in goldfish optic nerve during regeneration, Exp. Neurol. **25:**494-508, 1969.
29. Grant, G.: Neuronal changes central to the site of axon transection. A method for the identification of retrograde changes in perikarya, dendrites and axons by silver impregnation. In Nauta, W. J. H. and Ebbesson, Contemporary research methods in neuroanatomy, New York, S. O. E., editors: 1970, Springer-Verlag.
30. Griffin, J. W., Drachman, D. B., and Price, D. C.: Fast axonal transport in motor nerve regeneration, J. Neurobiol. **7:**355-370, 1976.
31. Guth, L.: Regeneration in the mammalian peripheral nervous system, Physiol. Rev. **36:**441-478, 1956.
32. Gutmann, E.: Histology of degeneration and regeneration. In Licth, S., editor: Electrodiagnosis and electromyography, Baltimore, 1961, Waverly Press.
33. Harkonen, M.: Carboxylic esterases, oxidative enzymes and catecholamines in the superior cervical ganglion of the rat and the effect of pre- and postganglionic nerve division, Acta Physiol. Scand. [Suppl.] **63**(237):1-94, 1964.
34. Harkonen, M. H. A., and Kauffman, F. C.: Metabolic alterations in the axotomized superior cervical ganglion of the rat. I. Energy metabolism, Brain Res. **65:**127-139, 1974.
35. Harkonen, M. H. A., and Kauffman, F. C.: Metabolic alterations in the axotomized superior cervical ganglion of the rat. II. The pentose phosphate pathway, Brain Res. **65:**141-157, 1974.
36. Haymaker, W.: Pathology of peripheral nerve injuries, Military Surg. **102:**448-459, 1948.
37. Hebb, C. O., and Waites, G. M. H.: Choline acetylase in antero- and retro-grade degeneration of a cholinergic nerve, J. Physiol. **132:**667-671, 1956.
38. Hirsch, H. E., and Obenchain, T.: Acid phosphatase activity in individual neurons during chromatolysis: a quantitative histochemical study, J. Histochem. Cytochem. **18:**828-833, 1970.
39. Hudson, A., Morris, J., Redman, F., and Waddell, G.: An electron microscopic study of regeneration in severed rat sciatic nerves anastomosed with silastic cuffs, Curr. Top. Surg. Res. **3:**187-190, 1971.
40. Hudson, A., Morris, J., and Waddell, G.: An electron microscopic study of regeneration in sutured rat sciatic nerves, Surg. Forum **21:**451-453, 1970.
41. Hudson, A., Morris, J. Waddell, G., and Drury, A.: Peripheral nerve autographs. An electron microscopic study, Surg. Res. In press.
42. Kauffman, F. C., and Albuquerque, E. X.: Effect of ischemia and denervation on metabolism of fast and slow mammalian skeletal muscle, Exp. Neurol. **28:**46-63, 1970.
43. Kline, D. G., Hayes, G. J., and Morse, A. S.: A comparative study of response of species to peripheral-nerve injuries. I. Severance. J. Neurosurg. **21:**968-979, 1964.
44. Kline, D. G., Hayes, G. J., and Morse, A. S.: A comparative study of response of species to peripheral-nerve injury. II. Crush and severance with primary suture, J. Neurosurg. **21:**980-988, 1964.
45. Kopin, I. J., and Silberstein, S. D.: Axons of sympathetic neurons: transport of enzymes *in vivo* and properties of axonal sprouts *in vitro*, Pharmacol. Rev. **24:**245-254, 1972.
46. Kreuzberg, G. W.: Changes of coenzyme (TPN diaphorase and TPN linked dehydrogenases) during axonal reaction of the nerve cell, Natute **199:**393-394, 1963.

47. Lieberman, A. R.: The axon reaction: a review of the principle features of perikaryal responses to axon injury, Int. Rev. Neurobiol. **14:**49-124, 1971.
48. Lieberman, A. R.: Some factors affecting retrograde neuronal responses to axonal lesions. In Bellairs, R., and Gray, E. G., editors: Essays on the nervous system, Oxford, 1974, The Claredon Press.
49. Matthew, M. R., and Raisman, G.: A light and electron microscopic study of the cellular response to axonal injury in the superior cervical ganglion of the rat, Proc. R. Soc. Lond. (Biol.) **181:**43-79, 1972.
50. McCaman, R. E., and Robbins, E.: Quantitative biochemical studies of Wallerian degeneration in the peripheral and central nervous systems. II. Twelve enzymes, J. Neurochem. **5:**32-42, 1959.
51. McQuarrie, I. G., and Grafstein, B.: Axon outgrowth enhanced by a previous nerve injury, Arch. Neurol. **29:**53-55, 1973.
52. Miani, N.: Metabolic and chemical changes in regenerating neurons. III. The rate of incorporation of radioactive phosphate into individual phospholipids of the nerve cell perikaryon of the C-8 spinal ganglion *in vitro*, J. Neurochem. **9:**537-541, 1962.
53. Moyer, E. K., Kimmel, D. L., and Winborne, L. W.: Regeneration of sensory spinal nerve roots in young and senile rat, J. Comp. Neurol. **98:**283-300, 1953.
54. Murray, M., and Grafstein, B.: Changes in the morphology and amino acid incorporation of regenerating goldfish optic neurons, Exp. Neurol. **23:**544-560, 1969.
55. Murray, M.: ^{3}H-uridine incorporation by regenerating retinal ganglion cells of goldfish, Exp. Neurol. **39:**489-497, 1973.
56. Nandy, K.: Histochemical study on chromatolytic neurons, Arch. Neurol. **18:**425-434, 1968.
57. Ochs, S.: Systems of material transport in nerve fibers (axoplasmic transport) related to nerve function and trophic control, Ann. N.Y. Acad. Sci. **228:**202-223, 1974.
58. Ochs, S., Sabri, M. I., and Johnson, J.: Fast transport system of materials in mammalian nerve fibers, Science **163:**680-687, 1969.
59. Oester, Y. T., and Davis, L.: Recovery of sensory function. In Woodhall, B., and Beebe, G. W., editors: Peripheral nerve regeneration, U.S. Government Printing Office, 1956, Washington, D.C.
60. Reis, D. J., and Ross, R. A.: Dynamic changes in brain dopamine β-hydroxylase activity during anterograde and retrograde reactions to injury of central noradrenergic axon, Brain Res. **57:**307-326, 1973.
61. Reis, D. J., Ross, R. A., and Joh, T. H.: Some aspects of the reaction of central and peripheral noradrenergic neurons to injury. In Fuxe, K., Olson, L., and Zotterman, Y., editors: Dynamics of degeneration and growth in neurons. (Wenner-Cren Symposium XII) Oxford, 1974, Pergamon Press Ltd.
62. Robbins, E., Kissane, J. M., and Lowe, I. P.: Quantitative biochemical studies of chromatolysis. In Folch-Pi, J., editor: Chemical pathology of the nervous system, Oxford, 1961, Pergamon Press Ltd.
63. Sjostrand J.: Morphological changes in glial cells during nerve regeneration, Acta Physiol. Scand. [Suppl.] **67**(270):19-43, 1966.
64. Strassman, R. J., Letourneau, P. C., and Wessells, N. K.: Elongation of axons in an agar matrix that does not support cell locomotion, Exp. Cell Res. **81:**482-487, 1974.
65. Sumner, B. E. H.: The effects of injury on two hydrolases in the hypoglossal nucleus, with quantitative data on N-acetyle-β-glucosaminidase, Brain Res. **68:**157-166, 1974.
66. Torvik, A., and Heding, A.: Effect of actinomycin D on retrograde nerve cell reaction. Further observations, Acta Neuropath. (Berl.) **14:**62-71, 1969.
67. Turner, R. S.: Chromatolysis and recovery of efferent neurons, J. Comp. Neurol. **79:**73-78, 1943.
68. Varon, S.: Neurons and glia in neural cultures, Exp. Neurol. **48:**93-134, 1975.
69. Watson, W. E.: An autoradiographic study of the incorporation of nucleic acid precursors by neurons and glia during nerve regeneration, J. Physiol. (Lond.) **180:**741-753, 1965.
70. Watson, W. E.: Observations on the nucleolar and total cell body nucleic acid of injured nerve cells, J. Physiol, (Lond.) **196:**655-676, 1968.
71. Watson, W. E.: Some quantitative observations upon the response of neuroglial cells which follow axotomy of adjacent neurons, J. Physiol. (Lond.) **210:**321-342, 1972.
72. Watson, W. E.: The binding of actinomycin D to the nuclei of axotomized neurons, Brain Res. **65:**317-322, 1974.
73. Weiss, P. A.: Neuronal dynamics and neuroplasmic flow. In Schmitt, F. O., editor: The neurosciences (second study program), New York, 1970, The Rockefeller Press.
74. Yamada, K. M., and Wessels, N. K.: Axon elongation: effect of nerve growth factor on microtubule protein, Exp. Cell Res. **66:**346-352, 1971.

Chapter 2

Functional microanatomy of the peripheral nerve

Julia K. Terzis

Easy access for experimental manipulation along with the development of sophisticated morphologic and electrophysiologic techniques has enhanced our knowledge and understanding of the functional anatomy of the peripheral nerve. Microsurgical expertise has allowed manipulation of the inner connective tissue sheaths of the peripheral nerve, improving the alignment of previously inaccessible bundles and facilitating excision of entrapping scar tissue. Much of the information obtained however is disseminated among a wide range of specialized fields and thus is not readily available to the clinician. Histochemical, biochemical, ultrastructural, and physiologic studies have reached a level of sophistication that escapes the understanding of the newcomer.

The following discussions serve two purposes: (1) to summarize the current concepts of the morphology and physiology of the peripheral nerve and (2) to present pilot data on the functional anatomy of one peripheral nerve, utilizing a novel and objective approach.

STRUCTURE

The building block of the nervous system is the neuron, a unique cell with capabilities of processing, assimilating, and conducting information. The neuron consists of a cell body or soma, one or more dendrites, and an axon. The dendrites are cytoplasmic extensions invading nearby areas, which serve as receiving antennae conveying incoming information to the cell body. The axon conducts the coded stimuli away from the cell body, making functional contact with other dendritic and neuronal surfaces or with effector sites at the periphery. The axonal processes external to the pial sheath that covers the central nervous system constitute the peripheral nerves.

The nerve fiber is the structural and functional unit of the peripheral nervous system; it consists of an axon with its associated Schwann cells. The Schwann cell is a nonexcitable cell that supports, nourishes, and maintains the enclosed axon. Peripheral nerve fibers enter or exit the spinal cord at the dorsal and ventral roots respectively. Both unite distal to the spinal ganglion of the dorsal root to form the spinal nerves (Fig. 2-1). The dural sheaths become confluent at the level of the ganglion and then merge with the epineurium of the spinal nerve. Soon after their formation each spinal nerve divides into a dorsal and ventral branch. The dorsal rami innervate the structures of the back, while the ventral rami supply the extremities and ventrolateral trunk. In the cervical and lumbosacral areas the anterior divisions merge and intermingle to form plexuses. There is an appreciable amount of reshuffling at the plexus level, although fibers destined to innervate the anterior limb maintain a stubborn independence from posteriorly destined fibers. Just at the root of the limb the major peripheral nerve trunks arise, which then course to their musculocutaneous terminations.

A peripheral nerve trunk is composed of neural and nonneural elements. The nonneural elements are all mesodermally derived structures serving the one function of the survival, preservation, and well-being of the enclosed nerve fibers. In essence there are three connective tissue sheaths associated with a peripheral nerve. These are the epineurium, perineurium, and endoneurium. The sheaths con-

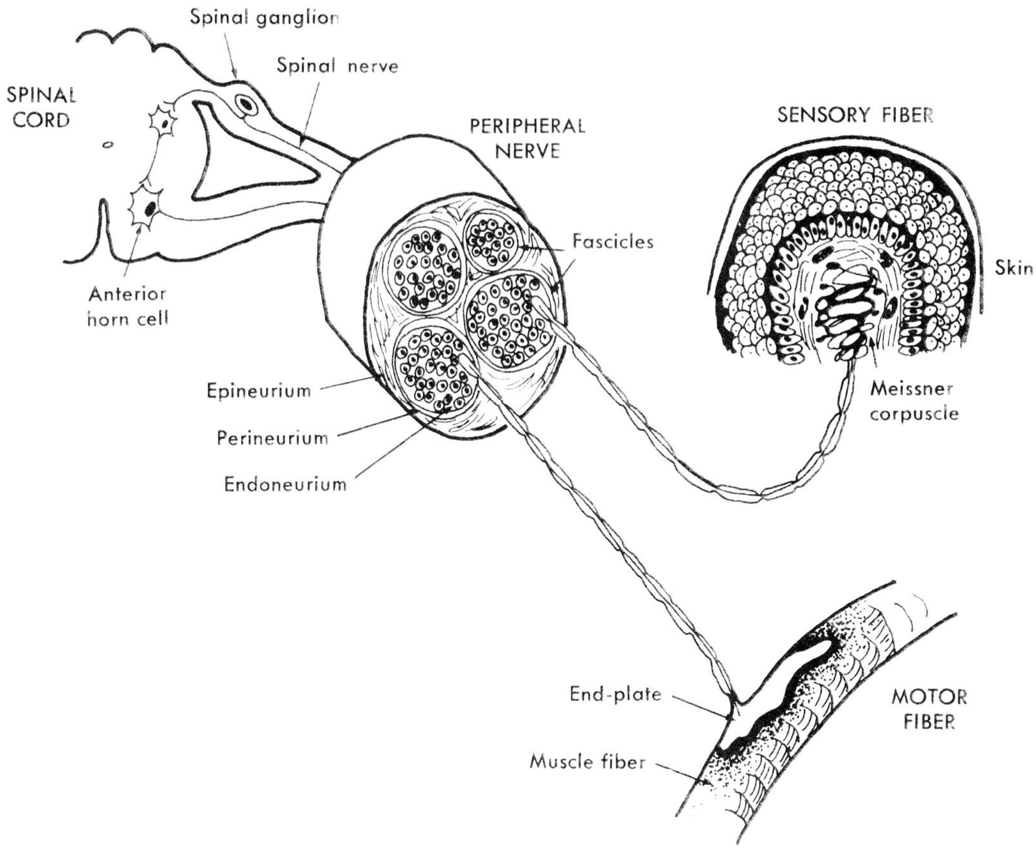

Fig. 2-1. Diagram of peripheral nerve depicting its proximal attachments and distal terminations.

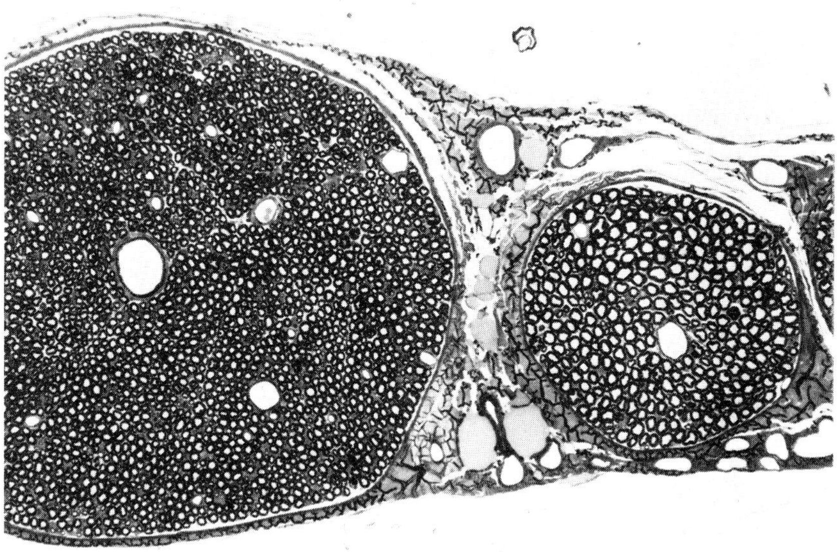

Fig. 2-2. Cross section of peripheral nerve. Note epineurial sheath that surrounds enclosed fascicles. Each fascicle contains nerve fibers, endoneurial collagen, and extensive capillary network; it is delimited by perineurium. Myelinated fibers stand out because of their size and staining properties. (Courtesy Dr. Peter S. Spencer.)

vey the intrinsic blood supply and lymphatic vessels, and the nervi nervorum that provide the nonneural structures with sympathetic and sensory innervation.

Each nerve fiber is individually surrounded by endoneurium, while large aggregates are enveloped by a sheath of perineurium. Such a bundle of fibers covered by a perineurial sheath constitutes a fascicle (fasciculus, funiculus). Groups of fascicles, held together by epineurial connective tissue, form the peripheral nerve trunk (Fig. 2-2). The epineurium is composed of loosely arranged, longitudinal collagen bundles, blood vessels, lymphatics, and adipose tissue. Its main function is to invest and support the enclosed nerve fascicles. The perineurium, the intermediate layer between endoneurium and epineurium, is the most cellular of the three sheaths and is composed of an outer dense collagenous layer and an inner cellular layer. The cellular portion consists of several layers of characteristically flattened squamous cells that are enveloped by a basal lamina and whose cytoplasm contains numerous pinocytotic vesicles. Functions ascribed to the perineurial sheath include active transport, diffusion barrier, maintenance of positive pressure, and structural support. The endoneurium consists of a loose collagenous matrix, a few fibroblasts and mast cells, and the intrafascicular capillary network.

These three morphologically distinct connective tissue sheaths provide a mechanical constraint for the enclosed nerve fibers, which nevertheless is not prohibitive enough to exclude intermingling. Repeated fasciculation along with numerous intraneural microplexuses continues to reshuffle and segregate axonal processes along the course of the peripheral nerve. Only very distally does ultimate fiber destination dictate some sort of provision for specific connections with receptor and effector mechanisms. Thus the initially mixed fiber population in the proximal level of the limb undergoes a progressive ordering by a process of divisions and reunions that seems to taper off only in proximity to the end organs. Even then, as we shall see later, pure uniformity among nerve fibers is never attained.

Nerve fibers are divided into one of two classes: myelinated and unmyelinated (Fig. 2-3).

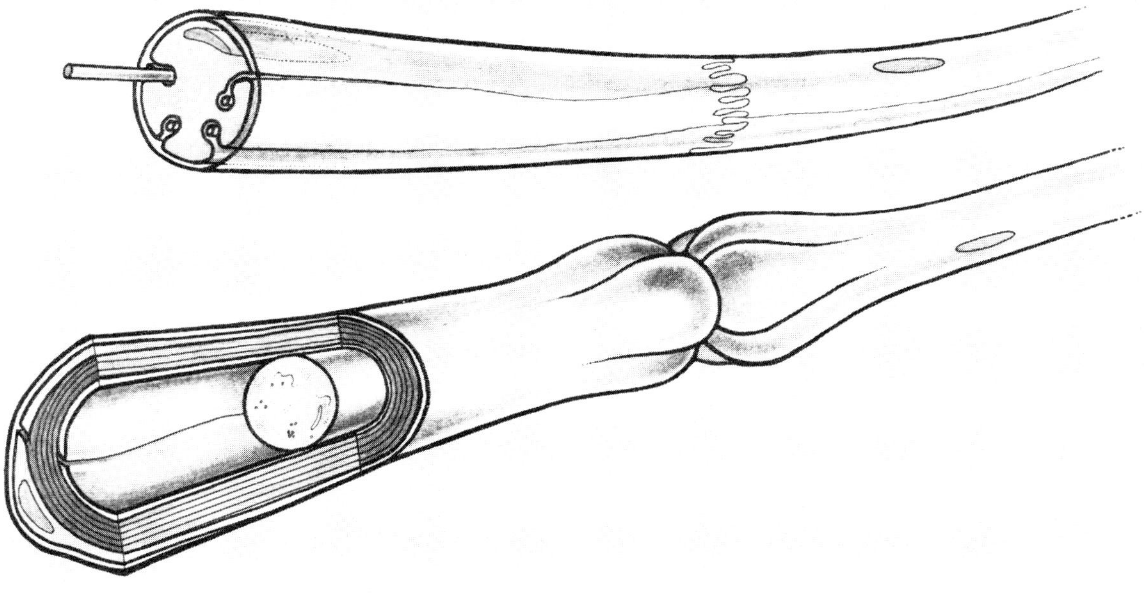

Fig. 2-3. Examples of myelinated and unmyelinated fibers. Note axon–Schwann cell relationships in each fiber. Myelinated fiber *(below)* has been transected at several levels to demonstrate enclosed axon, Schwann cell, and myelin sheath. Notched region between the two adjacent Schwann cells clearly defines node of Ranvier. Unmyelinated fiber *(above)* consists of four unmyelinated axons embedded in cytoplasm of single Schwann cell. Note that boundaries of two adjacent Schwann cells are not as clearly defined here. (From Daniel, R. K., and Terzis, J. K.: Reconstructive microsurgery, Boston, 1977, Little, Brown and Company.)

MORPHOLOGY

Myelinated nerve fiber

The giant unmyelinated axon of the invertebrates and the mammalian myelinated nerve fiber share as a common feature the rapidity of impulse transmission. Myelinization probably evolved to provide a structural economy to a system that required quick exchange of information. Thus the morphologic peculiarities of myelinated nerve fibers reflect their function as rapid signal mediators. The axon's satellite cells, the Schwann cells, elaborate and produce the myelin sheath, a highly regular structure composed of concentrically arranged lamellae. The mechanisms of myelin formation, first proposed by Geren[22] and later confirmed by others,[45,46] involve the rolling of the axon within a spiral of Schwann cell cytoplasm. These mechanisms are exceedingly complex and represent the intricate relationship between the axon and its satellite cells. There is evidence that the main stimulus for myelinization is simply the axon's attaining a certain critical diameter.[36] There remains considerable doubt, however, that this is so clearcut as there is considerable overlap between the sizes of some myelinated and unmyelinated fibers in man.[19,41] Whether the axon always dictates what the Schwann cell does is still a matter of controversy. Simpson and Young's experiments[48] in which they cross-united somatic with visceral nerves showed that the splanchnic Schwann cells, which previously were associated only with unmyelinated axons, were now able to produce fine myelin sheaths around the ingrowing somatic axons. However, remyelinization never approached the maturity and extent observed when similar axons were guided to their old somatic Schwann tubes.

There is always a one-to-one relationship between Schwann cells and axons destined to become myelinated both during normal development and during peripheral nerve regeneration. Schwann cells are arranged in a longitudinal manner along the length of the axon, each cell controlling a distinct territory known as an internode. There is one Schwann cell nucleus per internode, and any axonal branching takes place at this site. All internodes are bounded proximally and distally by a node of Ranvier, where the myelin sheath is interrupted. This node was first described by Ranvier in 1871, but its existence was later contested by others.[38] Proof of Ranvier's observations awaited ultrastructural examination. At the node of Ranvier the cytoplasm of the Schwann cell forms a collar of protruding fin-

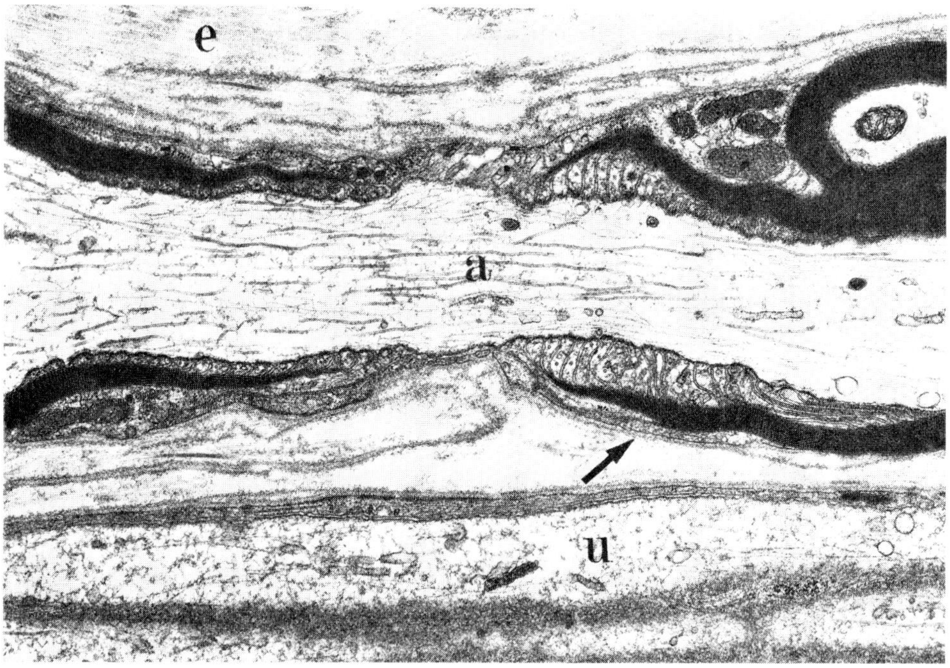

Fig. 2-4. Longitudinal section of node of Ranvier in vitro showing paranodal termination of black myelin sheath, axon, *a*, adjacent unmyelinated fiber, *u*, and endoneurium, *e*. Arrow points to basal lamina of Schwann cell. This figure is a transmission electron micrograph of thin epoxy section stained with uranyl acetate. (Courtesy Dr. Peter S. Spencer.)

gerlike processes that envelop the terminating myelin sheath (Fig. 2-4). These processes are thought to be active during injury or incipient demyelination,[3] and a "scavenger" activity has been attributed to them whereby damaged organelles or injured portions of axoplasm are sequestered and removed.[49] The importance of the node of Ranvier in saltatory conduction has been appreciated for over 30 years,[55] and it is generally accepted that propagation of nerve signals in myelinated fibers involves node-to-node transfer of rapid ionic fluxes.

Unmyelinated nerve fiber

The discovery of unmyelinated fibers is credited to Remak, who despite his use of very primitive microscopes and histologic techniques was able to observe their occurrence in practically all nerves. Although most common, unmyelinated fibers had been ill-defined prior to the early 1950s, as their axons are extremely slender neuronal processes, barely visible with the light microscope. With the advent of the electron microscope the precise relationship of unmyelinated axons and Schwann cells was clearly described, first by Gasser[21] and later by others.[2,14,16] It is clear today that in most peripheral nerves there exist large numbers of mature, fine caliber nerve fibers whose axons are permanently devoid of a myelin sheath. These fibers have to be differentiated from myelinated axons that temporarily lack myelin due to immaturity, as is the case in peripheral nerve regeneration. Myelinization to some degree depends on attainment of a critical axon diameter.[13,18,19] This concept led to the erroneous conclusion that unmyelinated axons remain devoid of myelin because they never reach the critical caliber for myelination.[13]

Recent evidence, however, shows that the diameter of many mature unmyelinated axons greatly exceeds the critical diameter for myelinization.[40,41] This evidence strengthens the argument that neurons which give rise to myelinated and unmyelinated axons probably have different influences upon their respective Schwann cells, and it seems reasonable to assume that unmyelinated axons lack the capability of stimulating myelin production.

In mixed peripheral nerves, unmyelinated fibers of different origin and diameter travel in groups and in proximity to myelinated fibers.[20,41] Schwann cells carrying unmyelinated axons are longitudinally arranged in columns, and a typical adult unmyelinated fiber may consist of three to six axons per Schwann cell. However, the number of axons within individual Schwann cell units varies from level to level due to constant interchange of axons between the Schwann cell chains. The intricate and dynamic relationships between unmyelinated axons and their satellite cells have been elegantly shown in three-dimensional reconstructions.[1]

FUNCTION

In the nervous system, information is transmitted in the form of signals or action potentials that consist of electric currents generated across the cell membrane. These currents result from ionic shifts that primarily reflect movement of charges carried by sodium and potassium ions. The basic mechanism of the action potential is well known and encompasses the phenomena of depolarization and repolarization. The former presupposes an increase in sodium conductance and, after some slight delay, an increase in potassium conductance. Repolarization occurs due to the transient nature of the depolarization process, and membrane permeability is restored to its resting level in a matter of milliseconds.

The first quantitative description of this process was offered in the 1950s,[26,27] and since that time there have been several reviews of the subject.[10,25,31,39,57] Once an action potential is generated, its transmission along a single nerve fiber is an all-or-none phenomenon. That implies a nondecremental propagation regardless of its direction. Thus centrifugal action potentials transmitted to peripheral effector organs (muscles) via the motor fibers behave in the same manner as do impulses that originate peripherally at the sensory receptors. Although the neural activity generated at the motor neurons or the sensory receptors is of little use to the clinician, the action potentials mediated within a nerve trunk can yield valuable information about the function of the peripheral nerve. This data can be of use only if the observer understands the meaning of the evoked signals.

Despite the fact that functional attributes (whether motor or sensory) do not influence the size or shape of the propagated action potential, anatomic parameters drastically affect its speed of transmission. Thus an action potential is conducted much more rapidly if it travels along a myelinated fiber than if it travels along unmyelinated fibers. That this should be the case encompasses the topic of saltatory conduction versus continuous spread. In unmyelinated fibers, impulse spread is continuous and is accomplished by sequential depolarization of the axonal membrane, progressively exciting neighboring inactive areas with the rate of spread proportional to the cross-sectional area of the axon. In myelinated fibers, the myelin sheath comprises a high-resistance, low-capacitance insulator that forces the nerve impulse to flow through the membrane only at the sites where the myelin sheath is interrupted, that is, at the nodes of Ranvier. Thus, in myelinated fibers the impulse jumps from one node of Ranvier to the next, a process known as saltatory conduction. This allows for much faster speeds of impulse conduction.

On a functional basis, peripheral nerves to the upper limb consist of both motor (efferent) and sensory (afferent) fibers. Motor impulses are conveyed by the motor fibers to neuromuscular junctions, while the sensory input is mediated by the afferent fibers to the spinal cord. Thus, the peripheral dendrites of dorsal root ganglia carry signals of pain, pressure, temperature, and stretch from free nerve endings or encapsulated receptors. These receptors are located in skin, muscle, tendons, joints, connective tissue, and bone.

A functional classification has been derived from the direct relationship that exists between total fiber diameter and conduction velocity.[28,47] Thus fibers in mixed peripheral nerves may belong to one of three groups: A, B, or C. Erlanger and Gasser[17] first defined these fiber groups by correlating the shape of the compound action potential with the fiber size histogram of the sciatic nerve. Group A comprises the largest fibers with the fastest conduction velocities; the large myelinated somatic motor and sensory fibers are included in this group. Group B consists of the finely myelinated preganglionic fibers of the autonomic system, and group C contains only unmyelinated fibers, both sensory and postganglionic autonomic efferents that have the smallest diameter and the slowest conduction velocity.

PHYSIOLOGY

Myelinated fiber

The largest myelinated fibers were investigated preferentially because of easier accessibility. Only recently are data accumulating on the smaller ones. In all cases fibers with the same function have similar diameters; however, the diameter range is quite wide, and thus there is appreciable overlap among functional fiber groups.[6]

The vibration sensibility is served by two encapsulated receptors, the pacinian and Meissner corpuscles, both of which provide input to large myelinated fibers (group A). The pacinian corpuscle is extremely sensitive to very small mechanical vibrations in the frequency range of 100 to 300 Hz.[24,54] It is the receptor that becomes activated by merely blowing a puff of air on the skin. It is situated deep in the hand, in dermis, in periosteum, and around joints and tendons. Often found in clusters, these receptors may number up to 200 per digit and several thousand in the entire hand.[9] The Meissner corpuscle is located characteristically in the dermal papillae of glabrous skin. It responds to low-frequency vibrations (5 to 80 Hz) and is probably responsible for the vibratory sensation of "flutter." Both of these myelinated fibers and their associated end organs appear to be rapidly adapting. Nerve fibers are said to adapt rapidly if after initial firing they stop sending impulses despite persistent stimulus.

The sensation of pressure presupposes the existence of receptors and parent fibers that can discharge for the duration of a sustained stimulus.[56] These slowly adapting fibers are relatively large myelinated fibers (5 to 15 μm in diameter) that emerge from the subpapillary nerve plexus to terminate in an array of nerve endings on the rete papillae of the dermal-epidermal junction in glabrous skin or at the dermal-epidermal interface in hairy skin under touch domes. The termination of these nerve fibers is embedded in specialized epithelial cells, probably of neural crest origin, known as the Merkel cells. These cells apparently function as mechanoelectric transducers.[29]

The myelinated fibers serving the modalities of vibration and pressure described thus far are of fairly large caliber (5 to 12 μm) and are usually referred to as Aβ fibers.[37] The smaller myelinated fibers have diameters ranging between 2 and 5 μm and are known as Aδ. Functionally these fibers serve the sensibilities of pain, temperature, and touch. The majority of the Aδ fibers are mechanoreceptors and mainly innervate hairs. The Aδ fibers that respond to sudden small increments in skin temperature are the thermoreceptors[11]; they comprise about 30% of these finely myelinated fibers. The remaining 20% of the Aδ fibers respond to noxious mechanical stimuli but remain silent when presented with noxious thermal or chemical stimuli.[42] Probably these fibers are responsible for the awareness of "pricking pain."[5]

Unmyelinated fibers

Unmyelinated fibers constitute a distinct group from myelinated fibers since they subserve specific functional modalities. This information is deduced from their preferential involvement in certain pathologic conditions. These neuropathies reflect disorders of autonomic and sensory function and include sweating abnormalities, postural hypotension, and impotence, as well as disturbances in appreciation of pain and temperature sensibilities. The high frequency of these manifestations should provide the impetus for further investigation of the pathophysiology of the unmyelinated fiber. Functional studies have been handicapped by the small size of the axons and the complexity of axon–Schwann cell relationships.

The C fibers are predominantly sensory and respond to innocuous tactile stimuli such as light touch, slight bending of hair, or moderate temperature changes. A small number of unmyelinated fibers respond to nonpainful pressure. Finally, one third are nociceptors and will fire if exposed to noxious heat, irritating chemicals, or damaging mechanical agents.[4]

These fibers are probably the mediators of the sensation of burning pain[5] and are important clinically since they probably are responsible for the phenomena of chronic neuralgia and hyperesthesias that at times accompany cutaneous reinnervation.

The motor C fibers are all of postganglionic autonomic origin, supplying sweat glands and vessels. They are responsible for maintenance of skin tone and regulation of peripheral blood flow. There is a remarkable lack of information regarding their electrophysiologic response characteristics.

In conclusion, it is evident from this discussion that the morphology and physiology of the peripheral nerve is exceedingly complex, and the surgical task of restoring normal connections following injury to this tissue is an impossible one. Distal axonal degeneration is the critical event and forms the basis of the unique problems associated with peripheral nerve reconstruction.

INTRANEURAL ORGANIZATION

Motor and sensory nerve fibers look deceptively alike, and at present their distinction, even under high ultrastructural observation, escapes our capabilities. Furthermore the intraneural organization of the peripheral nerve is confounded with plexuses and fasciculations so that nerve fibers undergo continuous intermingling and redistribution within the peripheral nerve trunk.

Past attempts to decipher intraneural topography included dissection and histologic examination,[33,50,52,53] electric stimulation and observation of the muscle response,[35] clinical examination following partial nerve injury,[12] and ascertainment of the fascicular distribution by plotting the degeneration secondary to partial nerve severance.[32] Of all these studies the morphologic work of Sunderland and his associates[50,52,53] is to be commended. They used histologic techniques to trace fiber groups along serially sectioned specimens of the major peripheral nerves and established the manner of fascicular plexus formations and how these modify the location of fiber groups from level to level.

Despite the elegance of these studies, physiologic correlates are missing. In an attempt to provide functional information we initiated a series of experiments in primates in which electrophysiologic techniques were utilized to depict the intraneural organization of the major peripheral nerves serving the upper limb. The following discussions

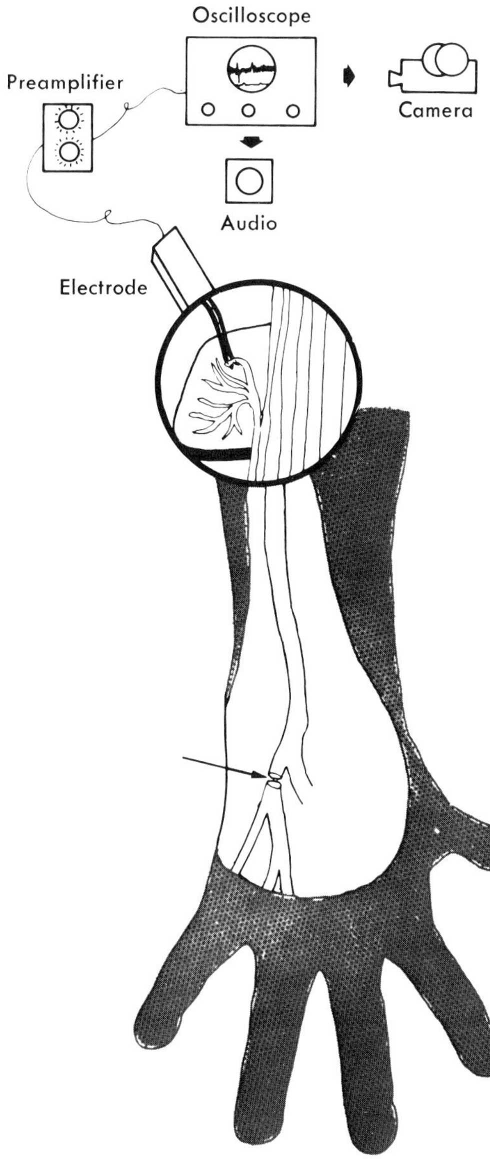

Fig. 2-5. Circle shows microdissection and recording arrangement. Arrow points to cut superficial branch of ulnar nerve.

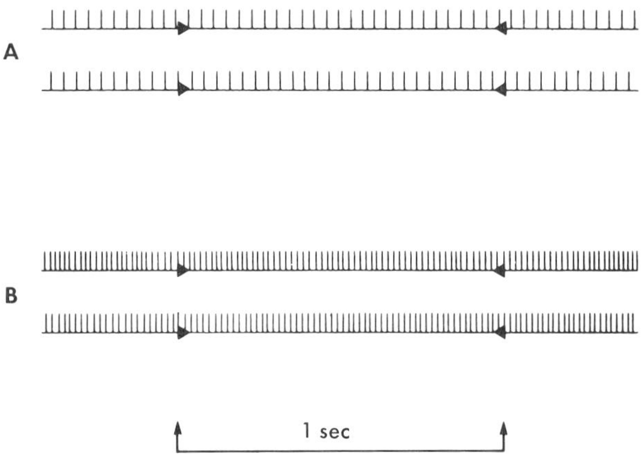

Fig. 2-6. A, Two 1-second samples of spontaneous discharge of an afferent fiber from flexor pollicis brevis muscle. **B,** Samples from same fiber obtained when thumb was held in extended position, thus stretching muscle. (Note increased discharge.) Each line is trace from computer-generated display, showing single fiber activity; vertical lines represent single impulses, while horizontal lines correspond to baseline. Arrows depict 1-second time intervals.

are limited to our experience with the functional anatomy of the deep motor branch of the ulnar nerve. This nerve was chosen for our pilot study because of the apparent controversies in the literature concerning its anatomic description.* The deep motor branch of the ulnar nerve is described in anatomic texts and papers as arising 4 to 20 mm below the radial styloid by the bifurcation of the ulnar nerve into a superficial and a deep branch. However, the many inconsistencies in the pattern of innervation of this nerve preclude the description of a representative case. Our own microdissection studies further emphasized this extensive variability. Probably the only general statement that can be made from all the anatomic data is that the ulnar nerve innervates the hypothenar muscles, all the interossei, and sends articular branches to carpometacarpal and metacarpophalangeal joints.

To provide physiologic correlation to the morphologic analysis and because of the total lack of information on the sensory role of this nerve, we conducted a series of experiments to demonstrate objectively the nature and variety of its sensory activity. Our findings suggest that the deep motor

*References 7, 8, 23, 30, 34, 51.

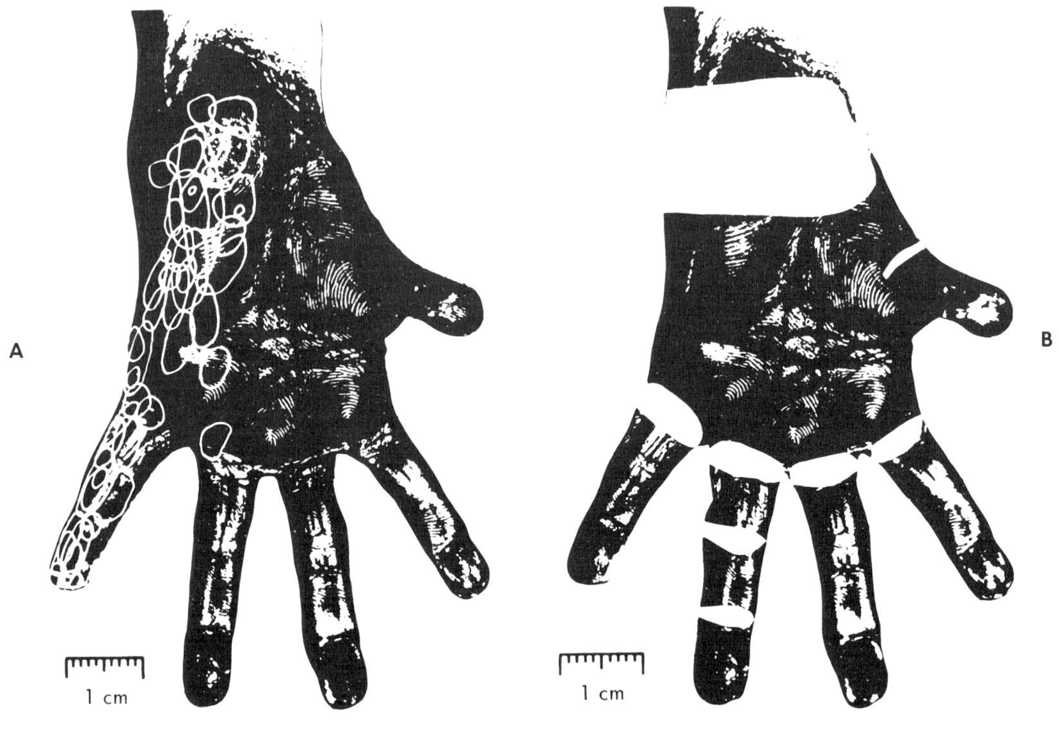

Fig. 2-7. Distribution of sensory fibers of deep branch of ulnar nerve from skin, **A,** and joints, **B.**

branch of the ulnar nerve is neither purely deep nor purely motor.

This investigation was performed on five hands from three monkeys. Each hand was immobilized by external fixation, and the ulnar nerve was exposed at distal forearm level. It was then traced distally, under the operating microscope, to its division into the superficial and deep branches. The superficial branch was then transected shortly after its origin from the ulnar nerve (Fig. 2-5). Thus, only the deep motor branch was left intact for physiologic examination. At the level of the lower forearm a small dissecting plate was lowered under the ulnar nerve. Subsequently under high magnification (25 to 40 ×) single fiber microdissection was performed. Dissection continued until single axon potentials were obtained when the fiber preparation was placed on the recording electrode (Fig. 2-5). Electrophysiologic assessment of each nerve fiber included the study of its receptive field, the adequate stimulus for excitation, and its mean discharge rate. Information was obtained from 627 single sensory fibers. Details of the recording arrangement are available elsewhere.[15] The most significant finding was that only 44% of the sensory fibers in the deep branch of the ulnar nerve arose from muscle spindles, while 33% came from deep tissues (joints, pacinian corpuscles, deep connective tissue) and 31% from skin. An example of the electrophysiologic data collected in these experiments is depicted in Fig. 2-6. Analysis of the muscle afferents in our sample showed that all the intrinsic muscles of the hand received contributions from the deep branch of the ulnar nerve. In the case of the first and second lumbricals, which according to anatomic literature are said not to be innervated by the ulnar nerve, our data showed that they received about one half the number of afferent fibers. The sensory fibers arising in joints and other deep structures emphasized once more the sensory role of the deep branch of the ulnar nerve and proved that the innervation of this nerve is far more extensive than previously defined. In our sample, afferent fibers were shown to arise from all the metacarpophalan-

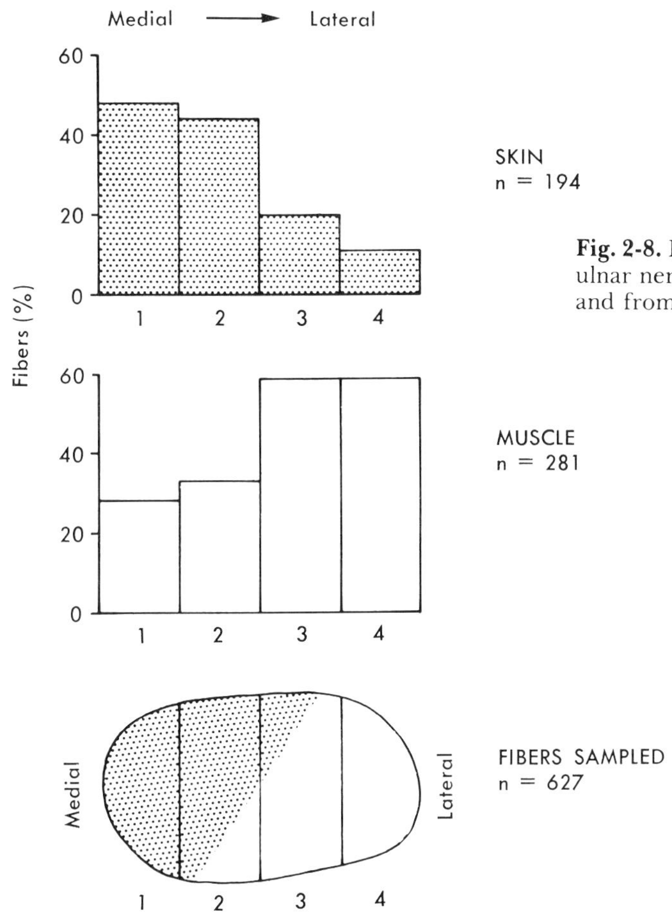

Fig. 2-8. Intraneural distribution of afferent fibers of the ulnar nerve in distal one third of forearm, from muscle and from skin.

geal joints, including the thumb, and from the interphalangeal joints of the fourth digit (Fig. 2-7).

Brushing the skin on the ulnar side of the palm activated 31% of the sensory fiber sample. This was a most surprising finding, since the deep branch of the ulnar nerve is not "supposed" to innervate skin. However, every ulnar nerve that was investigated neurophysiologically consistently revealed afferent fibers innervating skin (Fig. 2-7). The significance of this cutaneous sensory component must await future clinical documentation. These observations nevertheless may explain remaining sensibility in the autonomous ulnar zone following severance of the superficial ulnar branch. As the dissection of single fibers in the distal forearm proceeded from medial to lateral, it was observed that the contribution from muscle afferents gradually increased, whereas there was a corresponding decrease in the cutaneous afferents (Fig. 2-8). This finding was not expected and conflicts with previous anatomic work.[50]

Upon the completion of the physiologic assessment of the sensory fibers of the deep branch of the ulnar nerve, the ulnar nerve was transected in the lower forearm, and the distal stump was divided into several bundles. Electric stimulation of each bundle followed, and the hand was inspected for muscular contractions. All the intrinsic muscles that contributed to the sensory portion of the nerve were seen to contract. Furthermore, stimulation of one bundle optimally activated a specific muscle group, whereas stimulation of another bundle caused a different group of muscles to contract. In general, electric stimulation of the fascicular groups of the ulnar nerve at the forearm almost always produced a distal intrinsic contraction. These findings indicate that the motor component of the deep branch of the ulnar nerve at the distal forearm is distributed throughout and is not limited to a few fascicular groups as previously suggested.[50]

In conclusion, physiologic analysis provided novel information about the functional intraneural organization of the deep branch of the ulnar nerve and showed that there is a wide variety of sensory fibers not previously recognized. Furthermore, the motor component of this nerve was shown to be distributed throughout the entire ulnar nerve in the distal forearm and not restricted to specific fascicles. Contrary to previous assumptions, this nerve was proven to be mixed rather than purely motor; in fact, it is probably mostly sensory. This evidence questions the wisdom of considering any peripheral nerve as purely motor or purely sensory and emphasizes the need for a functional reappraisal of the intraneural organization of peripheral nerves.

REFERENCES

1. Aguayo, A. J., and Bray, G. M.: Experimental pathology of unmyelinated nerve fibers. In Dyck, P. J., Thomas, P. K., and Lambert, E. H., editors: Peripheral neuropathy, Philadelphia, 1975, W. B. Saunders Company.
2. Aguayo, A. J., Martin, J. B., and Bray, G. M.: Effect of nerve growth factor antiserum on peripheral unmyelinated nerve fibers, Acta Neuropathol. (Berl.) **20:**288, 1972.
3. Ballin, R. H. M., and Thomas, P. K.: Electron microscope observations on demyelination and remyelination in experimental allergic neuritis. 2. Remyelination, J. Neurol. Sci. **8:**225-237, 1969.
4. Bessou, P., and Perl, E. R.: Response of cutaneous sensory units with unmyelinated fibers to noxious stimuli, J. Neurophysiol. **32:**1025, 1969.
5. Bishop, G. H., and Laudau, W. M.: Evidence for a double peripheral pathway for pain, Science **128:**712, 1958.
6. Boyd, I. A., and Davey, M. R.: Composition of peripheral nerves, Edinburgh, 1968, Churchill Livingstone, pp. 1-57.
7. Brooks, H. St. J.: Variations in the nerve supply of the flexor pollicis brevis muscle, J. Anat. Physiol. (Lond.) **20:**641, 1886a.
8. Brooks, H. St. J.: On the morphology of the intrinsic muscles of the little finger with some observations on the ulnar head of the short flexor of the thumb, J. Anat. Physiol. (Lond.) **20:**645, 1886b.
9. Bushong, J.: A report on the frequency and distribution of the Pacinian corpuscle in a palm of a seven month human fetus, Master's thesis, Johns Hopkins University, 1963, p. 53.
10. Cole, K. S.: Membranes, ions and impulses, Berkeley, Calif., 1968, University of California Press.
11. Darian-Smith, I., and Dykes, R. W.: Peripheral neural mechanisms of thermal sensation. In Dubner, R., and Kawamura, Y., editors: Oral-facial sensory and motor mechanisms, New York, 1971, Appleton-Century-Crofts.
12. Dejerine, Mme., and Mouzon, J.: Les lesions des gros troncs nerveux des membres par projectiles de guerre, les differents syndromes cliniques et les indications operatoires, Presse Med. **23:**153, 1915.
13. Duncan, D.: A relation between axon diameter and myelination determined by measurement of myelinated spinal root fibers, J. Comp. Neurol. **60:**437-471, 1934.
14. Dyck, P. J., and Hopkins, A. P.: Electron microscopic observations on degeneration and regeneration of unmyelinated fibers, Brain **95:**223, 1972.
15. Dykes, R. W., and Terzis, J. K.: Functional anatomy of the deep motor branch of the ulnar nerve, Clin. Orthop. **128:**167, 1978.
16. Eames, R. A., and Gamble, H. J.: Schwann cell relationships in normal human cutaneous nerves, J. Anat. **106:**417, 1970.
17. Erlanger, J., and Gasser, H. S.: Electrical signs of nervous activity, Philadelphia, 1937, University of Pennsylvania Press.
18. Friede, R. L.: Control of myelin formation by axon caliber (with a model of the control mechanism), J. Comp. Neurol. **144:**233-252, 1972.

19. Friede, R. L., and Samorajski, T.: Myelin formation in the sciatic nerve of the rat. A quantitative electron microscope, histochemical and radioautographic study, J. Neuropathol. Exp. Neurol. **27:**546-570, 1968.
20. Gamble, H. J., and Eames, R. A.: An electron microscope study of the connective tissues of human peripheral nerve, J. Anat. **98:**655-663, 1964.
21. Gasser, H. S.: Discussion of paper by B. Frankenhaeuser, Cold Spring Harbor Symp. Quant. Biol. **17:**32-36, 1952.
22. Geren, B. B.: The formation from the Schwann cell surface of myelin, Exp. Cell Res. **7:**558-562, 1954.
23. Grant, J. C. B.: An atlas of anatomy. ed. 5, Baltimore, 1962, The Williams and Wilkins Company.
24. Gray, J. A. B., and Malcolm, J. L.: The initiation of nerve impulses by mesenteric pacinian corpuscles, Proc. R. Soc. Lond. [Biol.] **137:**96, 1950.
25. Hille, B.: Ionic channels in nerve membranes, Prog. Biophys. Mol. Biol. **21:**1-32, 1970.
26. Hodgkin, A. L., and Huxley, A. F.: A quantitative description of membrane current and its application to conduction and excitation in nerve, J. Physiol. (Lond.) **117:**500-544, 1952.
27. Hodgkin, A. L., Huxley, A. F., and Katz, B: Measurement of current voltage relations in the membrane of the giant axon of Loligo, J. Physiol. (Lond.) **116:**424-448, 1952.
28. Hursh, J. B.: Conduction velocity and diameter of nerve fibers, Am. J. Physiol. **127:**131-139, 1939.
29. Iggo, A.: Cutaneous receptors with a high sensitivity to mechanical displacement. In de Reuck, A. V. S., and Knight, J., editors: Ciba Foundation Symposium, Touch, heat and pain, Boston, 1966, Little, Brown & Company.
30. Kaplan, E. B.: The blood and nerve supply of the hand. In Functional and surgical anatomy of the hand, ed. 2, Philadelphia, 1965, J. B. Lippincott Company.
31. Katz, B.: Nerve, muscle and synapse, London, 1966, McGraw-Hill Book Co.
32. Kilvington, B.: A note on the distribution of myelinated nerve fibers within nerve bundles, Aust. J. Exp. Biol. Med. Sci. **18:**367, 1940.
33. Langley, J. N., and Hashimoto, M.: On the suture of separate nerve bundles in a nerve trunk and on internal nerve plexuses, J. Physiol. (Lond.) **51:**318, 1917.
34. Mannerfelt, L.: Studies on the hand in ulnar nerve paralysis: a clinical experimental investigation in normal and anomalous innervation, Acta Orthop. Scand. [Suppl.] **87:**1, 1966.
35. Marie, P., Meige, H., and Gosset, A.: Les localisations motrices dans les nerfs peripheriques, Bull. Acad. Med. **74:**798, 1915.
36. Matthews, M. A.: An electron microscopic study of the relationship between axon diameter and the initiation of myelin production in the peripheral nervous system, Anat. Rec. **161:**337-352, 1968.
37. Mountcastle, V. B.: Medical physiology, ed. 13, St. Louis, 1974, The C. V. Mosby Co., vol. 1, pp. 285-306.
38. Nageotte, J.: L'organisation de la matiere, Paris, 1922, Felix Alcau.
39. Noble, D.: Applications of Hodgkin-Huxley equations to excitable tissues, Physiol. Rev. **46:**1-50, 1966.
40. Ochoa, J.: The sural nerve of the human foetus: electron microscope observations and counts of axons, J. Anat. **108:**231-245, 1971.
41. Ochoa, J., and Mair, W. G. P.: The normal sural nerve in man. I. Ultrastructure and number of fibres and cells, Acta Neuropathol. (Berl.) **13:**197-216, 1969.
42. Perl, E. R.: Myelinated afferent fibers innervating the primate skin and their response to noxious stimuli, J. Physiol. **197:**593, 1968.
43. Ranvier, L. A.: Contributions a l'histologie et a la physiologie des nerfs peripherique, Acad. Sci. [D] (Paris) **73:**1168-1171, 1871.
44. Remak, R.: Observationes anatomical et microscopical de systematis nervosi structura, Berlin, 1938.
45. Robertson, J. D.: The ultrastructure of adult vertebrate peripheral myelinated nerve fibers in relation to myelinogenesis, J. Biophys. Biochem. Cytol. **1:**271, 1955.
46. Robertson, J. D.: The molecular structure and contact relationships of cell membranes, Prog. Biophys. **10:**343-418, 1960.
47. Rushton, W. A. H.: A theory of the effects of fiber size in medullated nerve, J. Physiol. (Lond.) **115:**101-122, 1951.
48. Simpson, S. A., and Young J. Z.: Regeneration of fibre diameter after cross-unions of visceral and somatic nerves, J. Anat. **79:**48-65, 1945.
49. Spencer, P.: Light and electron microscopic observations on localized peripheral nerve injuries, Ph.D. thesis, University of London, 1971.
50. Sunderland, S.: The intraneural topography of the radial, median and ulnar nerves, Brain **68:**243, 1945.
51. Sunderland, S., and Hughes, E. S. R.: Metrical and non-metrical features of the muscular branches of the ulnar nerve, J. Comp. Neurol. **85:**113, 1946.
52. Sunderland, S., Marshall, R. D., and Swaney, W. E.: The intraneural topography of the circumflex musculocutaneous and obturator nerves, Brain **82:**116, 1959.
53. Sunderland, S., and Ray, L. J.: The intraneural topography of the sciatic nerve and its popliteal divisions in man, Brain **71:**242, 1948.
54. Talbot, W. H., Darian-Smith, I., Kornhuber, H. H., and Mountcastle, V. B.: The sense of flutter-vibration: comparison of the human capacity with response patterns of mechanoreceptive afferents from the monkey hand, J. Neurophysiol. **31:**301, 1968.
55. Tasaki, I., and Takeuchi, T.: Der am Ranvierschen Knoten entstehende Aktionsstrom und seine Bedeutung fur die Erregungsleitung, Pfluegers Arch. **244:**696-711, 1941.
56. Werner, G., and Mountcastle, V. B.: Neural activity in mechanoreceptive cutaneous afferents: stimulus-response relations, Weber functions, and information transmission, J. Neurophysiol. **28:**359, 1965.
57. Woodbury, J. W., and Patton, H. D. In Ruch, T. C., and Patton, H. D., editors: Physiology and biophysics, Philadelphia, 1965, W. B. Saunders Company, ch. 1-3.

Chapter 3

Microsurgical repair of peripheral nerves: rationale and technique

Hanno Millesi

The goal of peripheral nerve surgery is to restore the continuity of as many axons as possible with maximal accuracy and minimal scar formation. Obviously the surgeon has no control over the central factors of nerve regeneration such as axonic sprouting. Even a technically poor repair may produce an excellent result if the patient has high regenerative powers such as those frequently seen in children. In patients with less favorable restorative potential the quality of the technical repair increases in significance. Rough surgical manipulation of the tissues and repairs under tension increase the tissue damage and lead to greater scarring. One must balance the accuracy of repair against the tissue trauma required to produce it.

Early surgeons were afraid to touch nerve tissue and thus repaired nerve by uniting the adjacent tissue ("cum carne"). In 1873 Hueter[13] first described epineural repair. This produced minimal trauma, permitted some tension, and soon became the technique of choice. Improved instrumentation and suture materials and the use of loupes for magnification followed. Even today there are many surgeons who still utilize this conventional repair as the method of choice.

In 1957 Nicholson and Seddon[24] published their results of epineural repair in civilian injuries. Patients had useful recovery in 70% of secondary median nerve repairs with gaps less than 2.5 cm. Only 50% of epineural repairs in patients with 2.5 to 5 cm gaps resulted in improvement. Defects of over 5 cm had a very poor prognosis. Sakellarides[27] reported similar results in 1965. Other authors have been more pessimistic. Önne[26] demonstrated that digital nerve repair in adults never resulted in useful two-point discrimination. This prompted Moberg[23] to develop the neurosensory island transfer for restoration of sensibility. My personal experience with conventional repair has also been less than satisfactory. I noted that useful motor recovery returned in most children but only in 50% of adults. The best sensibility I could obtain was protective, and no patient ever developed two-point discrimination.

Such poor results prompted a number of attempts at improvement in the 1950s and 1960s with such devices as Millipore filters, silicone sheaths, and glue instead of sutures. In the early 1960s the operating microscope became available, and Smith[32] in 1964 reported on its use in nerve repair. The magnification permitted more precise evaluation of the stump damage, more accurate debridement of scar and precision alignment and suturing of the ends. How much has this investment in equipment and operative time improved the results of epineural repair?

Braun[5] reported no detectable difference in animals whose nerves were repaired with and without the use of the microscope. My group[22] noted a marked difference but only in clean transections without any substantive tissue loss. Unfortunately such ideal patients are rare in clinical practice. It should of course be evident that microsurgery implies much more than the use of optical magnification. Its greatest value is in permitting the use of fine instruments and sutures that can delicately handle the tissue with a minimum of trauma. The improved mechanics lead to improved biology.

ABSOLUTE INDICATIONS FOR MICRONEURAL REPAIR

We must remember that a peripheral nerve consists of a varying number of fascicles embedded and surrounded by nonspecific connective tissue termed the epineurium. Each fascicle is wrapped in a specialized connective tissue, perineurium, that provides the tensile strength to the nerve and is the end point of the lymphatic vasculature. Tissue pressure is higher within the perineurium than in the surrounding substance. Nerve segments exposed to increased pressure or irritation contain much more interfascicular tissue than do others. The fascicular pattern continually changes throughout the course of the nerve. Nerve structure may consist of one large fascicle with a few satellites (the facial nerve at the stylomastoid foramen), a number of large fascicles, and many large fascicles oriented in groups or randomly distributed tiny fascicles.

In the proximal nerve the fibers to a specific area may be diffusely distributed, tending to arrange themselves according to their impending division as they move distally. It is the more frequently injured distal segments that tend to fascicular grouping.

Nerve lesions are classified according to the severity of the damage. Seddon[29] proposed three degrees: neurapraxia, axonotmesis, and neurotmesis. Sunderland[34] improved on this with five grades:

I. Conduction block with wallerian degeneration
II. Axolysis with wallerian degeneration
III. Damaged endoneurium with intact fascicles
IV. Fascicular disruption but epineural continuity
V. Loss of continuity

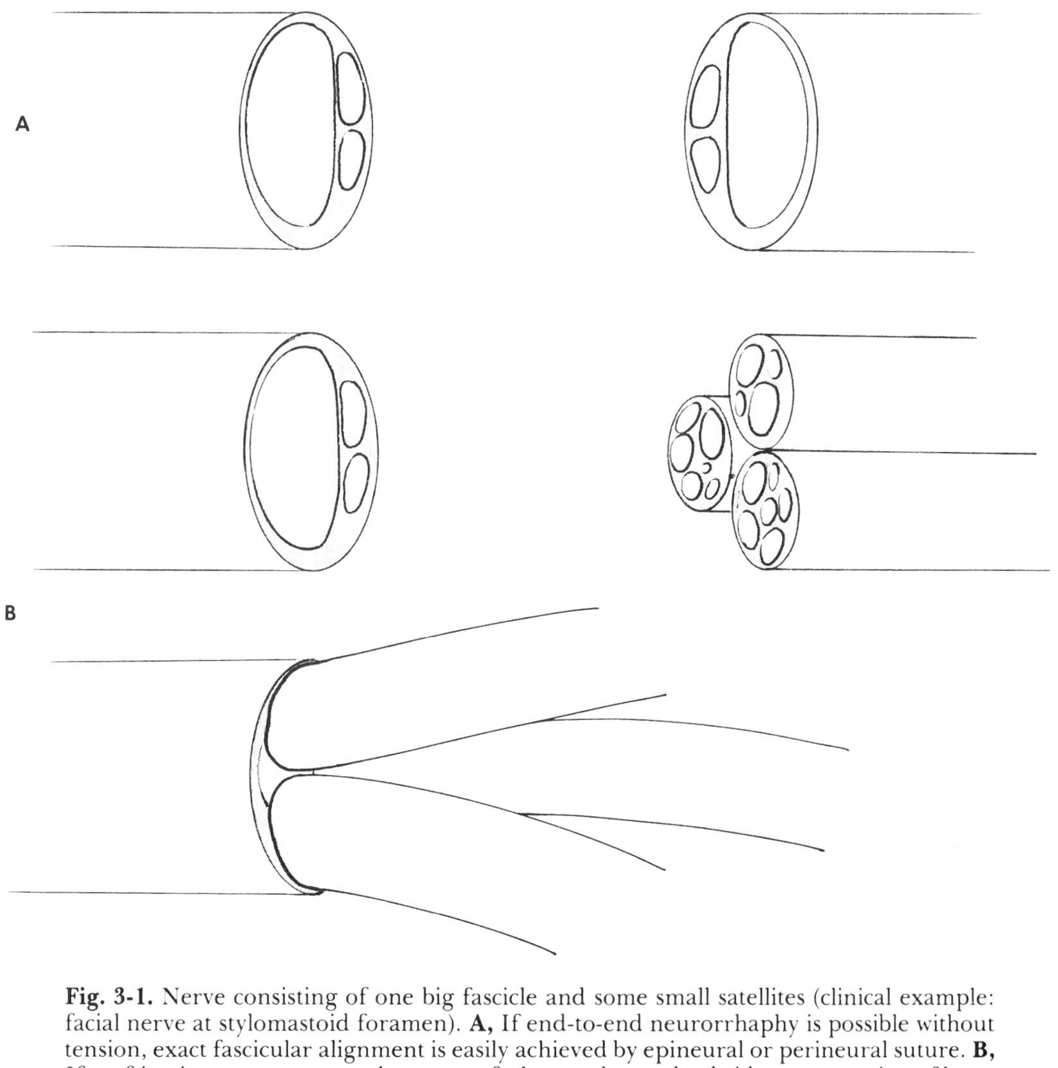

Fig. 3-1. Nerve consisting of one big fascicle and some small satellites (clinical example: facial nerve at stylomastoid foramen). **A,** If end-to-end neurorrhaphy is possible without tension, exact fascicular alignment is easily achieved by epineural or perineural suture. **B,** If grafting is necessary, several nerve grafts have to be used to bridge cross section of large fascicle (*fascicular grafting* 1:2, 1:3, or 1:4, etc.). Donor nerve fascicles are ignored.

Grades I and II almost always recover spontaneously. Grade III will occasionally recover without treatment.

Increased external pressure such as is seen from epineural fibrosis will impede nerve recovery and is a clear indication for neurolysis. After epineural neurorrhaphy, interfascicular fibrosis will obstruct the fascicles and interfere with the freedom required for individual bundles to move against each other as the nerve flexes. Perineural and endoneu-

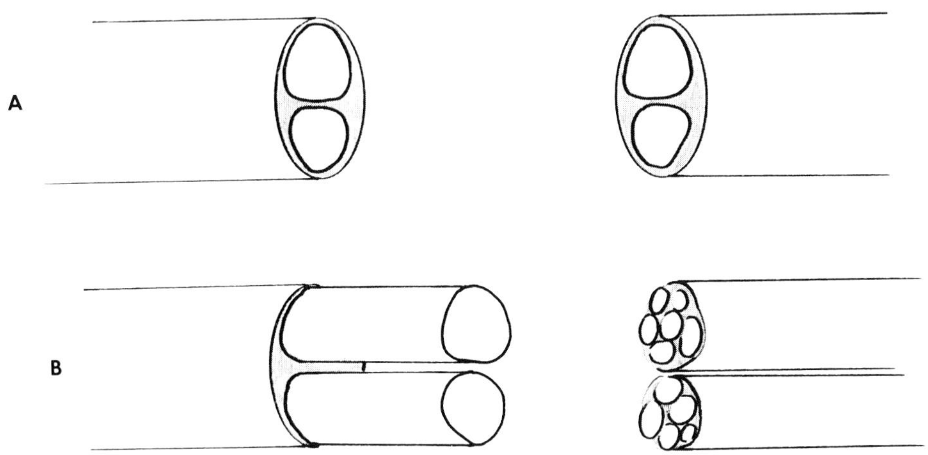

Fig. 3-2. Nerve with two large fascicles. **A,** With end-to-end nerve repair, good fascicular alignment can be achieved easily by whatever technique is used if malrotation is avoided. **B,** If grafting is indicated because of defect, each fascicle can be bridged individually by one nerve graft *(fascicular nerve grafting)* without splitting the graft.

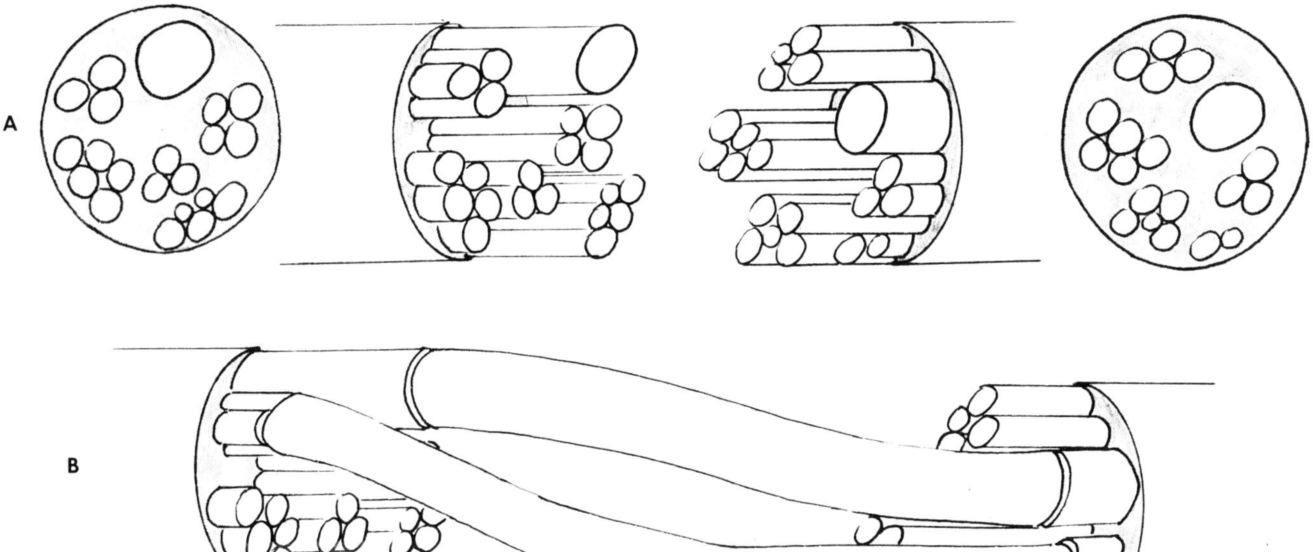

Fig. 3-3. Nerve containing many various-sized fascicles arranged in groups with much interfascicular tissue (clinical example: most peripheral nerves at their distal ends). **A,** By resection of strip of epineurium and interfascicular dissection, individual fascicle groups can be identified and united by direct coaptation if there is not tension. **B,** If there is a gap requiring tension for direct repair, fascicle groups are united by individual nerve grafts *(interfascicular nerve grafting).*

ral fibrosis complete the obstructive process. Scarring can result from almost any insult, including traction, compression, and devascularization (Volkmann ischemia), as well as direct trauma. External neurolysis produces dramatic results in grade I lesions due to external pressure. Before optical magnification and fine instruments were available, internal neurolysis was discouraged for fear of damaging intact fibers with recovery potential.

Modern microsurgical techniques have permitted accurate, safe interfascicular dissection and have been most beneficial in grade III lesions and in advanced severe compression syndromes.[9,28] When a failed epineural repair is reexplored each fascicle may be lysed and the decision for reresection and repair made on each one.

Classically the epineural suture has been the mainstay of nerve repair. Early attempts at fascicular repair date to 1917,[15] but the results were not impressive because the trauma of these early techniques negated the gains of increased anatomic accuracy. Epineural repair will tolerate some tension but cannot influence the fascicular alignment. The shortcomings of these repairs were demonstrated in the laboratory by Edshage[10] and in humans by the author.[20,21] Repair of the epineurium alone may result in buckled, malaligned fascicles. This is especially true in those nerves with many small fas-

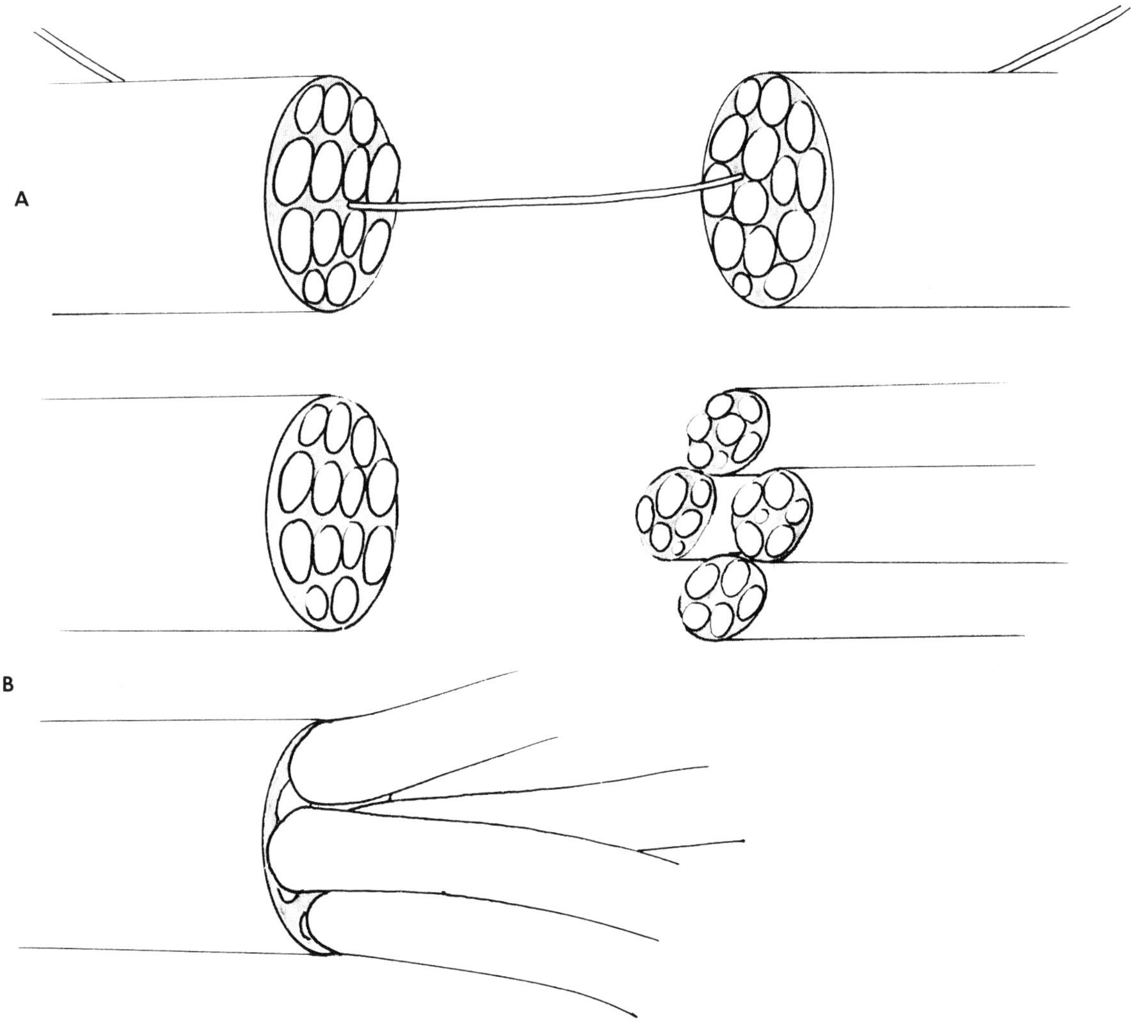

Fig. 3-4. Nerve with many small fascicles without group arrangement and minimal interfascicular tissue (clinical example: peripheral nerves in their central segments). **A,** Use of guide or end-to-end nerve repair sutures improves alignment. **B,** If there is a defect, several individual nerve grafts cover cross section, attempting to unite corresponding sectors. From studies of intraneural topography we know that sometimes nerve fibers of a specific function are concentrated in specific sectors *(sectoral nerve grafting).*

cicles. Thus, one cannot extrapolate the good results of epineural repair obtained in a nerve with only a few bundles with what one can expect from a polyfascicled nerve.[4] One must also be wary of results obtained from animals with high regenerative ability such as the cat or from those nerves that supply gross muscles as opposed to fine intrinsic muscles.[8] The applicability of such data to human lesions is questionable.[2,8]

Recent investigators have tried several approaches to fascicular alignment. Bora[3] emphasized the value of perineural suture. Smith[32,33] and Michon[17] used a central guide suture for alignment. Earlier Michon and Masse[18] suggested a combined perineural and epineural suture. Hakstian[12] used temporary intrafascicular sutures. O'Brien[25] also suggested perineural and epineural repair but advised leaving a large "window" in the epineurium. These techniques were traumatic and left much buried foreign material, albeit temporarily. Brunnelli[6] reported disappointing results with the intrafascicular suture.

Because of the differences in the anatomy of any given nerve at any given point it became apparent that repair must be individualized. In a nerve with only one or two large bundles such as the facial nerve at the stylomastoid foramen, alignment can be obtained by almost any repair. The microscope does, however, minimize malrotation. (Meissl[16] has shown that fibers innervating specific areas are anatomically discrete.) In nerves with several major fascicles the risk of malalignment is minimal. Those nerves with many fascicles of different sizes and groupings are most prone to misalignment, especially if there is much interfascicular tissue. This latter type does best with epineurial resection, interfascicular dissection, and coaptation of the bundles or bundle groups. The median and ulnar nerves in the forearm typically fall into this arrangement. Contrary to previous theory a watertight circumferential repair is not necessary. The sutures need not necessarily be anchored in the perineurium but are probably better placed in the interfascicular tissue as long as the bundles are well aligned. Nerves with small fascicles and minimal grouping do well with guide sutures and epineural repair as advocated by Smith,[33] Michon,[17] and Ishikawa[14] (Fig. 3-4).

We feel that the use of the microscope enhances the repair of all nerves. If the equipment is not available, then a conventional epineural repair is better than the trauma resulting from clumsy attempts at these more sophisticated techniques. One must, however, anticipate a failure rate of 30% to 50%. If secondary surgery is required, it should be referred to a center competent in microsurgery. Waiting too long for possible recovery considerably decreases the possible gains of secondary repair.

Nerve grafting

We have not as yet discussed the detrimental effect of tension on the suture line. Excess pull increases scar volume and produces fascicular separation. Even months later, connective tissue reaction at the suture line can damage axons that have already crossed.[20,21] We have shown experimentally that an axon will cross two atraumatic tensionless suture lines better than it will a single repair under tension,[21] and this has recently been confirmed by

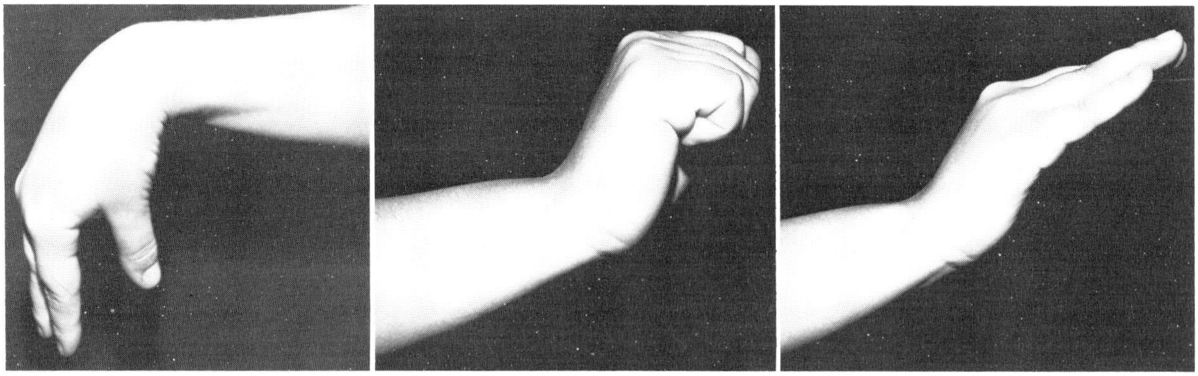

A B C

Fig. 3-5. A, Complete radial nerve lesion following fracture of humerus in 26-year-old woman. Several attempts to repair radial nerve over 2 years following original injury were unsuccessful. Restoration of continuity was accomplished by three 15 cm grafts from sural and cutaneous antebrachii medialis nerves. **B** and **C,** Results 3 years after surgery.

Terzis and associates.[35] In 1885 Albert[1] first described the use of nerve grafts. Attempts at using homologous grafts have been disappointing, but autogeneous cutaneous nerves have a long history of successful use.[7,11,29-31] They were used individually or combined as a cable for larger nerves. With the addition of microsurgical aids we have devised a new technique.[19, 22]Rather than the gross hit-and-miss cable technique we recommend epineural resection and dissection of each fascicle if it is large (Fig. 3-2, *B*) or each fascicular grouping about their intraneural vessel if they are multiple, small, and irregular (Fig. 3-3, *B*). Each bundle or bundle group should approximate the size of the donor cutaneous nerve graft. Large fascicles may require several graft segments (Fig. 3-1, *B*). Donor grafts

A B C D

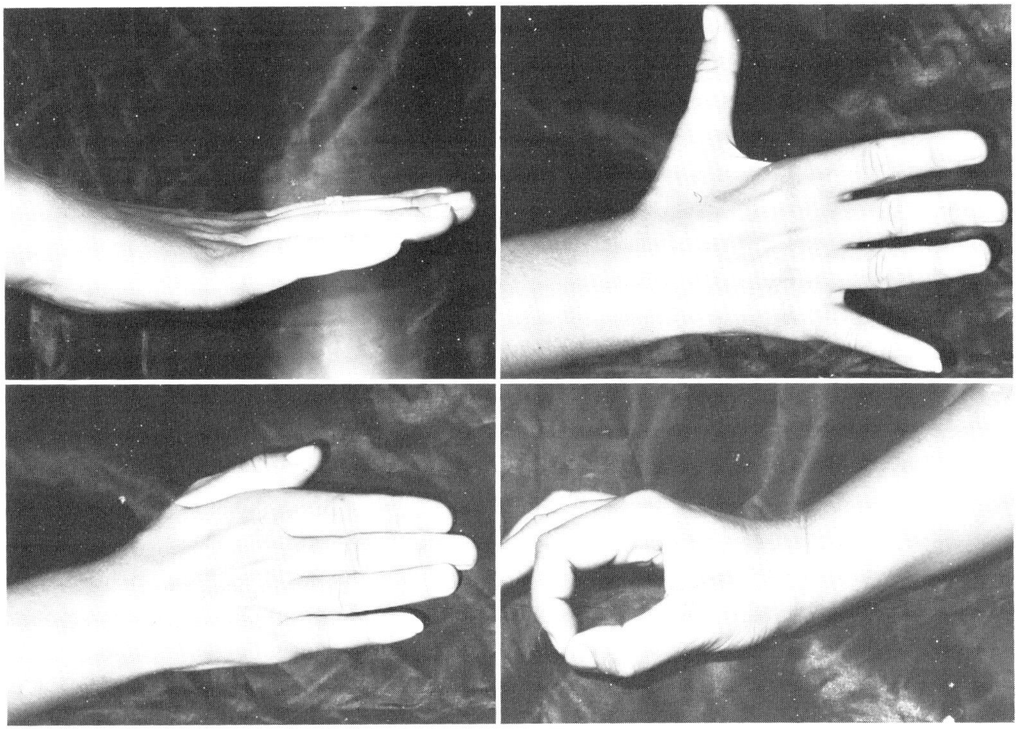

Fig. 3-6. Eighteen-month postoperative results of an ulnar nerve lesion from gun shot injury in 23-year-old woman. Continuity restored by five lengths of 5 cm grafts from sural nerve.

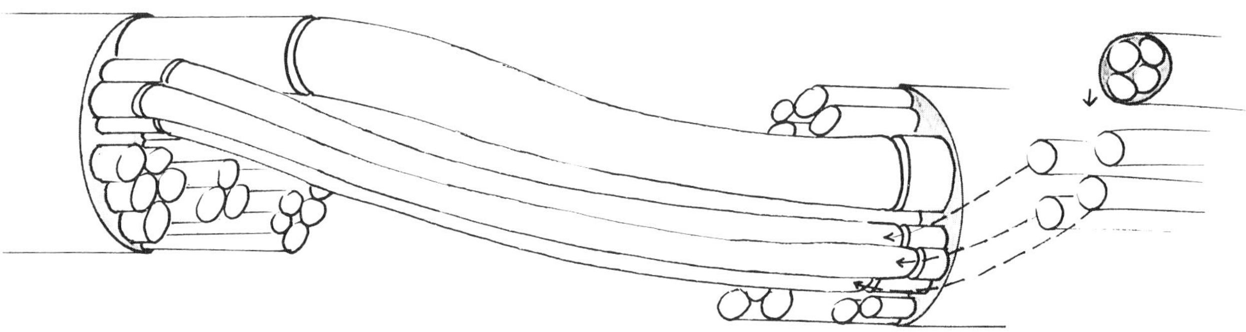

Fig. 3-7. Fascicular nerve grafting with splitting of grafts. Nerve as in Fig. 3-4. In contrast to interfascicular grafting technique, smaller fascicles of groups are isolated as well. Graft is split into its fascicles, and individual fascicles of grafts restore continuity to isolated small fascicles of the nerve.

can be obtained from the sural, the medial antebrachial cutaneous, the lateral femoral cutaneous, the greater auricular, or almost any convenient nonessential cutaneous nerve. The graft is cut into appropriate segments and may be split longitudinally to fit smaller fascicles. A single 10-0 nylon suture is sufficient to attach each end, but care must be taken to avoid prolapsing the epineurium across the repair. The graft must sit with absolutely no tension, thus minimizing the number of sutures required and the resultant increased foreign body reaction. The graft length should be judged with the limb in full extension, as flexion of a joint to overcome a gap risks failure. The fascicle groups are cut at different levels so that the staggering of the repair lends lateral stability (Fig. 3-3). Careful matching of the proximal and distal bundles is essential. Identification of the distal fascicles is aided by exposing the nerve to its division and tracing the bundles proximally. Skin closure must carefully avoid disruption of the repair, and the limb should be immobilized in plaster for 10 days.

Figs. 3-5 and 3-6 demonstrate representative cases. Confirmation of the success of this technique has been demonstrated in many centers.

Added experience has broadened our indications for grafting, and we now use grafts for any gap that is over 2.5 cm with the limb in full extension. We cannot overemphasize however the importance of using the entire armamentarium of microsurgery to obtain satisfactory results. Recently Tupper[36] has expanded this technique to individually graft each subunit (Fig. 3-7). This requires more dissection and graft splitting. Long-term results are not yet available.

SUMMARY

Microsurgical techniques are essential for improved results in peripheral nerve surgery if dissection at the fascicular level is required. It is indispensable for safe intraneural neurolysis or removal of intraneural tumors. Fascicular (for large fascicles) or interfascicular (for groups of smaller fascicles) dissection and repair can be accurately done with minimal trauma. Suture line tension is destructive to axonic growth and nerve recovery. Nerve grafting without tension produces superior results over simple neurorrhaphy under tension.

REFERENCES

1. Albert, E.: Einige Operationen am Nerven, Wr. Med. Presse **26:**1285, 1885.
2. Alnot, J. Y., Largier, A., Huten, B., and Hennie, D.:Suture nerveuse, expérimentale chez le rat, Reunion d'Automne du G.E.M., Nov. 26 1976, Paris.
3. Bora, W.: Peripheral nerve repair in cats, J. Bone Joint Surg. [Am.] **49**(4):659-666, 1967.
4. Bora, F. W., Jr., Pleasure, D. E., and Noubar, A.: A study of nerve regeneration and neuroma formation after nerve suture by various techniques, J. Hand Surg. **1**(3):138-143, 1976.
5. Braun, R. M.: Experimental peripheral nerve repair. Surg. Forum **15:**452, 1964.
6. Brunnelli, G.: Vortrag: Symposium über Mikrochirurgie der peripheren Nerven und Gefässe, Vienna, **18:**10, 1972.
7. Bunnell, S.: Surgery of nerves of the hand, Surg. Gynec. Obstet. **44:**145, 1927.
8. Cabaud, H. E., Rodkey, W. G., McCarroll, H. R., Jr., Mutz, St. B., and Niebauer, J. J.: Epineural and perineural fascicular nerve repair: a critical comparison, J. Hand Surg. **1:**(2):110-112, 1976.
9. Curtis, R. M., and Eversmann, W. W.: Internal Neurolysis as an adjunct to the treatment for the carpal tunnel syndrome, J. Bone Joint Surg. [Am.] **55:**733-740, 1973.
10. Edshage, S.: Peripheral nerve suture, Acta Chir. Scand. [Suppl.] **331:**1, 1964.
11. Förster, O.: Vortrag gehalten an der ausserordentlichen Tagung der Deutschen Orthopädischen Gesellschaft am February 8 and 9, 1916 in Berlin, Münch. Med. Wochenschr. **63:**283, 1916.
12. Hakstian, R. W.: Funicular orientation by direct stimulation. An aid to peripheral nerve repair, J. Bone Joint Surg. [Am.] **50:**1178-1186, 1968.
13. Hueter K.: Die allgemeine Chirurgie, Leipzig, 1873, Vogel Verlag.
14. Ishikawa, F.: Experimental studies on nerve suturing, especially in peripheral nerves, Med. J. Hiroshima Univ., 1966.
15. Langley, J. N., and Hashimoto, M.: On the suture of separate nerve bundles in a nerve trunk and on internal nerve plexuses, J. Physiol. (Lond.) **51:**318, 1917.
16. Meissl, G.: Die intraneurale Topographie des N. facialis, Acta Chir. Austr. [Suppl.] vol. 18, 1978.
17. Michon, J.: Vortrag gehalten auf dem 8th Symposium der Deutschsprachigen Arbeitsgemeinschaft für Handchirurgie, May 28-30, Handchirurgie **1:**75-76, 1969.
18. Michon, J., and Masse, P.: Le moment optimum de la suture nerveuse dans les plaies du membre supérieur, Rev. Chir. Orthop. **50:**(2):205-212, 1964.
19. Millesi, H.: Zum Problem der Überbrückung von Defekten peripherer Nerven, Wien. Med. Wochenschr. **118:**182-187, 1968.
20. Millesi, H., Berger, A., and Meissl, G.: Experimentelle Untersuchungen zur Heilung durchtrennter peripherer Nerven, Chir. Plast. **1:**174-206, 1972.
21. Millesi, H., Meissl, G., and Berger, A.: The interfascicular nerve grafting of the median-ulnar nerves. J. Bone Joint Surg. [Am.] **54:**727-750, 1972.
22. Millesi, H., Ganglberger, J., and Berger, A.: Erfahrungen mit der Mikrochirurgie peripherer Nerven, Chir. Plast. Reconstr. **3:**47-55, 1967.
23. Moberg, E.: In discussion of "The place of nerve grafting in orthopaedic surgery" by Donald Brooks, J. Bone Joint Surg. [Am.] **37:**305, 1955.
24. Nicholson. O. R., and Seddon, H. J.: Nerve repair in civil practice. Results of treatment of median and ulnar nerve lesions, Br. Med. J. **2:**1065, 1957.

25. O'Brien, B.: Personal communication, Melbourne, 1971.
26. Önne, L.: Recovery of sensibility and sudomotor activity in the hand after nerve suture, Acta Chir. Scand. [Suppl.] **300:**1-69, 1962.
27. Sakellarides, H.: A follow-up study of 173 peripheral nerve injuries in the upper extremity in civilians, J. Bone Joint Surg. [Am.] **44:**140, 1962.
28. Samii, M., and Wallenberg, R.: Tierexperimentelle Untersuchungen über den Einfluss der Spannung auf den Regenerationserfolg nach Nervennaht, Acta Neurochir. (Wien) **27:**87-110, 1972.
29. Seddon, H. J.: Three types of nerves injury, Brain **66:**237, 1943.
30. Seddon, H. J.: Restoration of function in peripheral nerve injuries, Lancet **1:**418, 1947.
31. Seddon, H. J.: Surgical disorders of the peripheral nerves, Edinburgh, 1972, Churchill Livingstone.
32. Smith, J.: Microsurgery of peripheral nerves, Plast. Reconstr. Surg. **33:**317, 1964.
33. Smith, F.: In Grobb, W. C., and Smith, J. W., editors: Plastic surgery, Boston 1968, Little, Brown and Company.
34. Sunderland, A.: A classification of peripheral nerve injuries producing loss of function, Brain **74:**491, 1951.
35. Terzis, J., Faibisoff, B., and Williams, H. B.: The nerve gap: suture under tension versus graft, Plast. Reconstr. Surg., **56:**166-170, 1975.
36. Tupper, J. W.: Panel discussion on microneurovascular transplantation and replantation, 32nd Annual Meeting of the American Society for Surgery of the Hand, Las Vegas, February 1977.

Chapter 4

Sensibility in reconstructive limb surgery

Erik Moberg

Sensibility, the "eye" of the skin, has been most highly developed, and consequently most studied, in the hand. Much of this chapter will refer specifically to hand sensibility, but the information can be directly related to other problem areas. While there are still many areas of controversy, all students of this subject must accept two premises: (1) only a disciplined, truly scientific method will lead to improved understanding of the problem, and (2) our ultimate goal is to provide improvements for our patients that are truly useful.

In the past there have been three obstacles to a truly objective, scientifically valid study of sensibility. First, the term "nerve repair" is semantically confusing. When we use the term we really mean that we are bringing the severed ends into gross anatomic proximity. The term makes no claim as to final function, which is the real reason for the "repair." Sensory nerve repair in an adult can be compared to the old car in Fig. 4-1. The horn still works and is thus protective, but does the vehicle function? Similarly, the patient's age, as shown by Seddon, Önne, and others, is still more important than the "repair" (even microsurgical) in determining final sensibility.[8,10] It is semantically more accurate and communicatively more reliable to describe our surgery as nerve suturing or grafting rather than as repair.

Second, the old science of neurology has been inappropriately applied to the study of the more youthful discipline of hand surgery. The purposes and tools of each are totally different. For the most part, the neurologist uses the peripheral nervous system as a window to examine more central pathology. The hand surgeon conversely usually encounters a normal central system with more distal pathology. The neurologist deals with the solution of diagnostic riddles, while the hand surgeon tries to provide utilitarian therapy. To quote Sir Russel Brain[1]: "The neurologist is concerned with sensibility primarily for the purpose of localizing lesions in the nervous system and determining their nature. His methods of investigation are therefore more 'rough and ready' . . . and have been adopted on account of their practical value for his immediate purpose." Adopted from whom? From physiologists who developed them for other purposes, but adopted by neurologists because of their practical value.

When hand surgeons tried to use the four modalities of touch, pain, heat, and cold to evaluate nerve sensory recovery, their results were disappointing. Seddon recognized this long ago when he distinguished between "academic" and "functional" recovery. To quote Goethe in Faust: "Grey, dear friend, is all theory, but green the golden tree of life."

When I compared results obtained by using all the known neurologic tests for the four modalities above (as well as vibration and electrophysiologic conduction tests) with true functional recovery, there was no correlation.[3]

For tasks to be accomplished with speed and skill, tactile gnosis is the essential sensory ingredient. This is rarely if ever obtained in adults by suturing severed sensory nerve ends together. Thus, only a small part of the sensory scale that can be determined by cotton wool and pinprick (Fig. 4-2) is of interest to the peripheral nerve surgeon. Although of course even protective sensibility is a worthy goal of repair, one must not lose sight of the possibility of troublesome paresthesia that frequently results from digital nerve anastomosis. This is especially common after joining severed distal radial nerves, with the resulting hyperesthesia frequently more disabling than anesthesia. Too often,

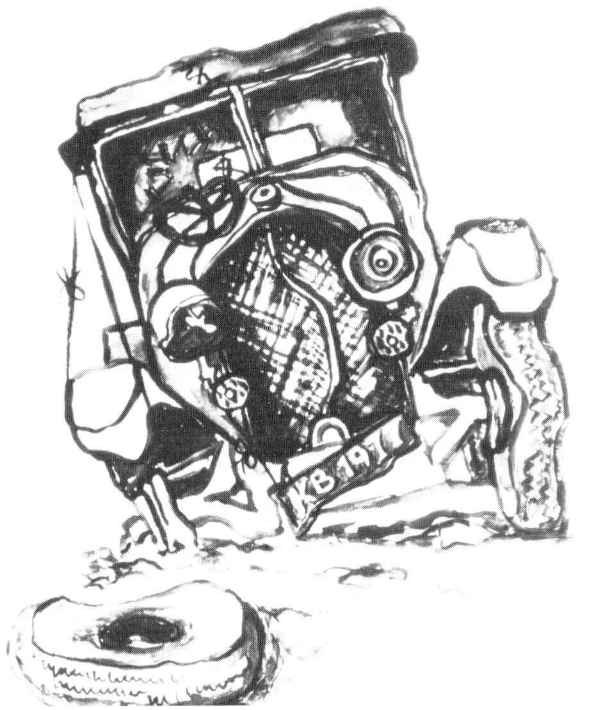

Fig. 4-1. Old car resembles adult sensory nerve repair. Horn still works as a protective device but does vehicle function?

lack of appreciation of these truths has resulted in erroneous reports of normal recovery when in fact function is limited. Such reports are unfair to the patients and misinform the unsophisticated. A properly scientific evaluation of sensibility requires the development of a new methodology and rejects the temptation to borrow from classic neurology.

Third, in 1954, the British Research Council adopted Highet's scheme for the evaluation of motor function. Five grades from M-0 to M-5 (normal) were used and have been generally adopted and stood the test of time. They also proposed a similar grading for sensibility from S-0 to S-4. However, for the reconstructive surgeon only the very top of this S scale is of real concern, and a more detailed distinction is needed. An additional plus or minus helps very little. Such a scale serves only to falsely satisfy the surgeon, but does little to describe the patient's real difficulty. This classification, however, still persists in the literature (especially in reimplantation reports) and to my mind is a serious deterrent to progress.

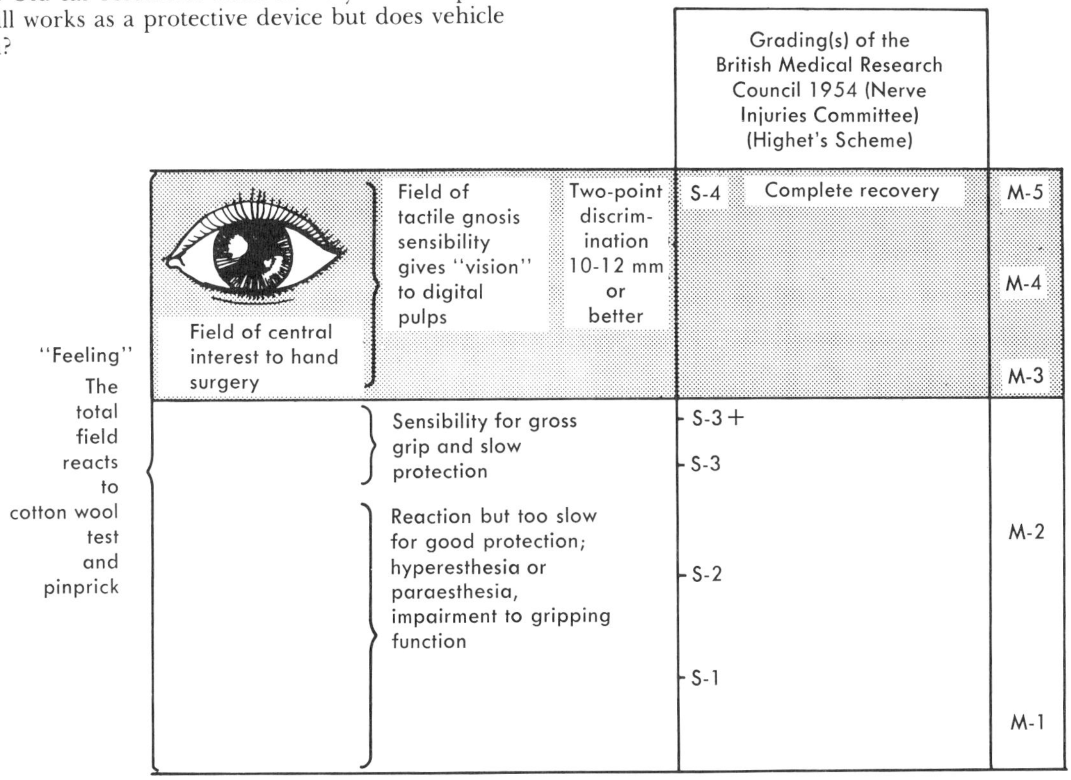

Fig. 4-2. Schematic relationship of some test methods used in neurology, qualities of sensibility of interest in reconstructive hand surgery, and corresponding grading according to Highet's scheme S adopted by British Medical Research Council in 1954. For comparison, scheme M is included. Observe how much more of its grades are in field of interest. It is obvious that cotton wool tests and use of pinprick and similar methods must be abandoned before evaluation of results for comparison can start and progress begin.

A B C

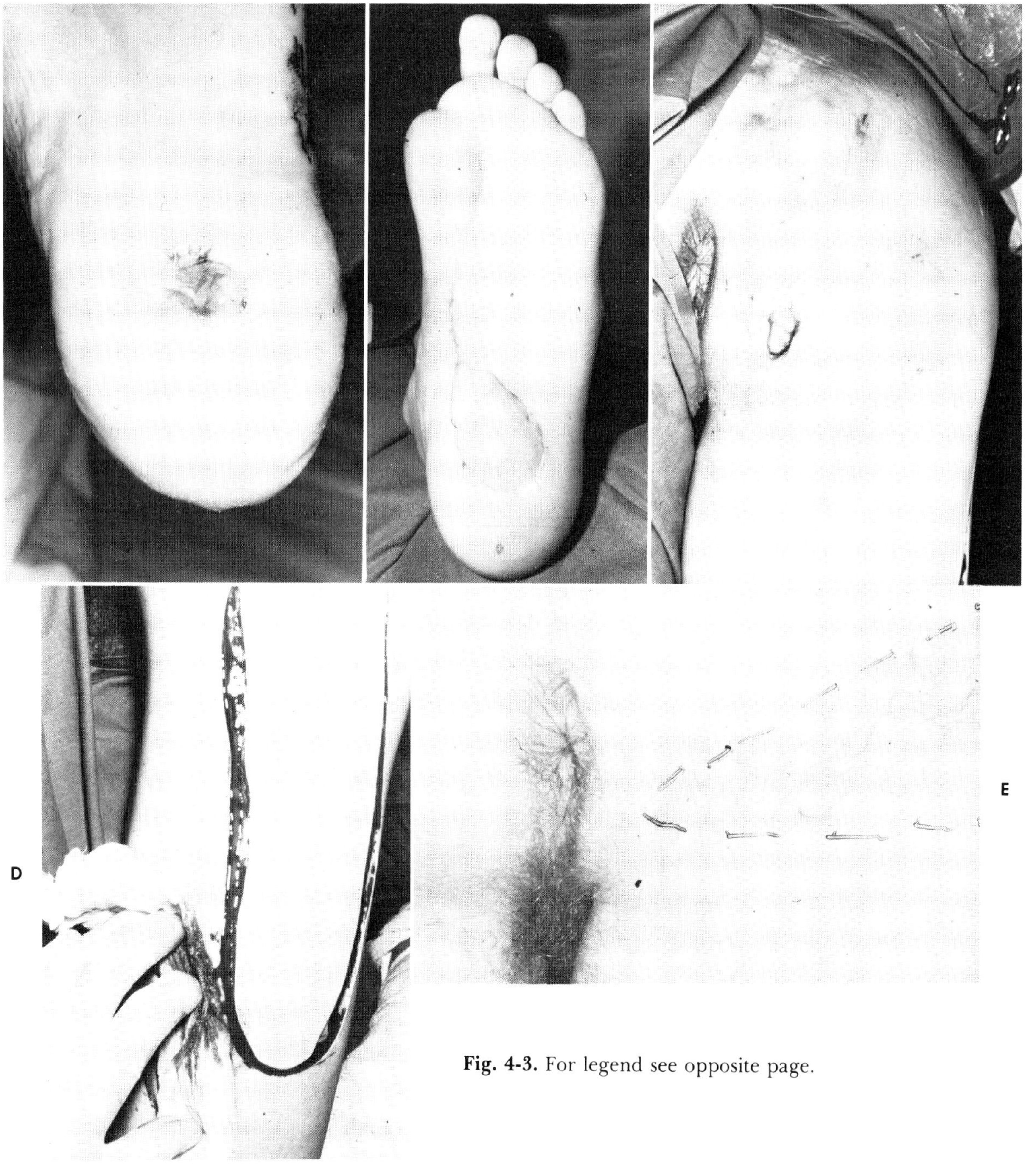

D E

Fig. 4-3. For legend see opposite page.

The subject of sensibility is best divided into four key queries: why, what, when, and how.

Why? All measurements must be made on a similar relevant scale in order to properly compare and evaluate results. The final function of neurovascular island flaps, reimplantations, and the myriad techniques of nerve suturing must all be evaluated by a single meaningful method to permit proper comparison. How good are our measuring tools? In 1907 German surgeons reported that about 70% of nerve "repairs" gave good results. Following World War I Davies and Pollock published identical figures, and Seddon found a similar proportion following civilian injuries 20 years ago. In 1975 Zilch and Buck-Gramcko[11] reported their results using sophisticated microsurgery, and again their "good" results approximated 70%.

Have all the advances in understanding and technique of the last five decades been of no real benefit to the patient? My own long professional experience belies this. While the current state of the art produces far from ideal results, it is still improved over what we could accomplish decades ago. Results have improved, but our current measuring tools have not been appropriate to appreciate the change.

To truly study the problem all the cases must be classified according to the patient's age, type of trauma, location of injury, time after injury, repair techniques, and so on. No one in the world has sufficient cases for statistically valid determinations. Only the pooled results from many centers can provide us with answers, but to be meaningful all must be measured on an identical scale with identical devices. Seddon[10] remarked: "It is doubtful if valid comparisons can be made unless the same observer assesses results; 'high church' investigators would say—impossible!" I would like to add that only "high church" investigators can claim scientific validity; subtle differences can only be detected by sensitive "tools." Therefore, the answer to "why" must be, because we know so little and have need to know so much more.

What? What should we look for to properly evaluate our patients? Fig. 4-2 tells us to look for the hand. We must first accept the fact, as also must our patients,—that the mere presence of "feeling" is of little concern. The word "feeling" is subject to the same semantic confusions as "repair." It is too broad and all encompassing to be of value. The most important sensory test for following the functional recovery of a sutured sensory nerve is that of *tactile gnosis*. Certainly qualities of sensibility below this are important (Fig. 4-3), but if the sophisticated problem of restoring tactile gnosis could be solved, the rest would follow with ease.

While tactile gnosis is the key factor in peripheral nerve disruption, proprioception must also be considered in proximal lesions such as stroke, cerebral palsy, and spinal cord injury. Fig. 4-4 describes a test to demonstrate that cutaneous receptors and afferents can precisely report position, motion, and force (i.e., proprioception) at a conscious level. This belies current physiologic concepts.

Thus tactile gnosis and proprioception could be reproducibly measured and the results pooled from many centers. A beginning toward a truly valid analysis could be made.

When? It seems basic to assume that postoperative results must be compared with the preoperative status to reveal the degree of improvement (or lack thereof) obtained. Yet most of our literature reports on the total postoperative result as a function of the surgery without any consideration to the contribution of preoperative residuals. The sensory contribution of the receptors preexisting in the flap

Fig. 4-3. Obviously qualities of sensory functions other than tactile gnosis and proprioception can be of interest in reconstructive work, as this case demonstrates. A young man had a low spinal injury with fewer calf muscles in one leg. Excess pressure of heel-only gait caused deep pressure ulceration with osteitis. Despite several surgical procedures this repair never did tolerate walking. When the patient was examined, it became obvious that posterior part of foot around ulceration had no two-point discrimination whatsoever. Pulp of great toe, however, had normal 15 mm two-point sensibility. It was useless for walking, and its loss was of no functional importance. Ulceration with bony base was excised, and pulp skin of great toe was transferred as a neurovascular island to heel. Dorsal artery was passed through first metatarsal interspace. After this successful result, **B,** patient requested treatment of ischial pressure sore, **C.** Examination also revealed total loss of sensibility over this area, but patient retained normal sensibility in distribution of lateral cutaneous femoral nerve. Flap was raised, **D,** and later brought around to sitting point, **E.** A decade later protective sensibility at both sites remains fully functional, recurrences have been absent, and two-point discrimination of toe pulp over heel shows just 2 mm lower value than originally.

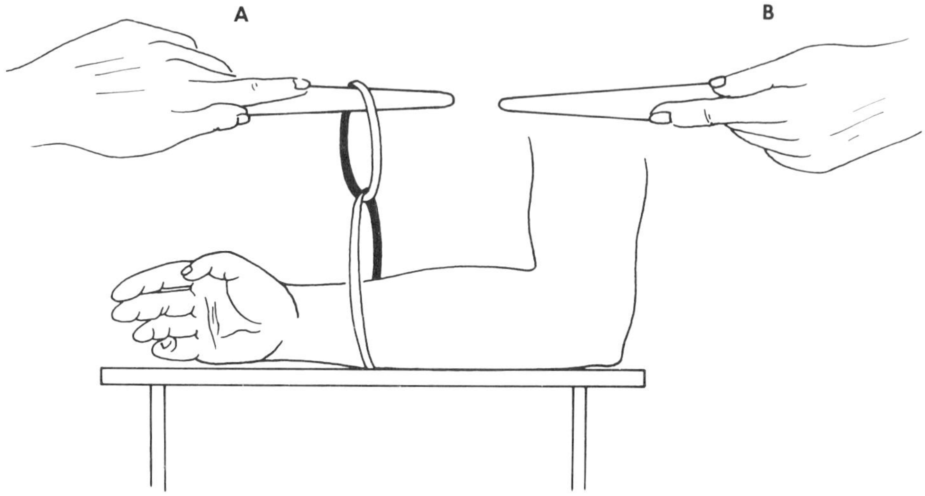

Fig. 4-4. Simple experiment shows how well cutaneous receptors alone, all information excluded, can provide proprioception to "artificial limb." Necessary prerequisites are the leader of experiment, a subject, two pens, and a few small rubber bands. Illustration shows correct setup. 1. Subject rests arm on table. He watches leader, **A,** move pen and "artificial limb" up and down (rubber bands are not attached to pen) and has, of course, no difficulty tracking its movement up and down with his own pen, **B.** 2. When subject's eyes are closed and rubber bands are not attached, this experiment is evidently impossible, due to lack of afferent impulses. 3. With rubber bands attached as shown in illustration, only cutaneous receptors from forearm can give information. With a pull of only about 50 g, all joint or musculotendinous afferents are excluded. Still, subject can follow pen, **A,** through proprioceptive control given by his skin. At start, his excursions are usually too small. But with rubber bands attached and his eyes open he will "program his computer" over his consciousness in a few minutes and then, even with closed eyes, be able to follow motion exactly. Proprioceptive skill is acquired.

or graft bed is never considered, nor is the effect of adjacent normal receptors. Patients do not always have classic anatomic nerve distributions. Now much of our supposed recovery is merely atypical innervation. When a single digital nerve is severed,[2] documentation of that patient's particular area of impairment requires a Ninhydrin map. Postoperative evaluation should also include blocking of adjacent nerves in order to document that "recovery" is from the "repair" and is not a misleading response to the test from adjacent areas with a normal nerve supply, never lost. The answer to "when" must therefore be, *before* as well as after the surgery. A detailed evaluation is required. This is certainly not standard care today but must be done if an accurate evaluation of results is to be available for comparison studies.

How? Do we have any useful and reliable test methods today? After much trial I have found that only the old Weber two-point discrimination test will give reliable reproducible data that corresponds to the true level of functional sensibility. All other tests are of little value. Even the Weber test, however, is not without pitfalls that could invalidate pooled data.

I have discarded calipers and now use a simple wire paperclip with a 0.9 mm diameter that is opened and bent to provide two points of adjustable distance. These are always available and are light enough so that their weight will not disturb measurements as do calipers, rulers, and so on. The blunt ends are less stimulatory to the frequently present hyperesthesia.

Improperly used, this test can be misleading and err on either side. Properly used, however, the results are reliable and reproducible. Both the patient's and the examiner's hands must be braced on a table as motion misleadingly improves two-point discrimination. Both prongs must touch the skin at the same instant. The pressure applied is critical. Too much force will depress adjacent skin and stimulate receptors far from the prongs. This gives a falsely optimistic reading. Proper pressure is achieved just at the point when blanching begins. (The American Society for Surgery of the Hand has recently recommended that the prongs be oriented in the longitudinal direction.) Further detail is available in a previous report.[6]

While not perfect, this is the best available test of tactile gnosis. Improved techniques await discovery.

It is now known that high-quality proprioception can be transmitted through cutaneous receptors. The evidence that muscle or tendon receptors in man can produce high-quality conscious proprioception is questionable. Thus, the deformation of the skin surface can be used for both proprioceptive and tactile gnostic testing—a fortuitous simplification. The scales are also similar. If the patient's injured digits can discriminate two points 10 to 12 mm apart, then proprioception is also present to a useful degree.

Seddon has perhaps done more than anyone else to advance the field of peripheral nerve surgery. In 1975 he said: "If . . . the recording of sensory recovery can be better defined and generally adopted, it will be a great step forward." Optimistic reports based on false analysis only clutter our literature and confuse the issue.

REFERENCES

1. Brain, R.: Disease of the central nervous system, London, 1962, Oxford University Press.
2. Fetrow, K. O.: Variations in sensory nerve supply to the hand. In Michon, J., and Moberg, E., editors: Traumatic nerve lesions of the upper limb, Edinburgh, 1975, Churchill Livingstone.
3. Moberg, E.: Criticism and study of methods for examining sensibility in the hand, Neurology (Minneap.) **12:**8-19, 1962.
4. Moberg, E.: Fingers were made before forks, Hand **4:**201-206, 1972.
5. Moberg, E.: Methods of examining sensibility of the hand. In Flynn, J. E., editor: Hand surgery, Baltimore, 1975, The Williams & Wilkins Company.
6. Moberg, E.: Reconstructive hand surgery. In Tetraplegia, stroke, and cerebral palsy: some basic concepts in physiology and neurology, J. Hand Surg. **1:**29-34, July 1976.
7. Moberg, E.: Future hopes for the surgical management of peripheral nerve lesions. In Michon, J., and Moberg, E., editors: Traumatic nerve lesions of the upper limb, Edinburgh, 1975, Churchill Livingstone.
8. Önne, L.: Recovery of sensibility and sudomotor activity in the hand after nerve suture, Acta Chir. Scand. [Suppl.] **300:**1-69, 1962.
9. Pollock, L. J., and Davis, L.: Peripheral nerve injuries, New York, 1933, Paul B. Hoeber.
10. Seddon, H.: Surgical disorders of the peripheral nerves, Edinburth, 1975, Churchill Livingstone.
11. Zilch, H., and Buck-Gramcko, D.: Ergebnisse der Nervenwiederherstellungen an der obere Extremität durch Mikrochirurgie, Handchirurgie **7**(1):21-31, 1975.

Chapter 5

Recovery of sensation following peripheral nerve repair

Michael E. Jabaley

Hands serve as grasping tools and as sensory organs. The nature of those tasks assigned to the hand is so precise and demanding that the hand robbed of feeling performs in clumsy fashion or not at all. To physically suture the divided ends of a peripheral nerve poses no great challenge to hand surgeons; to consistently recover a useful level of sensation in the territory supplied by such a nerve remains one of the most elusive challenges in all of hand surgery. The objectives of this chapter are to present relevant aspects of neuroanatomy and physiology, to relate this information to regenerating nerves, and to emphasize those aspects of nerve repair and wound care that appear to have an effect on the ultimate ability of the hand to function usefully.

ANATOMY

The hand and the fingertips are rich in sensory nerve endings.[1] These cutaneous endings are of three types (Fig. 5-1): (1) free endings, in which the bare nerve terminal lies among cells of the dermis or epidermis, (2) expanded tip endings, which are surrounded by dermal cells and occur throughout the dermis, and (3) encapsulated endings, which are enclosed by specialized and sometimes easily identifiable nonneural tissue.[10] When morphologists first described the various endings, it was common to assign a specific sensory modality such as light, touch, heat, and cold and an eponym such as Krause or Ruffini to each one. More recent evidence suggests that such a relationship is not valid, and these classifications are no longer used. First, there are more types of endings than sensory modalities to assign to them. Second, biopsies and serial section of skin spots associated with a specific modality, such as hot or cold skin spots, have not confirmed the presence of the appropriate receptor in the section corresponding to the sensation. Finally, a specific sensation is sometimes found in areas (such as the cornea) known not to contain the types of endings previously associated with that sensation.

Physiologists now consider that all sensory endings are either (1) *mechanoreceptors* (a synonym for touch and pressure), (2) *thermoreceptors,* or (3) *noci-*

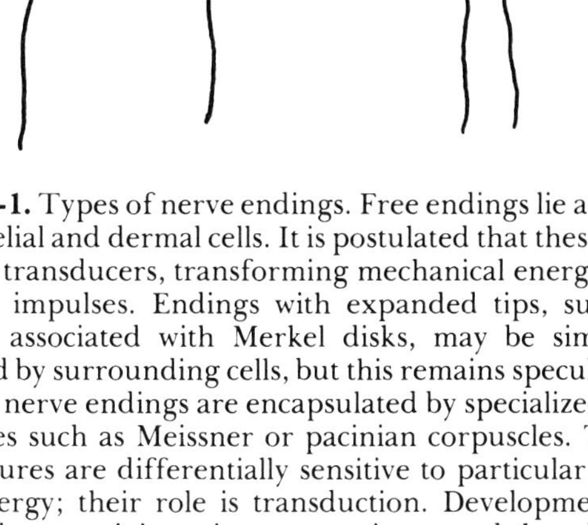

Fig. 5-1. Types of nerve endings. Free endings lie among epithelial and dermal cells. It is postulated that these cells act as transducers, transforming mechanical energy into nerve impulses. Endings with expanded tips, such as those associated with Merkel disks, may be similarly served by surrounding cells, but this remains speculative. Some nerve endings are encapsulated by specialized corpuscles such as Meissner or pacinian corpuscles. These structures are differentially sensitive to particular types of energy; their role is transduction. Developmentally they do not originate in nervous tissue, and they do not degenerate after injury as axons do.

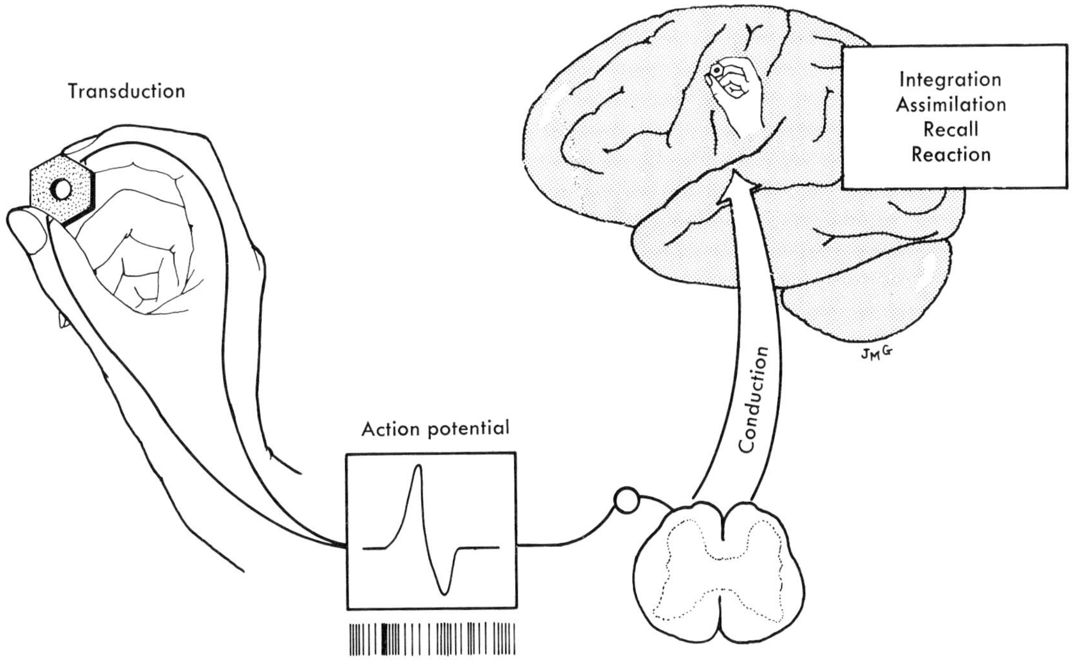

Fig. 5-2. Steps of sensation. Mechanical force of an object held between the fingers is transformed (transduced) by specialized endings in skin into an impulse that can be transmitted (and measured) along first-order afferent neurons. Sensibility is the reception and transmission of such impulses and their recognition in brain. Sensation embodies all those steps concerned with impulses reaching brain *plus* those processes concerned with their elevation to conscious level—integration with other incoming data, assimilation into past experience, recall of specific information, and finally, an appropriate response, such as motion or oral description.

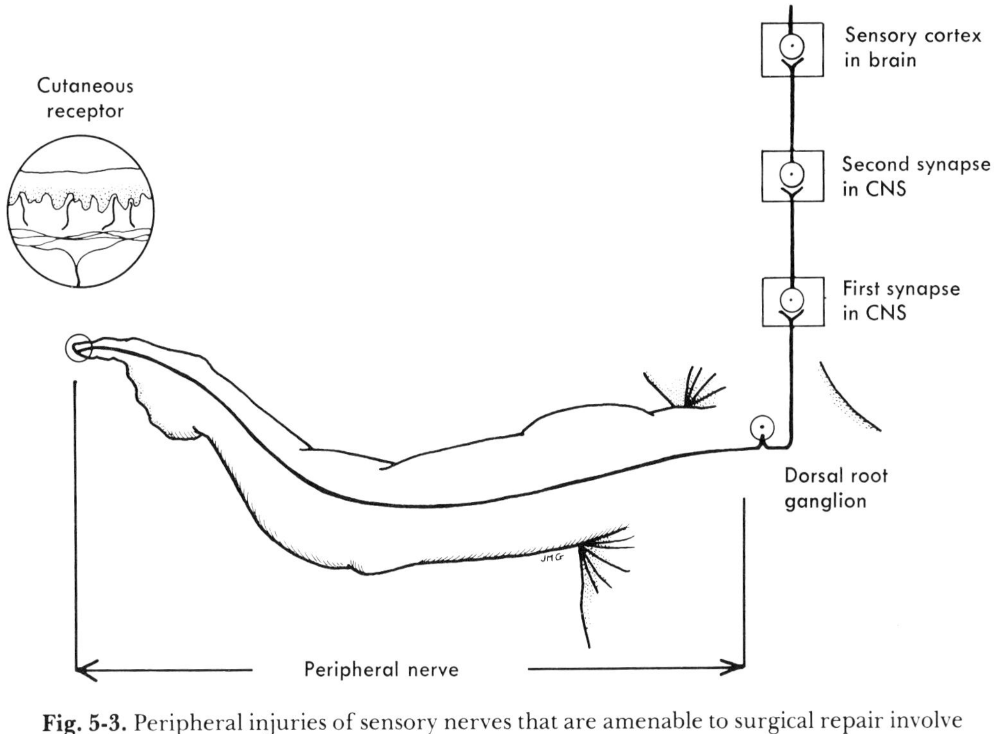

Fig. 5-3. Peripheral injuries of sensory nerves that are amenable to surgical repair involve axons of first-order afferent neurons. Remainder of sensory chain is in spinal cord and brain and is inaccessible. Goal of repair of peripheral nerves is accurate anatomic restitution of conducting units of first-order axons.

*ceptors.** Their endings are differentially sensitive to specific forms of energy that may be applied to the skin surface.[11] A common feature of sensory endings is that they are transducers; that is, they change the energy of external stimuli into conductible nerve impulses[9] (Fig. 5-2). These impulses proceed along a chain of three afferent neurons and ultimately arrive at the sensory cortex. *It should be apparent that all "peripheral nerve injuries" that are treated operatively involve and are limited to the axons of first-order afferent neurons.* For practical purposes, the remainder of the neuron chain is beyond the surgeon's reach (Fig. 5-3).

Major peripheral nerves contain several thousand axons. These may be myelinated (2 to 30 μm in diameter) or unmyelinated (smaller than 2 μm in diameter). Although such nerves are usually mixed, containing motor and sensory elements, this discussion will be limited to the sensory component. In sensory nerves the endings lie far in the periphery while the cell body is located in the dorsal root ganglia of the spinal cord. Afferent impulses from these cell bodies may proceed centrally to the brain by either of two systems: the lemniscal system or the anterolateral system.[12]

Lemniscal system

Large myelinated fibers of the dorsal roots travel the ipsilateral dorsal column and terminate in its nuclei. These nuclei project via the medial lemniscus (hence, the name) upon the contralateral ventrobasal thalamic complex and proceed to the postcentral gyrus of the sensory cortex. The distinguishing features of the lemniscal system are (1) that most of the fibers are large and myelinated and (2) that information concerning location, shape, quality, and temporal sequence of stimuli is transmitted rapidly and *with great fidelity* at each synaptic station. This characteristic of faithful transmission permits information to reach the brain in accurate detail; it is the basis for fine discrimination of mechanical stimuli.

Anterolateral system

First-order afferent neurons also connect by the interneuronal system of the dorsal horn of the spinal cord. Some fibers cross to the contralateral side and others continue on the ipsilateral side, but both proceed centrally in the anterolateral columns of the spinal cord. Fibers in this system characteristically are small myelinated or unmyelinated. Compared to the lemniscal system, these tracks are phylogenetically older and less precisely organized. Their cortical representation is less exact. They serve the modalities of pain and temperature as well as a general form of mechanoreception. The anterolateral system conducts more slowly, and its central representation is somewhat less precise that that of the lemniscal system. It is concerned more with a general level of sensation. Together, the lemniscal and anterolateral systems continually feed volleys of impulses to the brain. On the basis of this information the brain constantly updates its perception of the external world. This process of continuing input and modification is considerably more complex than the one ending–one modality concept.

The functional role of cutaneous sensory nerve endings appears to be the encoding of stimulus information received at the skin surface. There are a variety of possible codes. The simplest of these is an on-off system where an axon either develops and transmits an action potential or it does not. In this instance the combination of active axons determines the nature of the message. Other possible codes may be determined by rate, frequency, sequence, or other impulse characteristics. Whatever its nature, it is this transmitted code that reaches the brain and is interpreted as a specific sensation.

Very little is known about how messages that originate in the activity of ensembles of peripheral nerve endings are received and processed at the sensory cortical level. Nevertheless, it is this process of transduction, transmission, and interpretation, in its totality, that ultimately leads to conscious recognition. *Sensibility* can be defined simply as the ability to perceive an external stimulus. *Sensation* is infinitely more complex and includes other factors such as integration, association, enhancement, and recall. It is influenced by environment, experience, motivation, and other secondary objectives. For these reasons, sensation is infinitely more difficult to measure in the clinical setting. Nevertheless, sensation as well as sensibility must be recovered if a nerve repair is to result in useful function. In the repair of a nerve the simple restoration of axonal continuity is not suficient to produce satisfactory functional results; information must reach the brain in an interpretable fashion if orderly reaction is to result.

*The term "nociceptor" is preferable to pain receptor. The dual nature of "pain" refers both to the reception and interpretation of the sensation. The study of pain interpretation is necessarily limited to humans. The use of the term nociceptor refers to the reception of noxious stimuli and has nothing to do with the central interpretation of such sensations. Nociceptors and their function have been studied in animals and have provided considerable information and insight into the physiology of pain.

RESPONSE TO INJURY

Nerves contain two main structural components: the conducting neural tissue itself (axons) and the supportive nonneural structural apparatus (epineurium, perineurium, and endoneurium).[8] Considerable information exists concerning the events that occur following the division of a peripheral nerve.[4,15] For purposes of this discussion it is sufficient to recognize that neural tissue begins to degenerate distal to the site of injury shortly after injury occurs (wallerian degeneration). The changes that evolve in nonneural tissue, on the other hand, are slower, more subtle, and quite different. The supporting Schwann cells do not degenerate and die but rather remain intact for a long period of time. There is gradual and progressive fibrosis of the nerve trunk, clinically recognizable as a decrease in the diameter of the nerve. There appears to be a correlation between the time interval from injury to repair and the ability of regenerating axons to extend along the Schwann network. This is partly responsible for the poorer results seen when operating is delayed for long periods of time.

Although the axon and Schwann sheath response to injury has been carefully studied, less information is available about the fate of specialized cutanous endings. Recent morphologic studies of biopsies of skin in animals[2] and in patients[5] have shown that specialized encapsulated endings in denervated skin do not degenerate and disappear,

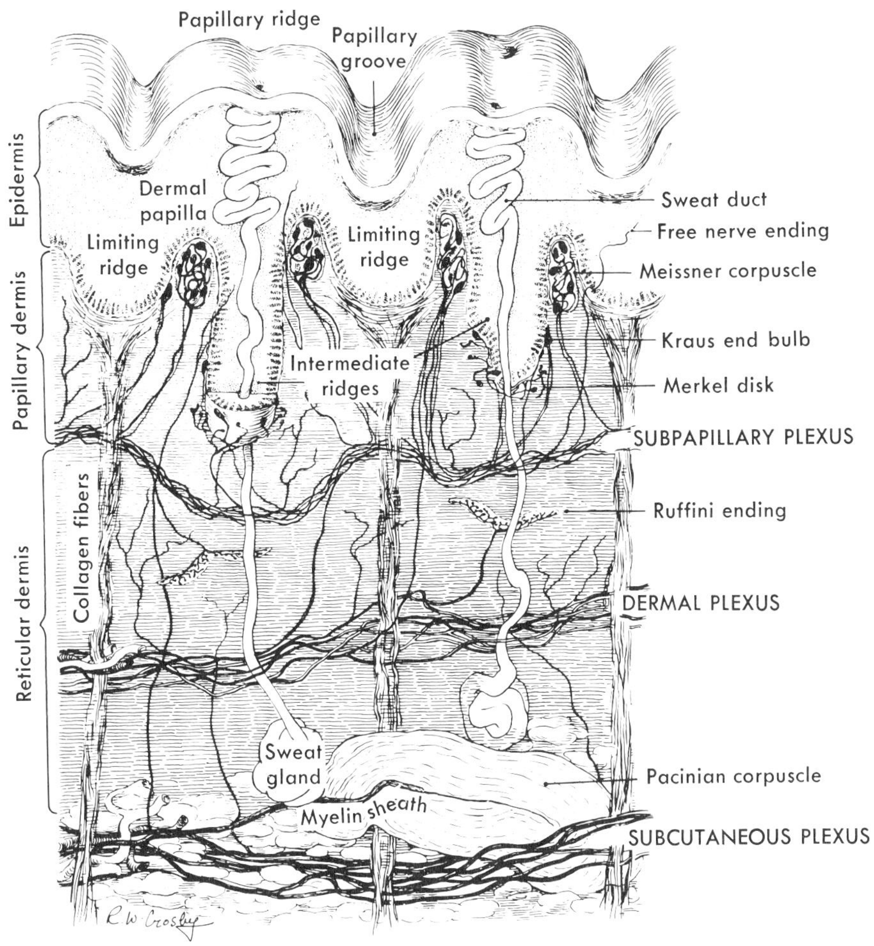

Fig. 5-4. Section of fingertip skin at right angles to papillary ridges. On left are layers of dermis and epidermis. Three main plexuses of nerve can be seen at subcutaneous, dermal, and subpapillary levels. Branches from each plexus go to upper level of dermis and epidermis where they terminate. Their endings may be free, expanded, or encapsulated. A large number of these endings serve as mechanoreceptors and are selectively sensitive to specific types of touch or pressure. It is unlikely that a naturally occurring stimulus would ever activate only one receptor. Numerous receptors act in concert to produce a composite descriptive code of external objects and events.

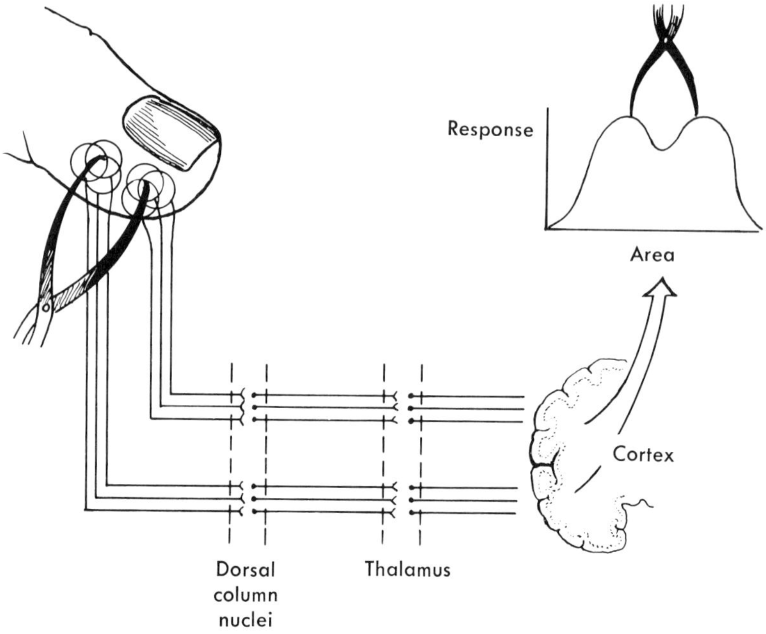

Fig. 5-5. Overlap of peripheral fields permits precise localization of mechanical stimuli and forms basis for two-point discrimination test. Each stimulus excites a number of receptors (small circles on thumb). Intensity of response depends on type of stimulus and its distance from each receptor. Each impulse that is generated provides a slightly different "fix" or localization of stimulus. Composite picture of all these impulses that is produced in sensory cortex is a precise representation of peripheral event and permits accurate description or reaction to it. Diagram *(upper right)* of an oscilloscope tracing shows two peaks, each corresponding to cortical area excited by a point stimulus. In normal circumstances, peaks are sharp. As points move closer together, peaks merge and two points are interpreted as one.

as some investigators had suspected. Instead, they undergo progressive atrophy but may remain in identifiable form for several months. They appear to be capable of reinnervation, a fact that is of great significance from the standpoint of ultimate recovery of function. There is no evidence to suggest that a regenerating axon can re-form a sophisticated nonneural capsule about its end once it has reached the skin level. If the transducer function of specialized organs is to be restored, the restoration must result from reinnervation of existing corpuscles or capsules.

RESPONSE TO NERVE REGENERATION

The ability of nerve axons to grow across a nerve juncture following successful suture has been documented; the factors that influence the quality of this regrowth have been carefully studied; and the rate of recovery has been investigated.[4,15] These aspects of recovery are easier to measure objectively in motor nerves than in sensory nerves. The clinician who repairs a sensory nerve must still monitor progress by an advancing Tinel sign, functional testing, or those tests based on known physiologic properties of receptors and fiber types. As noted above, specific information about the status of receptors in fingertip skin has not been available until recent years.[5] If surgeons are to consider nerve repairs in terms of the chain of neural events described earlier in this chapter, the need for specific information about the fate of cutaneous receptors and their possible reinnervation becomes clear.

Biopsies of fingertip skin of patients who have undergone successful nerve suture in our hospital have been examined for the presence of axons and nerve endings[6] (Figs. 5-4 and 5-5). Sections of these biopsies indicate that in every instance there is histologic evidence of nerve regeneration at least to the level of the intradermal plexus, and in a majority of cases, identifiable end organs are reinnervated as well (Fig. 5-6). Unfortunately, such morphologic studies do not correlate with clinical and functional recovery as it is usually measured. In our series, patients with a large volume of identifiable nerve sometimes performed poorly on clinical testing.[6] Conversely, some patients with a scant amount of

A

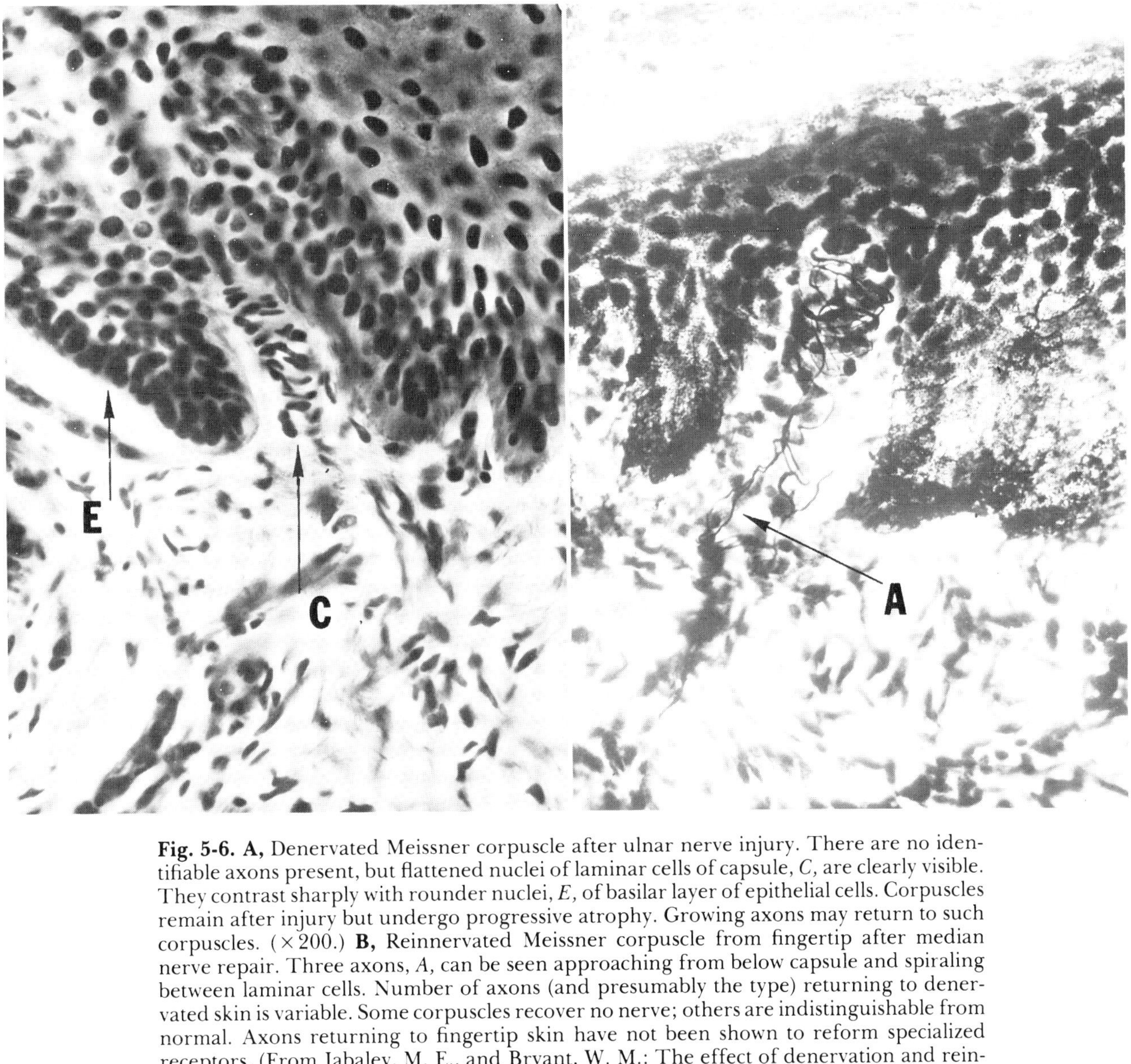

B

Fig. 5-6. A, Denervated Meissner corpuscle after ulnar nerve injury. There are no identifiable axons present, but flattened nuclei of laminar cells of capsule, *C,* are clearly visible. They contrast sharply with rounder nuclei, *E,* of basilar layer of epithelial cells. Corpuscles remain after injury but undergo progressive atrophy. Growing axons may return to such corpuscles. (×200.) **B,** Reinnervated Meissner corpuscle from fingertip after median nerve repair. Three axons, *A,* can be seen approaching from below capsule and spiraling between laminar cells. Number of axons (and presumably the type) returning to denervated skin is variable. Some corpuscles recover no nerve; others are indistinguishable from normal. Axons returning to fingertip skin have not been shown to reform specialized receptors. (From Jabaley, M. E., and Bryant, W. M.: The effect of denervation and reinnervation of encapsulated receptors in digital skin. In Marchac, D., editor: Transactions of the Sixth International Congress of Plastic and Reconstructive Surgery, Paris, 1976, Masson.)

nerve performed tests and used the part very well. This observation emphasizes that factors other than the regrowth of nerve axons are involved in the recovery of sensation. It explains, in part, why sensory reeducation may improve clinical performance following nerve repair.[3]

Paul and associates studied a group of monkeys in whom they divided a peripheral nerve at the wrist and repaired it immediately.[13,14] Repairs were performed with 8-0 silk and an operating microscope. Following a time interval sufficient to allow axon regeneration, the animals were studied by stimulating the cutaneous territory supplied by the nerve and simultaneously recording responses in the sensory cortex of the brain. The data obtained demonstrate that the normally orderly cortical pattern may be distorted to a considerable degree after axonal regrowth, in location, level, and type of response. A stimulus applied to an area of fingertip skin may be received in an area of cortex that was originally not associated with that digit at all.

Two clinical observations suggest that similar phenomena may occur in humans as well as monkeys. Following the successful repair of a peripheral nerve, transposition of sensory territories is sometimes noted. For example, stroking the index finger of a blindfolded patient who has undergone median nerve suture may be interpreted by the patient as stimulation of the middle finger, suggesting that the impulses originating at the index finger travel along axons that were originally destined for the middle finger. This can only be explained by a crossover of axons at the site of nerve suture. Conversely if a neurovascular island flap (with nerves intact) is transferred to another digit, stroking of the flap continues to be interpreted as stimulation of the original donor finger. The fact that skin resides on an alien digit does not directly influence the area of cortical reception since the conducting apparatus has not been interrupted. (The possibility of "retraining" such transplants is purposely omitted.) In both instances it seems clear that axons continue to feed into the cortical areas to which they were originally directed regardless of the location of the peripheral ending and stimulus. If this is so, it is incumbent on the surgeon to strive to direct regenerating axons along conduits to peripheral sites that correspond to their central destinations.

Summary

The sensory component of peripheral nerves serving skin may be analogous in one respect to other organ systems in the body: organs such as the lung, kidney, liver, and heart have considerable functional reserve and can perform in a more or less normal fashion despite the loss of much of their volume through injury or disease. Likewise, the sensory sheet of skin can function in a reasonably normal way with less than its full complement of axons and endings *so long as those that remain or re-*

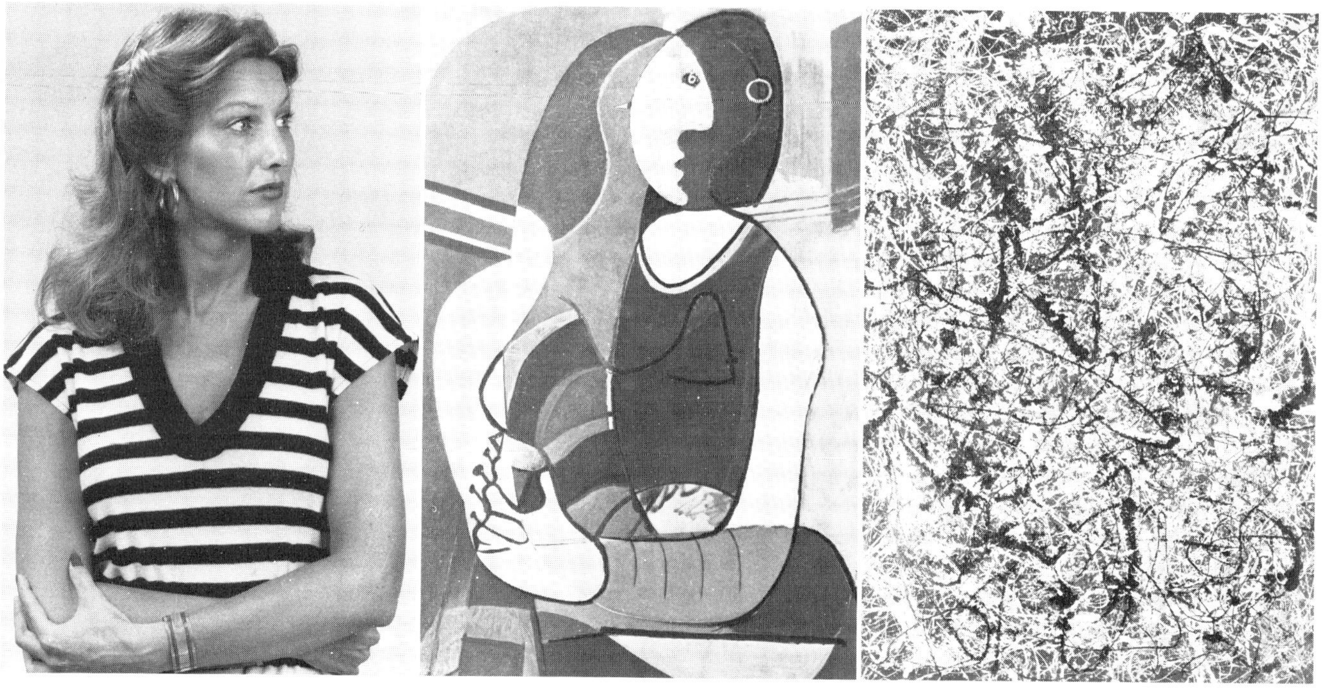

A B C

Fig. 5-7. Relationship between reality and perception. **A,** Under normal circumstances, external stimuli are received, transformed, and faithfully transmitted centrally. Image that is produced at conscious level is an accurate representation of stimulus. An appropriate response occurs. **B,** Picasso, *Seated Woman.* If there is significant crossover of axons at site of nerve juncture following a repair, external stimulus may still be normal, but image produced centrally may be distorted to point that identification is difficult and response slow or awkward. **C,** Jackson Pollock, *Mural,* 1950. In extreme instances image perceived in brain may not only be unintelligible but frankly distracting. Performance suffers accordingly. (**B** from Fox, M. S., editor: Picasso, New York, Harry N. Abrams; **C** from Mendelowitz, D. M.: A history of art, New York, 1970, Holt, Rinehart and Winston.)

cover terminate somewhere near their original cerebral cortical destination (Fig. 5-7). Since the more central portion of the nervous system (specifically, that portion proximal to a nerve repair) transmits faithfully the message code that it receives, the key to successful recovery or maintenance of function appears to be minimization of distortion of the distal signal. Axon crossover at the site of nerve suture must be kept to a minimum, as this is a major factor in the production of distorted impulses.

FACTORS AFFECTING THE QUALITY OF SENSORY RECOVERY

The objective of nerve repair is to rejoin the severed nerve ends accurately, with the formation of the least possible amount of scar at the juncture, and at a time that will allow the most rapid and orderly growth of axons along the distal Schwann system. Although a number of factors that come into play in this process are beyond the control of the surgeon, the decisions of the surgeon about the timing, technique, and choice of operation all have a definite effect.

Timing of repair

The timing of elective nerve repair has been debated since World War II.[4,7] There are several acceptable options. *Primary nerve* suture can be performed within the "golden period" of the first few hours following injury. Some clinical data has suggested that immediate nerve repair performed in tidy wounds results in better recovery of sensation than delayed repair, leading some authors to advocate this approach.

Some disadvantages to immediate repair are the following: The procedure must sometimes be performed at the end of a long day when the operating team is tired or some members may not be present. The wound is contaminated and risk of infection is somewhat higher. Additional trauma of surgical dissection is superimposed upon that resulting from the injury itself. Additional operating time must be added to that required solely for wound care. Most important is the difficulty in determining the degrees of injury that may be present in nerves damaged by crushing or gunshot wounds. Surgeons have sometimes sutured nerve ends that appeared normal at the time of repair only to find at a later exploration that a portion of a repaired end has become fibrotic and scarred because of unrecognized injury. Lastly, the role of axoplasmic flow in determining the eventual result must be considered. It is possible (but unproved) that nerves repaired after the cell body is in a positive metabolic state have a better chance of bridging the suture site than those repaired immediately. Immediate repair is clearly indicated in the clean, incised wound but should be used with caution if there is a crushing agent or penetrating missile involved.

Delayed primary nerve repair. A delayed primary nerve repair is performed a few days after injury but before the appearance of clinically recognizable scar in the wound. In practice this may be anywhere between 3 days and 3 weeks. When the patient is first seen, the wound may be cleansed and closed by suturing or it may be dressed open. If skin healing without infection appears likely, the nerve is repaired electively. The likelihood of infection in such wounds is extremely low. Bleeding has stopped, and any hematoma that is present can be evacuated. There is reduced edema and contusion; the nerve is in a positive metabolic state; and the degree of damage can be assessed accurately. The nerve ends can be excised if necessary. Delayed primary repair has all the advantages of immediate repair and few of the disadvantages. It does require a second operation, however, and many surgeons feel that it is simply unnecessary.

Early secondary repair. Early secondary repair is carried out several weeks after the time of injury. The skin wound is usually healed. Scar tissue surrounding the nerve must be excised, and structures to be repaired must be dissected free. The neuroma that is present must be excised and the nerve shortened. If an epineural suture is to be performed, many surgeons have found the thickened epineurium easier to suture than it might have been in the acute state, and this is offered as an argument for this type of repair. The reported results of early secondary repairs in some clinical series have been found to vary very little from the outcome of immediate repair utilizing similar technique. It is an acceptable alternative if other factors mitigate against earlier repair.

Late repair. Late repair of peripheral nerves is performed several months after injury and should be avoided if possible. The nerve shortens, and neuromas and gliomas form. This results in a sizable gap between the ends, which must be overcome by dissection and mobilization of nerve ends, flexion of joints, and stretching of nerve trunks. A graft is preferable if these manuevers must be carried to extremes. The quality of sensation that returns following repairs performed after delays greater than 3 weeks has been reported to fall at about the rate of 1% per week.[4] For this reason the interval from injury to repair should be kept to a few weeks if at all possible.

Technique of repair

The wound is the milieu in which the nerve ends must heal. For this reason the management of the wound is a vital aspect of nerve repair. The surgeon must carefully debride the skin edges and the deep wound, avoid desiccation, and remove all foreign bodies. He must avoid postoperative dead space and hematoma. The objectives of all these maneuvers are primary wound healing, avoidance of infection, and an absolute minimum of scar formation. The repaired nerve that lies in a well-vascularized bed will be least likely to be constricted by the encircling scar and will conduct better.[7]

Improvements in the manufacture of surgical instruments, sutures, and operating microscopes permit more accurate nerve repairs. The increased accuracy of suture placement that becomes possible with even low-power magnification is obvious to anyone who uses this adjunct and requires no comment. Modern-day suture is much less inflammatory than earlier material; it causes much less trauma to the nerve when swaged onto small sharp needles and placed with precision instruments. These technical advances result in more accurate axial alignment and less trauma and subsequent scar formation at the site of the nerve juncture. In terms of eventual recovery these are frequently the most important consideration of the repair.

When performing a secondary repair, the surgeon must excise neuromas and gliomas and identify healthy fascicles for suturing. There is a temptation to overcome resultant gaps between nerve ends by dissecting the proximal and distal segments for long distances. Although much of the blood supply of nerves appears to be longitudinal, some writers have questioned the wisdom of such extensive dissections, feeling that relative ischemia and increased scarring of the nerve may result. To overcome the gap between nerve ends, surgeons sometimes flex one or more joints. The joints must eventually be straightened, however, and a certain amount of tension inevitably results.

Millesi has stated that there is a direct relationship between tension and scar formation in the healing nerve (see Chapter 3). Scar at the site of nerve juncture is a mechanical barrier to axon growth, and he has recommended the use of nerve grafts as an alternative to extremes of flexion and lengthy dissection. His clinical results with grafts are superior to those obtained in patients with similar gaps treated by other means and appear to support his contention. If the tension of direct suture appears too great, a nerve graft is more likely to produce a statisfactory end result.

Whether one sutures nerve ends directly or interposes a graft, one must decide whether to perform an epineural or interfascicular suture. Although many excellent results have been obtained with epineural suture, our understanding of the microanatomy of nerves[8] and the importance of correct alignment suggests that an effort should be made to align individual fascicles as accurately as possible. This is most easily accomplished by direct suture of strategically located fascicles. Although proper alignment apparently occurs whenever a carefully performed epineural suture results in good functional recovery, direct suture of identifiable fascicles seems more likely to assure correct axial alignment.

In the past the entire nerve has been the smallest functional unit that could be satisfactorily manipulated and repaired; the epineurium was the cornerstone of nerve surgery. Now (and for the foreseeable future) the individual fascicle has become the functional working unit, and it is here that our hopes for improvement must lie. *Anyone who would repair peripheral nerves must align the fascicles as accurately as possible and hold them in a tension-free position until healing occurs.* Hand surgeons today are debating the relative merits of epineural suture, interfascicular suture, a combined suture, and a number of other techiques. Although the technique may for the present be undecided, the objective ought no longer to be in doubt.

Sunderland has focused attention on the problem of fascicular redistribution within a peripheral nerve by demonstrating that the cross-sectional relationship of fascicles changes continually at each level.[16] In addition, branches appear to travel from one fascicle to another. The practical consequence of this meandering of axons seems to be that removal of a section of a nerve will necessarily produce some fascicular malarrangement. For this reason we prefer not to shorten a transected nerve in a tidy wound; it appears preferable to excise contused epineurium and hematoma rather than arbitrarily shorten the nerve. In this manner the correct fascicular rotary relationship can be maintained. This technique cannot be used for late secondary repairs, of course. If these repairs are performed, resection of scar and neuroma must be adequate to leave healthy and viable fascicles for suturing.

The presence of the epineurium itself contributes to scar formation, and Millesi has suggested that results are likely to be better if this structure is dissected away from the area of the nerve juncture. To remove the epineurium increases dissection, makes suturing tedious, and adds to the difficulty of the repair. It remains to be seen whether the average surgeon will accept this concept and incorporate epineural excision into his technical repertoire. Epineurium is the strongest layer of the nerve, and many rely on it for strength. We have found that if the nerve is not shortened, the epineurium becomes a less important consideration and can be easily excised. When no nerve is removed, there is virtually no tension, and repairs can be performed with a minimum of sutures.

Skin at the receptor site

Whenever skin is transplanted to a fingertip, whether as a flap or graft, nerves must regrow into it. Similarly, patients undergoing nerve suture at a proximal level may sometimes suffer skin loss in the territory served by the repaired nerve. In both these instances, *the quality of sensation that can be recovered in such a territory can be no better than that of which the skin itself and the nerve endings therein are capable.*

When faced with skin loss, the surgeon must manage the wound so that it heals with the least possible amount of scar formation. Primary healing should be sought if at all possible. If it cannot be accomplished by direct suture, flaps or skin grafts are indicated. By all odds, local flaps of similar skin promise the best sensory results. If such flaps are unavailable and one must apply a graft, a donor site should be selected that has a high density of nerve endings. The more endings available for union with regenerating axons, the more likely one is to recover a high degree of sensation. Skin from the wrist crease, hypothenar eminence, or injured fingertips is probably superior to skin from the back or buttocks. When tested for two-point discrimination, the hand perceives at 2 to 4 mm, while the buttock and back do no better than 20 to 30 mm. Similarly, full-thickness or thick split-thickness grafts that contain the intradermal plexus as well as papillary dermal endings are a superior choice to thin split grafts (Fig. 5-4). (Thin split grafts have other advantages, however, that must be considered. Contracture reduces their size and passively draws adjacent normal skin into the area of the wound; because of their thinness, skin grafts permit stimulation of nerve endings that lie in deeper tissue beneath them.) Finally, flaps from distant sites such as the abdomen, chest, or groin seem least likely to accomplish satisfactory sensory results. Their thickness frequently works to their disadvantage, although well-thinned flaps sometimes manifest surprisingly good sensation. For example, we have sometimes noted that patients with flaps from hair-bearing areas easily detect movement of the hairs by stimuli that do not deform the skin. This suggests that nerve endings have regrown to the hair follicles themselves.

As pointed out earlier, however, considerations other than the potential for sensory recovery influence the choice of donor skin and method of use. A number of factors must be considered in selecting the type of operation for skin replacement. Surgeons who would reconstruct hands must be skilled in all the available techniques.

The inability to assess accurately the level of sensory recovery following nerve repair in patients makes it impossible to be dogmatic about sensory nerve surgery. The nature of the nerve itself is complex enough. The problem is compounded further by such major considerations as age, motivation, and individual biologic variation. Nevertheless, our understanding of normal physiology has progressed to the point that we can at least understand what we would *like* to have happen when a nerve is repaired. The challenge to clinical surgeons is to develop the judgment and surgical techniques to permit this sequence of events to occur at the most opportune time and in the most effective fashion.

REFERENCES

1. Cauna, N.: Nature and function of the papillary ridges of the digital skin, Anat. Rec. **119:**449, 1954.
2. Dellon, A. L.: Reinnervation of denervated Meissner corpuscles: a sequential histologic study in the monkey following fascicular nerve repair, J. Hand Surg. **1:**98, 1976.
3. Dellon, A. L., Curtis, R. M., and Edgerton, M. T.: Reeducation of sensation in the hand after nerve injury and repair, Plast. Reconstr. Surg. **53:**397, 1974.
4. Ducker, T. B., Kempe, L. G., and Hayes, G. J.: The metabolic background for peripheral nerve surgery, J. Neurosurg. **30:**270, 1969.
5. Jabaley, M. E., and Bryant, M. W.: The effect of denervation and reinnervation on encapsulated receptors in digital skin. In Marchac, C., and Hueston, J. T., editors: Transactions of the VI International Congress of Plastic and Reconstructive Surgery, Paris, 1976, Masson, pp. 103-106.
6. Jabaley, M. E., Burns, J. A., Orcutt, B. S., and Bryant, W. M.: Comparison of histologic and functional recovery after peripheral nerve repair, J. Hand Surg. **1:**119-130, 1976.
7. Jabaley, M. E., and Peterson, H. D.: Early treatment of war wounds of the hand and forearm in Vietnam, Ann. Surg. **177:**167-173, 1973.
8. Kuczynski, K.: Functional microanatomy of the peripheral nerve trunks, Hand **6:**1, 1974.
9. Lowenstein, W. R.: Biological transducers, Sci. Am. **203:**98, 1960.
10. Miller, M. R., Ralston, H. J., and Kasahara, M.: The

pattern of cutaneous innervation of the human hand, Am. J. Anat. **102:**183-218, 1958.

11. Mountcastle, V. B.: Sensory receptors and neural encoding: introduction to sensory processes. In Mountcastle, V. B., editor: Medical physiology, ed. 13, St. Louis, 1974, The C. V. Mosby Co.
12. Mountcastle, V. B.: The view from within: pathways to the study of perception, Johns Hopkins Med. J. **136:**109, 1975.
13. Paul, R. L., Goodman, H., and Merzenich, M.: Alternations in mechanoreceptor input to Brodmann's areas 1 and 3 of the postcentral hand area of Macaca mulatta after nerve section and regeneration, Brain Res. **39:**1, 1972.
14. Paul, R. L., Merzenich, M., and Goodman, H.: Representation of slowly and rapidly adapting cutaneous mechanoreceptors of the hand in Brodmann's areas 3 and 1 of Macaca mulatta, Brain Res. **36:**229, 1972.
15. Remensnyder, J. P.: Physiology of nerve healing and nerve grafts. In Krizek, T. J., and Hoopes, J. E., editors: Symposium on basic science in plastic surgery, St. Louis, 1976, The C. V. Mosby Co.
16. Sunderland, S.: Peripheral nerve trunks. In Nerves and nerve injuries, Edinburgh, 1972, Churchill Livingstone.

Chapter 6

Sensory reeducation after peripheral nerve injury

Raymond M. Curtis

The hand is unable to function without sensibility. Moberg[6,7] was one of the first to emphasize that hand function was dependent upon the degree of sensibility obtained following nerve repair. In adults with median and ulnar nerve laceration at the wrist, Önne[19] described poor recovery of two-point discrimination following repair. In reports by other authors[11,17,18,23] only 2% of adults obtained two-point discrimination of 3 to 5 mm following repair of median and ulnar nerve. Önne[19] reported excellent recovery of two-point discrimination in children. This could be based on the fact that the child has better nerve regeneration; however, it is undoubtedly due in part to the fact that the child has the ability to achieve a more perfect sensory reeducation pattern in the cerebral cortex following peripheral nerve repair.

Mitchell[10] described the phenomenon of false localization following nerve regeneration. This he refers to as the inability to accurately localize a point of stimulation on the skin despite good return of function of the basic modalities of sensation following nerve severance and regeneration. He cites, for example, that following the repair of a lacerated median nerve a point stimulus to the index finger will be clearly localized to another point in the distribution of this nerve. Increasing the intensity of the stimulation only makes the patient more convinced that it has occurred on the falsely localized area.

Mountcastle[14] in 1957 first proposed the unit column theory of cortical organization based on his electrophysiologic recordings and the previous work of Sperry.[22] This experimental work was done by stimulating a single neuron distally in the cutaneous nerve of the paw of the cat and recording with microelectrodes from the somatic sensory cerebral cortex (Brodmann's areas 3 and 1 of the postcentral gyrus of the brain). Mountcastle demonstrated that there was a discrete area of the brain that received the distal signal. This could be mapped as a specific localized area (such as the tip of the thumb or the tip of the index finger) on the cerebral cortex using a microelectrode.

Using adult rhesus monkeys, Paul and associates[19] in 1972 sectioned the median nerve and resutured it. Mapping experiments were carried out on both hemispheres of six operated monkeys 6½ to 7½ months following operations. The right hemisphere served as the control; the left hemisphere (contralateral to the denervated hand) served as the experimental model. Nerves of both hands were dissected out and photographed. Short sections of the digital nerve distal to the anastomotic site and sections from the anastomotic site were removed and stained with special myelin stains for histologic examination. In all six experiments following nerve section and repair there was a significant disorganization of the somatotopic representation of the skin of the monkey's paw in the cortex. This somatotopic experimental model demonstrated that the input to the cortical column in the brain is radically altered following peripheral nerve severance repair and regeneration.

In 1962 Vinograd and associates[24] described the use of common objects such as blocks, cubes, and triangles to reeducate sensibility in the hemiplegic hand. In 1966 Wynn Parry[25,26] demonstrated the usefulness of sensory reeducation using a similar technique. Dellon and associates[3,4] reported on a sensory reeducation program in which the patient was assigned a specific sensory exercise at the appropriate time in his recovery, that is, when specific clinical tests indicated he had reached the degree of recovery that would allow for reeducation of deep touch, light touch, movement, two-point discrimination, and the use of objects normally used in activities of daily living. Fragiadakis[5] observed that the results of nerve suture were better in patients who were dexterous rather than heavy manual laborers.

The blind have no greater capacity for touch than do the sighted, but their intensive training of tactile discriminating capacity reaches very high levels. Braille has each dot 1 mm above the surface separated by 2.5 mm. This is just above the two-point discrimination threshold for the fingertips. An experienced blind reader can read 100 words (approximately 600 letters) per minute. This is about the rate we read aloud. If the blind person presses his finger against the letter and prevents the scanning movements, his reading capacity is almost abolished. The practiced braillist uses the left index finger even when he is right-handed. In 1969 Heinrichs and Moorhouse[6] recorded two-point discrimination of 1.5 mm in blind diabetic patients. Bach y Rita[1] trained blind subjects to see by using a multipoint stimulator against the skin receptors of the skin of the back. The blind subject was taught to interpret the stimuli as sight, to recognize objects, and to operate an oscilloscope.

NEUROPHYSIOLOGY OF CUTANEOUS SENSATION

It has been estimated that there are as many as 2,500 nerve endings in 9 sq mm of the tip of the finger. These nerve endings are supplied by myelinated or nonmyelinated fibers. These nerve fibers may terminate free or in a specific structure such as a Meissner corpuscle, Merkel disk, or the pacinian corpuscle. The sensory endings possess a threshold; that is, there exists a physically definable stimulus of appropriate quality to which they respond with a discharge of a nerve impulse.[16] The large myelinated fibers (group A-β fibers) mediate the perception of touch and have been divided by

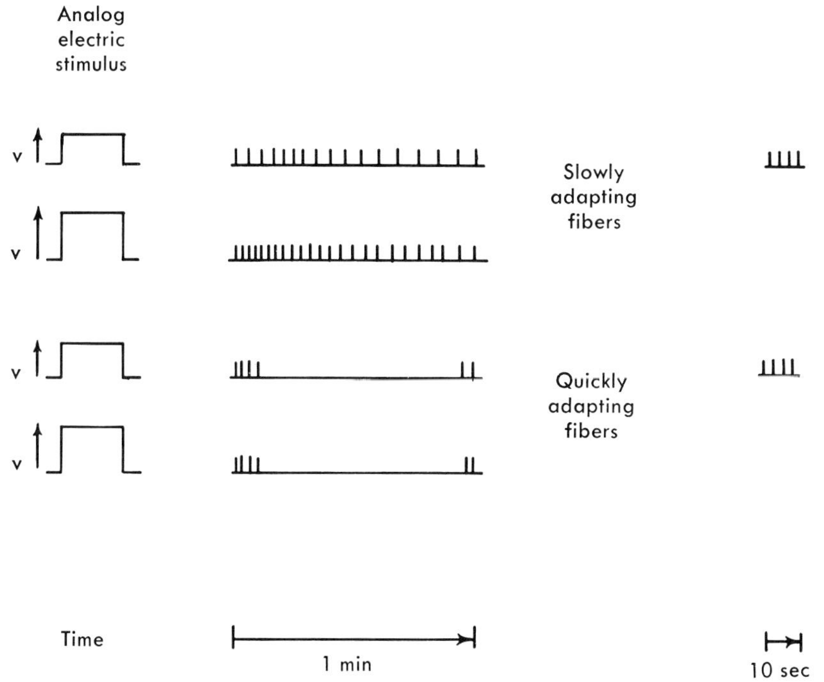

Fig. 6-1. Typical pattern of impulses in response to stimulus. Response patterns of slowly adapting and quickly adapting fibers to mechanical stimuli of constant duration. Both stimulus and response are illustrated by electric analog; square wave stimulus and spike-potential response from single fiber recordings. Each type of fiber is stimulated first with low intensity (voltage, *v*), and then with higher intensity, which is analogous to depth to which mechanical stimulus penetrated, and which corresponds to human experience of a constant-touch stimulus of two different pressures. Stimuli of both short and of long duration are used. (From Dellon, A. L., Curtis, R. M., and Edgerton, M. T.: Johns Hopkins Med. J. **130**:235-243, 1972.)

Mountcastle and associates[14] into two populations based on the way in which they respond to stimuli. These are the quickly adapting fibers and the slowly adapting fibers. The quickly adapting fibers are further divided into one group that responds maximally to a frequency in the range of 2 to 40 Hz, while the other responds best in the range of 60 to 300 Hz (Fig. 6-1). The large myelinated sensory fibers end in a mechanoreceptor (Merkel disk, Meissner corpuscles, and pacinian corpuscles). These latter structures transform the external stimulus into a conductible action potential that moves along the afferent neuron and is conducted finally to the postcentral gyrus of the sensory cortex.

Following nerve repair, axons regrow down the endoneural tube to its termination. These axons reinnervate the specialized nerve endings or end as simply free tips.

It is the A-β system that gives man the precision his hands possess. To understand these discriminating powers of human hand it is necessary to know that this system of intertwining fibers operates on the basis of "overlapping peripheral receptive fields."[12]

It is conceived that these receptive fields overlap since the afferent axons intertwine. Each unit has a small receptive field. In the hand we have the greatest number of units per body area. There is therefore a very high peripheral innervation density.

The perception of form and the direction of movement of a stimulus is not explained as an activation of isolated nerve fibers but rather as the cortical interpretation of profiles of the activities of partially overlapping peripheral receptive fields.[12]

METHOD OF REEDUCATION

The object of the sensory reeducation protocol is to improve sensibility by introducing the program as soon as possible in the recovery period. This is determined by the pattern of recovery of sensation. The pattern of sensory recovery is mapped at regular intervals, and the following are charted: Tinel sign, deep touch, light touch, movement, perception of vibration at 30 and 256 Hz by tuning fork, two-point discrimination, and pinprick.

The retraining session lasts 10 to 15 minutes and is carried out by the patient three to five times a day at home in a room with as few distractions as possible.

The patient observes what he is doing, thinks about how it feels, turns his head, closes his eyes, and verbalizes aloud what he is doing.

The therapist reevaluates the patient at regular intervals, introduces the appropriate exercise based on the degree of recovery, and reinforces the learning process by the interest shown in the improvement.

The therapist, when possible, should encourage the patient to use his forearm and hand muscles in the exercise. This enhances the learning process.

The patient is instructed to move the object back and forth between the thumb and the fingers in the normal hand, to shift the object to the injured hand, and to try to identify it, with his eyes opened and closed.

When the patient can detect vibratory sensation of 256 Hz at the fingertip, retraining for constant touch and movement should be introduced.

These objects are used for retraining:

1. Fingertip of normal hand for deep touch and movement
2. Soft object, such as an eraser on a pencil, for deep and light touch
3. Various sizes of square, hexagonal, and round objects, starting with an object about 3 cm in diameter (such as square and hexagonal metal nuts and washers)
4. Objects used in daily living, such as keys, coins, safety pins, screwdrivers, writing instruments, buttons on clothing, typewriters, nuts threaded on bolts, and tools used in work

Where there is hyperesthesia or pain over the distribution of the regenerating nerve, a procedure for desensitization must be carried out prior to sensory reeducation. It will not be possible to reeducate the hypersensitive hand. The technique consists of stroking the hypersensitive area with the finest piece of cotton that can be tolerated, progressing to wool fiber and felt.[9] In some instances treatment with a transcutaneous stimulator may be necessary.

DISCUSSION

Dellon and associates[4] reported recovery of normal or near-normal sensation in four adults, following sensory reeducation after nerve repair. In 1976 Wynn Parry and Salter[27] reported on sensory reeducation in 23 patients following median nerve repair. They were followed from 1 to 3 years, and an improvement in the time it took the patients to identify test objects and texture was noted. In almost all patients point localization returned to normal. The occupational therapist and workshop technicians reported a marked improvement in function once training began. Reid[21] reviewed the testing of 150 adult patients with median nerve injury 1 to 5 years after injury and found that these patients had nothing more than protective sensation. To retrain sensibility he used the Weber two-point test using a Boley gauge. The reeducation was begun after a preliminary battery of clinical tests had been carried out and when 256 Hz could be detected at the fingertip. There was an improvement in sensibility in all patients reeducated as evidenced by improved two-point discrimination, point localization, Moberg object identification, Moberg picking-up test, and Porter letter test. In addition the patients used the area of the hand supplied by the repaired median nerve.

The patients studied by Reid[21] maintained the improvement in two-point discrimination even after many years. One adult from the series, with a primary repair of a median nerve lacerated 12 cm proximal to wrist crease, was found to have two-point discrimination greater than 45 mm 6 months after repair. Following 6 weeks of sensory reeducation he had two-point discrimination of 11 to 15 mm. When he was examined 7 years later the two-point discrimination was 7 mm over the thumb and index finger. The patient used the area of the hand innervated by the median nerve for all functions without visual help.

SUMMARY

The nervous system faces the external world not directly but by an afferent input through a system of mechanoreceptors in the hand. When stimulated, these produce an electric impulse that travels by way of the nerve fibers to a specific area of the cerebral cortex. This area for the hand is massive, and consequently tactile acuity is very highly developed in the fingers.

Following the repair of a lacerated peripheral nerve, axons regrow down an endoneural tube to reinnervate the mechanoreceptors. This regrowth is not only disorderly but in most instances the same number of nerve endings are not reinnervated, and there is thus a reduction in the peripheral density. This produces an altered profile in the cerebral cortex of what exists distally.

A sensory reeducation program introduced at the appropriate time in the patient's clinical recovery can lead to an improvement in hand function as well as in the modalities of testing that are used to assess the recovery of sensibility.

REFERENCES

1. Bach y Rita, P.: Brain mechanisms in sensory substitution, New York, 1972, Academic Press.
2. Dellon, A. L., Curtis, R. M., and Edgerton, M. T.: Evaluating recovery of sensation in the hand following nerve injury, Johns Hopkins Med. J. **130:**235-243,1972.
3. Dellon, A. L., Curtis, R. M., and Edgerton, M. T.: Reeducation of sensation in the hand following nerve injury, J. Bone Joint Surg. [Am.] **53:**813, 1971.
4. Dellon, A. L., Curtis, R. M., and Edgerton, M. T.: Reeducation of sensation in the hand after nerve injury and repair, J. Plast. Reconst. Surg. **53:**297-305, 1974.
5. Fragiadakis, D. G., Lamb, D. W., and Honner, R.: An investigation of factors affecting the results of nerve division, Hand **2:**21-31, 1970.
6. Heinrichs, R. W., and Moorhouse, J. A.: Touch perception in blind diabetic subjects in relation to the reading of Braille type, N. Eng. J. Med. **280:**72-75, 1969.
7. Moberg, E.: Criticism and study of methods for examining sensibility in the hand, Neurology (Minneap.) **12:**1, 1962.
8. Moberg, E.: Methods of examining sensibility of the hand. In Flynn, J. E., editor: Hand surgery, Baltimore, 1966, The Williams and Wilkins Company.
9. Maynard, J.: Sensory reeduction after peripheral nerve injury. American Society for Surgery of the Hand. Symposium on Rehabilitation of the Hand. Phila., 1977.
10. Mitchell, J. K., Jr.: Remote consequences of injuries of nerves and their treatment. Examination of the present condition of wounds received 1863-65 with illustrative cases, Philadelphia, Lea Brothers and Co., 1895, 255 pp.
11. McEwan, L. E.: Median and ulnar nerve injuries, Aust. N.Z. J. Surg. **32:**89-104, 1964.
12. Mountcastle, V. B.: Sensory receptors and neural encoding: introduction to sensory processes. In Mountcastle, V. B., editor: Medical physiology, ed. 13, St. Louis, 1974, The C. V. Mosby Co. vol. 2, pp. 285-306.
13. Mountcastle, V. B., Talbot, W. H., and Kornhuber, H. H.: The neural transformation of mechanical stimuli, delivered to the monkey's hand. In de Reuch, A. V. S., and Knight, J., editors: Touch, heat and pain, Ciba Foundation Symposium, Boston, 1966, Little, Brown and Company, p. 325.
14. Mountcastle, V. B., Talbot, W. H., Darian-Smith, I., and Kornhuber, H. H.: A neural base for the sense of flutter-vibration, Science **155:**597, 1967.
15. Mountcastle, V. B., Modality and topographic properties of single neurons of cat's somatic sensory cortex, J. Neurophysiol. **20:**408-434, 1957.
16. Mountcastle, V. B., LaMotte, R. H., and Giancarlo, C.: Detection thresholds for stimuli in humans and monkeys: comparison with threshold events in mechanoreceptive afferent nerve fibers innervating the monkey hand, J. Neurophysiol. **35:**122, 1972.
17. Nicholson, O. R., and Seddon, H. J.: Nerve repairs in civil practice: results of therapy of median and ulnar nerve lesions, Br. Med. J. **2:**1065-1071, 1957.
18. Nielsen, J. B., and Torup, D.: Nerve injuries in the upper extremities, Dan. Med. Bull, **11:**92-95, 1964.
19. Önne, L.: Recovery of sensibility and sudomotor

function in the hand after nerve suture, Acta. Chir. Scand. [Suppl.] **300:**1-69, 1962.

20. Paul, R. L., Goodman, H., and Merzenich, M.: Alterations in mechanoreceptor input to Brodmann's areas 1 and 3 of the postcentral hand area of *Macaca mulatta* after nerve section and regeneration, Brain Res. **39:**1-19, 1972.
21. Reid, R. L.: Preliminary results of sensibility re-education following repair of median nerve, Am. Soc. Surg. Hand, Newsletter 15, 1977.
22. Sperry, R. W.: Cerebral regulation of motor coordination following multiple transection of sensorimotor cortex, J. Neurophysiol. **10:**275-294, 1947.
23. Stromberg, W. B., McFarlane, R. M., Bell, J. L., Koch, S. L., and Mason, M. L.: Injuries of the median and ulnar nerves, J. Bone Joint Surg. [Am.] **43:**717-730, 1961.
24. Vinograd, A., Taylor, E., and Grossman, S.: Sensory retaining of the hemiplegic hand, Am. J. Occup. Ther. **16:**246-250, 1962.
25. Wynn Parry, C. B.: Diagnosis and aftercare of peripheral-nerve lesions in the upper limb. Founders lecture, The American Society for Surgery of the Hand, J. Bone Joint Surg. [Am.] **48:**607, 1966.
26. Wynn Parry, C. B.: Rehabilitation of the hand, London, 1966, Butterworth and Co.
27. Wynn Parry, C. B., and Salter, M.: Sensory re-education after median nerve lesions, Hand, **8:**250-257, 1976.

Chapter 7

Neurovascular sensory island transplants

George E. Omer

The transplant of neurovascular cutaneous islands for the restoration of sensibilty has been utilized primarily by surgeons interested in restorative procedures for the hand. In 1955, during a discussion of tactile-sense restoration, Moberg[23] suggested the digital neurovascular pedicle sensory island as a method for sensibility redistribution in the hand. Littler[16,17] developed the techniques for making a vascular pedicle island incorporating a digital branch from either the median or ulnar nerve from single digits. Intact sensibility, peripheral circulation, and corniferous skin were restored by this method.[18,29,34] Subsequent techniques were developed to utilize double islands from two digits[22,27] and a radial-innervated island for the thumb.[12]

The hand is covered with thin, elastic skin on the dorsum and with nonslip grip pads on the volar surface, highly sensitive for precise prehension. There are three prime areas of the hand in which precision touch is critical: the ulnar-volar aspect of the thumb pulp, the radial-volar aspect of the index pulp, and the ulnar-volar aspect of the little finger.

Two general uses for the neurovascular sensory island transplant have developed: (1) reconstruction of the thumb distal to the level of the metacarpophalangeal joint level and (2) islands of sensibility over the radial half of the hand that has total median nerve loss distal to the volar carpal ligament.

THUMB PULP DEFECT

Many techniques have been devised for reconstruction following total thumb loss, such as pollicization of an available finger,[5,15,18] free great-toe transfers,[4] or the osteoplastic composite flap.[3,21] Several experienced surgeons[6,16,34] advocate osteoplastic reconstruction, including a neurovascular sensory island, when all fingers are normal in the presence of a mobile first metacarpal with distal avulsion. A thumb reconstructed by osteoplastic methods should be deliberately made shorter than normal. The neurovascular sensory island transplant is even more useful in providing a sensible, nonslip, durable surface for the volar pulp of the thumb with an avulsion injury.[10] However, the immediate application of a neurovascular island is not indicated. Wound healing should be obtained and the patient evaluated carefully before this elective procedure is performed.

Surgical considerations

The volar sensory supply of the digits of the hand is primarily from the median and ulnar nerves. These nerves terminate as common digital nerves that bifurcate into proper digital nerves, each supplying sensation to one hemidigit. The most common arrangement is for the median nerve to supply sensation on both sides of the thumb, index, and long finger and in the radial half of the ring finger. The ulnar nerve usually supplies both sides of the little finger and the ulnar half of the ring finger. The superficial radial nerve is important in the dorsal sensory supply of the fingers. The nerve is distributed to the radial-dorsal aspect of the hand, with one nerve branch tending to pass to each side of the dorsum of each digit. The superficial radial nerve fibers terminate over the proximal two thirds of the proximal phalanx.

The superficial palmar vascular arch of the hand is a continuation of the ulnar artery, and from this arch three common volar digital arteries arise and then bifurcate into the proper digital arteries on the ulnar side of the index finger, both sides of the long and ring fingers and the radial side of the little finger. The superficial palmar vascular arch underlies a transverse palmar line extending along the ulnar side of the widely abducted thumb. An Allen test should be done at the carpal level to evaluate the arterial supply of the hand. The superficial vascular arch may have to be interrupted and the radial portion freed to swing with the neurovascular pedicle attached to the cutaneous island. In patients over 40 years of age the prognosis is guarded due to circulatory impairment.[30]

Technique using the median nerve for sensibility

A paper pattern is made of the avulsed pulp area of the thumb or the new area of sensibility desired on the ulnar-volar aspect of the thumb pulp (Fig. 7-1). The completed pattern is outlined in sterile ink. It is then laid on the skin of the ulnar-volar aspect of the long finger or the radial-volar aspect of the ring finger. A large pattern includes more of the donor nerve and is not a disadvantage.[13] The

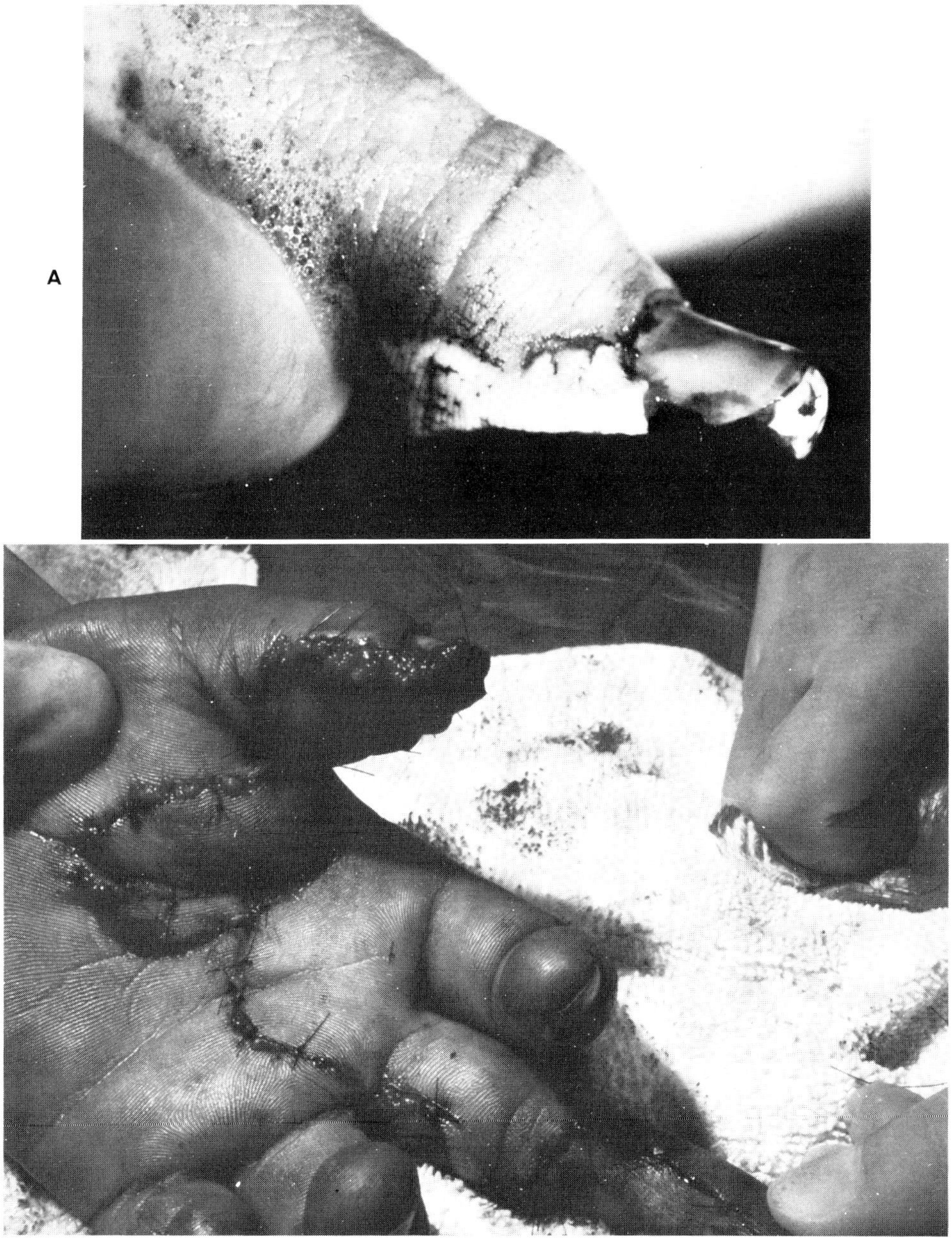

Fig. 7-1. A, Avulsed thumb pad. **B,** Median-innervated neurovascular island transplant from ulnar border of middle finger.

distance from the proximal edge of the pattern on the finger to the "swing-point" on the superficial vascular arch is measured, compared, and adjusted to the distance from the swing-point to the proximal edge of the original drawing on the thumb. These measurements should be made with the thumb widely abducted from the palm on a flat surface. Uneven distances indicate the superficial volar vascular arch will have to be interrupted and the radial portion freed to swing with the cutaneous island.

A zigzag longitudinal palmar incision, avoiding the pads over the metacarpal heads, is made along the course of the common digital nerve and vessels between the long and ring fingers. The incision extends proximally from the distal edge of the palm to the level of the superficial volar vascular arch. If there is abnormal vascular or nerve distribution, the palmar incision should be closed without further injury to the hand. If the anatomy is normal, the neurovascular pedicle distances should be measured again under direct visualization of the swing-point where the common digital artery leaves the superficial arch.

Liberation of the neurovascular pedicle requires cleavage of the common digital nerve in the palm into its two proper digital nerve components. This must be a meticulous procedure if loss of sensation is to be avoided. The nerve is dissected from its distal to its proximal end, beginning at the bifurcation in the web space. The proper digital arterial branch to the cutaneous island is freed, while the proper digital artery to the remaining finger is ligated. Perforating branches of the digital artery are tied. Ligation of a branch too close to the major trunk can distort the patent vessel and cause eddy currents with subsequent thrombosis.[30] Optical magnification is required for these procedures.

The cutaneous island is carefully dissected in a proximal-to-distal direction. The nerve branches should be superficial to the dissection. Sufficient subcutaneous tissue is removed to expose the flexor tendon sheath and perhaps the extensor mechanism, but a very thin transparent layer of tissue is left behind over the tendon structures. Small vessels are carefully ligated. A zigzag transverse palmar incision from the proximal portion of the initial palmar incision to the thumb recipient site is made through the palmar fascia just distal to the superficial volar arch, thus creating a fascial trough. The neurovascular pedicle is then placed in the fascial trough without tension, acute angulation, or constriction. The tourniquet is released to prove the viability of circulation to the cutaneous island and to obtain meticulous hemostasis.

If there is no avulsion of the thumb pulp, a full-thickness skin graft is removed from within the ink pattern outlined as the recipient site. This skin graft fits exactly in the island donor site on the long fin-

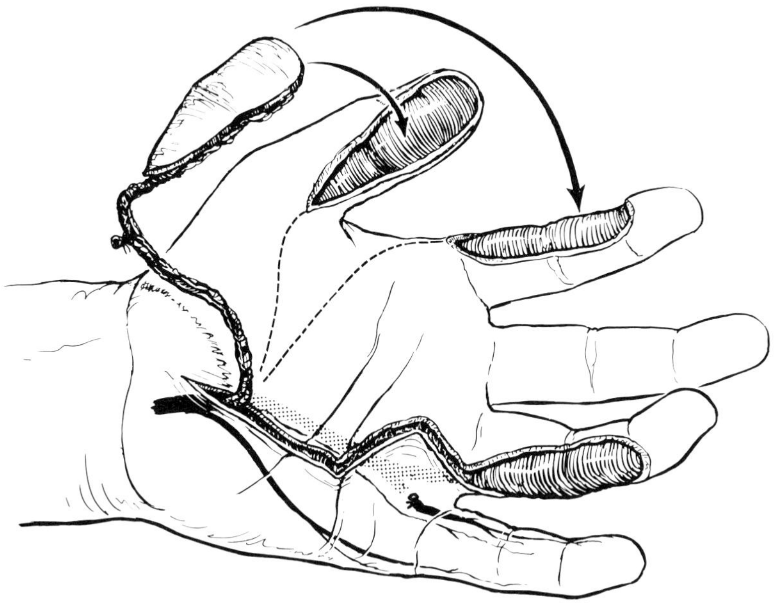

Fig. 7-2. Sensory cutaneous island transplant using ulnar-innervated skin to provide sensation following median nerve impairment.

ger. It is sutured into place with the ends of some of the sutures left long enough to tie around a glycerin and mineral oil–soaked cotton wedge compression dressing. If the thumb pulp is avulsed, the full-thickness skin graft can be obtained from the non-weight-bearing portion of the sole of the foot or from the hypothenar area of the hand.

The neurovascular island is then fitted into the recipient site on the thumb. The glycerin and mineral oil–soaked cotton wedge dressing is tied in place for even compression. The hand is immobilized for 3 weeks after surgery, but the extremity is free for an exercise program.

Technique using the ulnar nerve for sensibility

The procedure for the ulnar nerve is the same as for the median nerve, except the common digital nerve and vessels are exposed between the ring and little fingers, and the neurovascular cutaneous island is obtained from the ulnar-volar aspect of the ring finger (Fig. 7-2).

Technique using the superficial radial nerve for sensibility

When the superficial radial nerve is used, it is advisable to carry out preoperative evaluation by digital block of the proper volar digital nerves to the index finger. Occasionally the dorsal surface of the proximal phalanx of the index finger will be supplied by the median nerve.[1] Careful study with light touch and two-point discrimination distance is indicated after the appropriate nerve blocks.

If the preoperative evaluation proves favorable, a V-shaped skin incision is made, with one limb of the V at the level of the midlateral line on the radial side of the index finger and the other limb at the midlateral line on the ulnar side of the thumb. The point of the incision is near the first dorsal metacarpal branch of the radial artery. Gentle dissection will expose the longitudinal branches of the superficial radial nerve and vascular structures dorsal to the second metacarpal. If the vessels can be followed distally to the area of the proximal phalanx, a racquet-shaped cutaneous island with a neurovascular pedicle is dissected from the dorsal-radial surface of the index finger. This neurovascular island is then fitted into the volar-ulnar aspect of the thumb pulp. This procedure is precarious because the arterial supply to the cutaneous island is not constant. Consequently the procedure is usually modified in one of two ways: (1) a narrow dorsal strip of skin may be retained proximally from the index cutaneous island[12] or (2) a cross-finger flap from the index to the thumb may be used instead of the free cutaneous island.[1,2,11]

Results

Moberg[25] has indicated that all neurovascular sensory island transplants will have three negative aspects: (1) a loss of sensibility at the donor site, (2) a margin of hyperesthesia around the edges of the cutaneous island, and (3) a loss of the quality of sensibility secondary to cortical disorientation.

Murray and associates[26] reported their results in 16 patients who were seen 1 to 10 years after surgery. Based on two-point discrimination of distance and touch, the sensibility in the neurovascular island was less then normal. Of the 16 patients, 12 had continued intolerance to cold, and 7 had significant hyperesthesia at all times. Reorientation of sensation, so that stimuli on the cutaneous island were referred to the thumb and not to the donor finger, occured in four patients only after long periods ranging from 18 months to 8 years. Reid[31] reported deficient two-point discrimination in the neurovascular cutaneous islands of 14 patients. In contrast, Tubiana and Duparc[34] noted the gradual spread of protective sensibility into the tissue surrounding the transplanted cutaneous island, which may be related to the transferred nerve.

MEDIAN NERVE LOSS

The median nerve supplies the sensibility required for the precise prehension normally performed with the radial side of the hand. If there is an associated loss of motor function from a high (proximal) median nerve injury, the normal pattern of activity is reversed; the radial side of the hand is used for gross grip, while the ulnar side, with its intact muscles and ulnar nerve, is used for precise prehension. A neurovascular island transfer should not be considered in such cases until all possible tendon transfers have been accomplished.[27]

Surgical considerations

Only the common digital nerve between the ring and little fingers is available for a neurovascular cutaneous island, since sensibility along the ulnar aspect of the littler finger is essential in total median nerve loss. The usual technique is to transfer a neurovascular cutaneous island from the ulnar aspect of the ring finger to the ulnar-volar aspect of the thumb pulp. To obtain a greater area of sensation, a larger island can be dissected by using one half of the volar skin of the donor finger rather than only the distal volar skin from the tip of the donor finger.[13] This technique requires less dissection of the neurovascular bundle but also results in a shorter neurovascular pedicle. The superficial vascular arch may have to be interrupted and the radial portion freed to swing with the cutaneous island.

Technique using a double cutaneous island

The outline of the double island is drawn with a sterile skin marker along the ulnar aspect of the ring finger and the radial aspect of the little finger. The island on the ring finger extends to the pulp area, while the island on the little finger extends to the distal interphalangeal joint level. This preserves the distal pulp tip of the little finger for precise tactile activity. Both islands extend proximally to the distal edge of the palm. A narrow skin bridge is drawn on the web dorsal to its palmar edge. A pattern of the double island is made and traced on the skin at the selected recipient area along the ulnar-volar aspect of the thumb, and thumb–index finger web, and the proximal radial-volar aspect of the index finger.

A zigzag longitudinal palmar incision is made, avoiding the nonslip pads over the metacarpal heads and following the course of the common digital nerve and vessels between the ring and little fingers. If there is abnormal vascular or nerve distribution, the incision is closed without further surgery. The neurovascular pedicle distances are measured in the same way as for a single island transplant, and a decision is made concerning interruption of the superficial vascular arch. Interruption and extensive dissection of the vascular arch increase the danger of an ischemic flap, while the more proximal release of the common digital nerve threatens the sensibility of the cutaneous island.

The two islands are dissected free at the donor sites, and full-thickness skin grafts are developed at the recipient site. The skin graft from the thumb–index finger area fits exactly in the neurovascular cutaneous island site at the ring–little finger area. The free full-thickness graft is sutured into place with the ends of some sutures left long enough so that later a glycerin and mineral oil–soaked cotton wedge compression dresssing can be tied between the ring and little fingers.

A transverse palmar incision from the proximal point of the initial incision to the midpoint of the selected thumb–index finger recipient site is made through the palmar fascia just distal to the position of the superficial volar vascular arch. The neurovascular pedicle is placed in this fascial trough without tension, acute angulation, or constriction (Fig. 7-3). If the narrow skin bridge between the wide double islands does not fit without uneven skin tension, a small free split-thickness skin graft can be

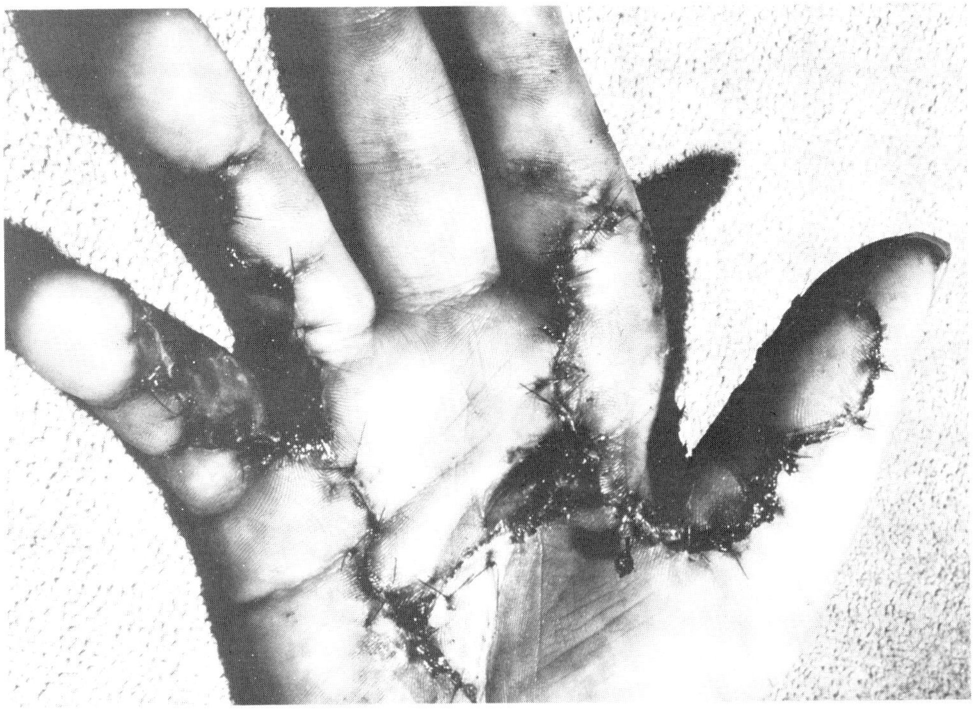

Fig. 7-3. Double neurovascular island pedicle.

added in the center of the thumb–index finger web along the dorsal margin of the neurovascular cutaneous islands. A bulky dressing without tie-over compression is used in the web space between the thumb and index finger. The hand is immobilized for 3 weeks after surgery.

Results

There is disorientation of sensitivity in all neurovascular sensory island transplants. For several months after transplant the patient recognizes stimulation in the island as coming from the original donor digit. Later, sensation is localized in both the recipient and donor sites. Finally some patients learn to interpret the sensibility to the recipient digit. If the hand is immobilized and nonfunctional for any period of time, however, the interpretation process must be repeated. Also in an emergency, such as a flame burn, the patient loses his interpretation ability and moves the original donor digit.[27]

My associates and I reported[27] our findings in 15 patients with median nerve loss that was followed with evaluation tests at 8-week intervals for 14 to 43 months after surgery. The two-point discrimination distance recognition and the von Frey light touch–pressure tests demonstrated a gradual reduction from normal sensation to merely protective sensation. I believed that this gradual loss of sensibility was directly related to the associated motor loss for the radial side of the hand, and without adequate motion and power for precise prehension, the sensibility for precise prehension must be lost.[28] Murray and associates[26] believed the sensibility loss to be caused by repeated traction on the transferred nerve pedicle.

WEIGHT-BEARING AREAS OF THE FOOT

In the patient with a neurotrophic ulcer of the foot a neurovascular cutaneous island transplant will enhance the circulation and stability of the weight-bearing area and afford protective sensation. Moberg[24] first utilized a cutaneous island transplant in the foot when he moved the pulp of the filleted great toe on a neurovascular pedicle to fill a neurotrophic ulcer of the heel.

Surgical conditions

The dorsalis pedis artery is the terminal branch of the anterior tibial artery. In midfoot the artery has two main branches, the medial and lateral tarsal arteries. Farther distally, the deep branch penetrates the second dorsal interosseous muscle to communicate with the deep plantar arch. The dorsal vein of the foot and the deep peroneal sensory nerve accompany the proper dorsalis pedis artery and the lateral plantar artery, which is the larger of the terminal branches of the posterior tibial artery. The planter metatarsal arteries run on the surface of the interosseous muscles and may pass dorsal or volar to the transverse metatarsal ligament. The medial plantar nerve divides into digital branches to the great toe, the second and third toes, and the tibial aspect of the fourth toe. The foot is more variable in its blood supply than the hand, and arteriography or a Doppler probe is most helpful in previewing the anatomic variations.

Technique using a toe for heel coverage

The neurotrophic ulcer on the heel is excised to the periosteum of the calcaneus. A zigzag longitudinal incision is then made on the non-weight-bearing medial aspect of the sole, extending from the medial aspect of the heel pad to the metatarsophalangeal joint level of the great toe. A flap is dissected, and the medial plantar neurovascular bundle is identified in the interval between the abductor hallucis and flexor digitorum brevis muscles. This dissection is continued to isolate the neurovascular bundle to the medial side of the great toe. Further dissection will identify the plantar metatarsal neurovascular bundle to the adjacent sides of the great toe and the second toe. The digital nerve to the tibial aspect of the second toe is dissected from the common digital nerve from the trunk of the medial plantar nerve, and the vascular branch to the tibial aspect of the second toe from the first metatarsal artery is ligated. If the first metatarsal artery is primarily supplied by the dorsalis pedis artery, then a long vascular pedicle is easily developed. If the major contributor to the first metatarsal artery is the lateral plantar artery, the dissection must be carried proximally into the sole of the foot between the first and second metatarsals to obtain an adequate vascular pedicle. The cutaneous island is developed from the volar skin and subcutaneous tissue overlying the phalanges and the metatarsophalangeal joint. The neurovascular cutaneous island is then rotated into the heel defect and sutured into position. The great toe is disarticulated through the metatarsophalangeal joint, and remaining dorsal skin provides the necessary flap to cover the donor defect.

Results. Toe-to-heel transplants of sensory cutaneous islands on neurovascular pedicles have been reported by Moberg and associates,[24] Snyder and Edgerton,[32] and Kaplan.[14] Detailed evaluations were not recorded by all these surgeons, but the follow-up to 2 years demonstrated that the cutaneous islands were well vascularized, and the patients appreciated sensation in the cutaneous islands. Sensibility was referred to the donor toe.

Technique using the dorsum of the foot

The entire dorsum of the foot can be safely elevated as an island flap if the deep branch of the dorsalis pedis artery is ligated and the distal dorsalis pedis artery is retained with the flap. McGraw and Furlow[20] state that the island elevation is begun medially, and only after identifying the deep dorsalis pedis branch, the proper dorsalis pedis artery, and the distal dorsalis pedis branch, should the deep branch be ligated. The dissection is then carried distally just superficial to the extensor tendons. Proximal to the deep branch of the dorsalis pedis artery, the proper dorsalis pedis artery is densely adherent to the tarsal bones, and one must dissect precisely on the surface of the tarsal bones. The cutaneous island cannot survive if it is separated from the vascular pedicle at this point. Further proximal, the lateral tarsal branch of the dorsalis pedis artery is ligated where it passes beneath the short-toe extensors. The extensor retinaculum can be divided, but the island cannot be extended more proximally, as the dorsalis pedis artery enters the island just distal to the extensor retinaculum. If possible, the entire dorsal venous arch should be included in the island. The dorsal venous arch has numerous intercommunications above the superficial fascia, and the arch communicates distally with the dorsalis pedis vein. The venous valves direct drainage into the greater saphenous vein from the distal venous arch.

Results. The full range of this island transplant has not been determined since it has usually been used as a flap. The flap has been used to resurface defects of the dorsum of the foot, both malleoli, the Achilles tendon, and the sole. When the flap is employed as a cutaneous island, coverage of portions of the weight-bearing area of the heel and the pretibial area should also be practicable.[19] McGraw and Furlow reported no complications at the donor site after nine cases, but the donor site has potential for problems.[8]

MICROSURGICAL FREE NEUROVASCULAR SENSORY ISLAND TRANSPLANTS

A neurovascular free sensory island has been defined as a skin flap isolated on a neurovascular stalk that is severed at the donor site and reanastomosed after direct transfer to the recipient bed. Its survival is dependent on reestablishment of a functioning intravascular circulation through the microvascular anastomoses and reinnervation of the flap's intrinsic nerve terminal through the microneural anastomosis.[8] The technique promises the restoration of protective sensation in weight-bearing areas of the lower extremity, the creation of pressure sensors for paraplegics, and tactile gnosis for sensory depleted hands.[7] However, cortical localization of sensation from the neural anastomoses is a problem and may require extensive reeducation. Several sites for microsurgical free neurovas-

Table 1. Follow-up report on microsurgical free neurovascular sensory islands

No. of cases	Donor sites	Less than 3 months			More than 3 months		
		Yes	No	Not done	Yes	No	Not done
7	*Web space and pulp of toes*						
	Protective sensibility	1			6		
	Light moving touch	1			6		
	von Frey filament (normal)	1			2		4
	Two-point discrimination (10 mm or less)		1		6		
6	*Dorsal pedis flap (dorsum foot)*						
	Protective sensibility	3			3		
	Light moving touch	3			3		
	von Frey filament (normal)			3	2		1
	Two-point discrimination (10 mm or less)		3		1		
11	*Groin (inguinal area), intercostal thoracic region, other regions*				2		
	Protective sensibility				11		
	Light moving touch				9	2	
	von Frey filament (normal)				3	3	5
	Two-point discrimination (10 mm or less)				3	8	
	TOTALS	9	4	3	55	15	10

cular sensory islands have been developed, including a dorsal foot flap,[9] a regional iliofemoral flap,[33] and an intercostal flap.[8]

Results

There are no published reports of long-term follow-up (5 years or longer) for microsurgical free neurovascular sensory islands. I have written recently to a selected cross section of 35 reconstructive surgeons to determine the current activity in this area. Replies were received from 86% of the surgeons, but only 23% of those who replied had experience with the microsurgical technique for free neurovascular sensory island transplants, and two or more procedures had been done by only 14% of the surgeons. There have been 24 procedures performed, and the longest follow-up was 3 years. The common areas selected for the donor sites were toe pulps and adjacent web spaces, the dorsum of the foot, the groin, and the thoracic wall (Table 1). The dominant recipient site was the hand, with a few transplants to the sole of the foot. The transplants from the toe pulps and adjacent web spaces demonstrated the best tactile gnosis in comparison to the other donor sites. The more experienced the surgeon, the more predictable the result for circulation and nerve regeneration. The potential for education of tactile gnosis in a donor site, such as the great toe pulp and adjacent web, has not been reported. With additional experience, the microsurgical free neurovascular sensory island transplant may become a consistent procedure of choice in areas requiring excellent sensibility.

ACKNOWLEDGMENT

I am indebted to Charles R. Ashworth, Harry J. Buncke, Joseph E. Kutz, Hanno Millesi, Richard J. Smith, Clifford C. Snyder, Morton Spinner, and Paul M. Weeks, for sharing their experience with these surgical procedures.

REFERENCES

1. Adamson, J. E., Horton, C. E., and Crawford, H. H.: Sensory rehabilitation of the injured thumb, Plast. Reconstr. Surg. **40:**53-57, 1967.
2. Bralliar, F., and Horner, R. L.: Sensory cross-finger pedicle graft, J. Bone Joint Surg. [Am.] **51:**1264-1268, 1969.
3. Broadbent, T. R., and Woolf, R. M.: Thumb reconstruction with contiguous skin-bone pedicle graft, Plast. Reconstr. Surg. **26:**494-499, 1960.
4. Buncke, H. J.: Free toe-to-hand transfers. In Daniller, A. I., and Strauch, B., editors: Symposium on microsurgery, St. Louis, 1976, The C. V. Mosby Co.
5. Bunnell, S.: Digit transfer by neurovascular pedicle, J. Bone Joint Surg. [Am.] **34:**772-774, 1952.
6. Chase, R. A.: An alternate to pollicization in subtotal thumb reconstruction, Plast. Reconstr. Surg. **44:**421-430, 1969.
7. Daniel, R. K., Terzis, J., and Schwartz, G.: Neurovascular free flaps: a preliminary report, Plast. Reconstr. Surg. **56:**13-20, 1975.
8. Daniel, R. K., and Terzis, J.: Neurovascular free flaps. In Daniller, A. I., and Strauch, B., editors: Symposium on microsurgery, St. Louis, 1976, The C. V. Mosby Co.
9. Daniel, R. K., Terzis, J., and Midgley, R. D.: Restoration of sensation to an anesthetic hand by a free neurovascular flap from the foot, Plast. Reconstr. Surg. **27:**275-280, 1976.
10. Frackelton, W. H., and Teasley, J. L.: Neurovascular island pedicle—extension in usage, J. Bone Joint Surg. [Am.] **44:**1069-1072, 1962.
11. Gaul, J. S., Jr.: Radial-innervated cross finger flap from index to provide sensory pulp to injured thumb, J. Bone Joint Surg. [Am.] **51:**1257-1263, 1969.
12. Holevich, J.: A new method of restoring sensibility to the thumb, J. Bone Joint Surg. [Br.] **45:**496-502, 1963.
13. Hueston, J.: The extended neurovascular island flap, Br. J. Plast. Surg. **18:**304-305, 1965.
14. Kaplan, I.: Neurovascular island flap in the treatment of trophic ulceration of the heel, Br. J. Plast. Surg. **22:**143-148, 1969.
15. Littler, J. W: The neurovascular pedicle method of digital transposition for reconstruction of the thumb, Plast. Reconstr. Surg. **12:**303-319, 1953.
16. Littler, J. W.: Neurovascular pedicle transfer of tissue in reconstructive surgery of the hand, J. Bone Joint Surg. [Am.] **38:**917, 1956.
17. Littler, J. W.: Neurovascular skin island transfer in reconstructive hand surgery. In Transactions of international society of plastic surgeons (Second Congress, London, 1959), Edinburgh, 1960, Churchill Livingstone.
18. Littler, J. W.: On making a thumb: one-hundred years of surgical effort, J. Hand Surg. **1:**35-51, 1976.
19. McGraw, J. B., and Furlow, T.: The dorsalis pedis arterial flap. In Grabb, W. C., and Myers, M. B., editors: Skin Flaps, Boston, 1975, Little, Brown and Company.
20. McGraw, J. B., and Furlow, L. T.: The dorsalis pedis arterialized flap. A clinical study, Plast. Reconstr. Surg. **55:**177-185, 1975.
21. McGregor, I. A., and Simonetta, C.: Reconstruction of the thumb by composite bone-skin flap, Br. J. Plast. Surg. **17:**37-48, 1964.
22. McGregor, I. A.: Less than satisfactory experiences with neurovascular island flaps, Hand **1:**21-22, 1969.
23. Moberg, E.: In discussion of "the place of nerve grafting in orthopaedic surgery" by Donal Brooks, J. Bone Joint Surg. [Am.] **37:**305, 1955.
24. Moberg, E.: Evaluation and management of nerve injuries in the hand, Surg. Clin. North Am. **44:**1019-1029, 1964.
25. Moberg, E.: Useful surgical arrangement of skin with normal sensibility to mutilated hands. In London, S. B., editor: Accident surgery and medicine, London, 1970, Butterworth.

26. Murray, J. F., Ord, J. V. R., and Gavelin, G. E.: The neurovascular island pedicle flap, J. Bone Joint Surg. [Am.] **49:**1285-1297, 1967.
27. Omer, G. E., Jr., Day, D. J., Ratliff, H., and Lambert, P.: Neurovascular cutaneous island pedicles for deficient median-nerve sensibility, J. Bone Joint Surg. [Am.] **52:**1181-1192, 1970.
28. Omer, G. E., Jr.: Neurovascular island flaps and fillet of finger. In Grabb, W. C., and Myers, M. B., editors: Skin flaps, Boston, 1975, Little, Brown and Company.
29. Peacock, E. E., Jr.: Reconstruction of the hand by the local transfer of composite tissue island flaps, Plast. Reconstr. Surg. **25:**298-311, 1960.
30. Peacock, E. E., Jr.: Island pedicle gymnastics. In Cramer, L. M., and Chase, R. A., editors: Symposium on the hand. St. Louis, 1971, The C. V. Mosby Co.
31. Reid, D. A. C.: The neurovascular island flap in thumb reconstruction, Br. J. Plast. Surg. **19.**234-244, 1966.
32. Snyder, G. B., and Edgerton, M. T.: The principle of the island neurovascular flap in the management of ulcerated anesthetic weightbearing areas of the lower extremity, Plast. Reconstr. Surg. **36:**518-528, 1965.
33. Taylor, G. L., and Daniel, R. K.: The anatomy of several free flap donor sites, Plast. Reconstr. Surg. **56:**243-253, 1975.
34. Tubiana, R., and Duparc, J.: Restoration of sensibility in the hand by Neurovascular skin island transfer, J. Bone Joint Surg. [Br.] **43:**474-480, 1961.

Panel discussion on neurophysiology and sensory nerve injuries

MICHAEL E. JABALEY, Moderator
RAYMOND M. CURTIS
THOMAS B. DUCKER
HANNO MILLESI
ERIK MOBERG
GEORGE E. OMER

Question: Dr. Ducker, given ideal circumstances, is there anything about the metabolism of peripheral nerve healing that should influence the timing of repair?

Ducker: The neuron begins axonic sprouting 3 or 4 days after injury, and theoretically this should be the opportune time for repair. However, that is not a particularly good time to be reopening a wound. A delayed repair is best done at 17 to 21 days as far as the peripheral tissues are concerned. Practically speaking, it would be better to do a primary repair on the day of injury than delay until the wound is secure.

Question: On what do you base your statement that day 3 is ideal?

Ducker: Axonic sprouting can be demonstrated to begin on day 3 to 7. There is an initial degenerative reaction in the anterior horn cell which then "shifts gears" to send repair elements to the periphery, traversing the axon in a single day. Much depends on the initial injury. If you cut 2 miles off a $2^{1}/_{2}$ mile long axon, that neuron is pretty sick. It will have to spend the first 3 weeks just trying to survive before it has the resources to initiate regeneration. Now, practically, what do you do for a brachial plexus injury? That is a complex problem, as different percentages of the nerve cell are amputated in the different nerve segments. Ideally, you would like to repair the comparatively distally severed nerves to the shoulder and upper arms on day 1. However, the longer median and ulnar nerves represent a very proximal injury, and one would like to permit the cells to recover somewhat so that the repair can coincide with the delayed sprouting. We know that nerves rarely regenerate across two joints except in the very young. Thus, the prognosis for distal recovery is poor under any circumstances. At best one can expect some sensory ability to appreciate pain and 30 to 40 cycle vibration but little more. All of this must be weighed in your final decision.

Question: Dr. Ducker, is there any information on what happens to the nerve when it is recut 21 days after the initial injury?

Ducker: This is very complex and presently under study. According to some work done at Cornell, the unmyelinated fibers seem to regrow faster when recut. The heavily myelinated fibers that we are most interested in seem to grow at the same rate or perhaps slightly slower. The actual processes are much more complex, but in practical terms, *if the wound is clean, do a primary repair, and if it's a mess, don't.*

Question: In view of the recent military experience with delayed primary wound repair, would it be advisable to do the definitive repair at 3 to 5 days if this is the ideal time for nerve regeneration?

Omer: In Vietnam most wounds were considered dirty, and thus the repair was delayed until we were certain that the initial debridement was adequate. It seemed to be very little problem waiting 3 to 5 days, but I would be less enthusiastic waiting 7 to 10 days. I agree with Tom (Ducker) that going back at 3 weeks in a high lesion is frightening, especially if there was an initial vascular repair or graft. I would make every effort to do a primary or delayed primary repair.

Question: Dr. Millesi, would you describe how you manage the nerve ends in this early period before there is scarring? Specifically, please discuss the fascicular and epineural management.

Millesi: The major problem of primary repair is the difficulty in judging adequate debridement in other than sharply incised injuries. It is too easy to unite two damaged ends that will later fibrose. If the nerve is cleanly cut, then I would do a conventional epineural repair and expect satisfactory results. If it fails, then the nerve can be reexplored with little lost. If the injury is untidy, then I would wait several weeks. We have seen little difference in results from intervention at 3, 4, or 5 weeks.

Question: Is there a visible neuroma at 5 weeks?

Millesi: Yes.

Question: Assuming a delayed repair, 6 weeks or later, how much gap in the nerve endings are you willing to overcome by flexion of the joints?

Millesi: Much depends on the repair used. Epineural repairs are strong and can be used to securely overcome a gap of up to 2.5 cm by flexing the joint. This is confirmed by the reports of Seddon who noted a marked drop in success rates of median nerve repairs if the gap was over 2.5 cm. If you do a fascicular repair then tension is poorly tolerated and even small gaps must be bridged by grafts.

Question: We know from Sunderland's work that the fascicular interweavings continually change their alignment. If the nerve endings must be trimmed, what hope is there of any reasonable surgical realignment and recovery of sensibility?

Moberg: If we expect that only chance determines the alignment, then we would expect no real recovery at all. However, our results are far better than chance realignment can explain. One can theorize some chemotatic or other influence.

Millesi: While the fascicular arrangements do indeed continually change, the fascicular groups are fairly constant over short distances. Thus even in longer defects, staying in the correct quadrant will increase the chance of proper alignment.

Ducker: I would like to place the issue of timing of repair in perspective. Delayed repair received its impetus in World War II. Initially everyone tried to sew nerves together immediately, but the failure rate was over 50%. With the many untidy and high velocity injuries the surgeons simply could not predict the correct level of demarcation. The judgment must be based on the level of the injury, the mechanism of injury, adjacent tissue damage, and so on. There are no hard and fast rules, and each case must be evaluated in the light of our understanding of wound physiology and repair mechanisms.

Question: If the Schwann cell is ultimately responsible for the mechanical strength of a nerve repair, how long should one immobilize the part?

Ducker: My experience is mainly with the major proximal trunks. We circularly cast the part for 3 weeks and then splint it for another 3 weeks. By the time the stiff joint recovers mobility, regeneration has begun, and the repair is secure. We once marked our nerve repairs with wire sutures and then measured the distraction by x-ray. In 104 anastomoses (some done under perhaps more tension than recommended here today) we had only one that was pulled apart.

Millesi: If you repair your nerves without tension in the extended position, or even fascicular repairs with grafts, then 10 days of immobilization is sufficient. While the strength of the nerve trunk comes from the peripheral mesenchymal tissue rather than the neural elements, tension can stretch the repair as well as disrupt it. It may retain mechanical continuity, but the long scar is a poor bed for neural regeneration.

Question: How long would you wait for sensory recovery before considering reexploration?

Omer: In an adult I wait from 12 to 24 months, depending on the level. I'm not sure, however, that our surgical technique is the key to success. One must always consider the effects of reeducation and the ability of the patient to reeducate himself or to be assisted by a formalized program. For example, we studied some patients who had no nerve repair but immediately began a program of reeducation. After a few months they could recognize the majority of a nine-object Moberg picking-up test, *without any repair.* When the objects were changed they no longer recognized them. Therefore, how can you judge 2 years after a repair whether the recovered sensibility was due to your surgical skills or the patient's educability?

Curtis: Again, each patient must be judged on his merit. I recall Dr. Bunnell saying that he wouldn't hesitate to repair a motor nerve up to 3 years after injury and a sensory nerve up to 10 years later.

Ducker: The best statistics we have are from Woodall and Beebe's study in World War II. They followed 3,565 motor nerve repairs and found that after a 2- to 3-week wait there was 1% less success for every 6 days' delay. Thus after 600 days or about 2 years there was no chance of recovery. Even after 1 year the results are discouraging. The same study showed that some sensory recovery occurred even after marked delays. Children, as we have said before, are of course an exception to these statistics and should be treated with greater optimism.

Part II

Motor nerve injuries: pain and reflex dystrophy

Chapter 8

Timing and objectives of tendon transfers after nerve injury

Paul W. Brand

The timing of tendon transfers depends on the objectives of tendon transfers. Most of us develop objectives that are too narrow. "Management by objectives" has proved to be so effective in industry that it has invaded many other fields such as agriculture and health care. The trouble is that in dealing with life systems it is much more difficult to define single clear-cut measurable objectives in order of priority, so that they can be used as indices of progress. The result is that objectives are sometimes chosen because they can be measured easily rather than because they are more important. In agriculture, for example, much serious irreversible soil erosion has resulted from the single-minded pursuit of maximizing the harvest each year. A long-term unmeasured loss is accepted without thought in exchange for a transient measurable gain. In health, also, major long-term objectives are hard to quantify, while short-term goals are measurable if they are narrow enough.

When a person has an industrial accident resulting in a nerve injury he has to put himself into the hands of a number of specialists, each of whom has his own objectives. The patient has a lawyer, and the lawyer's objective is to gain the maximum financial settlement for the patient. The fact that the lawyer may keep a third of it for himself ensures a single-minded pursuit of this objective. He wants the patient to convince a jury that he has severe disability. The neurosurgeon has the objective of maximum sensory and motor recovery. He also wants to be able to demonstrate and measure the recovery. The therapist wants good reeducation of the affected limb. He also wants to be identified with the success of that reeducation and recovery of sensation and motor power.

What about the patient? Does he have an objective for himself? If he has a high nerve injury it may take 2 full years of his working life to satisfy the objectives of his lawyer, his surgeon, and his therapist. The surgeon may want the patient to return to work while he waits for his nerve to grow down to the fingertips, but the lawyer insists that he must not work till his case is settled, and that must wait till no further recovery can be expected. The hand surgeon may want to transfer tendons to compensate for the residual paralysis, but the neurosurgeon insists that the nerve may still recover a little more. By the end of 2 years the patient may have good financial compensation and a fair sensation and some motor recovery, but he may now look upon himself as a cripple. His hand is probably stiff. He has forgotten how to work and has become habituated to receiving welfare or disability payments. He has convinced himself that the world owes him a living. There are a few obstinate patients who have the same high nerve injury but who refuse doctors and lawyers and therapists and go right back to work. They use the uninjured hand and the good part of the bad hand, and they continue to have pride in their independence. At the end of 2 years such a patient may have more measurable disability in his hand, but he has minimized its significance. In terms of the real goals of a *good life,* maybe he is ahead.

The answer, of course is that neither extreme is good. It should be possible for a case of nerve injury to be managed with the patient's own overall best interest as the goal of all the specialists who advise and help him. For this to happen we really need a wise old man, perhaps a family physician, who has no direct involvement in the special techniques that are used. He may listen to all the advice and then help the patient to determine the plan to follow. In the absence of such an ombudsman, the physician who carries out the first operation has a real responsibility to attempt a detached evaluation of the patient's priorities and goals. He must take time to listen to the patient and consider his job, his home and family responsibilities, and his own image of himself and then try to judge the effect on him of the available alternative programs. We have to realize that the most important single asset that any patient has is his spirit. He will emerge from this traumatic period of his life with his will and courage and spirit intact only if he is allowed to understand his total problem and accept responsibility for it. It is so easy for us with all the paraphernalia and scientific jargon of our profession to convince a patient that he is inadequate and incompetent to have any part in the management of his own hand. The patient becomes passive, and from then on he deteriorates.

We should be willing sometimes to do tendon transfers and muscle balance operations early, in order to free a patient from splints and get him back to activity, even though in a few cases such patients may recover the use of the muscles later and thus demonstrate that the tendon transfer could have been avoided. I have had this happen, but have never regretted the fact that the patient has had a year or so of activity that he would otherwise have missed.

The time to do a tendon transfer is not necessarily when recovery has progressed as far as it can possibly go. It may be done either when the final result can be predicted, or even sometimes to serve mainly until recovery occurs, to shorten the temporary disablement that may result in permanent harm to the total person.

To justify doing a muscle balance operation before the nerve has had time to recover as fully as possible, one has to be able to (1) identify a benefit and (2) assess the possible harm that will result from the procedure.

The benefit will be in two major categories: (1) shortening the time of actual functional disablement and (2) avoiding the results of disuse or misuse of the hand that might otherwise occur; harm would result if a muscle or muscles were transferred that would leave a significant defect in their original function. Harm would also result if muscles that might later recover were to be inhibited by the earlier operation.

I like to divide muscle balance operations into two categories: (1) those that cause no significant defect and can be used early even if more recovery is expected and (2) those that should ordinarily be done only if paralysis is demonstrably irreversible. I will give examples of typical cases of high median, ulnar, and radial nerve injury. Low injury, near the point of innvervation of the muscles, gives good results so quickly that early tendon transfers are rarely indicated.

HIGH MEDIAN PALSY

Muscle balance operations for high median palsy should be considered in two parts. The forearm muscles are innervated relatively close to the nerve injury and thus have a fair chance of recovery and also a shorter waiting time. The thenar muscles and lumbricals are far from the injury; thus they are much less likely to have a good recovery and have much longer to wait. Therefore in many cases it would be reasonable to provide an early transfer for abduction and opposition of the thumb. A transfer of the extensor indicis, taken through the interosseus space between radius and ulna or around the ulnar border would leave adequate index finger extension and would allow the hand to be used for effective grasp between the thumb and the ulnar side fingers until the median side fingers recovered. The thumb would probably flex adequately with the ulnar-supplied part of the short flexors until its flexor pollicis longus recovered. To restore flexion to the index and middle fingers and thumb would involve major transfers and side-to-side suture in the forearm that would have to be undone later if recovery took place, so this should not be done early unless the median nerve injury were so gross that recovery was unlikely.

HIGH ULNAR NERVE INJURY

The disability of a high ulnar nerve injury is frequently minimal at first, but it increases as time passes because the volar plate and anterior capsule of the metacarpophalangeal joints become stretched, and there is unopposed hyperextension of the metacarpophalangeal joints. The proximal interphalangeal joints become chronically flexed after this and then become stiff in flexion. Once this happens the chance of a good final result is greatly diminished. Thus there is much to be gained by early operation. Moreover the recovery of the intrinsic muscles after high ulnar nerve injury is usually very poor indeed, so that tendon transfer will be needed ultimately anyway.

A many-tailed graft, using the extensor carpi radialis brevis as the motor and plantaris or fascia lata femoris as graft material, is suitable for this condition. Although the extensor carpi radialis brevis may seem too important a muscle to use for intrinsic replacement, it loses none of its original wrist extensor function if it is passed along its own fascial space after attachment of the grafts, and then the grafts are passed through the second and third interosseus spaces between the second, third, and fourth metacarpals to be attached either to lateral band or to the flexor sheath in the first segment of each finger. The extensor carpi radialis brevis is a wrist extensor because it crosses on the dorsal side of the wrist in a certain position. The fact that it may then go on to stabilize the metacarpophalangeal joints in flexion need not change its prime function.

The other ulnar-supplied function of the intrinsic muscles is thumb adduction. The loss of this results in flexion of the tip of the thumb while pinching. To correct this it is best to use a flexor superficialis tendon, and this is a more serious loss to the hand. Thus unless the thumb is seriously disabled, I prefer to leave this until I am sure the adduction will not recover.

HIGH RADIAL NERVE INJURY

The prognosis for motor recovery is good in many cases of radial nerve injury. However, there is one operation that I like to do in some cases to get the patient active early. This is the attachment of the pronator teres to the extensor carpi radialis brevis in continuity.

This operation allows the patient to extend his wrist immediately and therefore to use his hand without a splint. It does not prevent the pronator's being used for pronation with or without wrist extension, and it does not prevent the extensor's being used for its original function when it recovers.

The patient can wait for the recovery of his extensor digitorum until the nerve grows down, because his intrinsic muscles will extend his interphalangeal joints enough to open his hand wide enough to grasp most objects. Then his pronator stabilizes the wrist so that the flexors of the fingers can make an effective grasp.

Whatever type of tendon transfer is planned, it must be fully understood by the patient.

The most important aspect of the whole program of rehabilitation is that the patient accept the responsibility and the initiative for his own recovery. All aspects of the program must be explained to him, preferably with the therapist and a key member of the family present. There should be some avenues of choice left open to the patient so that he or she may take a definitive position. If it proves impossible to get the patient back to work, because of legal difficulties, it is good to outline some very positive work objectives to be carried out at home or in the rehabilitation setting. The time off from work is an opportunity to build that greenhouse or paint the boat or take a course in dressmaking. This too must be thought about in advance and planned as a project that the patient wants and in which he or she can take pride. The goals of the work project should be integrated with the goals of surgery and reeducation. For example, if the home project is to develop a vegetable garden, the first 3 months while the hand is weak might be devoted to attending a university extension course on home gardens. By that time the hand might be ready for the heavier tasks of controlling the tiller and planting and weeding. The whole creative effort of learning a new skill and tasting the fruits of his labor (or wearing the clothes that have been produced) gives the period of disability the flavor of new ability. This may be as important for the patient as the two-point discrimination test is for the surgeon.

Chapter 9

Brachial plexus injuries

Hanno Millesi

Prototypically, the patient who sustains a brachial plexus injury is a young motorcyclist with a blunt injury sustained either from compression of the plexus between the calvicle and first rib or by traction on the hyperextended arm. The full spectrum of nerve injury may occur. Simple conduction block (Sunderland grade I) and axonic damage with wallerian degeneration but intact endoneural structures (grade II) has an excellent chance of spontaneous recovery. Grade III lesions with endoneural disruption but intact fascicles may also spontaneously recover, but this is somewhat less likely.[1,2] Grade IV (fascicular disruption but continuity intact) and grade V (complete nerve section or root avulsion) have poor to zero chance of recovery without treatment. Mixed lesions are frequent.

Past attempts to surgically correct these lesions have had little success.[6] The recommended approach was to wait for any spontaneous recovery and then to maximize function with palliative reconstructive surgery. In permanent complete plexus palsies amputation above the elbow, shoulder joint arthrodesis, and a prosthesis have been suggested.[2] Few of these patients really used their prosthesis.

Three factors have detracted from direct surgical intervention:

1. It was often difficult to differentiate preoperatively between root rupture and avulsion. Avulsions of course have a hopeless prognosis.
2. There was concern that structures with recovery potential might be further damaged and destroyed by surgical exploration. Even internal neurolysis was considered hazardous.[6]
3. Frequently the gaps between the nerve ends were too great for direct repair.

The recent development of microsurgery and all that it encompasses have helped to overcome some of these problems. Our experience with 54 cases has delineated the surgical indications and improved the prognosis in select cases.

We recommend exploration when there is no sign of recovery after 3 or 4 months. This saves time and helps salvage muscles before they have become irreversibly atrophied. The plexus is exposed by a zigzag incision without clavicular osteotomy. The operative details have been described in a previous paper.[3-5]

Careful delicate dissection with optical magnification will avoid trauma to still functioning fibers. In our series only three patients noted temporary postoperative weakness, and none had permanent functional loss. Nerve grafting has permitted the bridging of even large gaps and allows one to bypass heavily scarred areas. Grade III lesions have been improved by internal neurolysis with optical assistance.

Total avulsion of all roots has been rare (2 out of 56 cases). Root level lesions frequently showed both avulsion and disruption. Most had at a least one root with a usable proximal stump. Intercostal nerve transfers have been sucessful in partially neurotizing the distal stumps of avulsed roots so that avulsion should no longer be considered an absolute contraindication to exploration.

Physiotherapy is extremely important in the postoperative care while awaiting nerve recovery, as 12 to 18 months is the usual recovery period. Following repair, patients with grade IV and V lesions in our series have usually recovered biceps or triceps function. Shoulder mobility has been improved and joint subluxation prevented. Some patients have even recovered the use of their forearm muscles, but intrinsic function is rare. Most of our patients have less atrophy and at least protective sensation post repair.

Thus grade IV and V lesions can be improved to grade III with direct nerve repair, graft, or transfer. This may seem minimal, but for a patient with a disturbingly useless flail limb, recovery of elbow flexion and forearm function can be most meaningful. Subsequently, palliative procedures such as wrist arthrodesis and tendon transfers further enhance the patient's rehabilitation.

Modern microsurgical techniques have improved peripheral nerve surgery to permit safe neurolysis and improved recovery rates from nerve repair, grafts, and transfers, thus improving the prognosis of the more severe brachial plexus injuries.

REFERENCES

1. Alnot, J. Y., Cadre, N., Frot, B., and Sedel. L.: Etude clinique et parachirurgie puis, évolution spontanée des paralysies plexus brachial, 50ième Réunion Annuelle, Soc. Francaise de chirurgie orthopédique et traumatologique, Paris, Nov. 4-7, 1975.
2. Merle D'Aubigne, R.: Conference at the Symposium on Brachial Plexus Injuries, Vienna, Nov 17, 1976.
3. Millesi, H.: Die Eingriffe an der Hand und Fingernerven Allgemeine und Spezielle Operationslehre X. Band, Springer Verlag Heidelberg, 1972, Springer Verlag, pp. 226-253.
4. Millesi, H., Meissl, G., and Katzer, H.: Zur Behandlung der Verletzungen des Plexus brachialis. Vorschlag einer integrierten Therapie, Bruns' Beitr. Klin. Chir. **220:**429-446, 1973.
5. Millesi, H.: Microsurgery in the managment of brachial plexus. In Daniller, A. S., and Strauch, B., editors: Symposium on microsurgery, Saint Louis, 1976, The C. V. Mosby Co.
6. Seddon, H. J.: Surgical disorders of the peripheral nerves, Edinburgh, 1972, Churchill Livingstone.

Chapter 10

Brachial plexus injuries in children

M. Mark Hoffer
Roger Wickenden
Bryan Roper

DEVELOPMENT OF TREATMENT REGIMENS

Brachial plexus injuries were first described by Smellie in 1765. By the middle of the nineteenth century, Duchenne, one of the fathers of neurology and electrodiagnosis, described the upper root lesions due to stretch occurring during trauma in adults.[6] This most productive man refused to accept academic or prestigious hospital appointments, for he felt they would take time from his life's work.[5] He also began using galvanic current to avoid atrophy of recovering muscles. This stimulation continues to be used by some, although it is difficult to prove its worth.

Twenty-five cases of brachial plexus palsies were recorded in the American Civil War, out of a documented 5,000 cases of neck injuries (Fig. 10-1). Many patients were treated with galvanism, and some were examined during an attempt to ligate adjacent bleeding vessels.[3]

Further battlefield experience with such nerve injuries was documented by one of the fathers of American neurology, Mitchell.[13] As a Democrat in Civil War Philadelphia, Mitchell was out of academic favor and oddly enough, became a Civil War battlefield surgeon. His descriptions of the discomfort of traumatic nerve injury are still classics. (Fortunately this "injured-nerve" pain rarely occurs in children, but it is very common in adults with brachial plexus palsies and in amputees.) The battlefield horror witnessed by Mitchell made a deep impression upon him. It is said that his last hours in life were spent in reveries of those tragic times.

In 1874 the brilliant German neurologist, Erb, redescribed the upper root palsy that bears his

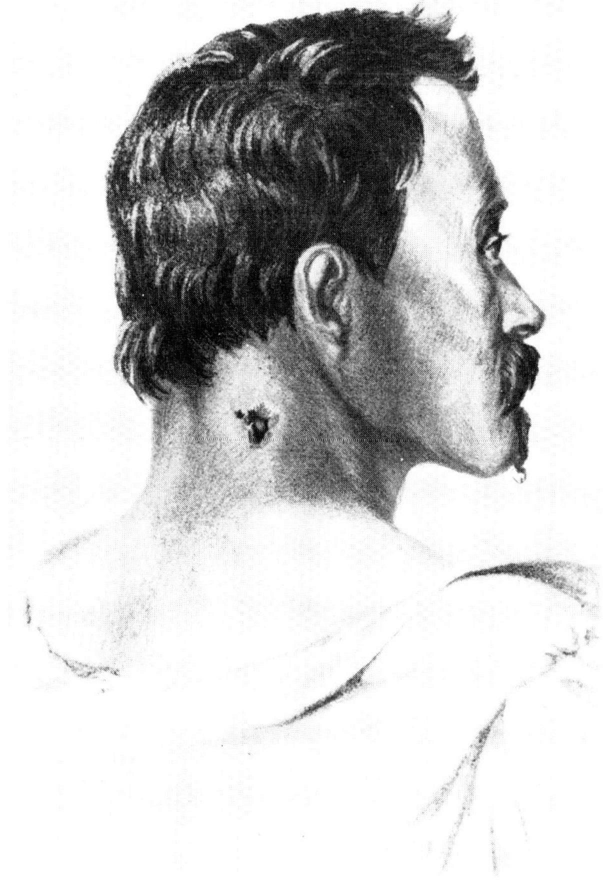

Fig. 10-1. Entrance wound, producing brachial plexus injury in Civil War casualty. (From Barnes, J. K., and Otis, G. A., editors: Medical and surgical history of the war of the rebellion, 1870, Surgeon General's Printing Office, part 1, vol. 2, p. 402.)

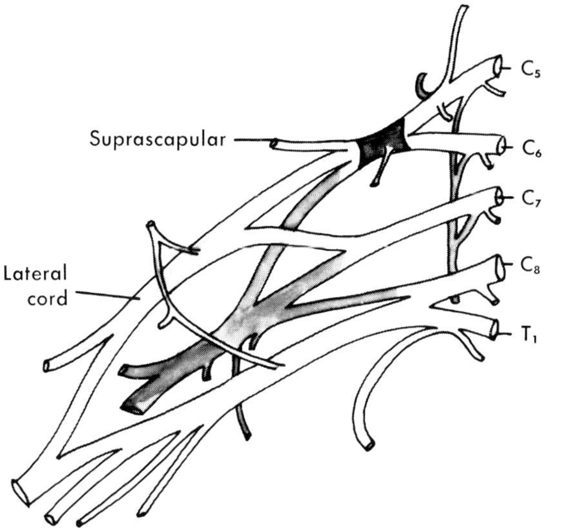

Fig. 10-2. Erb palsy of C_5-C_6 nerves.

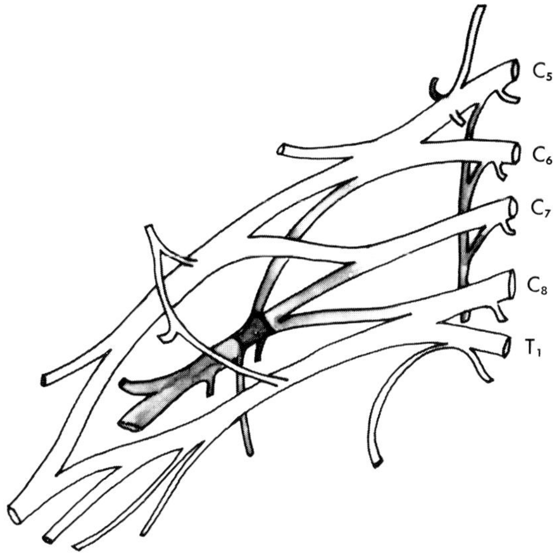

Fig. 10-3. Posterior cord palsy.

name.[14] The point at the junction of the fifth and sixth cervical roots from which the suprascapular nerve emerges is called Erb point. Erb emphasized that stretch of this point by contralateral head motion with the shoulder fixed during a delivery or accident could cause the typical palsy. This palsy affected shoulder abduction, external rotation, and elbow flexion (Fig. 10-2).

In 1885 Klumpke, while a medical student in Paris, described the lower root palsies caused by severe abduction of the after-coming arm in breech or other difficult deliveries (Fig. 10-3). Klumpke was an American woman who so impressed Professor Charcot that he kept her in his neurology training program. She married another prominent student of Charcot, Dejerine. This marriage resulted in many subsequent publications coauthored by the husband and wife team.[14]

Fairbank[8] in 1913 and Sever in 1924[16] emphasized the problems with shoulder internal rotation contractors in upper root palsies. Sever was the son of a Mayflower Pilgrim family, and cousin of Bradford, the chief of the Boston Children's Surgical Program. Sever was able to accumulate 1,100 cases of birth palsy early in the twentieth century in that most prestigious citadel of medical care. He began surgically releasing these tightly contracted internal rotation deformities. The pectoralis major and subscapularis muscles were severed in most cases.

L'Episcopo in 1934[9] and Zachary in 1947[19] popularized the transfer of latissimus dorsi and teres major to the lateral aspect of the proximal humerus to convert these internal rotators to external rotators. Roper modified this approach by transferring the muscles into the posterior rotator cuff, thus achieving both rotation and the stabilizing effect of the cuff.[15]

The operative procedures designed for polio in the early twentieth century were applied to patients with brachial palsies.[1,4,5,17] These procedures included shoulder fusions, humeral osteotomies, elbow flexoplasties, wrist tendon transfers, and wrist fusions.

INITIAL THERAPY

It has been our experience that most palsies spontaneously resolve themselves in the first year. We have seen new muscles return even up to age four. In these first four years our general plan is passive range of motion of all paralyzed joints and use of dynamic orthotic devices. We use dynamic abduction and flexion orthoses for the upper root palsies to substitute for shoulder abduction and elbow flexion. Dynamic wrist extension and metacarpophalangeal flexion assists are employed for the various hand palsies found in the lower root and posterior cord problems. We avoid rigid-positioning orthoses during this period.

SURGICAL THERAPY

By age four to seven, a clear stable neurologic picture should be identified. Either an upper root (Erb) (Fig. 10-2), cord (medial, lateral, or posterior) (Fig. 10-3), lower root (Klumpke) (Fig. 10-4), or mixed lesion will be defined.

Erb palsies are by far the most frequent and

represent a lesion secondary to abnormal stretch of the plexus by lengthening the relative position of the head and shoulder beyond physiologic limits. The typical patient will have secondary contractures with arm adduction and internal rotation, elbow extension, and forearm pronation (Waiter tip deformity). This deformity is due to loss of elbow flexors and forearm supinators and to graded muscle paralysis of (1) the deltoid therefore losing abduction; (2) the supraspinatus, thus losing humeral stabilization; and (3) the infraspinatus and teres minor losing external rotation.

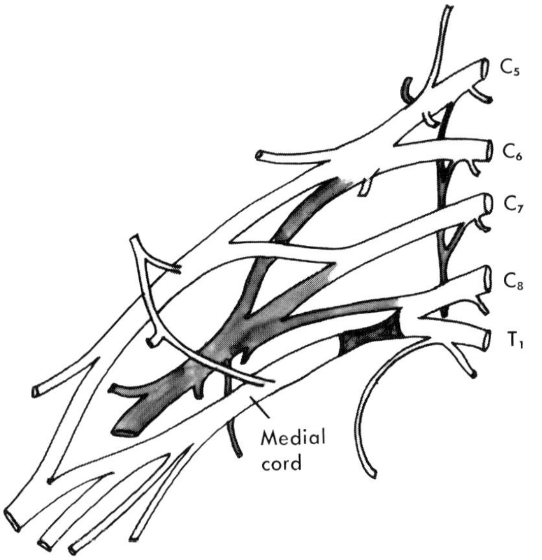

Fig. 10-4. Klumpke palsy of C_7-T_1 nerve.

We have followed 25 such Erb palsies. In 11, progressive internal rotation contracture of the shoulder developed despite therapy, requiring release and tendon transfers as described by Roper.

In Roper's procedure the pectoralis major is released anteriorly, and through a posterior incision the conjoined tendons of the latissimus dorsi and pectoralis major are transferred from their normal position to the rotator cuff. Postoperatively the patients are maintained in a shoulder spica for 4 weeks. The cast is then bivalved, and reeducation of the transfer and strengthening gradually progress. As the transfer achieves greater strength, the arm is gradually brought down to the patient's side. The patient wears an airplane splint for at least 6 months postoperatively, as a positioning device. It has been our experience that both external rotation and abduction are increased by this transfer (Figs. 10-5 and 10-6). Details of the procedure and results are reported elsewhere.[8a]

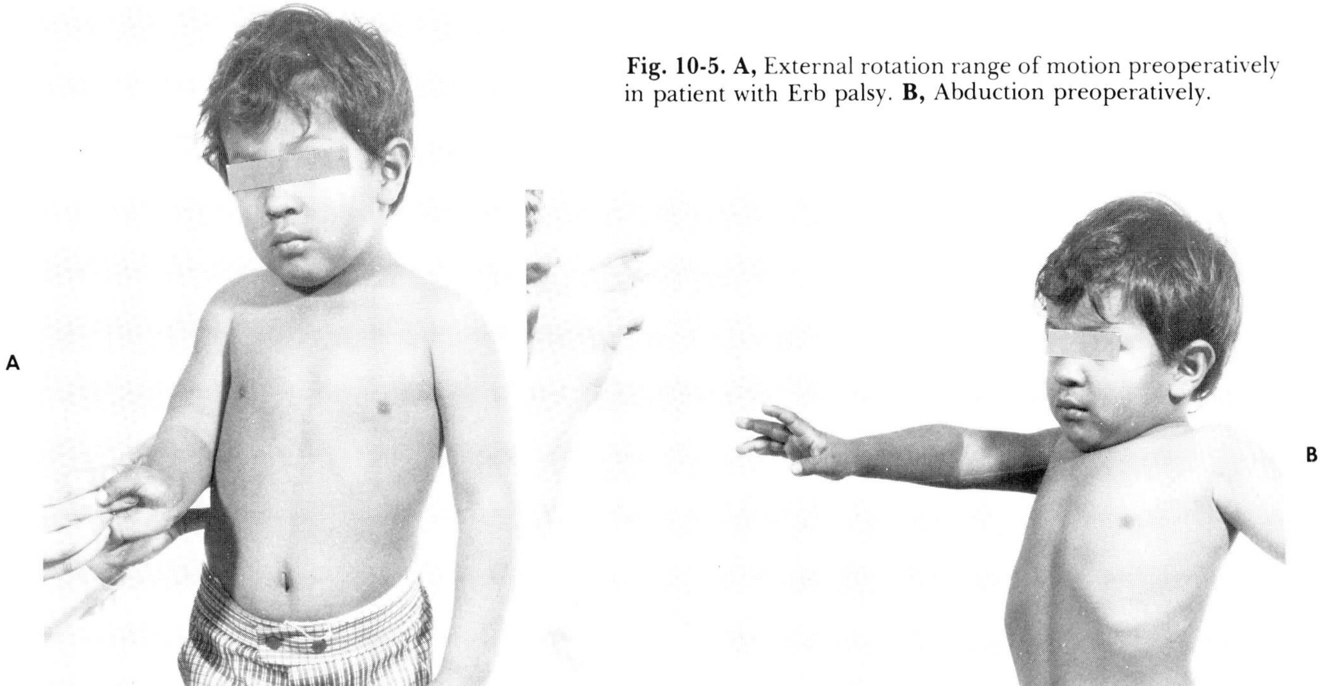

Fig. 10-5. A, External rotation range of motion preoperatively in patient with Erb palsy. **B,** Abduction preoperatively.

Fig. 10-6. A, External rotation range of motion postoperatively. B, Abduction postoperatively.

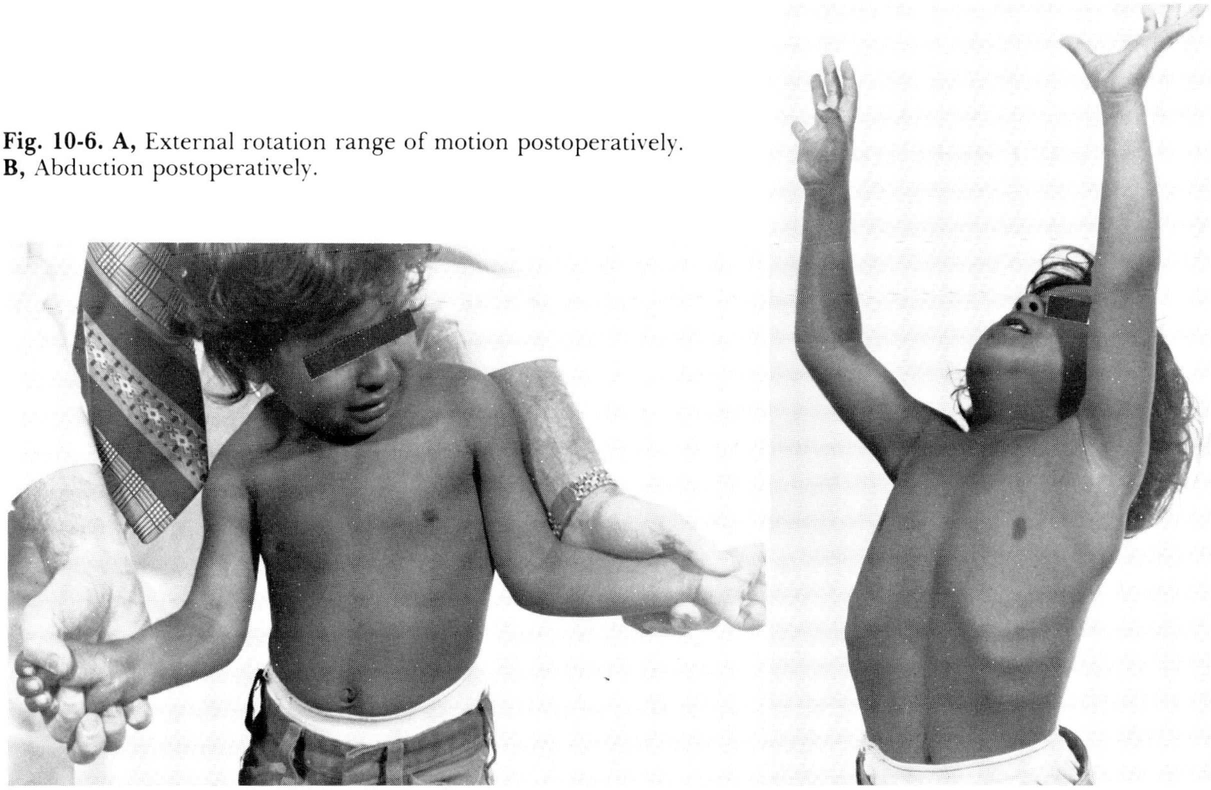

A

B

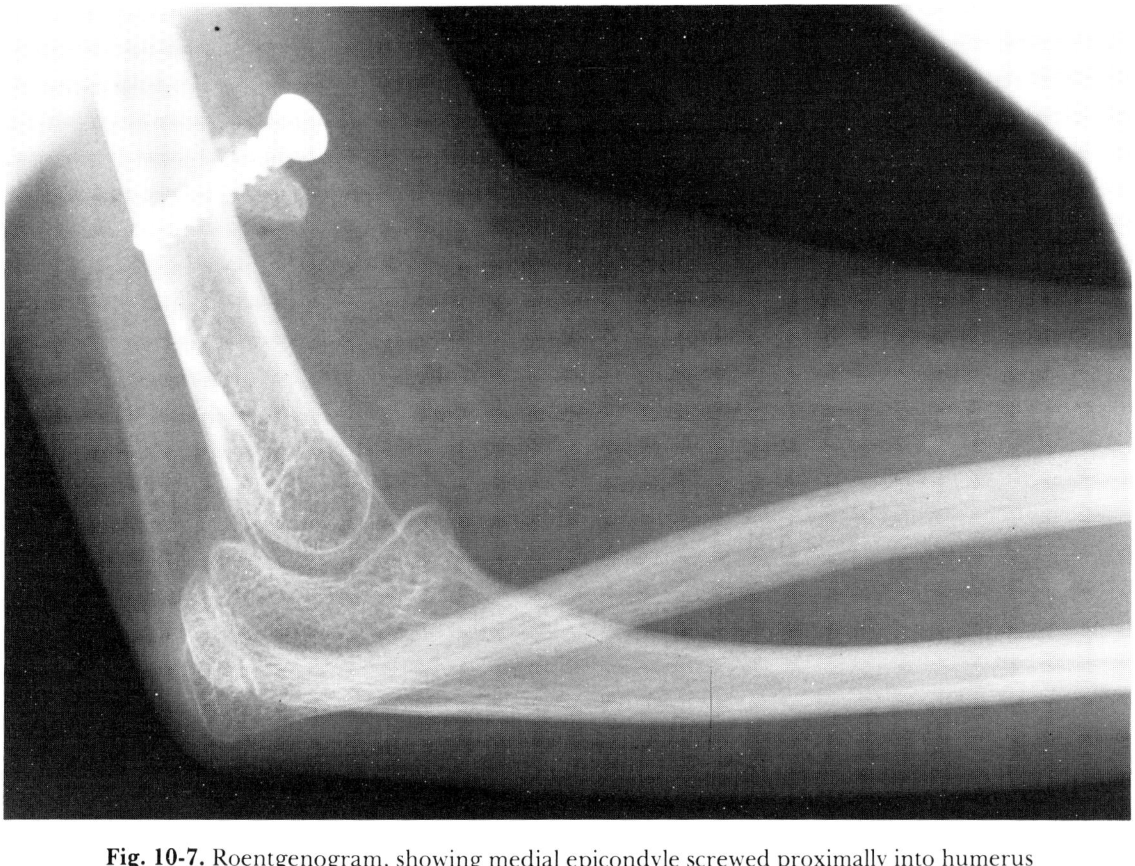

Fig. 10-7. Roentgenogram, showing medial epicondyle screwed proximally into humerus after flexorplasty. Note posterior dislocation of radial head, for which no treatment is advised.

Four of our Erb palsy patients have required elbow flexorplasty for weak elbow flexion. The entire medial epicondyle is advanced to the center of the distal third of the humerus, anteriorly, and held in place with a compression screw (Fig. 10-7). This should limit passive extension by at least 30 degrees. The collateral ligament of the elbow is carefully preserved. Early motion in a dynamic brace that prohibits extension beyond 90 degrees is utilized.

The posterior dislocation of the radial head noted in this type of palsy is due to unopposed pronation[2] and should not be treated unless it becomes symptomatic. If posterior dislocation of the humeral head has been allowed to occur,[8,11,18] tendon transfers are not advised, but osteotomy or glenohumeral fusion may be necessary.

We have followed four posterior cord palsies. This type of palsy is characterized by paralysis of the deltoid, triceps, and wrist and finger extensors. All four of our patients have required transfers of the wrist flexors and pronators to the finger and wrist extensor as described in radial nerve palsies.

Two of the patients with posterior cord palsies have had anterior dislocating radial heads due to unopposed biceps action. The resulting unstable joint makes active flexion difficult. In these cases we have transferred the biceps to the ulna with good results.

Two of the posterior cord patients have required glenohumeral fusions. This is performed only in patients with good hands and excellent scapulothoracic muscle control (trapezius and serratus anterior action). The position of fusion is very slight abduction, forward flexion, and internal rotation. No more than 30 degrees of each of these positions should be accepted. The fusions are done after all other reconstructive procedures have been completed.

Klumpke palsies occur less frequently as they are often associated with breech deliveries. They typically involve the lower two roots of the plexus. Patients may or may not have an associated Horner syndrome. Bilaterality does occur in the Klumpke palsy. The paralysis includes intrinsics of the hand as well as wrist and finger flexors. Sensibility is frequently lost in the entire hand and proximally along the ulnar border of the extremity. We have followed seven such cases. Two of them were breech births and bilateral. Unfortunately, useful reconstructive surgical procedures cannot be performed for these upper extremities because of lack of sensation. These children have utilized dynamic orthoses for limited periods of time, but they then adapt to one-handed and assisted patterns of hand use.

Although we understand that amputation and prosthetic devices have been tried in palsied adults, we do not advocate their use in children. Our children have not had skin problems or nerve causalgias described in the adult trauma palsies, and they have been very threatened by the thought of loss of a limb and body image effects. The children adapt to loss of single limb function so effectively that they rarely would use the prostheses even if offered.

In the last few years, we have also seen 13 trauma-induced, non-birth-related, brachial palsies in young children. Three of these had myelographic evidence of pseudocysts, indicating root sleeve damage in C5, C6, C7, C8, and T1. Yet these three have made significant recovery in the muscles about the shoulder, elbow, and hand. This test is thus not prognostic for children.[10]

Brachial plexus palsies from birth are certainly markedly declining[7] with modern obstetrical care. With the increased number of head injuries suffered by children in our mechanized society, we may see more and more of the acquired palsies.

REFERENCES

1. Adler, J. B.: Erb's palsy: long term results of treatment in 88 cases, J. Bone Joint Surg. [Am.] **49:**1052-1064, 1967.
2. Aitken, J.: Deformity of the elbow joint as a sequel to Erb's obstetrical paralysis, J. Bone Joint Surg. [Br.] **34:**352-365, 1952.
3. Barnes, J. K., and Otis, G. A., editors: Medical and surgical history of the war of the rebellion, 1870, Surgeon General's Printing Office, part 1, vol. 2, pp. 408-410.
4. Chung, S. M. K.: Obstetrical paralysis, Orthop. Clin. North Am. **6:**393-399, 1975.
5. DePalma: Surg. Shoulder, pp. 523-533, 1973.
6. Duchenne, G. B.: Physiology of motion, (translated by Kaplan, E. B.), Philadelphia, 1949, J. B. Lippincott Company.
7. Eng, G. D.: Brachial plexus palsy in newborn infants, Pediatrics **48:**18-28, 1971.
8. Fairbank, H. A. T.: Birth palsy: subluxation of shoulder joint in infants and young children, Lancet **1:**1217, 1913.

8a. Hoffer, M. M., Wickenden, R., and Roper, B.: Brachial plexus birth palsies: results of tendon transfer to the rotator cuff, J. Bone Joint Surg. [Am.], 1978. In press.

9. L'Episcopo, J. B.: Tendon transplantation in obstetrical paralysis, Am. J. Surg. **25:**122, 1934.
10. Leffert, R. D.: Brachial plexus injuries, N. Engl. J. Med. **291:**1059-1067, 1974.
11. Liebolt, F. L.: Obstetrical paralysis with dislocation of the shoulder, J. Bone Joint Surg. [Am.] **35:**227-230, 1953.

12. Major, R. H.: A history of medicine, vol. 2, Springfield, Ill., 1955, Charles C Thomas, Publisher.
13. Mitchell, S. W.: Gunshot wounds and other injuries to nerves, Philadelphia, 1864, J. B. Lippincott Company.
14. Rang, M.: An anthology of orthopedics, New York, 1969, Longman.
15. Roper, B.: A new operation to improve weakness of the abductors and external rotators of the shoulder, Orthopedic Seminars, Rancho Los Amigos Hospital, Downey, Calif. **4:**347-353.
16. Sever, J. W.: Obstetric paralysis, report of 1100 cases, J.A.M.A. **85:**1862-1865, 1925.
17. Wickstrom, J.: The surgical management of residual deformities of the shoulder following birth injuries of the brachial plexus, J. Bone Joint Surg. [Am.] **37:**27-36, 1955.
18. Wickstrom, J.: Birth injuries of the brachial plexus, treatment of defects in the shoulder, Clin. Orthop. **23:**187-195, 1962.
19. Zachary, R. B.: Transplantation of the teres major and latissimus dorsi for loss of external rotation at shoulder, Lancet **2:**757-758, 1947.

Chapter 11

Myoelectric assists and feedback in the upper extremity

Vert Mooney
James B. Reswick

HISTORY AND DEVELOPMENT OF SENSORY FEEDBACK SYSTEMS

It is generally recognized that the success of functional substitution and the rate of successful patient fitting is far better for lower limb protheses than for upper limb devices. Certainly the function of grasp and release is more difficult to replace and control than are the swing and stance phases of lower limb prosthetic function. But perhaps a more devastating loss in the upper limb amputee is the absence of sensation that provides the normal hand with the feedback necessary for manual dexterity. This chapter records the current state of attempts to provide a substitute sensory feedback through the peripheral nervous system.

In the United States the first attempt to provide an electronic system of sensory feedback for the upper limb amputee was by a group at Duke University headed by Dr. Frank Clippinger. His work had been built upon the experience of several previous investigators who had utilized various transducers at the prosthetic terminal device and translated this signal into proportional feedback. In 1969 Pfeiffer and associates [4] used audio feedback. Feedback by way of electric stimulation to the skin was first reported by Beeker and associates [1] in 1967. A self-contained system wherein the terminal device activity was proportionally transmitted to vibration at the residual limb within the socket of the prosthesis was reported from Japan in 1969 by Kawamura and Sueda.[3]

Improvement in electronic technology, however, provided the opportunity for the use of an inductively coupled signal to be translated from the terminal device, through the intact skin to a buried receiver, which transmitted this electric signal to circumferential electrodes on the peripheral nerves. In their first publication on this approach (1974) Clippinger and associates[2] indicated that this system originally had been utilized as a method of treating phantom limb pain. With the technical success of the electronic system the original report noted the experience in nine patients with neuroelectric feedback from the terminal device.

The systems they described used a cable-driven, voluntary-closing, APRL hook in which the locking cam had been removed and fitted in reverse so that the thumb was on the ulnar side of the forearm. The transducer was a strain gauge located in the cable and thus varied according to the force of closing.

According to the Duke report, patient acceptance of this system was extremely gratifying. None of the patients abandoned the system, although service problems sometimes did interfere with continued usuage. Many of the patients reported not only a perception of the amount of pressure necessary to hold an object, but also recorded a qualitative component to the perception, that is, a sensation of the consistency of the object being held. One of the most important findings of this study was that pain was not a significant factor in the patient's perception of electric input. Electric input into the peripheral nervous system as increasing frequency from 0 to 100 Hz could be interpreted not just as a "buzz" but as truly functional "sensation."

As clinicians caring for a significant number of amputees, we were aware of the need to improve

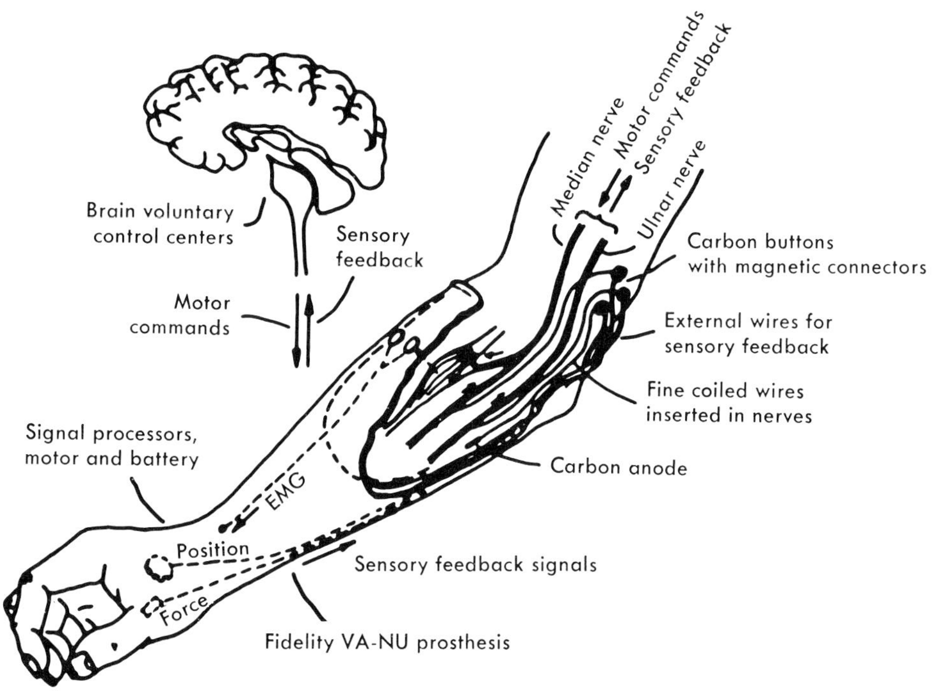

Fig. 11-1. Conceptual illustration of sensory feedback system in a Rancho-VAPC EMG hand applied to a powered, myoelectrically controlled prosthesis, the Fidelity VA-NU prosthesis.

upon the functional acceptance of upper limb prostheses. We were greatly encouraged by the success and acceptance reported from the Duke study. Several questions remained to be clarified before we could identify the role of a sensory feedback system in the fitting of upper extremity amputees.

First, since all the patients had been previously fitted with cable-controlled prostheses, to what extent were their subjective views of improved function based on the new fitting system? These patients now had a voluntary-closing hook with proprioceptive feedback secondary to the cable control as well as electronically. However, perhaps a voluntary-closing system is indeed more appropriate for enhanced feedback than the more typical voluntary-opening system.

Another question concerned the technical equipment. The induced signal system (Avery Laboratories) required a coupled system that had to use a fixed signal. Was this the most ideal electric signal to be perceived by the central nervous system? If the pulse width were varied, amplitude varied, or the signal further manipulated, would there be a change in perception of the signal? Furthermore, although the induced signal system has demonstrated itself to be extremely reliable and has already demonstrated success in clinical applications for other diseases, such as pain control and peripheral motor nerve stimulation, it is expensive and complicated. Is there a simpler system to provide a direct electronic link with the peripheral nervous system?

Finally, since myoelectrically controlled and electronically powered systems have improved greatly, would the neuroelectric feedback system offer a unique advantage to these more technically advanced power and control systems that do not have the benefit of cable proprioceptive feedback?

In animal and human studies a coiled wire neuroelectrode has been demonstrated to be successful. This particular electrode design offered the potential advantage of being able to discontinue the implant without the need of an extensive surgical procedure. Merely pulling the wire would remove the whole electrode. The conceptual framework for these ideas is presented in Fig. 11-1.

METHOD

Since this study was conceived to identify the applicability of neuroelectric feedback systems to the upper limb amputee using myoelectrically con-

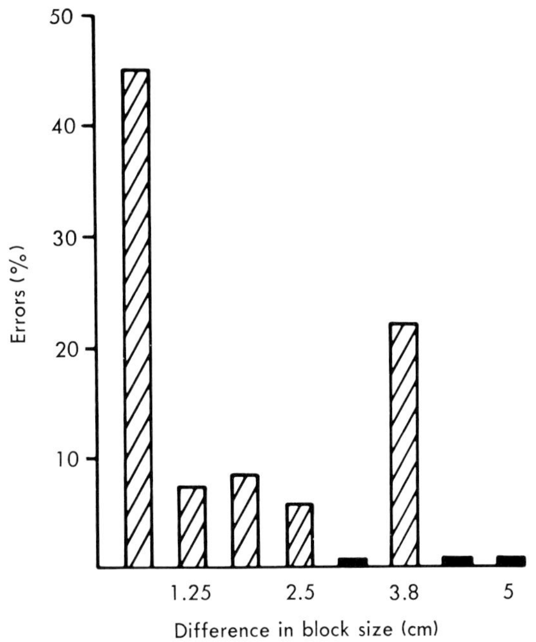

Fig. 11-2. Using conventional prosthesis, patient was requested to discriminate block sizes without visual feedback. Although there were frequent errors below the 1.25 cm size, patient was excellent in differentiating sizes greater than 1.25 cm.

trolled and electronically powered prostheses, it was decided to challange the question of applicability to various types of amputee problems.

Three different types of amputees were studied. The first amputee was already an experienced and truly functional user of a cable-driven below-elbow porsthesis. He was tested to objectively identify the amount of nonvisual feedback of terminal device position that is inherent in a functional user. This amputee was also used to verify the technical feasibility of the transcutaneous neuroelectric feedback system. The second amputee fitted with the system was a recent below-elbow amputee who had not yet become expert in the use of any prosthesis. He was fitted with the VA-NU–powered prosthesis with the neuroelectric feedback system. He was also fitted with a standard prosthesis for comparison. The third subject was a recent bilateral below-elbow amputee who had the neuroelectric feedback system applied to the nondominant limb (left), and specific comparisons concerning the use and function of the two prostheses were made. A description of each fitting and results follow.

The first patient is a 45 year-old junk dealer who has been a left, below-elbow amputee for 8 years. He bas been accustomed to using a standard below-elbow fitting with a voluntary-opening, cable-driven, hook-type terminal device. The patient had

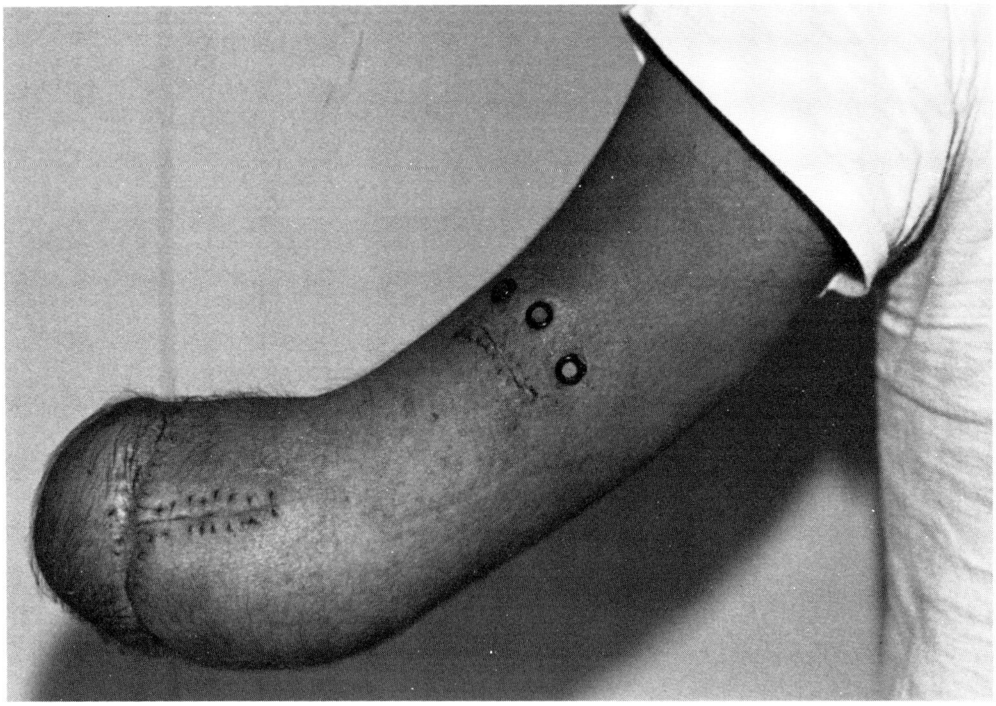

Fig. 11-3. Magnetic core carbon buttons with intraneural electrodes.

a history of routine servicing over the past several years, indicating hard use of the prosthesis. The patient's proficiency in differentiating block size without visual feedback (Fig. 11-2) was tested the week before the surgical procedure.

Three carbon buttons utilizing a magnetic connector system were surgically implanted proximal to the antecubital fossa in March 1975. One electrode was inserted into the median nerve, one into the ulnar nerve, and the third terminated in a ground electrode fabricated from pyrolytic carbon (Fig. 11-3). The use of carbon button connector systems had been confirmed by previous clinical experience.

The intraneural electrodes were of coil wire, free of insulation, and were passed through the nerve by means of a needle that had been crimped to the end of the coiled electrode. Once through the nerve, the needle was cut away, leaving the coiled electrode indwelling within the nerve. Thus, with the completion of surgery, connectors had been placed in the skin proximal to the antecubital fossa with wire connections to the median and ulnar nerves. The connectors were placed through the skin by subcutaneous dissection and the use of a tubular boring instrument to make a hole for their portrusion through the dermis.

Healing of the tissues occurred within 10 days. The patient felt no discomfort and could wear his standard prosthesis comfortably. The patient was also fitted with an APRL voluntary-closing hook with a transducer to identify position. Thus position was translated to variable frequency signals.

Although the device was functional and pain free, the patient was unwilling to pursue any efforts at retraining. He indicated that he could identify no improvement of function using the APRL hook with neuroelectric feedback versus his original equipment.

The second patient was a recent below-elbow amputee. He had no prior prosthetic experience. He had neuroelectric implants as decribed for the previous patient. In addition, he was fitted with a VA-NU specially instrumented myoelectric hand. Although there were some initial technical problems in its use, the patient rapidly became adept and could comfortably use the myoelectric system (Fig. 11-4) with feedback as supplied by VAPC.

When the two electronic systems were used together, however, considerable interference was discovered. The electronic signal used for sensory feedback created interference with the signal for the myoelectric hand, and thus "chatter" was developed with the use of the hand. The interference was even at low amplitudes below those that produced sensation. At higher levels where sensation was evi-

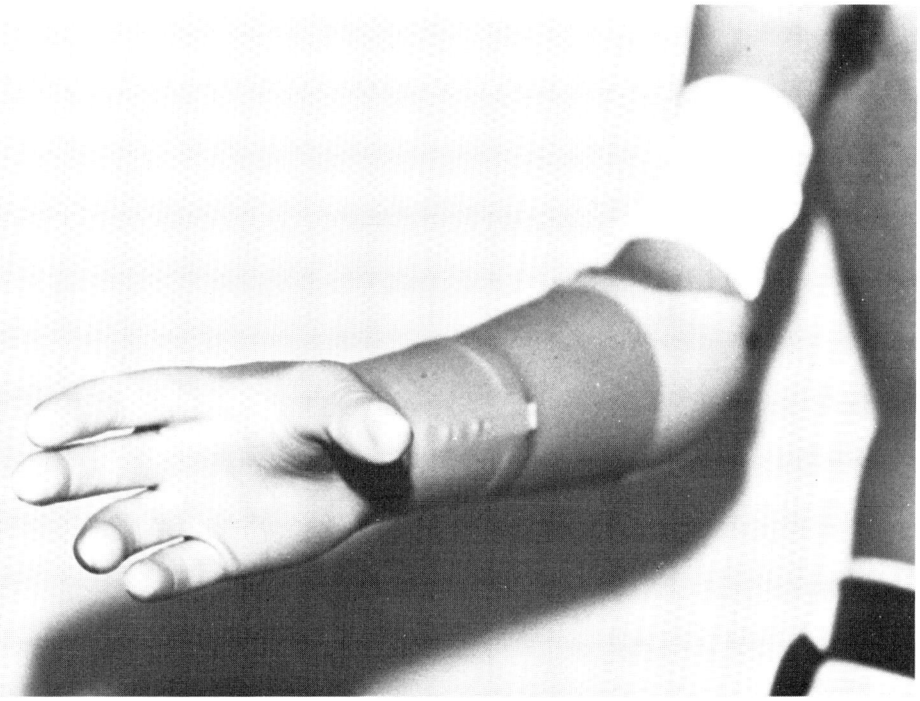

Fig. 11-4. Patient using VA-NU prosthesis.

dent, the hand would open involuntarily because of the interference. Because of frequent downtimes with the myoelectrically controlled prosthesis, the patient was also fitted with a conventional hook-and-cable mechanism.

He gradually began to rely more on the hook-and-cable prosthesis. He did use the myoelectrically controlled hand for social occasions and was extremely adept as its use. He would only connect the neuroelectric system for test purposes and in occupational therapy training. Because of the apparently insurmountable technical problems related to the electric interference between neuroelectric feedback and myoelectric control, the patient was given the option of converting from a myoelectrically controlled hand to a neuroelectric feedback cable-driven hook. The patient preferred to keep his myoelectrically controlled hand and not pursue the neuroelectric fitting further.

The third patient is a 47-year-old recent bilateral below-elbow amputee; his amputation was secondary to an electric burn. He had no prior prosthetic experience before entering this study. He was right-hand dominant and was fitted with an APRL voluntary-closing cable-driven prosthesis on that side. On the left he had a similar prosthesis but, in addition, had electrode implants as did the previous two patients and position and force transducers located in his terminal device. He has been equipped with this system since November 1975. He has become a proficient user of his prosthetic devices and definitely prefers the neuroelectric feedback system on the left. Initially, he had feedback into both median and ulnar nerves, but 4 months postimplant one of the subcutaneous wires broke, and thus feedback was only to the ulnar nerve. He has had extensive testing with and without neuroelectric feedback and has demonstrated objectively an improvement of function with the neuroelectric system (Fig. 11-5).

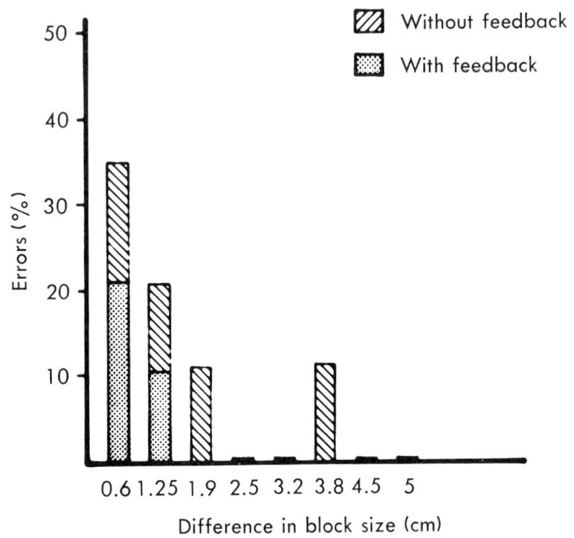

Fig. 11-5. Comparison of ability of patient to differentiate block sizes with and without neuroelectric feedback. Errors decreased by 40% to 50% when neuroelectric feedback system was utilized.

The patient now states that he definitely preferred the left upper extremity function compared to the right. The aspect that is most pleasing to him is the constant input from the left terminal device, which he states "gives me the sensation that the prosthesis is part of me." He routinely keeps the hook slightly open so that the input is constant, as the feedback turns off when the hook is completely closed.

DISCUSSION

Several significant things have been learned from this study, some positive and some negative. On the negative side, there is a nearly insurmountable technical problem concerning simultaneous neuroelectric input of feedback from the terminal device conflicting with myoelectric output for control of the powered terminal device. Multiple attempts at manipulating the electric circuitry through various filters and timing of signals have been unsuccessful in the clinical sense. In the one patient where this problem has been challenged, he chose to continue with a myoelectrically controlled hand without feedback rather than to further pursue the intricacies of neuroelectric feedback.

A second negative finding from this study concerns the applicability of enhanced neuroelectric feedback to a practiced functional prosthetic user. From the experience with our first patient it was apparent that through continued use and training he was quite adept at estimating sizes of objects without visual feedback as an advantage to function, when compared to the additional gadgetry required to achieve this additional dimension. It is quite possible that his negative response was based on imperfections of our system, as we also went through a learning phase. He possibly did not find improved function in switching to a voluntary-closing system from a voluntary-opening system. This was not a problem in the experience from the group at Duke, and our lack of correlations with their experience is confusing. It is apparent, however, from the lack of favorable response in the first two patients that additional neuroelectric feedback is not an overwhelming addition to functional use for some patients.

On the positive side, several strides forward in the fitting of amputees have been made. The achievement of transcutaneous neuroelectric input into the sensory system has been demonstrated. The system is quite simple and generally has worked well. There was no incidence of lack of tolerance for the carbon buttons or technical failure with the magnetic connector system. One buried wire electrode broke, and in one patient the stimulus was perceived as painful following trauma to the forearm. The implanted system was discontinued simply under local anesthesia in the outpatient unit when the first patient decided that the additional gadgetry was of no value to him.

The third patient demonstrated a successful fitting and application of the enhanced feedback by neuroelectric connection. Being a bilateral amputee without prior prosthetic experience, he was in the best position to give an objective evaluation of the advantages and disadvantages of the system. The neuroelectric feedback system was fitted to the nondominant left side; however, he so much preferred to use the feedback that he is now left-hand dominant.

Because of the simplicity of the neuroelectric implanted system, the input signal can be manipulated as desired. On this basis an innovative mechanism that varies the input signal simultaneously on two parameters (frequency and pulse duration) has been demonstrated. Additonal experience will be necessary to fully identify the idealized mode of stimulation for the best perception of functional "sensation." Nonetheless, depending on the system utilized, continued manipulation of the signal is available.

The question yet remains whether an implanted system is truly necessary. The patients' comments as to the desirable features of the neuroelectric system constantly concern not so much the signal change in proportion to force or position of the terminal device, but rather the presence of the signal itself. The patient identified the constant input from the terminal as making him feel that the prosthesis was more a part of him. Perhaps a less sophisticated system, such as a mechanical vibratory system on the skin surface to provide continual feedback, would be appropriate.

Certainly the experience with this preliminary study has identified large areas of ignorance, that can only be solved by greater experience and more astute and objective observation.

SUMMARY

1. Experience with three below-elbow amputees utilizing a transcutaneous neuroelectric feedback system has been reviewed.
2. In two of our patients there was insufficient advantage from the implanted system to warrant continued effort on their part to utilize the feedback system.
3. Technical considerations greatly limit the potential of simultaneous neuroelectric sensory input with myoelectrically controlled systems.
4. In the bilateral patient the desirability of neuroelectric feedback systems has been clarified. A system that presents simultaneous input for both force and position has been utilized successfully.

REFERENCES

1. Beeker, T.W., During, J., and de Hertog, A.: Artificial touch in a hand-prosthesis, Med. Biol. Eng. **5**:47-49, 1967.
2. Clippinger, F. W., Avery, R., and Titus, B. R.: State of effort—a sensory feedback system for an upper-limb amputation prosthesis, Bull. Prosthet. Res. pp. 247-257, Fall 1974.
3. Kawamura, Z., and Sueda, O.: Sensory feedback device for the artificial arm, Monograph presented at 4th Pan Pacific Rehabilitation Conference, 1969.
4. Pfeiffer, E. A., Rhode, C. M., and Fabric, S. I.: An experimental device to provide substitute tactile sensation from the anaesthetic hand, Med. Biol. Eng. **7**:191-199, 1969.

Chapter 12

Neuromas: diagnosis and management

H. Bruce Williams

A significant number of symptomatic neuromas occur in patients following injuries of peripheral nerves. These neuromas may follow partial or complete nerve severance, and they present a variety of problems to the treating surgeon, both in diagnosis and treatment. The terminal or stump neuroma and the neuroma in continuity will be discussed to indicate the changes that occur following these nerve injuries and how these might be managed in clinical cases.

STRUCTURE OF NERVES

A peripheral nerve is composed of many thousands of axons carrying motor, sensory, and automatic impulses to and from the various end organs (Fig. 12-1). The nuclei of the motor nerve cells are located in the anterior horn of the spinal cord and in the posterior root ganglia for the sensory nerves. Axons vary from a few millimeters to over a meter in length and from 0.5 to 30 μm in diameter. They must be connected with the cell body to survive.

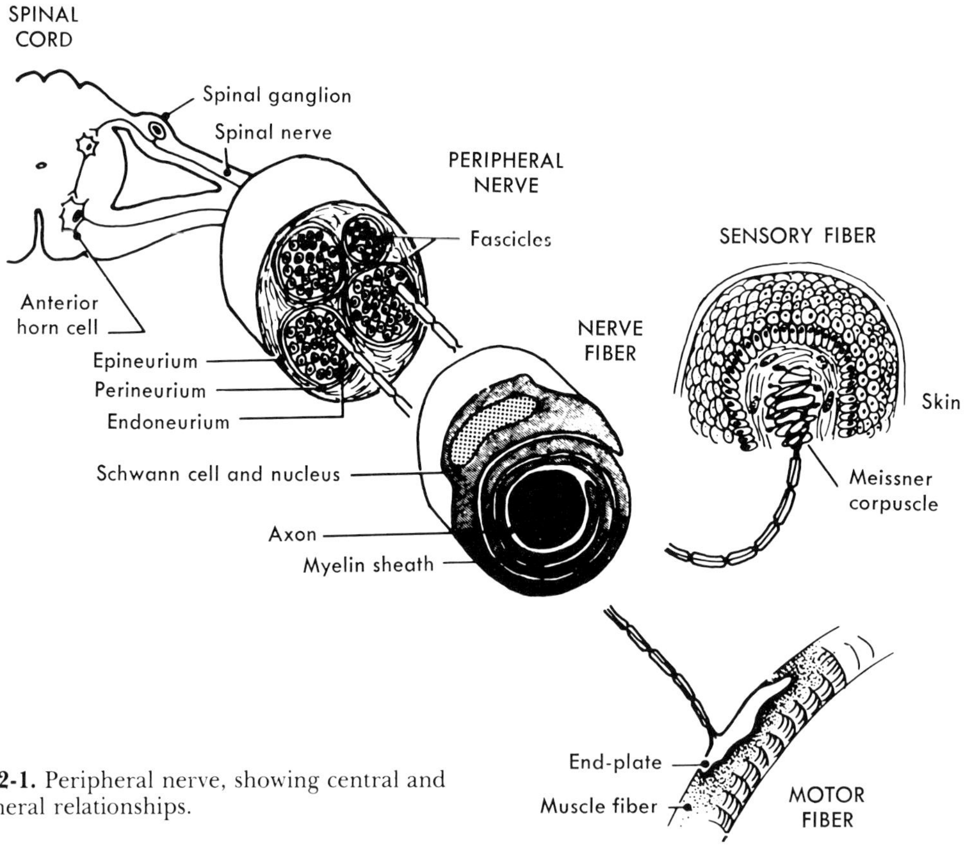

Fig. 12-1. Peripheral nerve, showing central and peripheral relationships.

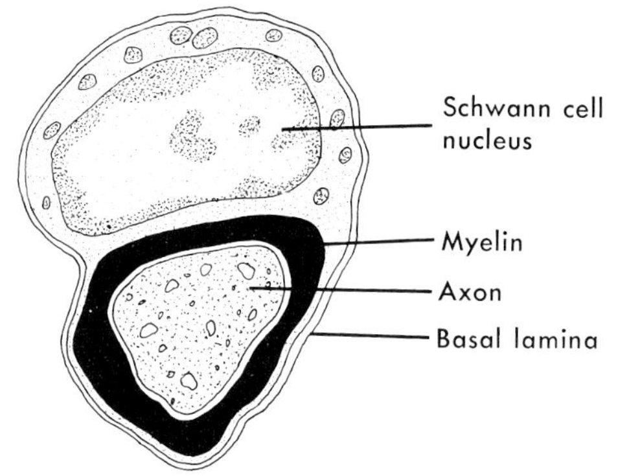

Fig. 12-2. Myelinated single axon with Schwann cell and sheath. (× 3,000.)

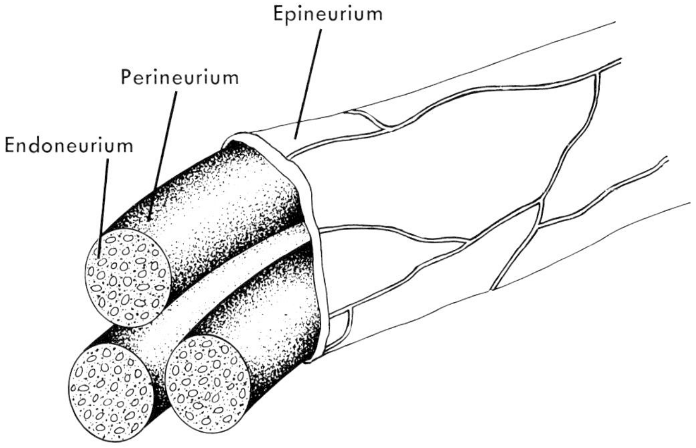

Fig. 12-3. Fibrous layers of peripheral nerve. Note well-vascularized mobile epineurium.

Each axon is surrounded by a multi-layered Schwann sheath, and there are both myelinated and unmyelinated fibers. There is a relationship of one Schwann cell to each axon in the myelinated group, but in the unmyelinated fibers, one Schwann cell may surround several axons. Myelin is a complex lipoprotein produced by the Schwann cell, and the nodes of Ranvier separate each Schwann cell at regular constant intervals throughout the length of the nerve. In general, fibers less than 2 μm in diameter are considered to be unmyelinated, while fibers of 2 to 30 μm in diameter are considered to be myelinated. Around each Schwann cell layer is the endoneurium, a protective delicate investment of loose collagen fibers with sparse fibroblasts. The basal lamina separates the nerve fiber from the surrounding endoneurium. This, together with the axon myelin sheath and Schwann cell, forms the endoneurial tubes (Fig. 12-2).

These endoneurial tubes containing the axons are grouped together and are surrounded by flattened cells, arranged in concentric layers, separated by collagen and elastic fibrils. This structure is the perineurium, and it acts as a barrier to diffusion of various substances.[10,19] This collected bundle of nerve fibers within the perineural sheath is called a fascicle or funiculus. A loose, areolar type of connective tissue richly supplied with blood vessels surrounds and separates the fascicles and is called the epineurium. This loosely arranged layer allows free movement of the nerve in joint excursions and yet provides an adequate blood supply (Fig. 12-3).

NERVE INJURIES

Nerve injuries may be grouped according to severity and range as in Seddon's[13] classification from neurapraxia, which is a temporary loss of conduction without loss of continuity, through axonotmesis, complete axonal severance with preservation of endoneurial sheaths, to neurotmesis, complete nerve severance with loss of continuity of the nerve sheath.

Sunderland[15] further subdivided nerve injuries into five grades according to severity:

I. Loss of conduction in the axons
II. Loss of continuity of the axons without affecting the endoneurium
III. Loss of continuity of the nerve fibers (endoneurium affected)
IV. Loss of continuity of the fascicles (perineurium affected)
V. Loss of continuity of the nerve itself

This classification can be compared to Seddon's classification: grade I injuries correspond to neurapraxia, grade II injuries to axonotmesis, and grades III, IV, and V injuries are variations in severity of neurotmesis.

CHANGES IN THE NERVE FOLLOWING INJURY AND NEUROMA FORMATION

With neurapraxia, recovery usually takes place within 6 weeks. This likely represents a conduction block, perhaps associated with demyelinization with return of function. Very little histologic material of this type of injury is available for study.

In more severe injuries with axonotmesis and neurotmesis and actual severance of the nerve, the changes can be discussed as they apply in the proximal and distal segments.[11]

Proximal segment

The parent cell, either in the anterior horn of the spinal cord or in the posterior root ganglia, shows changes in the cell body, the nucleus, and the

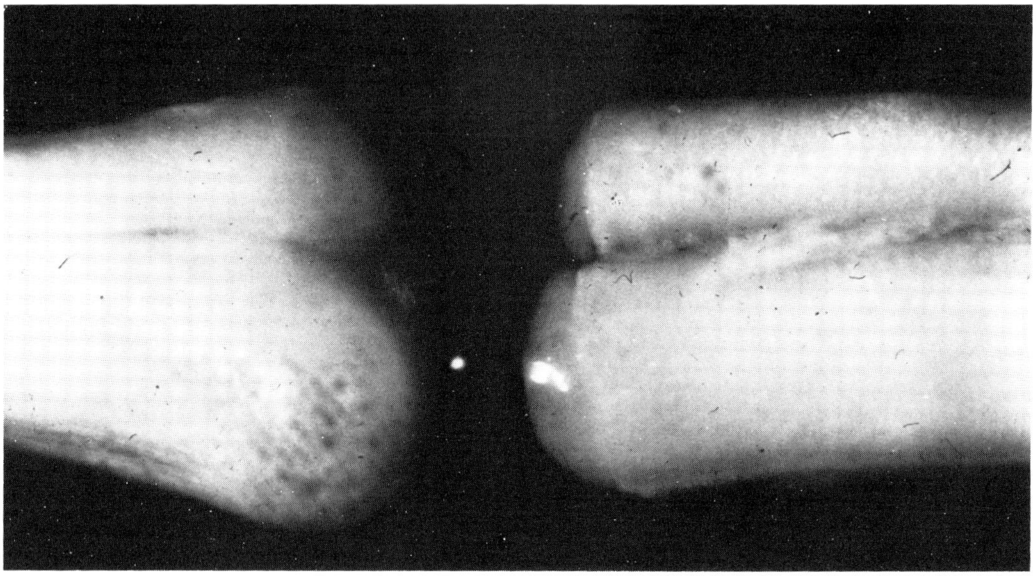

Fig. 12-4. Cut nerve that was not repaired for 3 weeks. Note bulbous proximal neuroma (left) and more symmetric distal end (right).

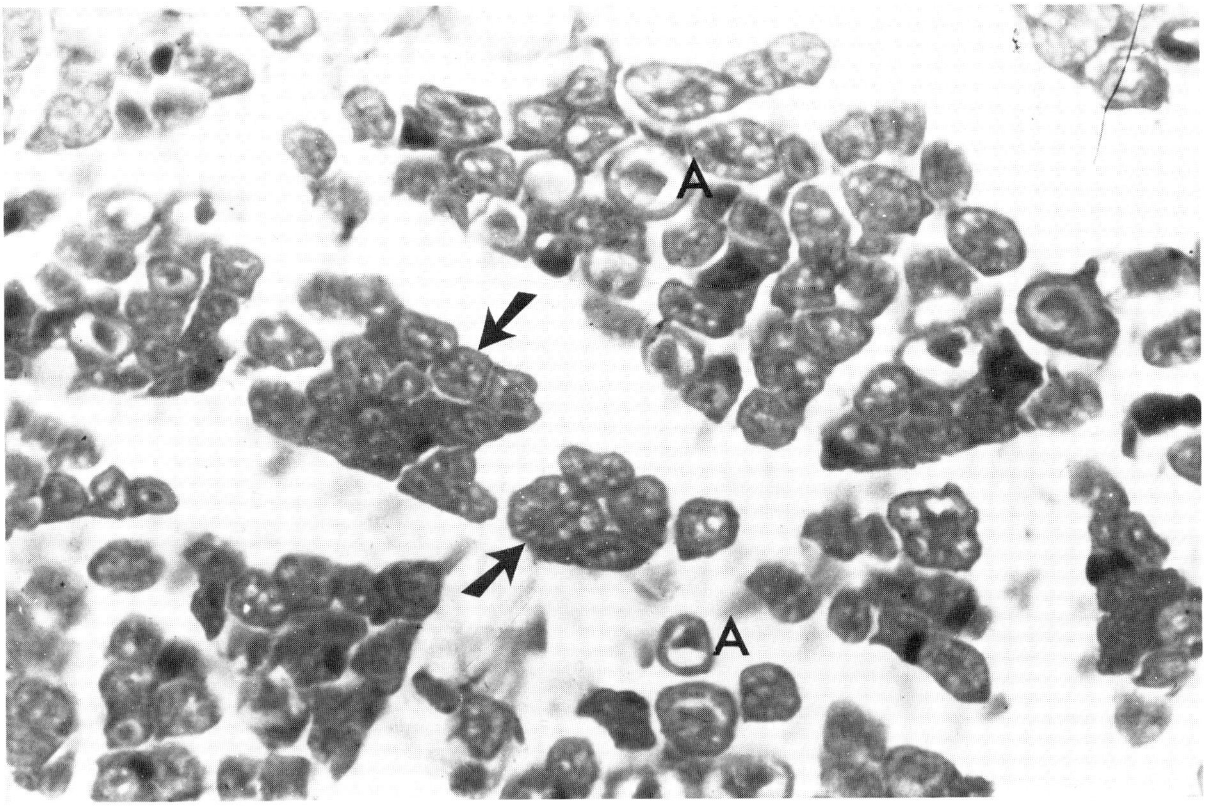

Fig. 12-5. Histologic section of distal end after 3 weeks (H & E stain). Only a few axonal fragments remain, *A*, while most endoneurial tubes are filled with fatty vacuoles *(arrows)*.

nucleolus. The cells swell, the Golgi apparatus fragments, and the Nissl granules may dissolve. The fiber itself degenerates retrograde to the next intact node of Ranvier. Within a few days, fibroblasts and Schwann cells proliferate, forming a bulbous proximal neuroma (Fig. 12-4).

Distal segment

Following nerve severance, changes are clearly evident in the axon within 24 hours. In the early stages, there is swelling followed by fragmentation of the neurofibrils and separation of the myelin sheath. All traces of the axon disappear by the second or third week. The myelin sheath fragments into droplets, and the Schwann cells show proliferation within 48 hours. The myelin fragments, axonal remnants, and debris are removed in the process of phagocytosis by either the Schwann cells or by macrophages; this process is called wallerian degeneration. All that survives is a syncytial strand of cells, reinforced by the endoneurial connective tissue sheath (Fig. 12-5).

RECOVERY IN INJURED NERVES

When the injured nerves recover, the process is reversed with return of the nerve cell to normal size and shape with accumulation of nucleoproteins into the pattern of Nissl bodies. At the cut end, the axons branch and begin to grow distally.[12] This is under the influence of the cellular changes and axoplasmic flow. The regenerating axons will branch and grow distally and find their way into intact endoneurial tubes.[12] Usually all other branches will resorb if one portion of the axon enters an intact distal tube. A short delay will exist at the cut end, and again this will be prolonged if scar is present.

With accurately repaired nerves, when each proximal fascicle is carefully sutured to its corresponding distal end the flow should continue to proliferate distally down the nerve and give satisfactory recovery. As the axon grows distally, a myelin layer between the Schwann cell and axon reappears, and this also progresses distally. Eventually the regenerated nerve closely resembles the anatomy seen before injury. However, if the nerve ends

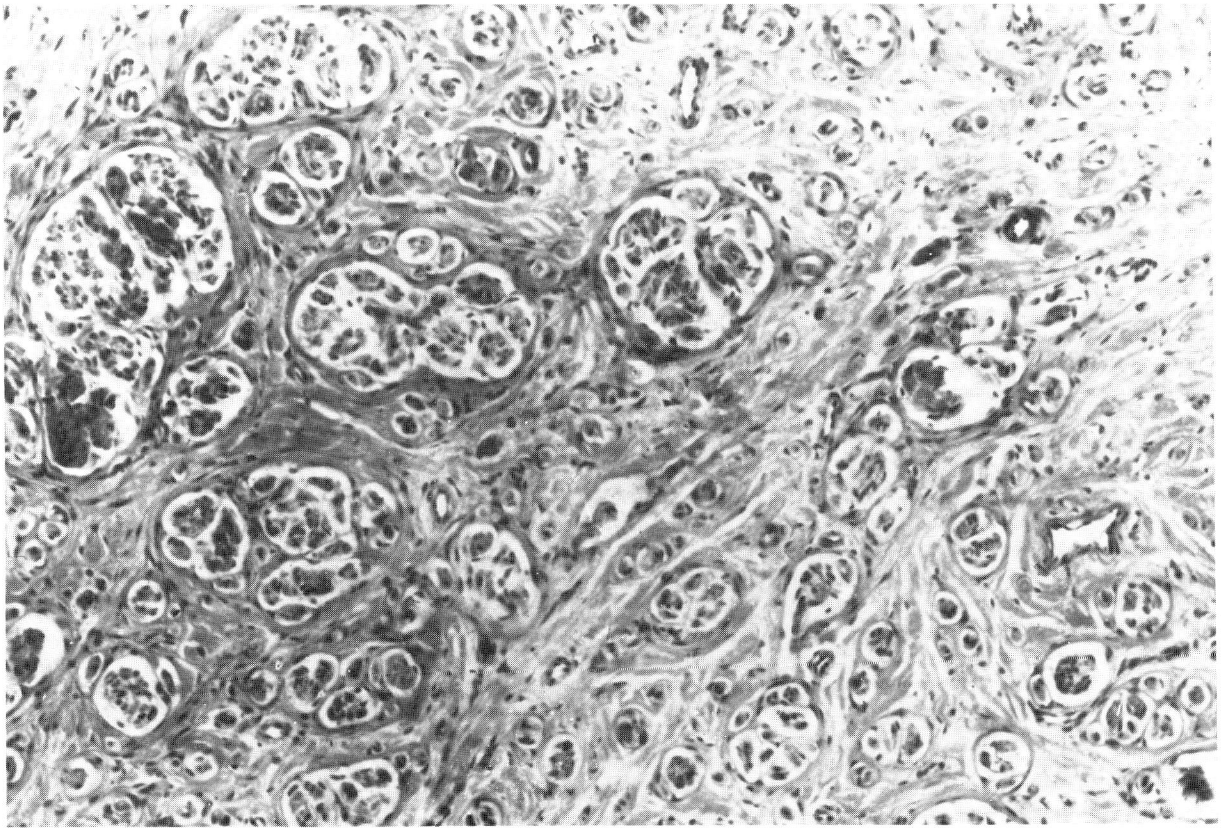

Fig. 12-6. Neuroma. Haphazard arrangement of nervous elements admixed with fibrous tissue.

are allowed to separate as naturally occurs with elastic recoil, or at an amputation site, then the proximal nerve budding and growth will be unsatisfied and will grow, proliferate, and branch into all surrounding tissue. Depending on the type of injury, a terminal neuroma or a neuroma in continuity, either partial or complete, will be formed.

TERMINAL OR STUMP NEUROMAS

Neuromas form at the proximal cut end of a severed nerve or at the ends of divided nerves at amputation sites. The unsatisfied axonal fibers intermingle in a haphazard fashion with proliferating fibroblasts, Schwann cells and collagen fibers, leading to a bulbous mass of disorganized scar (Figs. 12-6 and 12-7). The neuroma may become attached to surrounding tissue such as bone, tendon, or skin, or it might become fixed to adjacent scar. A certain percentage of neuromas become painful, and others might show reflex sympathetic dystrophic changes. This pain mechanism is difficult to explain, but there is a great patient specificity as some patients show various gradations of pain while others remain completely asymptomatic. The pain might be described as burning, sharp, or aching, but usually a trigger area can be identified, which is the central focus for the pain stimulus.

Prevention

Careful surgical management of the amputation stump or severed nerve will decrease the common occurrence of neuromas. Dissection and freeing of the severed nerve end and then allowing it to retract into healthy tissue is probably the most successful manner of reducing the chances of neuroma formation. Methods such as crushing, coagulation, injection of chemicals, or ligation of the nerve end likely add very little in prevention.

Treatment

Local: massage, percussion tapping, and use of the part will often help in the alleviation of symptoms.

Release of scar: a careful neurolysis with freeing of the nerve from adherent scar and surrounding structures, allowing proximal retraction, will give relief in well over 60% of cases.

Nerve capping: various materials have been used

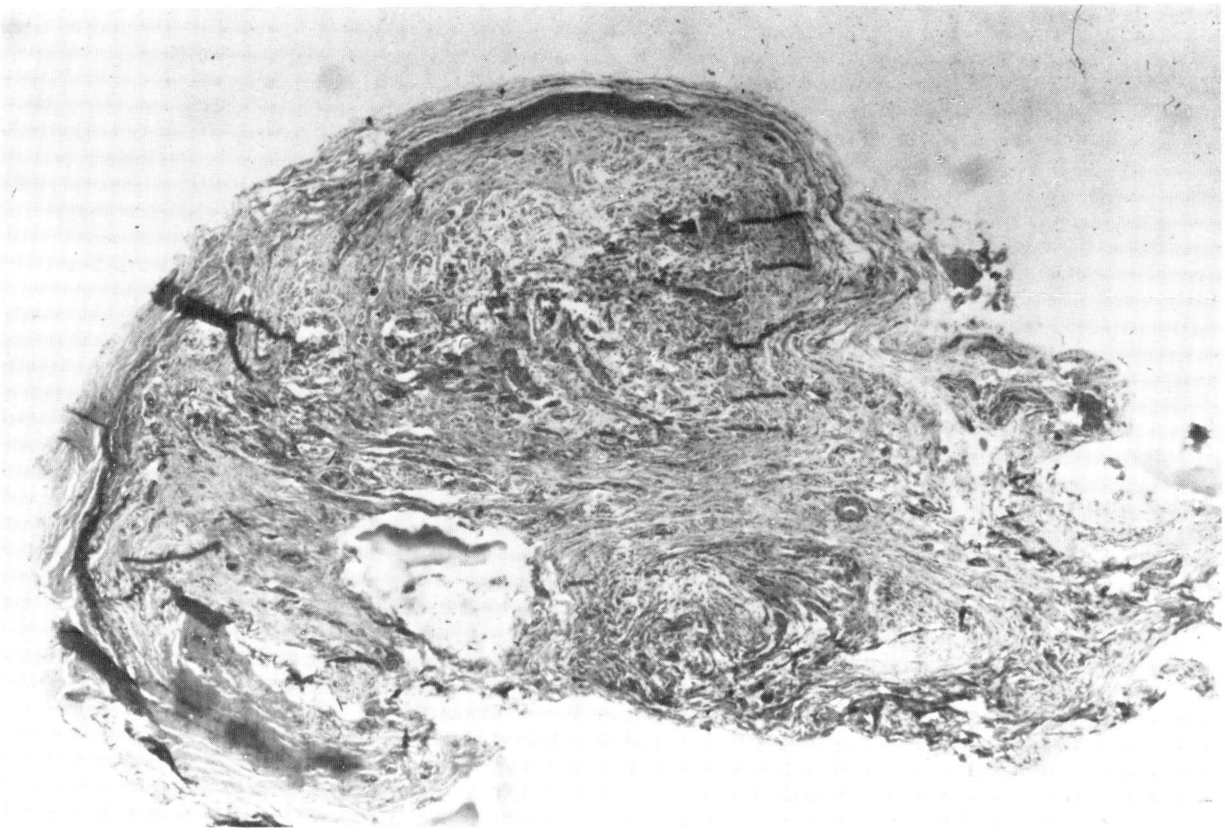

Fig. 12-7. Stump neuroma under lower magnification, showing similar structure as in Fig. 12-6.

in the past in an attempt to prevent recurrence of neuromas and to wall them off from surrounding tissues. Millipore was used by Campbell and associates[1] and Micropore by Freeman and associates[5,6] for nerve injuries in continuity. Gold foil and tantalum[21] have been used in the past. More recently, Tauras and Frackelton,[17] Frackelton and associates,[4] and Swanson and associates[16] have reported on the use of silicone caps to allow epineurial healing over the severed perineurial tubes and hopefully to decrease the chances of painful neuroma formation. This method has been successful in about 70% of reported cases. The nerve is dissected free from all adjacent scar, and the epineurium is brought over the ends of the fascicles and passed into the silicone cap and anchored (Fig. 12-8). This is shown schematically in Fig. 12-9, experimentally in a rat in Fig. 12-10, and in a patient with stump neuroma following partial amputation of the middle finger in Fig. 12-11.

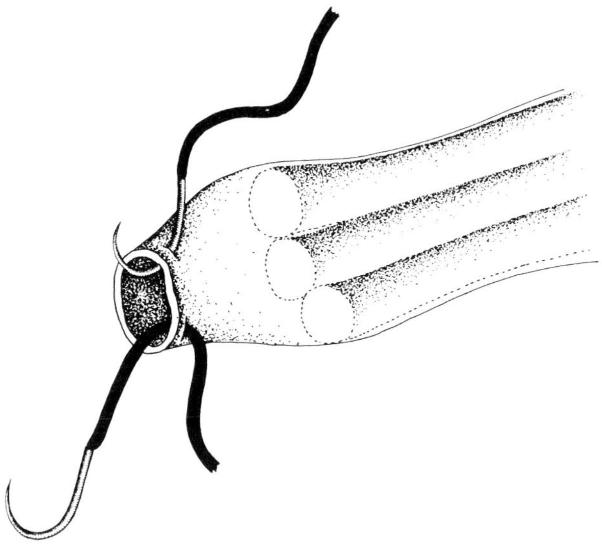

Fig. 12-8. Epineurial suture placed, which will be passed into silicone cap.

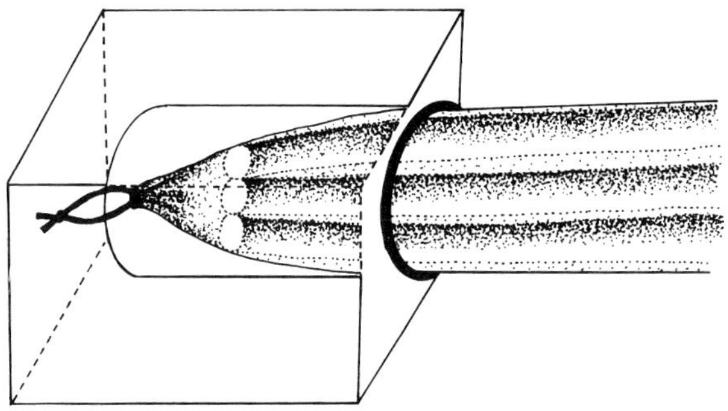

Fig. 12-9. Nerve brought into silicone cap and epineurial suture passed through cap (silicone cap may be round, square, or rectangular).

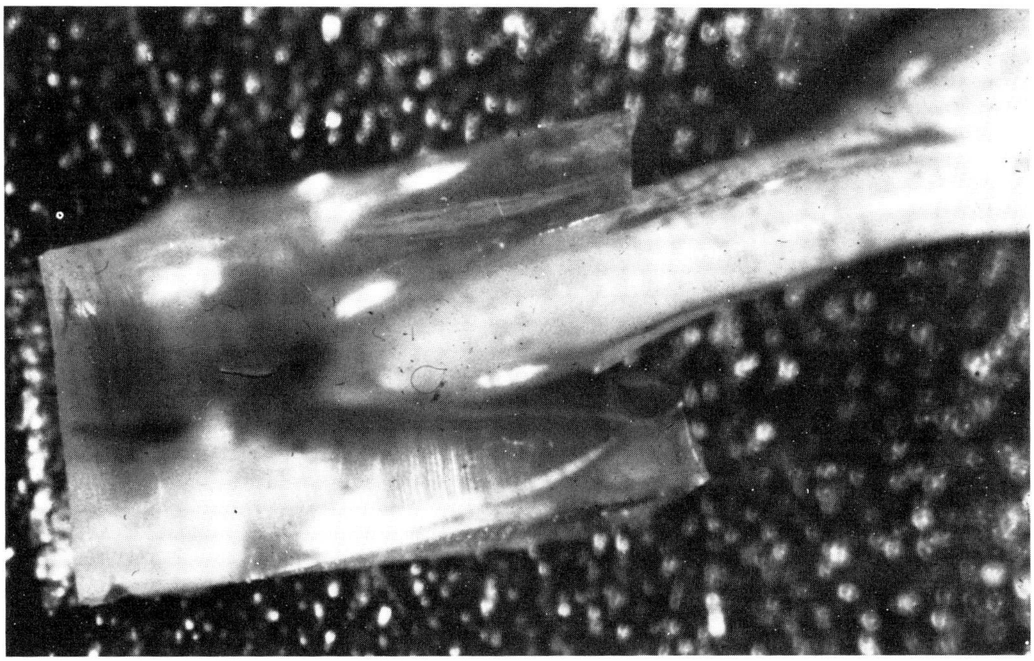

Fig. 12-10. Rat model, showing cut nerve in silicone cap.

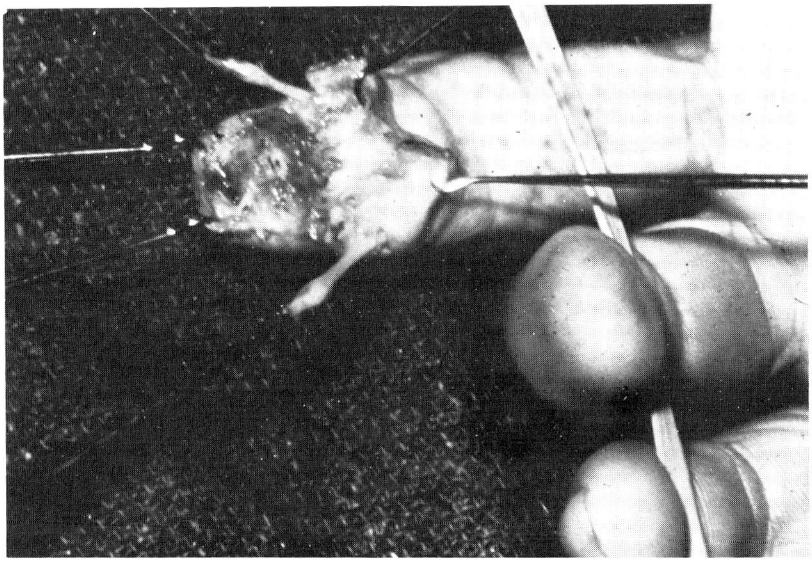

Fig. 12-11. Bilateral digital nerve neuromas in preparation for silicone capping.

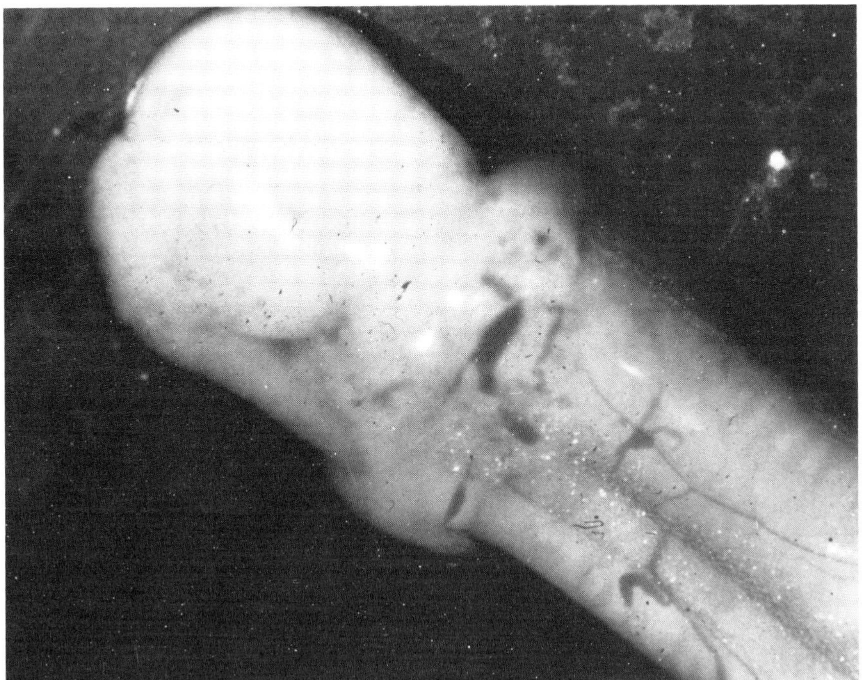

Fig. 12-12. Stump neuroma with epineurium dissected proximally and obvious coning.

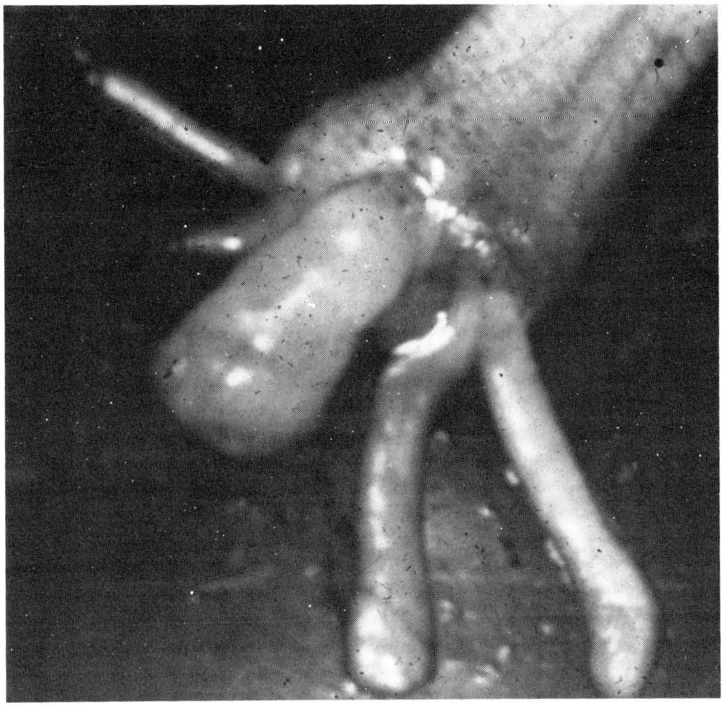

Fig. 12-13. Separate fasicles dissected free. These will be excised, allowing epineurium to be brought distally.

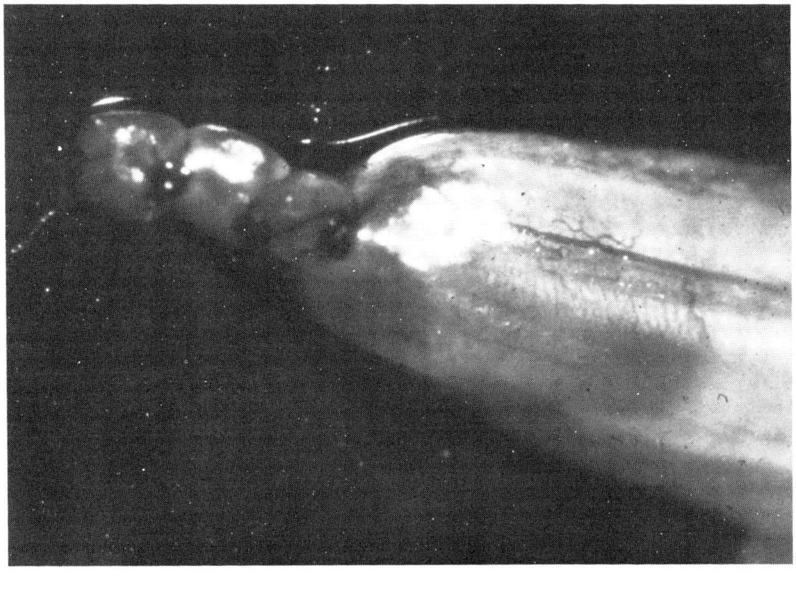

Fig. 12-14. Double-suture ligation of epineurium after funiculectomy.

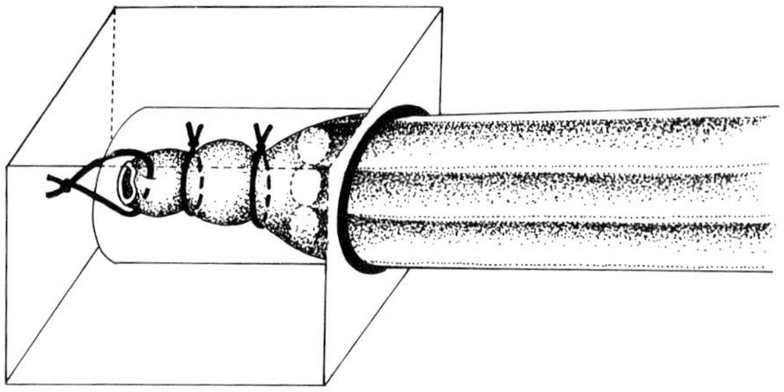

Fig. 12-15. Combination of capping and funiculectomy techniques.

Funiculectomy and epineurial sleeves: Chapple[2] reported on epineurial sleeves in 1918. More recently, Tupper[20] reported on the combination of epineurial sleeves after funiculectomy and compared these with treatment using silicone caps. He reviewed 172 patients with 348 painful neuromas. Excisional neurectomy alone was successful in 65% of patients, and silicone caps did not improve the results. Funicular resection with epineurial ligation in 45 patients gave as good results as excisional neurectomies. This method is illustrated in Figs. 12-12 to 12-14 to indicate ligation of the epineurial sleeve over the shortened fascicles after adequate dissection under microscopic control.

In the management of stump neuromas, great importance should be placed on adequate freeing of the nerves from surrounding structures, excision of scar, shortening of the nerve, and replacement in healthy tissues. Adjunctive procedures such as capping with silicone or funiculectomy and epineurial sleeves should likely be reserved for treatment of recurrent neuromas. Perhaps a combination of both capping with funiculectomy and epineural sleeves could be considered for difficult problems (Fig.12-15).

NEUROMAS IN CONTINUITY

A neuroma in continuity might indicate partial or complete severance of the nerve. Sunderland[15] and Spencer and associates[14] have demonstrated the importance of the perineurium. If the perineurium is violated, the neurons will escape, causing a

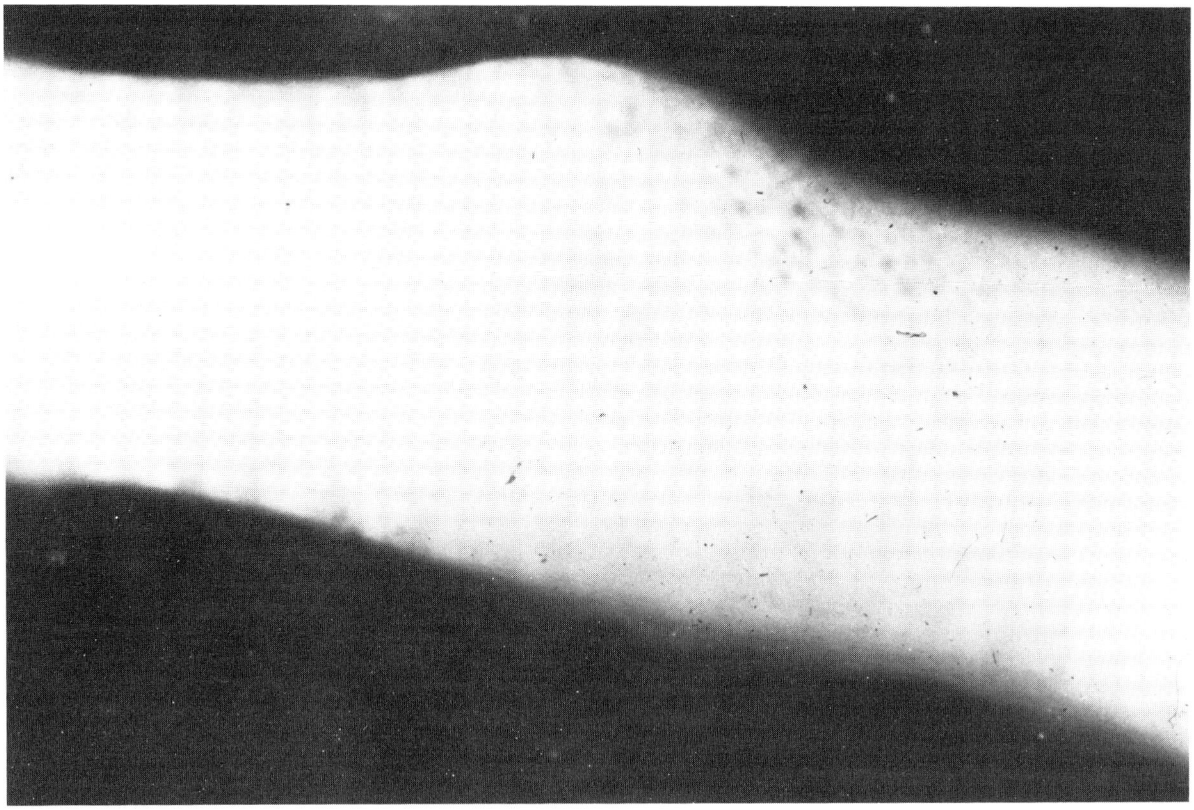

Fig. 12-16. Small lateral swelling in nerve after longitudinal incision through perineurium.

bulge at the periphery of the nerve (Figs. 12-16 and 12-17). Although it has never been recorded, this might occur with injudicious intraneural neurolysis for nerve compression injuries and compound the problem. Similar changes might occur in other neuromas.[3,7] Surgical exploration of the neuroma in continuity is often difficult, and it may be impossible to discern, either by gross inspection or by using microsurgical magnification, whether a nerve is completely severed or only partially damaged. With this dilemma, it is often impossible to state which part of the nerve requires resection and repair and which part can be left to regenerate spontaneously.

In recent years, with use of fascicular dissection and electrophysiologic recording techniques under operating room microscopic magnification, it has been possible to separate the injured portion of the nerve into the partially and completely damaged portions.[22] If the fascicles are not in continuity and are separated with scar tissue alone, then resection and nerve repair or nerve grafting is obviously required. However, if the fascicles are damaged but obviously in continuity, then following dissection and with electrophysiologic techniques an intraoperative diagnosis can be made to assist in the management of individual problems.[22] Kline and associates[8,9] performed whole nerve recordings in the operating room and studied the compound action potential with amplitude and conduction velocity. This method determines if there is conduction through the entire injured nerve, but more recently with fascicular recordings[18] it has become possible to divide the problem into smaller individual segments of the nerve, preventing unnecessary resection. With this method of electrophysiologic fascicular recordings the damaged portion can be separated from the remaining nerve, and appropriate measures such as fascicular repair, fascicular nerve graft, or neurolysis can be performed. Two cases are described to indicate the application of this method in diagnosis.*

*The peripheral nerve recordings in the two cases were done by Dr. Julia K. Terzis with technical advice from Dr. Robert K. Dykes.

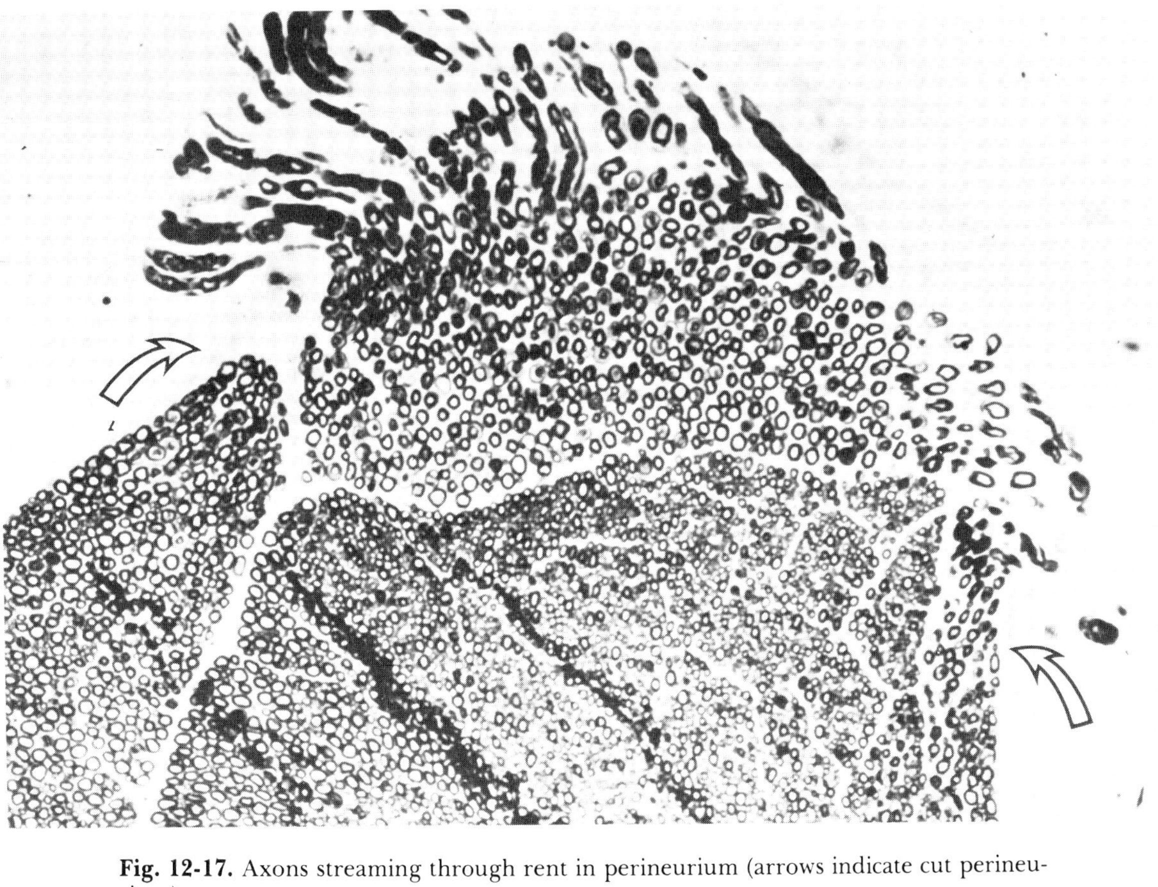

Fig. 12-17. Axons streaming through rent in perineurium (arrows indicate cut perineurium).

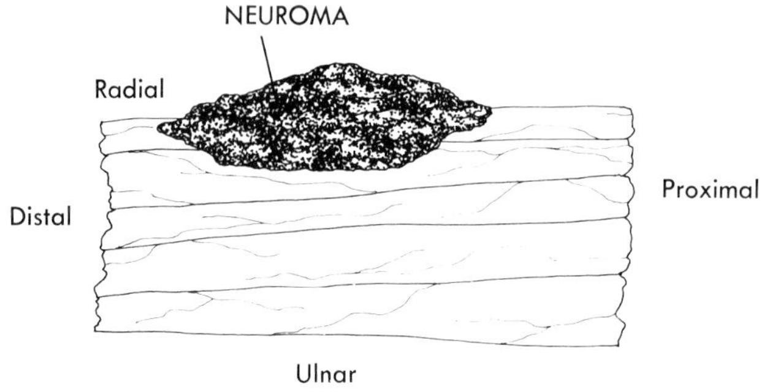

Fig. 12-18. Neuroma in continuity situated over radial aspect of median nerve.

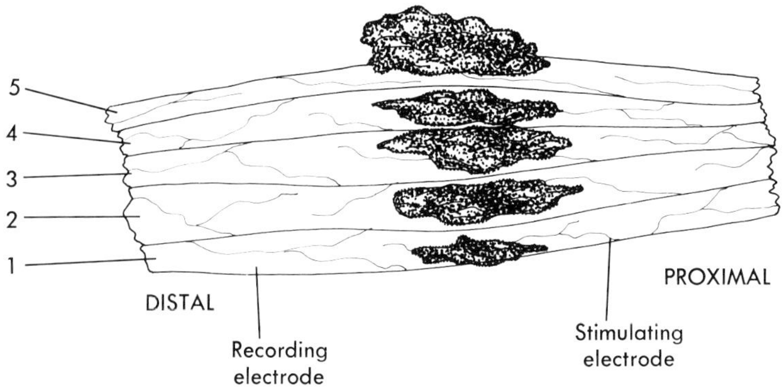

Fig. 12-19. Five fascicles involved in neuroma.

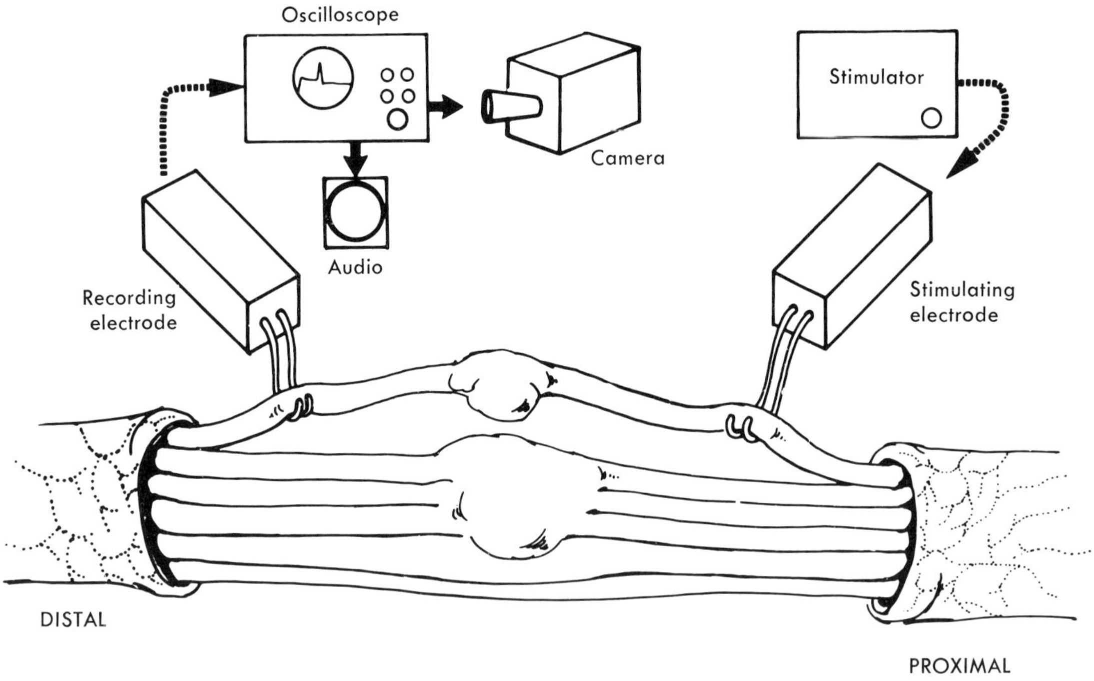

Fig. 12-20. Electrophysiologic recording from involved fascicle.

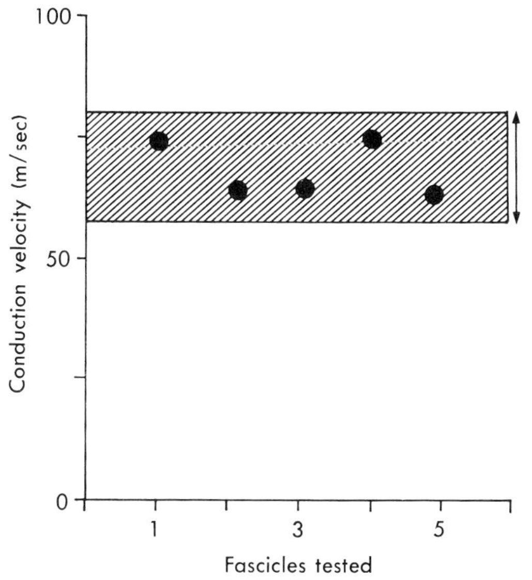

Fig. 12-21. Graph indicating conduction velocities of five fascicles, all within normal range.

Case 1. A 35-year-old man presented with a painful neuroma at the wrist level following an injury with broken glass 2 months prior to his admission. He had hypoesthesia over the thumb and index finger, and sensory testing revealed decreased sensibility to light, touch, and pinprick. Pseudomotor activity was minimal, and his two-point discrimination over the involved digits was 8 mm.

Exploration of the median nerve revealed a neuroma in continuity situated over the radial aspect (Fig. 12-18). Further dissection under the operating microscope revealed that five fascicles were involved in the neuroma, and each was tested individually by electrophysiologic techniques for conduction across the damaged area (Figs. 12-19 and 12-20). A recording from a normal fascicle served as the control. The resulting conduction velocities were all within normal range (Fig. 12-21). The loss of amplitude of the evoked responses of each fascicle compared to the control ranged from 25% to 75%. An intraneural neurolysis only was performed, and no resection of the neuroma was necessary. One year later, the patient was free of pain, and he stated that his hand felt normal. Two-point discrimination ranged from 4 to 5 mm (his normal two-point discrimination was 3 mm).

Case 2. A 22-year-old man presented with a 2-year history of a severed median nerve at the right wrist (Fig. 12-22). Initial repair was performed at another institution, and he showed recovery of protective sensation only over the involved median nerve distribution. The thenar muscles were atrophied, and he had absent opposition. His two-point discrimination was greater than 15 mm. On exploration, a large neuroma in continuity of the median

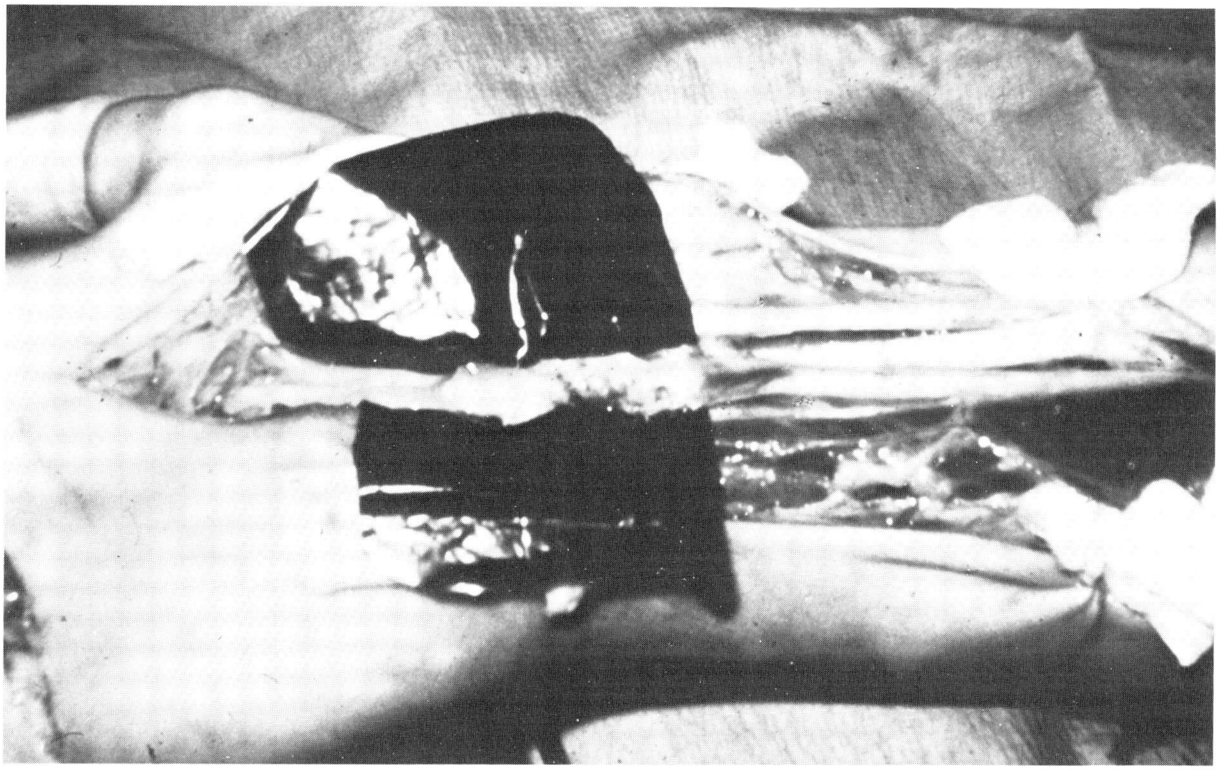

Fig. 12-22. Dissection of severed median nerve, right wrist.

nerve was found 1 inch above the wrist. Marked scarring was present, and following dissection under the operating microscope the major portion of the nerve was found to be involved in the neuroma. Only two fascicles could be dissected free from the involved mass (Fig. 12-23). A whole nerve recording was performed and action potentials were negative. The two small fascicles were then tested separately, and a low-amplitude action potential was recorded indicating the usefulness of this fascicular recording in contrast to whole nerve testing. The level of resection was then determined by nerve recordings, and it was necessary to extend this level 6 cm proximal to the area of neuroma in order to obtain a normal electrophysiologic response (Fig. 12-24). The change in progression proximally is indicated by a 100% drop-off in conduction at the neuroma with increasing improvement in amplitude as one progresses proximally from the neuroma (Fig. 12-25). This electrophysiologic diagnosis indicated that a normal appearing nerve in cross section does not necessarily respond normally to electric stimuli. A sural nerve graft was then used to fill the 7 cm deficit, and five fascicles were used in the graft (Fig. 12-26). At 3 months postoperatively, the patient showed an advanced Tinel sign in the midpalmar area, but it is too early to assess his final result.

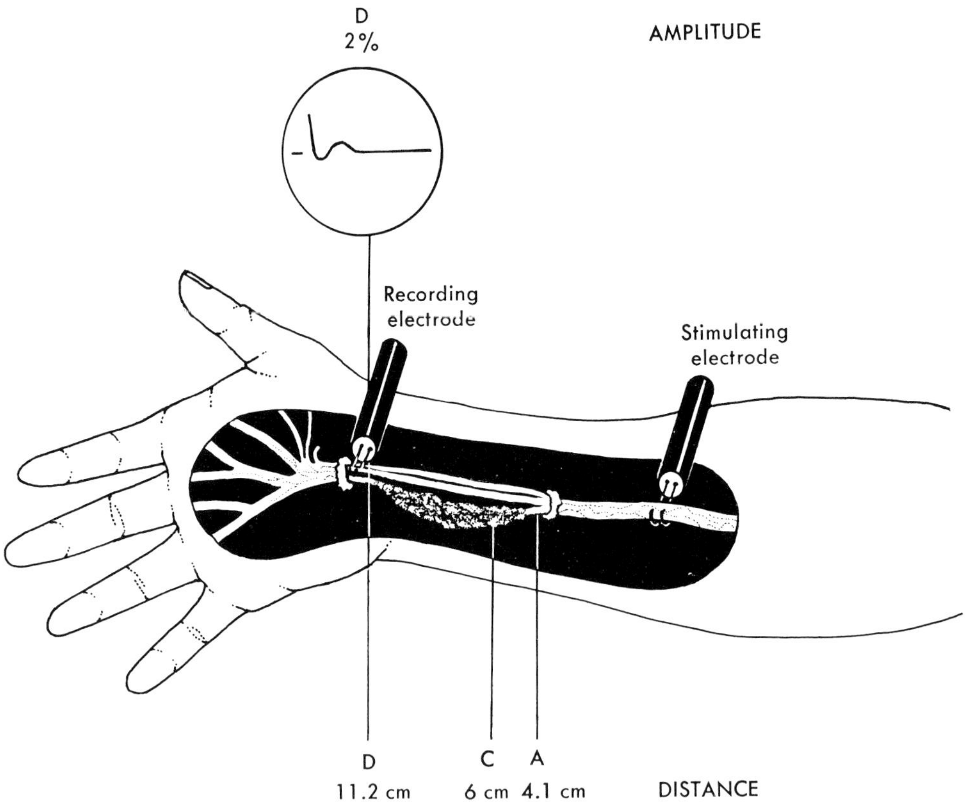

Fig. 12-23. Recording from two small intact fascicles, showing only 2% response in amplitude.

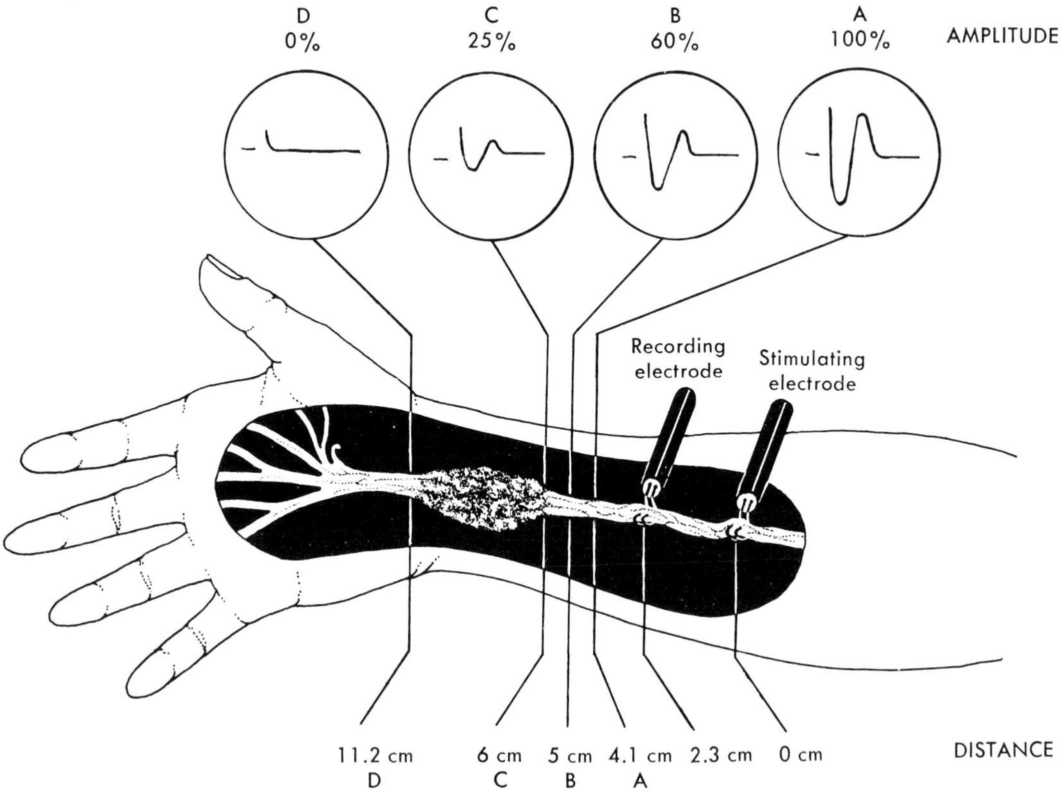

Fig. 12-24. Results of electrophysiologic recordings. **A,** Amplitude of 100% at 4.1 cm from proximal recording electrode (1.9 cm proximal to neuroma). **B,** Amplitude of 60% at 5 cm. **C,** Only 25% amplitude at 6 cm from proximal electrode (just proximal to neuroma). **D,** No response with full nerve recording.

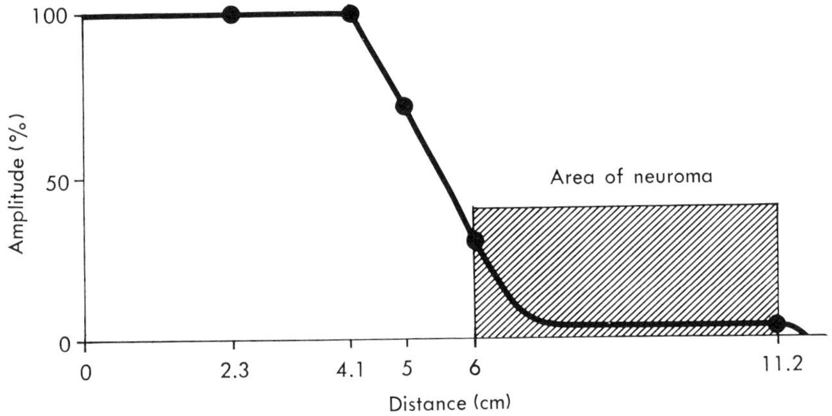

Fig. 12-25. Graph showing percentage amplitude at different distances (same as Fig. 12-24) from neuroma.

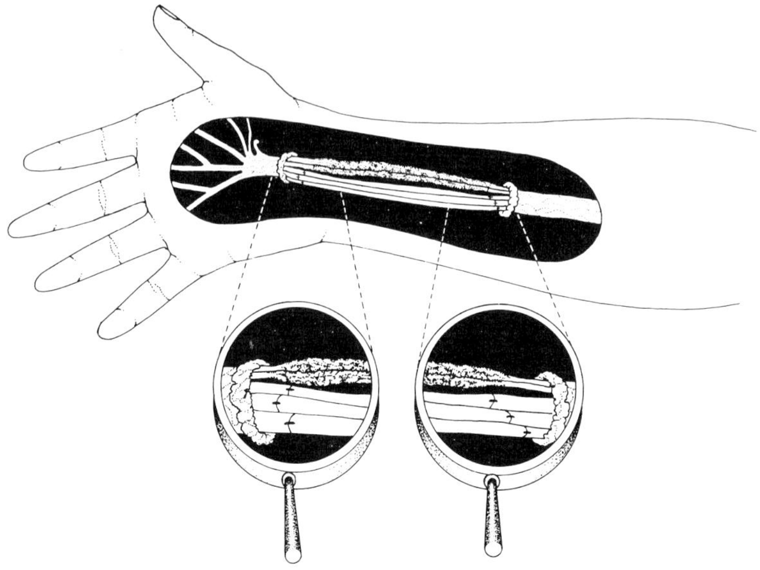

Fig. 12-26. Diagram showing sural nerve grafts in place and two small fascicles left intact on radial aspect.

SUMMARY

Neuromas continue to be a problem in clinical practice. Prevention is the key in stump or terminal neuromas, but in established cases, careful dissection is required with excision of scar tissue, thus allowing the nerve end to retract into normal surroundings. Additional procedures with capping or funiculectomy and epineurial sleeves are useful in recurrent cases.

Neuromas in continuity require careful diagnosis, dissection, and repair. In selected cases, electrophysiologic recordings and assessment in the operating room are of assistance in determining an accurate diagnosis so that proper treatment methods can be performed.

ACKNOWLEDGMENT

I would like to express my appreciation to Drs. Julia K. Terzis and Robert K. Dykes for their assistance in the clinical management of the reported cases.

REFERENCES

1. Campbell, J. G., Bassett, C. A. L., and Bohler, J.: Frozen irradiated homografts shielded with microfilter sheaths in peripheral nerve surgery, J. Trauma **3:**303-311, 1963.
2. Chapple, W. A.: Re-amputation, Br. Med. J. **2:**242, 1917.
3. Dobyns, J. H., O'Brien, E. T., Linscheid, R. L., and Farrow, G. M.: Bowler's thumb: diagnosis and treatment, J. Bone Joint Surg. [Am.] **54:**751-755, 1972.
4. Frackelton, W. H., Teasley, J. L. and Tauras, A.: Neuromas in the hand treated by nerve transposition and silicone capping. In Proceedings of the American Society for Surgery of the Hand, J. Bone Joint Surg. [Am.] **53:**813, 1971.
5. Freeman, B. S.: Adhesive neural anastomoses, Plast. Reconstr. Surg. **35:**167-176, 1965.
6. Freeman, B. S., Perry, J., and Brown, D.: Experimental study of adhesive surgical tape for nerve anastomosis, Plast. Reconstr. Surg. **43:**174-179, 1969.
7. Howell, A. E., and Leach, R. E.: Bowler's thumb: perineural fibrosis of the digital nerve, J. Bone Joint Surg. [Am.] **52:**379-381, 1970.
8. Kline, D. G., Hackett, E.R., and May, P. R.: Evaluation of nerve injuries by evoked potentials and electromyography, J. Neurosurg. **31:**128, 1969.
9. Kline, D. G., and Nulsen, F. E.: The neuroma in continuity: its preoperative and operative management, Surg. Clin. North Am. **52:**1189, 1972.
10. Lundborg, G.: Structure and function of the intraneural microvessels as related to trauma, edema formation and nerve function, J. Bone Joint Surg. [Am.] **57:**938-948, 1975.
11. Omer, G. E.: Assessment of peripheral nerve injuries, In Cramer, L., and Chase, R., editors: Symposium of the hand, St. Louis, 1971, The C. V. Mosby Co.
12. Orgel, M., Aguayo, A., and Williams, H. B.: Nerve regeneration in skin grafts, J. Anat. **111:**121, 1972.
13. Seddon, H.: Surgical disorders of the peripheral nerves, Churchill, Livingstone, Edinburgh, 1972.
14. Spencer, P. S., Weinberg, H. J., et al.: The perineurial window—a new model of focal demyelination and remyelination, Brain Res. **96:**323, 1975.

15. Sunderland, S.: Nerves and nerve injuries, Baltimore, 1968, The Williams and Wilkins Company.
16. Swanson, A. B., Boeve, N. R., and Lumsden, R. M.: The prevention and treatment of amputation neuromata by silicone capping, J. Hand Surg. **2:**70-78, 1977.
17. Tauras, A. P., and Frackelton, W. H: Silicone capping of nerve stumps in the problem of painful neuromas, Surg. Forum, **18:**504, 1967.
18. Terzis, J., and Williams, H. B.: Functional aspects of reinnervation of skin grafts, Surg. Forum **25:**518, 1974.
19. Thomas, P. K.: The connective tissue of peripheral nerve, an electron microscope study, J. Anat. **97:**35, 1963.
20. Tupper, J. W.: Treatment of painful neuromas of sensory nerves in the hand: a comparison of traditional and newer methods, J. Hand Surg, **1:**144-151, 1976.
21. White, J. C., and Hamlim, H.: New uses of tantalum in nerve suture, control of neuroma formation, J. Neurosurg, **2:**402, 1945.
22. Williams, H. B., and Terzis, J.: Single fascicular recordings: an intraoperative diagnostic tool for the management of peripheral nerve lesions, Plast. Reconstr. Surg. **57:**562, 1976.

Chapter 13

The reflex sympathetic dystrophies and other pain syndromes

George E. Omer

PAIN

Pain can be totally incapacitating following many nerve injuries. Free nerve endings serve as the receptor structures for pain, and pain can arise from all stimuli that produce sensation: mechanical, electrical, thermal, or chemical. Pain has many conscious levels and is described in many ways: aching, burning, cutting, dull, evil, gnawing, hard, itchy, knifelike, lightning, mean, penetrating, quick, radiating, shooting, tearing, ugly, or vicious. These and many other words attempt to describe the intensity, temporal length, spatial dimension, relationship with other sensory modalities such as temperature or pressure, or the emotional response that is associated with pain.

Cutaneous pain has a temporal pattern related to axon diameter.[6] First pain is conducted by larger diameter A axons (δ group). It is brief, pricking, sharp, relatively localized in character, and elicits a prompt withdrawal reaction. Second or delayed pain is related to the slow-conducting smaller diameter unmyelinated C axons and is persistent, spreading, and burning in character. In contrast, pain from deep tissues has no obvious time pattern and is aching and dull. Periosteal tissues are more sensitive than muscle, but deep pain is difficult to localize. Deep pain is prolonged and enforces immobilization of the affected extremity. Deep pain produces reflex complications such as sweating, bradycardia, hypotension, and nausea.

Stimulation of a peripheral sensory axon evokes impulses that are transmitted to three spinal cord systems: the substantia gelatinosa in the dorsal horn, the dorsal column tracts that project directly to the brain, and the first central transmission cells in the dorsal horn that project toward the anterolateral tracts. Within the substantia gelatinosa are many axon branches and short tracts, allowing maximum interaction between the A and C axons. Similar interaction may occur at successive synapses at any level of the central nervous system. The thalamus, limbic system, hypothalamus, brain stem reticular formation, parietal cortex, and frontal cortex are all involved in pain perception. Other brain areas are involved in the motor and automatic response in the behavior sequence. A chronic pain syndrome is an ongoing process of perception and response influenced by psychologic factors, such as attention or emotion.

The spinal cord is continuously bombarded by incoming sensory and outgoing sympathetic impulses, even without apparent stimulation. The base level of sensory activity is transmitted predominantly by the small unmyelinated C axons, which tend to be tonically active and adapt slowly. Melzak and Wall[13] have proposed an "interacting gate control system" with spatial and temporal summation that accounts for the hyperalgesia, spontaneous and referred or spreading pain, and the delayed pain after stimulation that is characteristic of reflex sympathetic dystrophy. Large myelinated A axons carry precise tactile impulses to the dorsal column tracts and also transmit impulses into the first central transmission neurons (T cells) in the dorsal horn. Dorsal column impulses trigger the motor responses and central efferent impulses to influence afferent information still arriving over slower conducting axons. Small unmyelinated C axons carry pain, temperature, and crude touch impulses totally into the T cells. The T cells are presumed to signal the conscious recognition of pain. Sustained activity in these afferent impulses gives rise to feedback effects mediated by the "gating cells" of the substantia gelantinosa, which exert presynaptic inhibition on both the large myelinated and small unmyelinated sensory axons. It is hypothesized that prolonged sensory activity or disproportionate numbers of small unmyelinated axons, as happen during regeneration of neurons following a traumatic peripheral nerve trunk injury, would inhibit the gating cells and thus increase pain perception. This would also permit the sympathetic outflow to be unchecked by presynaptic inhibition. In contrast, activity in the large myelinated axons excites the gating cells and thus decreases summation and pain perception. Treatment techniques utilizing physical medicine procedures or electric stimulation for amplification of the inhibitory mechanisms are based on these considerations.

The hypothesis that an external high-velocity physical injury can produce a breakdown of normal biophysical insulation in a nerve trunk with resulting abnormal cross stimulation between sympathetic and sensory axons has clinical support,[10] and motor axon interaction with sensory axons has been demonstrated in the laboratory.[7] Impulses are constantly passing peripherally in sympathetic axons and could initiate impulses at the site of injury that might pass either centrally or peripherally in the sensory axons. The centrally directed impulses (orthodromic) would be interpreted directly as pain, and the peripheral impulses (antidromic) might also cause pain by chemical reaction. Electric stimulation of the distal end of a divided peripheral nerve trunk causes the release of a relatively stable vasodilator substance named neurokinin.[3] Neurokinin can be obtained also be perfusion of the tissues supplied by the stimulated peripheral nerve, and when it is injected into the skin elsewhere, it causes burning pain. Treatment techniques tnat interrupt the appropriate sympathetic axons at any level are based on these considerations.

The innervated vessels serving thermoregulation of the body are irritated by a pain response and convert the corresponding vascular area into a "target zone."[16] Signs of target zone irritation are vasomotor changes such as abnormal vasoconstriction or dilation that show a vascular rather than a dermatome pattern, with accompanying trophic changes and pain. The sympathetic ganglion chain, with extensive synapses to all levels of the nervous system, may participate in these alterations, and the abnormal vasomotor changes may spread in the homolateral side of the sympathetic system. This may account for the unpredictable spread of pain and the development of new "trigger zones" in chronic pain syndromes.

PAINFUL NEUROMA

A distorted quality of sensation, or altered sensibility, is a transient experience in almost all nerve injuries and may be related to the preponderance of unmyelinated fibers during the period of regeneration. Pain can be a prominent feature of the experience and may be related to neuroma formation, either a terminal bulb or an intraneural neuroma from compression. In a susceptible individual the established syndrome has these characteristics: (1) a high threshold to light touch with an increased distance for two-point discrimination, (2) a long latent period between stimulus and response, (3) the explosive appearance of a peculiarly unpleasant pain that is poorly localized, and radiates to a wide area, and outlasts the stimulus, and (4) vigorous protective movements by the patient.[25] A variety of terms have been used to describe the disagreeable pain: dysesthesia, hyperalgesia, hyerpathia, irritation, neurodynia, overresponse, painful neuroma, paresthesia, peripheral neuralgia, and wicked pain. Since transient distortion of sensibility is common after nerve injury, the surgeon should institute measures to prevent the development of an established or prolonged syndrome: (1) during surgery there should be meticulous approximation of sensory nerves, such as the superficial radial nerve, that have been divided accidently during elective surgery or disrupted by trauma and observed during debridement; (2) during the immediate posttrauma period, such as after reduction of a fracture-dislocation, there must be careful evaluation of extremity compression, and tests such as the two-point discrimination distance should be utilized at regular intervals; circular plaster casts must be removed, and surgical release of fascial sheaths performed when indicated; (3) the surgeon must initiate early active motion and functional activities for the patient; every patient who suppresses voluntary movement because it is painful should be placed on an enforced supervised program of active function; (4) the surgeon should unemotionally discuss with the patient the fact that some distorted sensibility with pain is to be expected as the usual course of events during the period of nerve regeneration; the pain should not be the basis for apprehension but the signal for increased voluntary activity.

A neuroma can become the trigger spot for prolonged spontaneous pain with narcotic addiction and emotional deterioration of a susceptible individual. Nonsurgical treatment methods have been local injections to relieve pain and sensory reeducation by percussion. Percutaneous injection of triamcinolone acetonide (Kenalog) about the neuroma after a cutaneous anesthetic block with 2% lidocaine hydrochloride (Xylocaine) has been reported to relieve the pain symptoms in 50% of patients after one injection and in 80% of patients after multiple injections.[20] It was surmised that softening the fibrous tissue about the neuroma was the basis for the relief of pain. Percussion or massage of painful neuromas has been a clinical procedure in military amputees since World War I. Controlled clinical studies[8] have indicated the technique is very useful in selected cases. Rubber mallets, mechanical vibrators, and ultrasonic treatments can be utilized to provide the repetitious percussion. Local anesthesia may be necessary over the area of trigger pain at the beginning of the treatment program; later the percussion or massage can be done without local anesthesia.

A variety of physical and chemical methods have been used during surgery to prevent the formation of a painful neuroma. Ligation of the proximal stump with silk, wire, fascia, or other suture materials has not been successful. The proximal nerve stump has been implanted under fascia or into muscle, bone, and veins, and even into its own proximal nerve trunk (neurocampsis).[22] The proximal stump has been capped with sheaths of glass, gold foil, tantalum, silver, Millipore, methyl methacrylate, and silicone. Initial clinical success was reported with all ensheathing materials, but all except silicone have been abandoned.[24,25] Electrocoagulation, freezing, steroids, or injection with phenol, alcohol, nitrogen mustard, tannic acid, gentian violet, and many other chemicals has not prevented painful neuromas. Snyder[21] has estimated that more than 150 physical and chemical methods have been used, but none have had consistent success.

The nerve trunk has been divided at one or more sites proximal to the terminal neuroma and resutured with an epineural technique. The rationale for proximal neurotomy is axon degeneration at several levels and a resulting inability to form the terminal neuroma. This is effective only if there is considerable length of nerve distal to the neurotomy.[12]

The best surgical approach for a painful neuroma is transfer of the entire neuroma and the proximal nerve stump to a new tissue bed where compression is unlikely and traction is minimal. The neuroma should be placed in an area of good circulation with a thick subcutaneous layer that is free of scar. Success has been reported in 82% of patients treated with this technique.[9] A repeat excisional neurectomy is indicated one time in those cases with continued pain.[22,25]

A painful neuroma in continuity can occur following contusion or compression of a peripheral nerve. The traumatic episode may be isolated, as in radial nerve compression from "Saturday night palsy" or the deep peroneal neuroma in continuity following a fracture of the proximal tibia. More often the trauma is repetitious, as in Morton metatarsalgia, bowler's thumb, or the cubital and carpal tunnel syndromes.[12] Often a nerve-ligament crossing is the point where the neuroma forms, such as the inguinal ligament and the lateral femoral cutaneous nerve in meralgia paresthetica. Surgery for a neuroma in continuity can be either neurolysis or excision of the neuroma. Meticulous intraneural neurolysis is helpful if the cause is repeated compression with retention of distal function, as in medial nerve pain from a carpal tunnel syndrome.[25] When there is significant paralysis distal to the lesion, it is best to excise the neuroma in continuity and suture the nerve trunk under minimal tension. The resection must be complete.

The best objective guide in selecting patients whose painful neuroma can be relieved by local surgery is a diagnostic nerve block. The local anesthetic can be injected about the neuroma or more proximal about the nerve trunk. The pain must be completely relieved. One should do a short series of nerve blocks, using a placebo of normal saline for one block to evaluate the patient's emotional reaction. Diagnostic blocks are also valuable in amputees with both a painful trigger point and an associated reflex sympathetic dystrophy.

If there is no relief from local surgery, an anterolateral cordotomy is indicated in the patient threatened with permanent dysfunction and narcotic addiction. However, White and Sweet[25] have found that postcordotomy analgesia cannot be expected to last longer than 6 months, with somewhat better results in those cases involving the lower extremity than in those cases involving the upper extremity. Rhizotomy, posterior column tractotomy, postcentral gyrectomy of the sensory cortex, and frontal leukotomy have all been ineffective for sustained relief of pain. Initial success has been reported after cingulectomy,[12] but evaluation of sustained relief of pain after this procedure is incomplete. Most of the surgical procedures for the central nervous system interrupt the spinothalamic tract, which projects pain to the ventroposterolateral nucleus of the thalamus and to the parietal cortex. The return of pain after surgery is related to the increased activity of polysynaptic systems (paleospinothalamic system or spinoreticulothalamic system) that are present in the spinal cord, and highly developed and widespread in the brain stem and thalamus. These polysynaptic systems conduct pain impulses.

REFLEX SYMPATHETIC DYSTROPHY

Pain, like all sensibility, is subjective, individual, and modified by degrees of attention, emotional stress, and the conditioning influence of past experience. Posttraumatic pain with functional impairment can vary in intensity from annoying to total disability. There is no direct relationship between the injury and the amount of pain that is experienced by the susceptible individual. Reflex sympathetic dystrophy usually develops in the patient with a low threshold of pain and a dependent personality. The pain syndrome often does not develop immediately but gradually dominates the clinical condition. A variety of clinical states have been described that demonstrate pain, abnormal vasomotor response, and dystrophy. Some examples include Raynaud disease, traumatic hard edema of Secretan (peritendinous fibrosis), painful phantom limb, shoulder-arm-hand syndrome, Sudeck atrophy, and Leriche posttraumatic pain syndrome (minor causalgia).

When a peripheral nerve is injured, the loss of vascular, sudomotor, pilomotor, and muscle tone controls will cause profound nutritional (trophic) changes. Lack of use and an inadequate blood supply will cause atrophy of subcutaneous tissue, skin, muscle, and bone, with production of inelastic fibrous tissue. The usual vascular response to trauma is vasoconstriction for a few hours and then vasodilation until the reparative process has been completed. In a susceptible individual the vasospastic reflex is severe and prolonged. It is postulated that an abnormal reflex arc is initiated from the peripheral pain stimulus through afferent sensory nerve roots, across the spinal cord and out the anterior horn, through the white rami to the sympathetic ganglion, where the impulses are passed through a synapse into a new efferent fiber, out of the gray rami, and back into the peripheral nerve as a motor fiber supplying sympathetic control to the peripheral blood vessels. Continuation of the painful stimuli causes this abnormal vasomotor reflex arc to become a vicious cycle. The vasospasm causes tissue anoxia and edema, and therefore more pain, which continues the abnormal cycle. The pallor of the first few days gives way to a deeper coloration, which may be either red or blue. The red hue indicates vasodilation of all vessels, while cyanosis indicates venospasm and pooling of blood in the smaller venules. In either case, there is decreased circulation and resulting anoxia. The extremity becomes, pale and cool with marked hyperhidrosis. Joint stiffness is produced by increased fibrosis secondary to tissue anoxia, poor nutrition, and extravascular protein. Osteoporosis is not visible by x-ray examination until the process has continued for 5 to 8 weeks. Even when the injury is adequately immobilized, the patient continues to have an exaggerated degree of pain, is anxious, and shows great concern over his condition. The pain often does not conform to the distribution of peripheral cutaneous nerves but instead is generalized or follows the course of major blood vessels. Tenderness and increased sensitivity to touch are the common objective findings.

There are two principles in a treatment program for reflex sympathetic dystrophy: (1) relief of the pain and (2) active use of the involved extremity.

In those patients with pain associated with Raynaud-like symptoms, it is important to measure digital blood flow. We follow Porter and associates'[17] method: the patient sits quietly for 30 minutes in a warm room (approximately 24 C). The digital pulp temperature is determined with an electronic telethermometer. The patient's hands are then immersed in an ice water mixture for 20 seconds, following which the hands are blotted dry on a towel, and the digital pulp temperature is measured for 45 minutes or until the temperature returns to the baseline value. Normal temperature recovery time is 10 minutes, with a range from 5 to 20 minutes. The digital temperature test can be supplemented with arteriography to differentiate arterial spasm from organic obstructive disease. The arteriovenous communications and the precapillary arterioles of the extremities are sympathetically innervated, and a variety of drugs that decrease sympathetic activity should be beneficial for the patient with painful Raynaud symptoms. A variety of drugs have been proposed, including the alpha-receptor blocking drugs tolazoline hydrochloride (Priscoline) and phenoxybenzamine hydrochloride (Dibenzyline), the beta-adrenergic–receptor blocking drug propranolol hydrochloride (Inderal), and the neuronal norepinephrine depletors reserpine (Serpasil), methyldopa (Aldoril), and guanethidine (Esimil). Griseofulvin (Grisactin) has also been used because it has a direct vasodilator action exclusive of sympathetic innervation. Porter and associates obtained excellent patient response with repeated brachial artery injections of reserpine (0.25 mg) at approximately 2- to 3-week intervals.[17] They also treated 23 patients with guanethidine, 10 mg daily, and then increased the level 10 mg each week until there was hypotension or symptomatic improvement. Two patients could not tolerate guanethidine even at the minimal dose of 10 mg daily because of hypotension and were changed to phenoxybenzamine, 10 mg daily. After an average follow-up of 12 months, 19 of the 23 patients had significant reduction in the frequency and severity of the Raynaud attacks. Similar results have been reported for propranolol hydrochloride in dosages of 40 mg, every 4 hours over a 3-month period.[19] Surgical sympathectomy has yielded only minimal improvement in patients with marked Raynaud-like symptoms.

Vitamin B_{12} has been reported to improve the burning paroxysmal pain. Verdan and Narakas [23] administer 10,000 IU by intramuscular injections, several times a day, to maximum dosage of 60,000 IU daily. When effective, the pain is reported to diminish after 2 or 3 days. The treatment is maintained with one or two injections per day for 1 or 2 weeks.

It is worthwhile to relieve the patient's anxiety during treatment. Trifluoperazine (Stelazine), 1 to 2 mg twice daily, is effective, or one can use diazepam (Valium) or chlordiazepoxide hydrochloride (Librium) in younger patients.[11] Salicylates should also be given to relieve any inflammatory reaction. Narcotics are dangerous in these chronic problems and should be withheld. A static splint will relieve pain and should be changed periodically as deformities are progressively improved.

When the patient is first examined, the involved extremity should be palpated and tapped very gently from distal to proximal to demonstrate any trigger points of extreme irritation. If a trigger point is found, the area is surgically prepared and marked with a sterile pen. After local cutaneous anesthesia is administered, a 16-gauge needle is inserted into the area of irritation. The needle is aspirated to avoid blood vessel penetration, and a flexible 18-gauge polyethylene intravenous catheter is inserted through the 16-gauge needle. If the procedure is performed in this manner, the intravenous catheter should not penetrate a nerve or blood vessel. The large-bore 16-gauge needle is then removed, leaving the catheter in place. Next, 0.5 ml of 0.5% lidocaine hydrochloride (Xylocaine) is injected into the intravenous catheter for anesthetic effect. If the trigger point pain is relieved, the catheter is capped and taped in place. The anesthetic block usually is insufficient for complete motor or sensory paralysis, and the pain-free patient is asked to exercise the extremity, to walk, and to perform assigned physical therapy. If the anesthetic block is not effective, then one additional milliliter of lidocaine is injected, and if this also is not effective, the intravenous catheter is withdrawn. If the anesthetic block is effective, then additional periodic injection of lidocaine solution is based on the time of pain-free activity. The patient decides the frequency of injection, dependent upon pain relief. Our usual regimen has been 0.5 ml of 2% lidocaine hydrochloride (Xylocaine) solution with 1:100,000 epinephrine or mepivacaine hydrochloride (Carbocaine) every 4 hours. The volume for each injection has ranged from 0.5 to 1 ml, and the time range between injections has been 1 to 10 hours. The average time range between injections was 2 hours 12 minutes during the acute stage, lengthening to 3 hours 24 minutes as the effect of the periodic peripheral infusion decreased pain and muscle strength improved. The periodic infusion is injected through the catheter without need for further skin puncture and has been continued for 2 weeks in a few cases.[16] If there is more than one area of irritation, separate catheters should be used for each trigger point. In contrast to a central chemical stellate block, the periodic peripheral infusion is a ward procedure that can be performed simultaneously with other modes of treatment and should block the formation of neurokinin more effectively than the central chemical block. The peripheral infusion will relieve painful symptoms for a variable period of time but will not produce permanent relief of pain. It is much less effective in those cases where the pain has been untreated and unrelieved for 3 or more months after injury.

Transcutaneous electric stimulation is used as a peripheral method for the production of local analgesia. The technique attempts to selectively stimulate large myelinated sensory fibers (A axons) and control pain (small unmyelinated C axons) by activating the inhibitory mechanisms. The direct current stimulator delivers a modified square wave pulse with controllable frequency, pulse width, and voltage. When relief is obtained, it should last for 2 to 3 hours after 2 minutes of stimulation. The intensity should be varied by the patient because stimuli that are too intense overcome the inhibition mechanism and produce additional pain. The best results are obtained when the treatment is given within 3 months of the onset of pain. In our patients with established pain for 3 months or longer, the percutaneous electric stimulator has produced subjective improvement if it is operated continuously but has not been effective enough to produce objective improvement such as increased grip or pinch strength or endurance pull without supplemental analgesia, and it has not produced pain relief for 2 or 3 hours when stimulation is stopped. At Massachusetts General Hospital, operative placement of the electrodes directly involved on peripheral nerves and prolonged stimulation has resulted in lasting relief of pain in 30% of 44 patients who were observed for at least 6 months. An additional 31% had initial pain relief, but pain returned as scar tissue formed around the electrodes.[25] Another study at Duke University[14] reported lasting relief of pain in 36% of 20 patients observed for 30 months after surgical implantation of the electrodes directly on involved peripheral nerves.

These patients often have basic emotional problems, and a psychiatric consultation is indicated. Psychotherapy should be concurrent with other diagnostic and treatment procedures. The attending physician must take additional time to reassure the patient while simultaneously enforcing the need for the patient to actively participate in the treatment process. A battery of psychometric tests, such as the Minnesota Multiphasic Personality Inventory, may be valuable in management of the whole patient.

Acupuncture has recently become popular in the United States and seems to be effective in the susceptible individual. However, there is no scientific evidence, anatomic or physiologic, that acupuncture points or meridians exist.[2] In the latter part of the 18th century the German physician Franz Anton Mesmer developed the modern technique for hypnosis. Experiments in hypnosis have shown that subjects can distort perception as well as motor movements, and through hypnosis one can produce partial to total anesthesia. Successful acupuncture and hypnosis both require the cerebral cortex to activate complex conditioned reflexes that lower pain thresholds, remove anxiety and tension, and relieve depression.

Frazier and Kolb[5] emphasize the element of psychopathology in the painful phantom limb. They distinguish the patient with phantom pain resulting from physical disease from the patient with psychogenic pain. The phantom limb with physical disease has had a period of no pain, and when pain develops, it follows anatomic nerve distribution. The patient with psychogenic pain has immediate intermittent episodes of pain that do not follow anatomic nerve distribution. He makes poor use of prostheses and is maladjusted in his home and society.

The second principle in the treatment program for reflex sympathetic dystrophy is use of the involved extremity. We divide available physical modalities into passive and active assistors. The passive activities will improve circulation, decrease edema, and prepare the patient for active voluntay participation in the active exercise program. Passive modalities include elevation, traction, plaster casts, static splints (Orthoplast), faradic muscle stimulation, ice packs, hot paraffin packs, combined contrast baths, massage, and inflatable splints* with positive-negative pressure. Some passive modalities may be contraindicated in some cases, such as the whirlpool bath, which is heat dependent and may increase edema and inflammatory reaction. The more important phase is active exercise, which can be assisted with dynamic splints, supportive exercising slings, and special handles for tools. Special care has to be directed to key circulation areas, such as the rotator cuff muscles in a shoulder-arm-hand syndrome. General body conditioning is important, and the patient should be ambulatory, if at all possible, to meet his environment. Function can be developed with diversional games, assigned work, and activities of daily living. It is most imortant that physicians, physical therapists, occupational therapists, and other attendants be compassionate and yet obtain maximal effort by the patient. The best functional activity is the patient's return to his usual work. In general, approximately 20% of patients have combined and emotional problems that elude immediate therapy.[16]

CAUSALGIA

Causalgia is a systemic process of "burning pain" initiated by a physical injury to a peripheral nerve. The clinical syndrome represents a constellation of symptoms and signs that have been recognized since Mitchell's description following the American Civil War.[18] In 1920 the Nerve Injuries Committee of the British Medical Research Council defined causalgia as having the following characteristics: (1) it is spontaneous; (2) it is hot and burning in character, intense, diffuse, persistent, and subject to exacerbations; (3) it can be excited by stimuli that do not necessarily produce a physical effect on the limb; and (4) it tends to lead to profound changes in the mental state of the patient. Causalgia develops in 2% to 5% of patients with injuries to peripheral nerves. The syndrome usually results from a high-velocity missile injury involving the proximal portion of the extremity. The median and tibial nerves,

---

*Jobst, PO Box 653, Toledo, Ohio 43694.

both containing a high percentage of sympathetic neurons, are most often involved in the clinical syndrome. There is usually incomplete severance of the injured nerve, with retention of partial sensory and motor function. There is an associated injury to a major artery in more than one third of the cases. In our experience, pain is the immediate and dominant feature. Half of our patients had characteristic symptoms on the day of injury, and two thirds of the patients by the end of the first week after injury.[15]

Treatment should be instituted as soon as the syndrome is suspected, and chemical central sympathetic block is performed promptly to serve as a diagnostic test as well as a therapeutic procedure. The blocks are performed with solutions of either 1% lidocaine hydrochloride (Xylocaine) or 1% mepivacaine hydrochloride (Carbocaine) and should produce prompt peripheral warming and loss of sweating, as well as relief from the peripheral hyperesthesia. The anterior approach is preferred for a stellate block, using the technique described by Kleinert and associates[11] and a paravertebral injection of the lumbar sympathetic chain as described by Moore.[25] An adequate block should be obtained with 10 to 20 ml, and while the patient is free from pain, an accurate physical examination of the extremity can be performed. Subsequent blocks may utilize an anesthetic agent with a longer duration of action, such as prilocaine hydrochloride (Citanest) or bupivacaine[1] as a 1% solution. If necessary to relieve pain, a continuous chemical central sympathetic block can be performed using the same technique as the periodic peripheral infusion with an intravenous catheter that is taped in place and attached to an intravenous stand; however, the diagnostic goal is to evaluate the length of pain-free time between blocks. A series of four or five blocks should be given on consecutive days; one placebo of normal saline solution should be given during the series to confirm the diagnosis. An adequate block will indicate the degree of pain relief to be expected from surgical sympathectomy. The prognostic effect of a chemical sympathetic block is uncertain, but some generalizations have been made[16]: (1) one block may give total relief; (2) one block may reduce residual pain to a tolerant level; (3) the effective duration of the first block may exceed that expected of the agent used, and subsequent blocks may give progressively longer pain-free periods; (4) the effective duration of the first block may exceed that expected of the agent used, but subsequent blocks may give progressively shorter pain-free periods; and (5) the block gives relief only for the duration expected from the anesthetic agent used. If the blocks produce effects 1 through 3, the prognosis for permanent improvement is excellent. If the blocks produce effects 4 or 5, permanent improvement should not be expected. A series of chemical central sympathetic blocks instituted early in the course of treatment may lead to resolution of the pain syndrome, and further treatment, other than physical medicine procedures and active mobilization, will not be necessary.

The great majority of reported cases of causalgia require surgical sympathectomy, and surgery should be performed when the burning pain completely responds to central chemical sympathectomy but requires repeated blocks for the long-term relief of pain. The effectiveness of sympathectomy is not related to interrupting a sensory pathway from the extremity but to eliminating the sympathetic efferent discharge to the peripheral arteries and sweat glands. Sympathectomy will relieve only burning pain; associated painful neuromas or arthritic pain will not be altered. We favor the transaxillary approach over the posterior transcostal approach, with removal of the sympathetic chain from the fourth thoracic level superior to include the lower half of the stellate ganglion. Horner syndrome often is not present after the transaxillary approach, which permits removal of only the lower half of the stellate ganglion, but it is more often present following the supraclavicular approach and can be most annoying to the patient. In the lower extremity a retroperitoneal approach through a lateral flank incision, as described by White and Sweet,[25] allows removal of the sympathetic ganglions from the second to the fifth lumbar level. For a satisfactory result, postoperative precise sudomotor function tests should demonstrate complete sympathetic denervation of the involved extremity.

Curtis advocates internal neurolysis in treatment of causalgia that has followed compression of the median nerve at the carpal level,[4] for example, fracture-dislocations of the proximal carpal row. To be effective, the transverse carpal ligament must be released completely and a meticulous longitudinal release done between the thickened epineurium and the compressed funiculi. Magnification is required to identify the involved structures.

The two treatment objectives in all pain problems are relief of discomfort and use of the involved extremity. The passive modalities that are utilized in a painful neuroma or reflex sympathetic dystrophy may need to be preceded by very delicate passive techniques in the apprehensive causalgic patient. The skin can be lightly stroked with a feather, followed by very gentle massage, and then hot paraffin baths, before inflatable splints* and similar passive modalities will be tolerated. However, the patient must progress to functional activity as soon as he can tolerate active use of the extremity.

PAIN MANAGEMENT PROGRAM

The important principle in the management of pain as a complication of peripheral nerve injury is prompt recognition and vigorous treatment. Pain may be relieved by transcutaneous electric stimulation, by peripheral nerve blocks or central chemical sympathetic block, or by systemic medication to decrease sympathetic influence upon the vascular system. The patient's anxiety and pain deserve medication, but not a prolonged program of narcotics and sedation. Psychiatric consultation is helpful in the majority of patients with chronic pain. Treatment aims to develop independent use of the involved extremity and utilizes both passive and active modalities. Passive techniques include elevation, traction, static splints, muscle stimulation, massage, percussion, ice packs, paraffin baths, and inflatable splints with positive-negative pressure and a fluid cuff for contrast baths. Independent use of the involved extremity demands active exercise, which can be assisted with dynamic splints or slings, and special designs for tools. Function can be developed with diversional games, activities of daily living, and everyday work. Surgery has a minor role in comparison to therapeutic physical modalities. A painful neuroma can be transferred to a thick layer of scar-free soft tissue. Surgical sympathectomy is indicated very early in the treatment of causalgia. Surgical procedures on the central nervous system, such as cordotomy or postcentral gyrectomy of the cerebral cortex, have all been demonstrated to be ineffective for sustained relief of pain.

---

*Jobst, PO Box 653, Toledo, Ohio 43694.

REFERENCES

1. Bromage, P. R.: Nerve physiology and control of pain, Orthop. Clin. North Am. **4**:897-906, 1973.
2. Cantrell, J. R.: Acupuncture: A form of psychologic healing, South. Med. J. **63**:14-17, 1975.
3. Chapman, L.F., Ramos,A.O., Goodell, H., and Wolff, H. G.: Neurohumoral features of afferent fibers in man. Their role in vasodilation, inflammation and pain, Arch. Neurol. **4**:617-650, 1961.
4. Curtis, R.: Internal neurolysis in nerve compression syndromes, Am. Soc. Surg. Hand Newsletter, January 19, 1970.
5. Frazier, S. H.,and Kolb, L. C.: Psychiatric aspects of pain and the phantom limb, Orthop. Clin. North Am. **1**:481-495, 1970.
6. Geldard, F. A.: Human senses, ed. 2, New York, 1972, John Wiley and Sons.
7. Granit, R., Leksell, L., and Skoglund, C. R.: Fiber interaction in injured or compressed region of nerve, Brain **67**:125-140, 1944.
8. Grant, G. H.: Methods of treatment of Neuromata of the hand, J. Bone Joint Surg. [Am.] **33**:841-848, 1951.
9. Herndon, J. H., Eaton, R. G., and Littler, W.: Management of painful neuroma in the hand, J. Bone Joint Surg. [Am.] **58**:369-373, 1976.
10. Kleiman, A.: Causalgia: evidence of the existence of crossed sensory sympathetic fibers, Am. J. Surg. **87**:839-841, 1954.
11. Kleinert, H. E., Cole, N. M., Wayne, L.: Post-traumatic sympathetic dystrophy, Orthop. Clin. North Am. **4**:917-927, 1973.
12. Mathews, G. J., and Osterholm, J. L.: Painful traumatic neuromas, Surg. Clin. North Am. **51**:1313-1324, 1972.
13. Melzak, R., and Wall, P. D.: Pain mechanisms: a new theory, Science **150**:971-979, 1965.
14. Nashold, B. S., Jr., Goldner, J. L., and Bright, D. S.: Direct electrical stimulation of the peripheral nerves for relief of intractable pain, J. Bone Joint Surg. [Am.] **57**:729, 1975.
15. Omer, G. E., and Thomas, S.: Treatment of causalgia, review of cases at Brooke General Hospital, Tex. Med. **67**:93-96, 1971.
16. Omer, G. E., and Thomas, S. R.: The management of chronic pain syndromes in the upper extremity, Clin. Orthop. **104**:37-45, 1974.
17. Porter, J. M., Snider, R. L., and Bardana, E. J., et al.: The diagnosis and treatment of Raynaud's phenomenon, Surgery **77**:11-23, 1975.
18. Richards, R. L.: Causalgia: a centenial review, Arch. Neurol. **16**:339-350, 1967.
19. Simson, G.: Letter: propranol for causalgia and sudeck's atrophy, J.A.M.A. **227**:327, 1974.
20. Smith, J. R., and Gomez, N. H.: Local injection therapy of Neuromata of the hand with triamcinolone acetonide, a preliminary study of twenty-two patients, J. Bone Joint Surg. [Am.] **52**:71-83, 1970.
21. Snyder, C.: The surgical handling of tissue, Proceedings of seventh annual convention, American Association Equine Practitioners, Fort Worth, Tex., December 1961.
22. Tupper, J. W., and Booth, D. M.: Treatment of painful neuromas of sensory nerves in the hand: A comparison of traditional and newer methods, J. Hand Surg. **1**:144-151, 1976.
23. Verdan, C. and Narakas, A.: Nerve surgery of the hand. In Goldwyn, R. M., editor: The unfavorable result in plastic surgery. Avoidance and treatment, Boston, 1972, Little, Brown, and Company.
24. Weeks, P. M., and Wray, R. C.: Management of acute hand injuries: a biological approach, St. Louis, 1973, The C. V. Mosby Co.
25. White, J. C., and Sweet, W. H.: Pain and the neurosurgeon: a forty-year experience, Springfield, Ill., 1969, Charles C Thomas, Publisher.

Chapter 14

Occupational therapy for the treatment of reflex sympathetic dystrophy and posttraumatic hypersensitivity in the injured hand

Lois M. Barber

REFLEX SYMPATHETIC DYSTROPHY

Moberg has stated that the important central feature of the reflex dystrophy syndrome is impairment of the pumping mechanism of the arm and the hand. Whereas the arterial supply depends on blood pressure, a significant portion of the venous and lymphatic return against gravity depends on external factors such as active muscle function in the arm and hand.[1] The effects of sustained hydrostatic edema to the limb can be catastrophic and irreversible.

The treatment regimen described here is based on this principle and has been consistently successful with patients who have had late edema and stiffness out of proportion to their injury. Therapeutic techniques have been aimed at three basic objectives: the control of swelling, establishment of an active exercise routine, and support of painful or weak parts by splinting.

When the patient with advanced involvement cannot initially move vigorously enough to accomplish effective pumping, edema control begins with elevation. The patient is encouraged to elevate the arm as much as possible during exercise and rest. Exercises and therapeutic crafts are contrived to be performed in the elevated position, all the while aiming to reestablish the pumping mechanism by encouraging motion. When edema limits the joint motion and thus the pumping action, a vicious cycle may be established. It may then be helpful to mechanically force hydrostatic edema out of the hand by a variety of custom-made devices. A device such as the one shown in Fig. 14-1 should hold the hand in a functional position and give as uniform a pressure distribution as possible. In the construction of such equipment various combinations of Temper Foam* and pressure systems can be used. Air splints plus Temper Foam forms have been combined to provide fairly uniform pressure and simplify application. Wearing time is established according to each patient's clinical picture, generally for hourly periods twice daily prior to exercise. Such devices are time consuming to apply properly and must be custom constructed, but they can effectively reduce the swelling enough so that the patient can accomplish some active motion and begin to reverse the vicious cycle of edema and inactivity. These devices do not allow active motion while being worn. A new device consists of a double air compression bag that allows some movement of the fingers, maintains constant adjustable pressure, is quick and simple to apply, and is portable and economical (Fig. 14-2).

Most patients who have developed the reflex dystrophy syndrome have been very passive when first moving the extremity following injury. Moberg states, "The active patient is not able to keep his

*A viscoelastic polyurethane material; tends to flow and mold itself to distribute pressure; sold as Temper Foam by Edmont-Wilson and as T-Foam by Alimed.

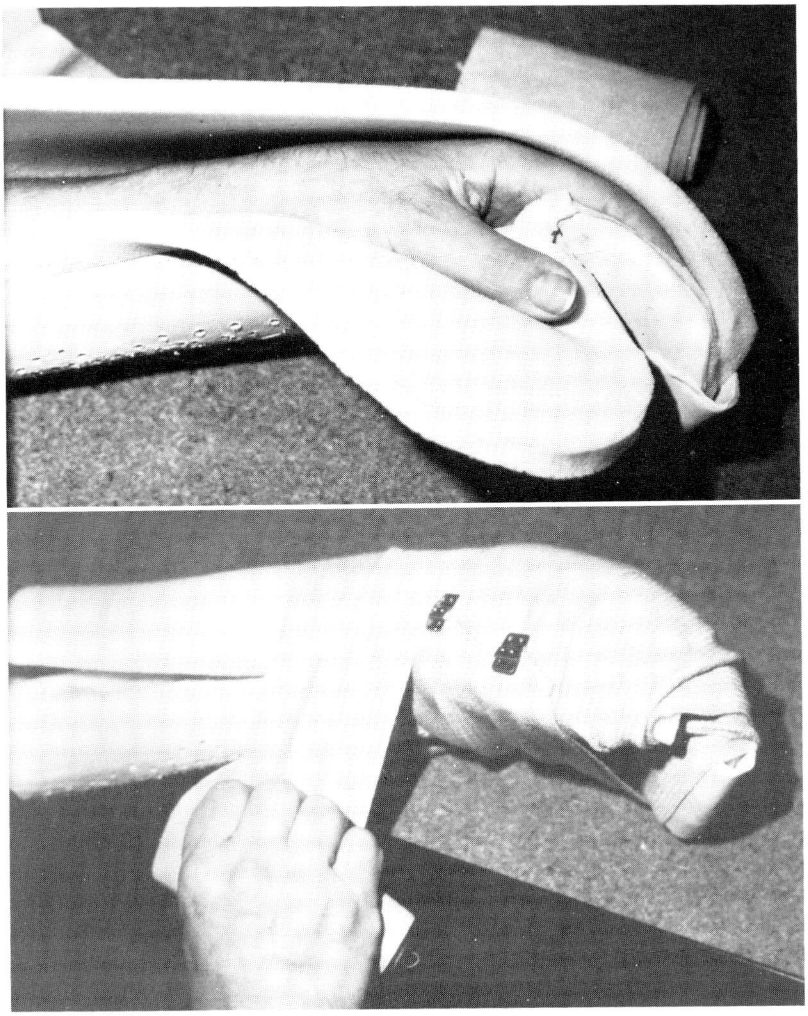

Fig. 14-1. Individually tailored Temper Foam and Orthoplast device for control of swelling.

damaged arm strictly immobilized even if he attempts to do so. Therefore, the function of the pumping system is retained. On the other hand the passive patient, especially the hypersensitive one, will immobilize himself completely even following slight trauma."[2] Thus it is extremely important to begin to instill a habit of exercise on the very first day of treatment. It is necessary to monitor and encourage the patient frequently and for extended periods of time. Exercises to increase strength and range of motion of the shoulder are begun immediately. The patient is taught the standard pendulum-and-wand exercises, which he can do at home or during treatment time. The mobile arm support that was developed as a functional aid has been an excellent therapeutic exercise device to give the patient relatively frictionless shoulder and elbow ranging (Fig. 14-3). The "skateboard" is used to give more resistance in the horizontal plane and is encouraged as strength increases (Fig. 14-4). Reciprocal pulleys are useful for aiding vertical motion and can be easily adapted for home use (Fig. 14-5).

It is imperative to take time to be sure that the patient know exactly what he is to do and to be specific in instructing the patient in all exercises. This requires individual attention and enough time and repetition to actually instill a habit of motion. These passive patients need continual reinforcement.

Many patients have limited elbow motion, and most have decreased forearm rotation. When elbow flexion is limited, a piece of foam against which the patient flexes is a simple idea that encourages increased elbow flexion range. This can be trimmed

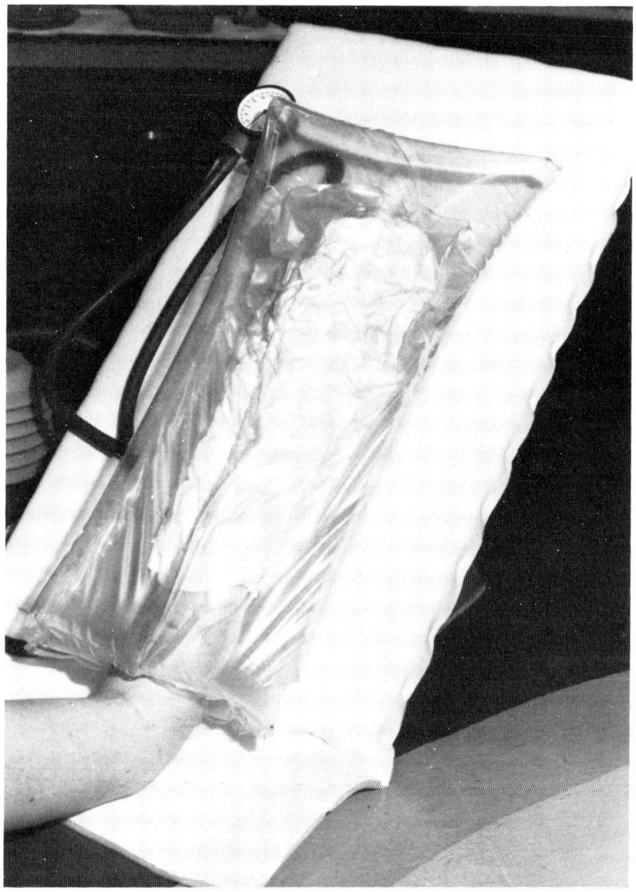

Fig. 14-2. Double plastic pressure bag with Temper Foam insert and flexible inner bag to allow movement.

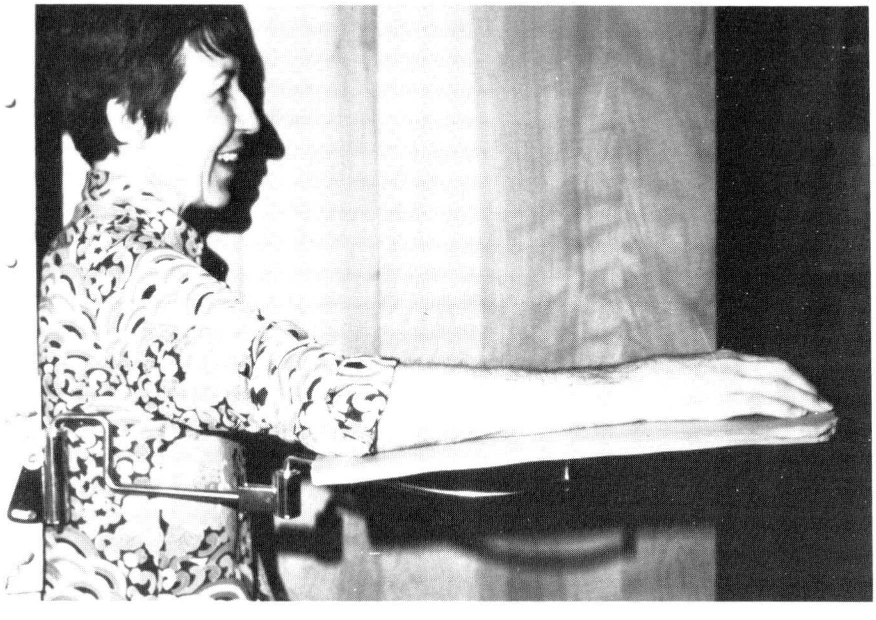

Fig. 14-3. Mobile arm support to encourage free shoulder and elbow motion.

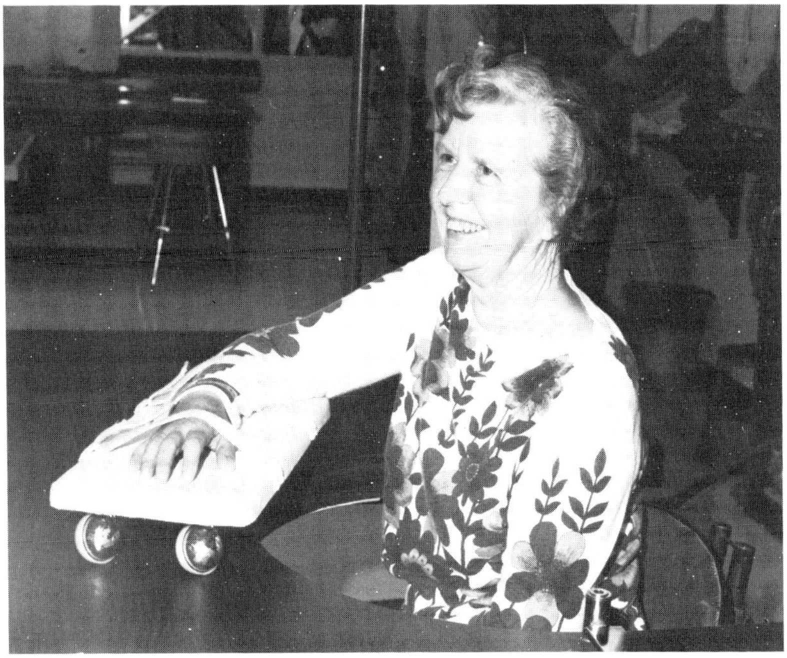

Fig. 14-4. Skateboard exercises to encourage shoulder and elbow motion with slight resistance.

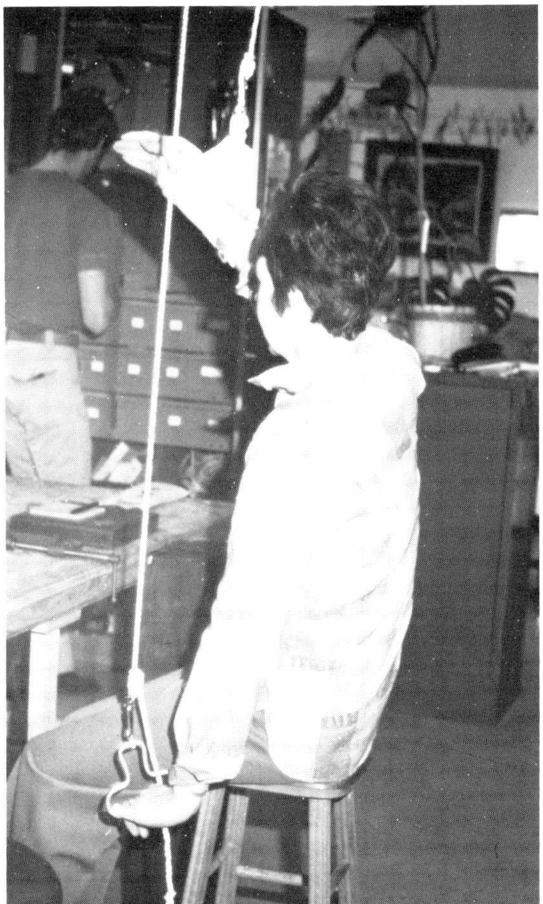

Fig. 14-5. Reciprocal pulley system for active, assistive shoulder exercise.

as range increases. A molded plastic forearm cuff with rubber band assistance encourages forearm rotation. The patient can also take this device home. It is reasonably inexpensive and simple to construct (Fig. 14-6). Care must be taken to get a good purchase on the forearm proximal to the wrist to avoid excessive strain at the wrist joint.

While occasional rest periods on a regular basis may be necessary, the goal repeatedly instilled in the patient both verbally and by example of other patients is to move. Exercises are devised to encourage the patient to always perform to his limit. A home program is initiated so that the habit of moving is consistent and so that exercises are continued at home during weekends and later when supervised treatment frequency is decreased.

Meaningful, well-directed handicraft exercises are most beneficial both for their versatility and their ability to motivate the patient to move without having to do boring repetitive calisthenics. Since all joints of the upper extremity are usually affected to varying degrees in most patients with this problem, full limb motion is encouraged. The patient is instructed to relax between motions in order to gain the maximum pumping action. Resistive sanding, for example, involves both grasp and release and shoulder and elbow motion (Fig. 14-7) and can be easily graded in both time and resistance.

A device called the weight-well uses a single dowel in a frame with a rope and weight attached. It can be adapted with a variety of handles for hand

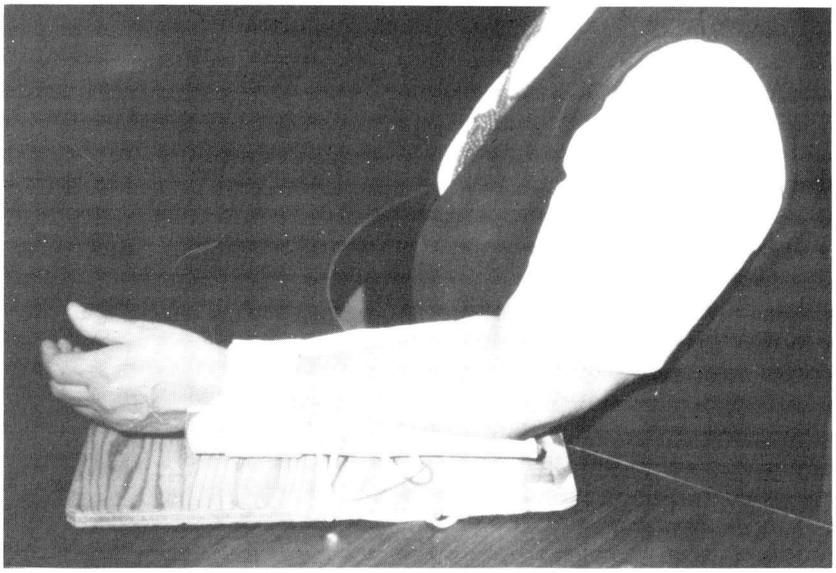

Fig. 14-6. Molded plastic forearm cuff to position forearm in rotation.

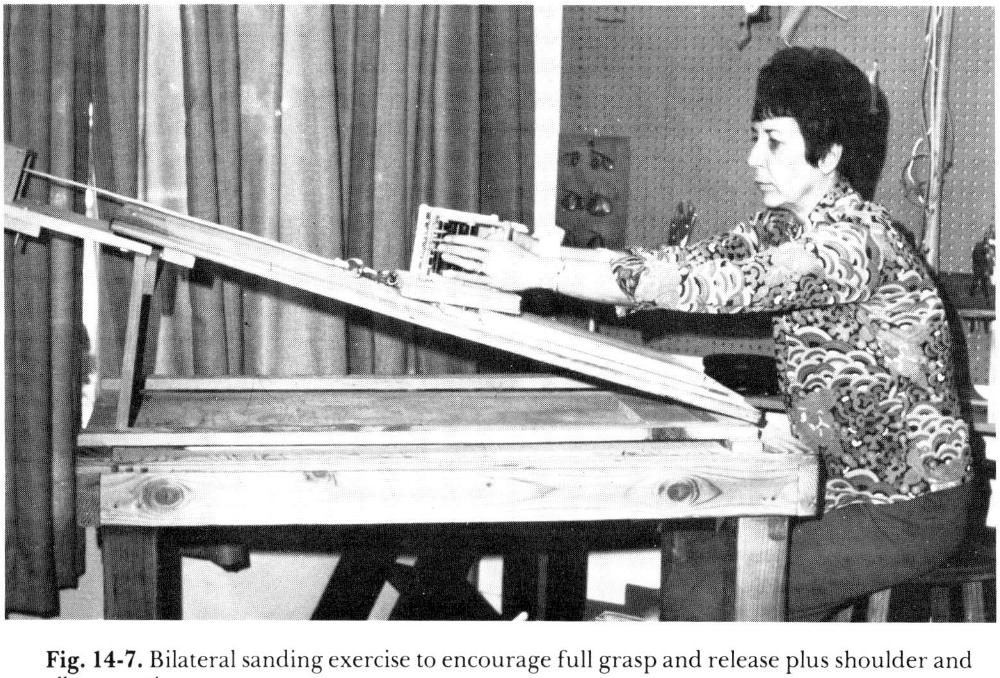

Fig. 14-7. Bilateral sanding exercise to encourage full grasp and release plus shoulder and elbow motion.

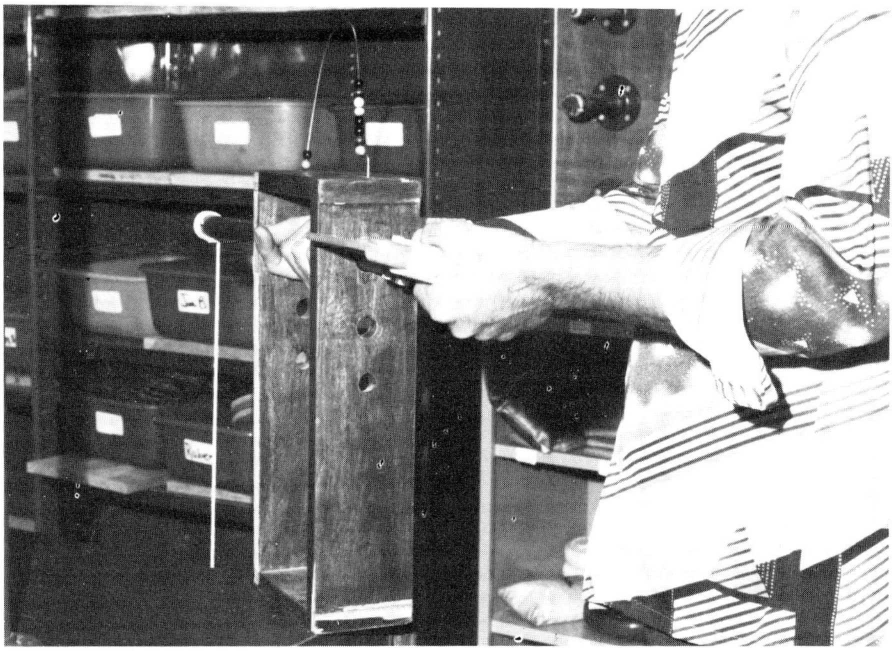

Fig. 14-8. Weight-well designed to strengthen forearm rotators.

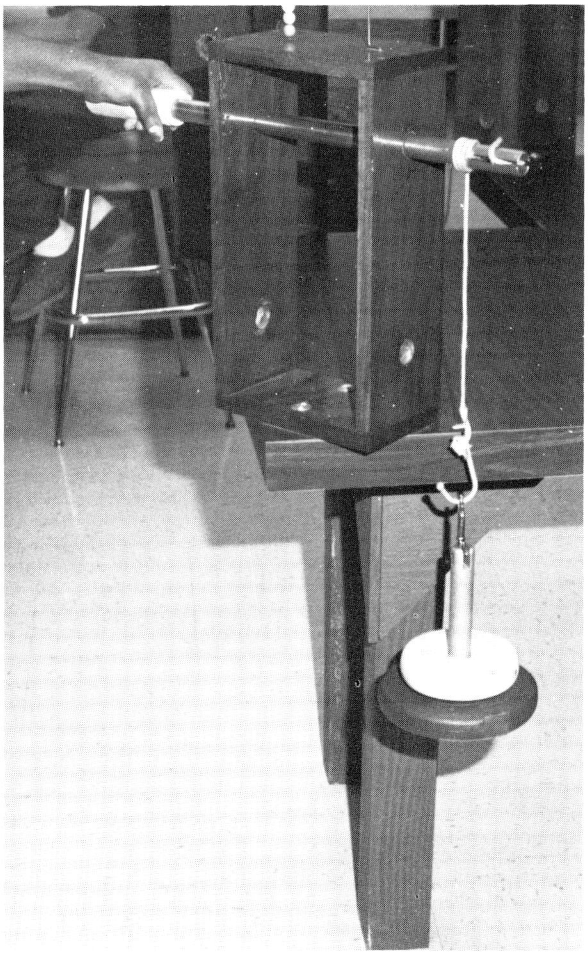

Fig. 14-9. Weight-well exercise, encouraging full release of grip as well as full grasp on each rotation.

and forearm exercises. As the patient rotates the forearm, grips, or pinches, a weight is lifted. A certain number of repetitions are performed during each stage of the exercise, and resistance is changed as strength increases. The standard weight-well exercise with the forearm in the pronated position and the patient grasping and releasing fully as the dowel is rotated is excellent for gaining range of motion and strength (Fig. 14-8). Forearm rotation can be actively encouraged by means of a different handle on this device which can similarly be rotated against resistance (Fig. 14-9). In all exercises the patient is encouraged to move through a full active range of motion and to exert his maximum effort. Full flexion and extension of the wrist and the fingers in the natural reciprocal pattern are encouraged. The weight-well exercise is excellent for establishing the pumping action that is desired. It can be adapted for use in the vertical plane when forearm rotation or wrist range or both are limited (Fig. 14-10). The device is simply constructed and can easily be used at home.

Patients frequently develop the habit of extending the wrist with the common finger extensors (Fig. 14-11). This contributes to metacarpophalangeal joints that are stiff in extension and to claw deformity of the fingers. To prevent this the wrist should be splinted in as near-functional position as possible, and the splint worn at all times except while doing specific wrist motion exercises (Fig. 14-

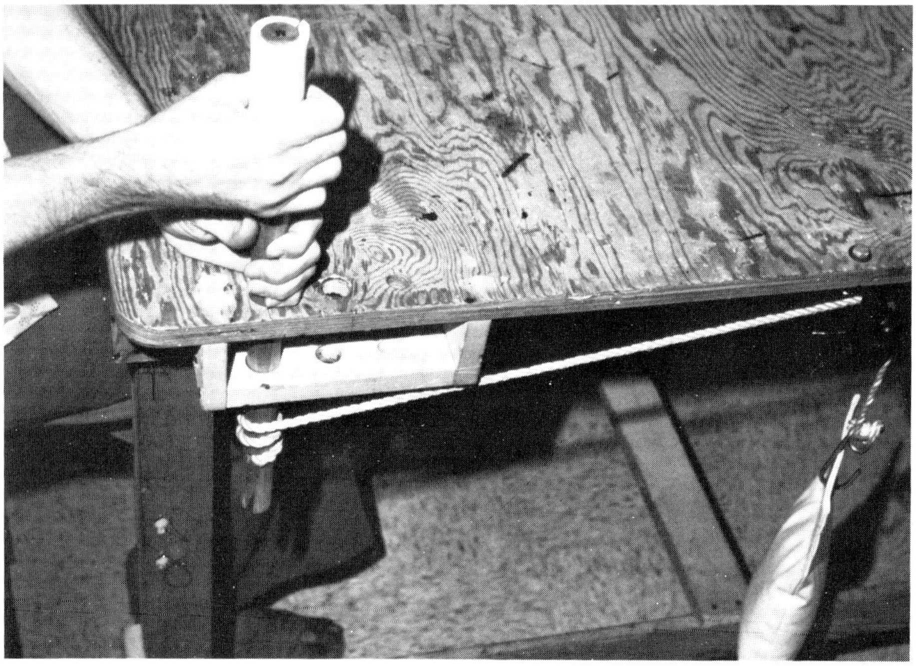

Fig. 14-10. Weight-well adapted for use on vertical plane.

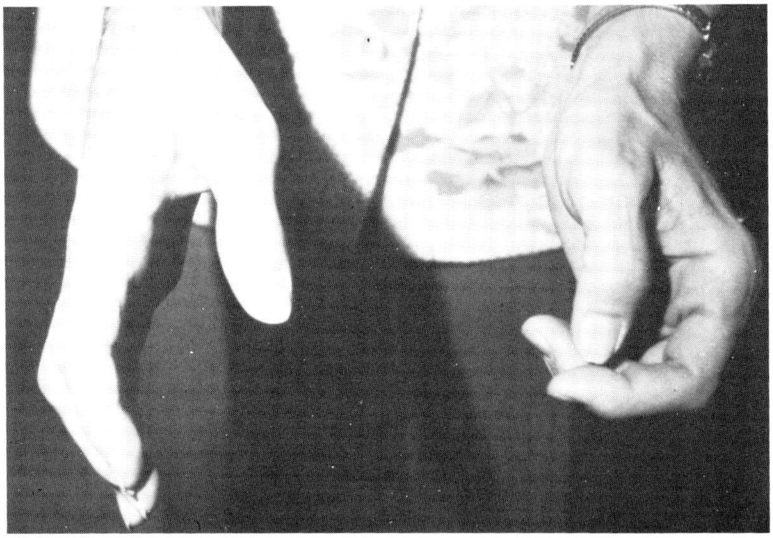

Fig. 14-11. Patient attempting to extend wrist of involved right hand. Note extension at metacarpophalangeal joints.

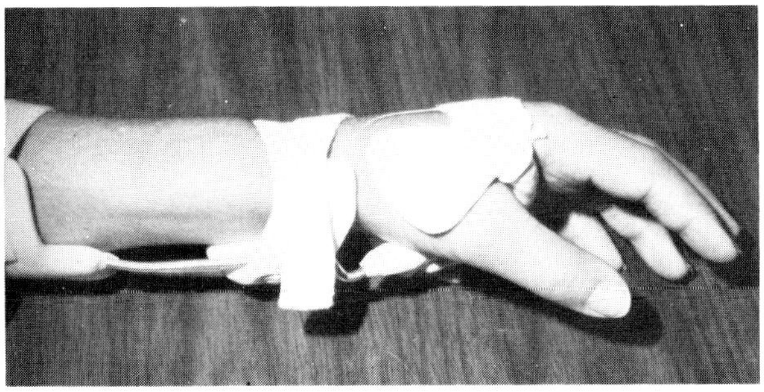

Fig. 14-12. Splint to support wrist, allowing independent finger movement.

12). Dynamic hand splinting is frequently helpful. Positioning of the fingers may be graded by means of leather loops and a cuff over the dorsum of the hand attached to the splint by means of rubber bands. This is useful between exercises and at night to increase flexion range. Electromyographic biofeedback devices are also helpful for reeducation in the appropriate use of the wrist extensors.

Progressive resistance exercises are used for wrist strengthening as soon as the patient can lift the wrist against gravity. As the wrist musculature strengthens and substitution of long-finger extensors is corrected, the splint time is decreased and reserved for performance of heavier tasks or when the wrist needs support because of pain. Because many patients like the feeling of compression around the wrist, occasionally a snug gauntlet or simple Ace wrap is used.

The patient is encouraged to move in spite of pain. Analgesics are sparingly prescribed if indicated. The patient is treated in a gentle manner in therapy so as not to have him develop an aversion to exercise and perpetuate the vicious cycle of inactivity and immobility. Most importantly the patient is helped to establish a routine of exercise that does not increase the pain beyond tolerance but permits gains in strength, range of motion, and ultimately function; that is, the patient is helped to "work through the pain." The group environment of many patients actively involved in therapy has been a positive influence on the activity level of most patients. The patients support each other in working through the painful state. The individual patient's social environment must be evaluated, and overly accommodating family members discouraged from assisting the patient. From the very beginning, use of the hand for functional activities is encouraged, and the patient is weaned to full independence as soon as possible. In general, progress is gradual, especially in older people with established joint stiffness and the patient must be forewarned that improvement may be frustratingly slow.

The treatment regimen described has been successful with a series of eight patients analyzed, who developed reflex sympathetic dystrophy following Colles fracture. Their treatment periods ranged from 2 to 10 months, gradually decreasing in frequency near the end of treatment. The only patient who did not improve had significant pain and was primarily concerned with suing the first doctor who treated her.

THE TREATMENT OF HYPERSENSITIVITY IN THE TRAUMATIZED HAND

Hypersensitivity is a common sequela of many hand injuries. It may be localized to an area such as a healing wound or nerve repair or may include a larger skin surface sometimes remote from the site of trauma such as in sympathetic dystrophy. Patients understandably avoid touching the sensitive area, and this may result in disuse of the entire hand.

Long-standing experience has shown that the most effective way to diminish hypersensitivity is repeated touching of the sensitive area, in effect bombarding the area with stimuli, resulting in decreased sensitivity. The desensitization program described below is based on this experience.

Technique

The patient is first introduced to a number of different particulate materials ranging from soft to hard, nonirritating to irritating. They are arbitrarily sequenced as follows: cotton balls, foam rubber particles, terry cloth particles, beans, rice, plastic particles, buckshot, and ball bearings. By trial and error the patient chooses a texture that produces only slight discomfort. He is instructed to repeatedly submerge his hand in containers of this material for 5-minute periods twice daily and to progressively increase his time to 20 minutes. When this is tolerated and no longer seems irritating he selects another slightly irritating texture and repeats the process. This is continued until improvement is maximal (Fig. 14-13).

In addition to these tasks the patient is given a textured dowel to carry with him, and he is urged to touch the sensitive area approximately 5 minutes an hour. The dowels range in texture from soft and smooth to hard and rough (Fig. 14-14). As tolerance increases the patient is encouraged to habitually tap the tender area for further stimulus bombardment.

Aside from this specific program, further activ-

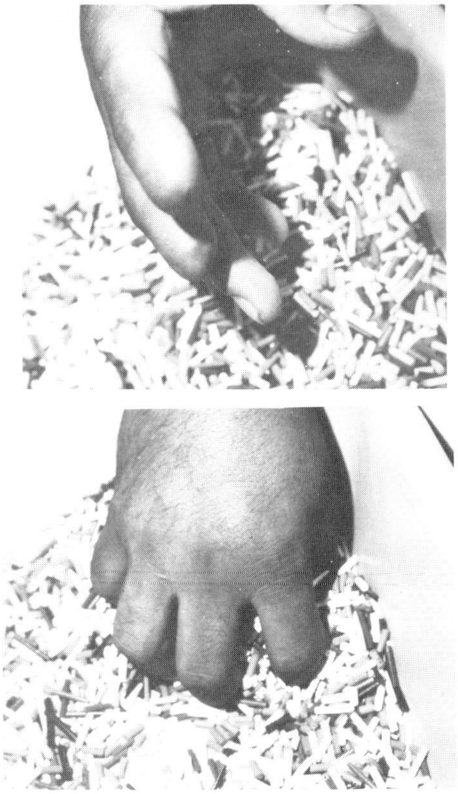

Fig. 14-13. Patient with sensitive amputation stumps repeatedly contacting slightly irritating particles.

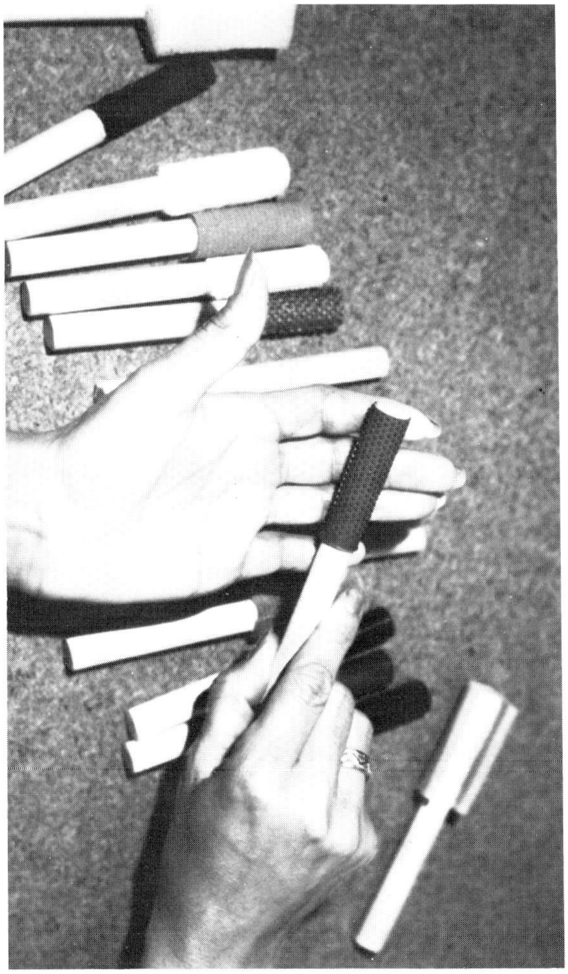

Fig. 14-14. Patient contacting sensitive area with dowels covered with various degrees of textured material.

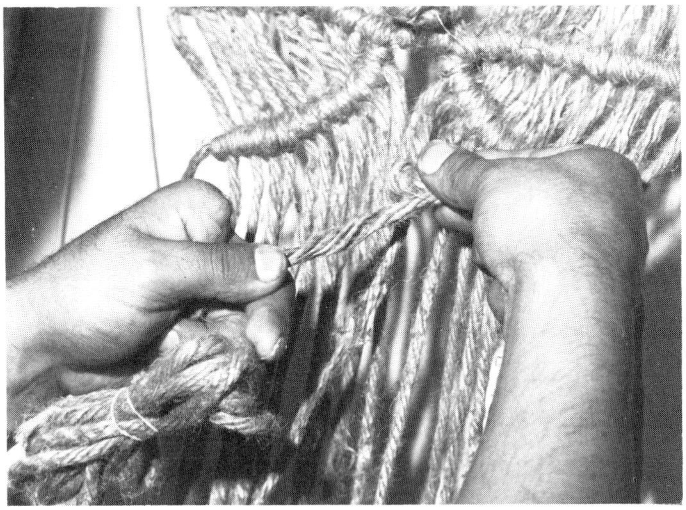

Fig. 14-15. Patient doing knotting craft as means of desensitization.

ities and exercises are designed to aid in desensitization. The staff observes and encourages the patient to use the sensitive part for contact in all exercises and daily living activities (Fig. 14-15).

The programs outlined have a high rate of success with patients who do not have overwhelming secondary gain concerns. After successful treatment most patients will admit to continued hypersensitivity but do not have the marked avoidance response that inhibits use of the digits. The hypersensitive area can then be used for most tasks and is minimally disabling.

SUMMARY

Successful treatment programs using a structured therapy environment alone have been outlined for the care of patients with reflex sympathetic dystrophy and posttraumatic hypersensitive scars and neuromas.

REFERENCES

1. Frykman, G.: Fracture of the distal radius including sequelae—shoulder-hand-finger syndrome, disturbance in the distal radioulnar joint and impairment of nerve function, Acta Orthop. Scand. [Suppl.] **108:**3, 1967.
2. Moberg, E.: The shoulder-hand-finger syndrome, Surg. Clin. North Am. **40:**367-373, 1960.
3. Steinbrocker, O.: The shoulder hand syndrome: present perspective, Postgrad. Med. **49:**888-895, 1968.

Panel discussion on injury to motor nerves, pain, and dystrophy

H. BRUCE WILLIAMS, Moderator

PAUL W. BRAND
M. MARK HOFFER
HANNO MILLESI
VERT MOONEY
GEORGE E. OMER

Question: Dr. Hoffer, you have stated that 90% of congenital brachial plexus injuries recover. Is there ever an indication to explore the remaining 10%?

Hoffer: We feel that recovery is not complete for 4 years. After waiting that long we are pessimistic that exploration would be of value. I have never explored such a patient.

Millesi: I agree with Dr. Hoffer, unless I have some evidence of direct trauma, such as an associated clavicular fracture.

Question: Dr. Mooney, does a child with a unilateral amputation successfully wear a prosthesis?

Mooney: Forceful parents can induce a child to wear the device up to age 5 or 6. After that the unilateral prosthesis is rarely accepted until the patient perceives some value in it. In boys that is usually in their late teens when they start messing with cars.

Question: Dr. Brand, in what percentage of patients would you do an early tendon transfer, that is, within a month or two of injury?

Brand: The important thing is to give the patient enough capability to get back to activity. Therefore, I try to find a transfer that will overcome any obviously irreducible deformity without sacrificing a vital original function. For example, in a high radial nerve injury I try to correct the wrist drop with nonessential donors and even if motor recovery occurs, nothing is lost. In a high median nerve injury, replacement of the long thumb and index flexors usually requires transfer of two significant donor muscles. I would prefer to be certain that recovery will not occur before sacrificing these motors. In the same high median injury, intrinsic recovery is unlikely so that an early opponen's transfer is judicious. Certainly with a functioning opponens transfer the patient is more likely to oppose against the innervated ring and little fingers than against the insensitive index and middle fingers.

Millesi: I would not do such a transfer on the high radial nerve lesion, as the recovery potential is high and dynamic splinting provides effective temporary function. I would also consider procedures such as a Zancolli for ulnar nerve lesions to prevent clawing while awaiting motor return.

Omer: I am now doing early tendon transfers in almost all high lesions more frequently. These should probably be considered, as Bill Burkhalter has pointed out, as nothing more than internal splints. For example, an early opponens transplant not only preserves joint motion but keeps the patient in a proper pattern of movement and permits early sensory reeducation. Thus you are not only assisting the functional anatomy but teaching the patient as well.

Question: Dr. Spinner, you have collected over 100 posterior interosseus nerve lesions. Do these ever require tendon transfers?

Spinner: Yes, on three occasions I have encountered a case of tardy posterior interosseus nerve paralysis due to childhood osteomyelitis of the proximal one third of the radius. Twenty years later digital extensor function was lost because of scar fixation of the nerve. A second patient had a failed repair of the nerve due to a shotgun injury and ulnar nonunion. I would like to comment on early tendon transfers for opposition. Remember that in 40% of patients enough of the thenar muscles are sufficiently ulnar nerve innervated to function satisfactorily without tendon transfers. Also many civilian patients that I see would prefer to wait before considering a possibly unnecessary procedure.

Question: Dr. Brand, in the procedure you described for ulnar nerve palsy, do you still insert the palmaris longus graft into the extensor hood?

Brand: Lately I have been inserting the tendon in the volar sheath to try to get better momentum but only if I am using a tendon with excursion to spare. However, I cannot comment on this modification as I have done too few of them for proper evaluation.

Hoffer: Dan Reardon has told me that some of these patients develop a late swan-neck deformity. I would support Dr. Brand's approach but would think the insertion should be in the bone of the proximal phalanx.

Omer: Depending on the resulting balance, insertion into the hood can produce swan necking, while insertion into the sheath can produce a flexion contracture at the proximal interphalangeal joint. I am now placing the tendon end into the insertion of the central slip at the middle phalanx. I'm not sure which is correct for if patients are followed long enough a certain number of them do not do well when you are trying to balance three or four muscle functions with a single insertion.

Question: Dr. Williams, when a nerve is sectioned it always forms a neuroma. Yet why are only a small percentage painful? Secondly, you state that 70% of painful neuromas respond to surgically placing them out of the field of contact. In the residual 30% do any of the other modalities really help?

Williams: No one really knows why some neuromas are painful. I do think that pain develops in neuromas trapped in scar and adherent to skin, bone, tendon and so on. I am not at all positive that procedures such as capping, sleeves, and funiculectomy really do help except perhaps by properly dissecting the nerve free of the adherent scar.

Curtis: By way of prognostication, beware of the patient who in addition to complaining of sensitivity on pressure describes a constant burning pain. This is the patient who frequently starts with a small amputation and may still have his pain after nine different procedures.

Omer: While running a large amputee center we have done over 800 below-knee amputations and 300 Syme amputations. None have had neuroma problems so that symptomatic neuromas seem to be unknown when the amputation is done for vascular disease. We have followed approximately 20 other patients who have been referred because of painful neuromas, frequently after several procedures. All had secondary gain potential, with many involved in litigation. These patients therefore should also be considered poor risks for surgical improvement.

Part III

Upper motor neuron and congenital muscular disorders

Chapter 15

Surgery of the hemiplegic hand

Robert L. Waters

Most stroke-related hemiplegic patients have both motor and sensory involvement. Upper extremity dysfunction is usually the result of infarction in the region of the cerebral cortex, which is supplied by the middle cerebral artery or one of its branches. An ascending frontal branch supplies the motor cortex anteriorly, and an ascending parietal branch supplies the sensory cortex posteriorly.

Patients with relatively intact motor control and sensation, but with restricted extension at the wrist, fingers, or thumb as a result of mild flexor spasticity, are candidates for hand surgery to improve function. Those with bilateral hemiplegia due to multiple strokes have a poor rehabilitation prognosis and are not candidates for surgery. An exception to this general principle is the patient with intact cognition whose bilateral hemiplegia is due to brain stem infarction.

MOTOR RECOVERY

Recognition of the characteristic patterns of motor impairment allows the surgeon to select those patients who will predictably benefit from surgery. Motor recovery in the paralyzed upper extremity typically follows a consistent pattern, with the greatest amount of spontaneous recovery occurring in the first 6 weeks following the stroke.[6] Return of motor function depends primarily on the extent of the lesion and amount of collateral circulation.

In the completely paralyzed extremity, voluntary movement returns first as flexion of the shoulder. Further recovery appears as flexion of the elbow, wrist, and fingers and as supination of the forearm. Flexor spasticity is greatest at this stage. Any voluntary movement of the affected extremity results in simultaneous flexion of all joints. If there is no further recovery, contractures commonly occur unless the joints are passively extended as part of a daily exercise program.

In general by the time flexor synergy includes the wrist and fingers there is also extensor motion present at the shoulder and elbow. At this stage of recovery there is normally a delay of several seconds between the command to execute movement and the time that muscle contraction or relaxation occurs.

Selective motion (the ability to move a joint independently without involving the entire flexor or extensor synergy) usually returns first at the shoulder and elbow. With the development of selective extension there is marked improvement in the speed and precision of flexor motor control as well as reduction in flexor spasticity.

Simultaneous flexion and extension of all fingers precedes the ability to selectively flex and extend one finger at a time. Independent control usually occurs first in the index and middle fingers. Thumb opposition, at first, is to the side of the index finger (key pinch). Full opposition returns later.

Most hemiplegic patients will not use the affected hand, even as an assist, unless they can selectively extend the fingers or thumb without eliciting a simultaneous mass extensor synergy. When it has been determined that recovery has ceased at a point where some selective extension of the fingers or thumb is present but is incomplete due to mild flexor spasticity, surgery to improve function may be indicated.

SENSORY IMPAIRMENT

Even if the cerebral infarct involves the entire sensory cortex the patient will respond to the basic modalities of touch, temperature, and pain, although he will have difficulty appreciating changes in intensity. Depending on the extent of the lesion he may be unable to discriminate higher aspects of sensation such as shape, size, texture, point localization, and proprioception. If the infarct extends posteriorly to the parietal lobe the patient will have additional perceptual problems involving motion of the limb in space and awareness of the limb itself.

Functional use of the hand is dependent on sensory awareness as well as motor control.[3] The patient without sensory perception may use the affected hand on request, relying on visual feedback, but will not routinely use it even as an assist. Hemiplegic patients prefer to use the uninvolved extremity alone rather than grope with a hand that lacks sensation.

The most important test of sensory function is careful observation to determine if there is spontaneous purposeful use of the hand. The two-point discrimination test is easily performed and quantitated and, in our experience, correlates closely with the patient's overall sensory status.[3] Most patients will use the hand as an assist if motor function is intact, and two-point discrimination is less than 5 mm. We have not observed significant functional use when proprioception is absent, and two-point discrimination is greater than 10 mm at the fingertips or palm.

PROCEDURES TO IMPROVE HAND FUNCTION

The surgeon will be aided in selecting hemiplegic patients who will predictably benefit from surgery by following these general rules:

1. It is at least 9 months since the patient's stroke, and he has good cognition and motivation.
2. There is some selective extension of the fingers or thumb.
3. The patient uses the hand spontaneously to perform some functional activities.
4. Proprioception is intact, and two-point discrimination is less than 10 mm, preferably 5 mm at the palm or fingers.
5. The patient has no fixed joint contractures.

Surgery is performed to improve extension of the wrist, thumb, or fingers when hand opening is restricted by mild spasticity or myostatic contracture. Preoperatively, local anesthetic block of the median or ulnar nerves will permit the differentiation of spasticity from contracture. If the restriction is due to spasticity, improved extension will occur following the block, demonstrating that the patient will benefit from surgery.

Fingers

When finger extension is restricted by mild spasticity or contracture, the surgeon may improve function by lengthening the flexors to increase active extension (Fig. 15-1). Release of the flexor pronator origin has been advocated as a method for treatment of spastic wrist and finger flexion deformities.[4] This procedure requires extensive dissection, and in our experience supination deformity often results. We have found that individual tendon lengthening is a more reliable procedure.

Lengthening of spastic flexor tendons results in some loss of voluntary flexor strength. If myostatic contracture is present there is a decreased active range of muscle contraction. Hence the amount of tendon lengthening, which is determined preoperatively, is only one half the amount necessary to extend the finger from the point of restriction of voluntary extension to full extension.[4] Usually lengthening 1 cm to 1.5 cm is sufficient.

A

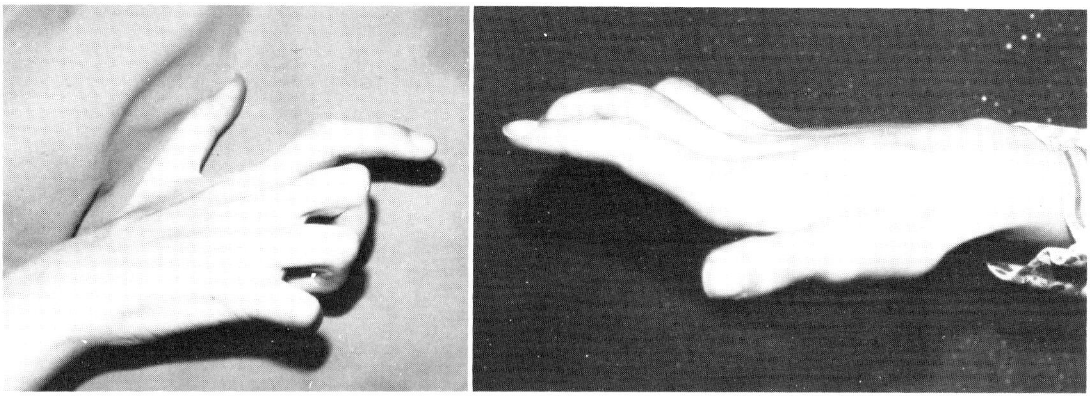

B

Fig. 15-1. A, Finger extension restricted for long, ring, and small fingers. **B,** Finger extension improved following 1 cm lengthening of sublimis and profundus tendons.

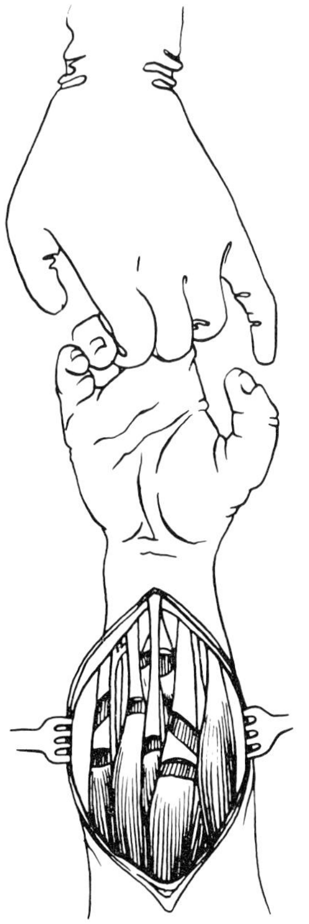

Fig. 15-2. Fractional flexor tendon lengthening is performed by making one or two transverse cuts on volar surface of flexor tendon overlying muscle fibers and inserting further distally on same tendon. Extension of fingers causes separation of cut ends. Muscle fibers underlying severed tendon preserve continuity.

Frequently on passive extension of the fingers only the sublimis tendons appear tight. However, lengthening of these tendons generally unmasks restrictive spasticity in the profundus tendons. Consequently both tendons are lengthened an equal amount.

If only one or two fingers are involved, tendon lengthening is performed either by fractional lengthening or multiple Z-plasties of the individual tendons (Fig. 15-2).[5] Thereafter, the hand is splinted in a functional position for 3 weeks before active motion is allowed.

Thumb

For some patients with voluntary key pinch between the thumb and the side of the index finger there may be restricted extension due to adductor pollicis or flexor pollicis longus spasticity. Contracture of the web space and the first dorsal interosseous muscle web is uncommon unless the deformity is long-standing. Determination of whether adductor pollicis spasticity is causing limited function is obtained by anesthetic block of the ulnar nerve. If improved extension occurs, release of the adductor is indicated (Fig. 15-3). This is performed distally at the metacarpophalangeal joint. The thumb is splinted in extension for 3 weeks following surgery. We have not observed a functionally significant loss of key pinch strength or late metacarpophalangeal instability following this procedure.

A

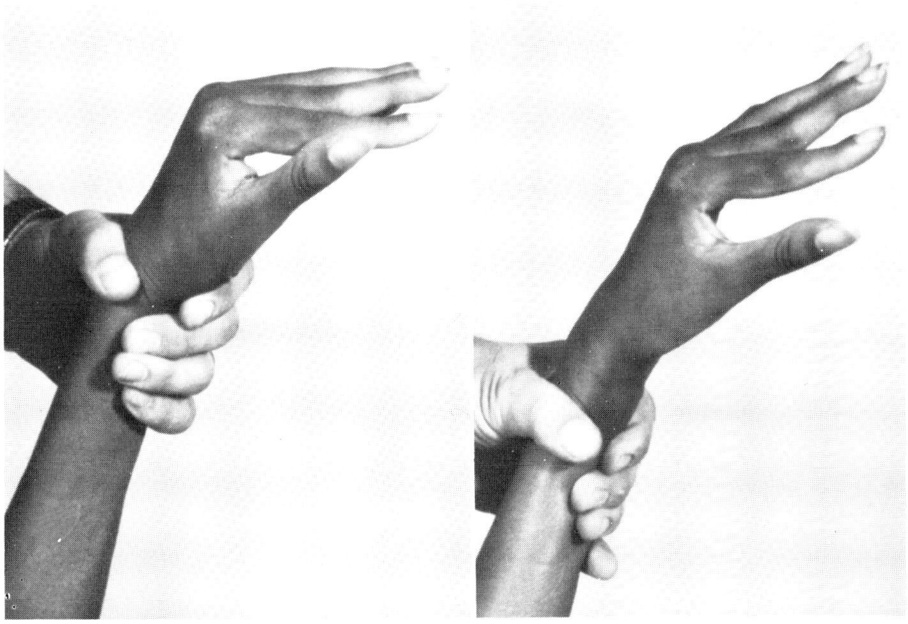

B

Fig. 15-3. A, Limited thumb opening, preventing useful hand function. **B,** Anesthetic block of ulnar nerve temporarily paralyzed adductor pollicis, enabling patient to extend thumb.

If the interphalangeal joint of the thumb is flexed during attempted extension, the flexor pollicis longus is restricting terminal extension and should be lengthened. Lengthening is in the forearm, by Z-plasty. The interphalangeal joint is fused in neutral to ensure stability. In patients with paresis of the flexor pollicus longus and hyperextension at the interphalangeal joint, hindering pinch, fusion of this joint is also indicated.

Wrist

Inadequate wrist extension may be present despite satisfactory finger extension. However, before a decision is made to lengthen the wrist flexor tendons, it must be determined whether the patient will be able to extend the fingers after the wrist flexor tendons are lengthened. If the finger flexors are shortened due to spasticity or myostatic contracture, finger extension may be lost if the wrist flexion deformity is corrected. A preoperative check should be done, with the wrist held manually in the corrected position to determine if satisfactory finger extension occurs. If it does, then wrist flexor tendon lengthening may be safely performed.

If surgery is deemed necessary, it should first be determined which wrist flexor tendons are to be lengthened. Manual palpation usually reveals the flexor carpi ulnaris is active during attempted hand opening. The contribution of the flexor carpi ulnaris can be determined by anesthetic block of the ulnar nerve. If satisfactory extension occurs, then only this tendon is lengthened. If the wrist remains flexed, then the flexor carpi radialis is lengthened also, and the palmaris longus is sectioned.

We have not found it advisable to transfer the wrist flexors to the wrist extensors in hemiplegic patients. The degree of spasticity, active range of contraction, and the pattern of activity in the individual tendons vary in each patient. No guidelines have as yet been established to allow an accurate determination of how to secure a transferred tendon under the proper amount of tension. If it is secured too tightly, wrist hyperextension will occur. Fortunately tendon transfer is seldom necessary. Most patients with selective finger extension will have sufficient wrist extensor strength if the wrist flexors are lengthened.

SURGERY IN THE NONFUNCTIONAL HAND

Surgery is indicated to correct spasticity deformities that cause pain or prevent adequate hygiene. In these instances the general guidelines for the surgeon in selecting hemiplegic patients who will benefit from surgery to improve functional use of the hand do not apply.

The surgeon should not attempt to release all finger and wrist flexors. If there was any wrist extensor tone present prior to surgery, the wrist may hyperextend postoperatively and may even dislocate dorsally.

When there are both wrist and finger flexion deformities, the sublimis to profundus transfer is a reliable method of achieving the amount of tendon lengthening necessary to extend the wrist and fingers to neutral without tension.[2] Through a volar approach in the distal forearm, all sublimis tendons are divided distally, and all profundus tendons are divided proximally. The proximal ends of the sublimis tendons are sutured en masse to the distal ends of the profundus tendons. The wrist flexor tendons and the flexor pollicis longus may be lengthened through the same incision, provided the wrist and interphalangeal joint of the thumb were flexed prior to surgery.

Unless the finger flexion deformities are long-

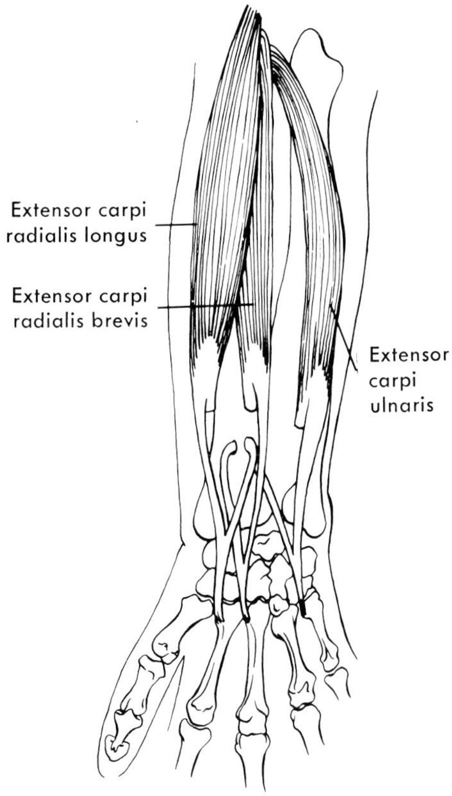

Fig. 15-4. Extensor tenodesis is performed by inserting one half of extensor carpi radialis longus, extensor carpi radialis brevis, and extensor carpi ulnaris through two drill holes in radius and suturing muscles to themselves.

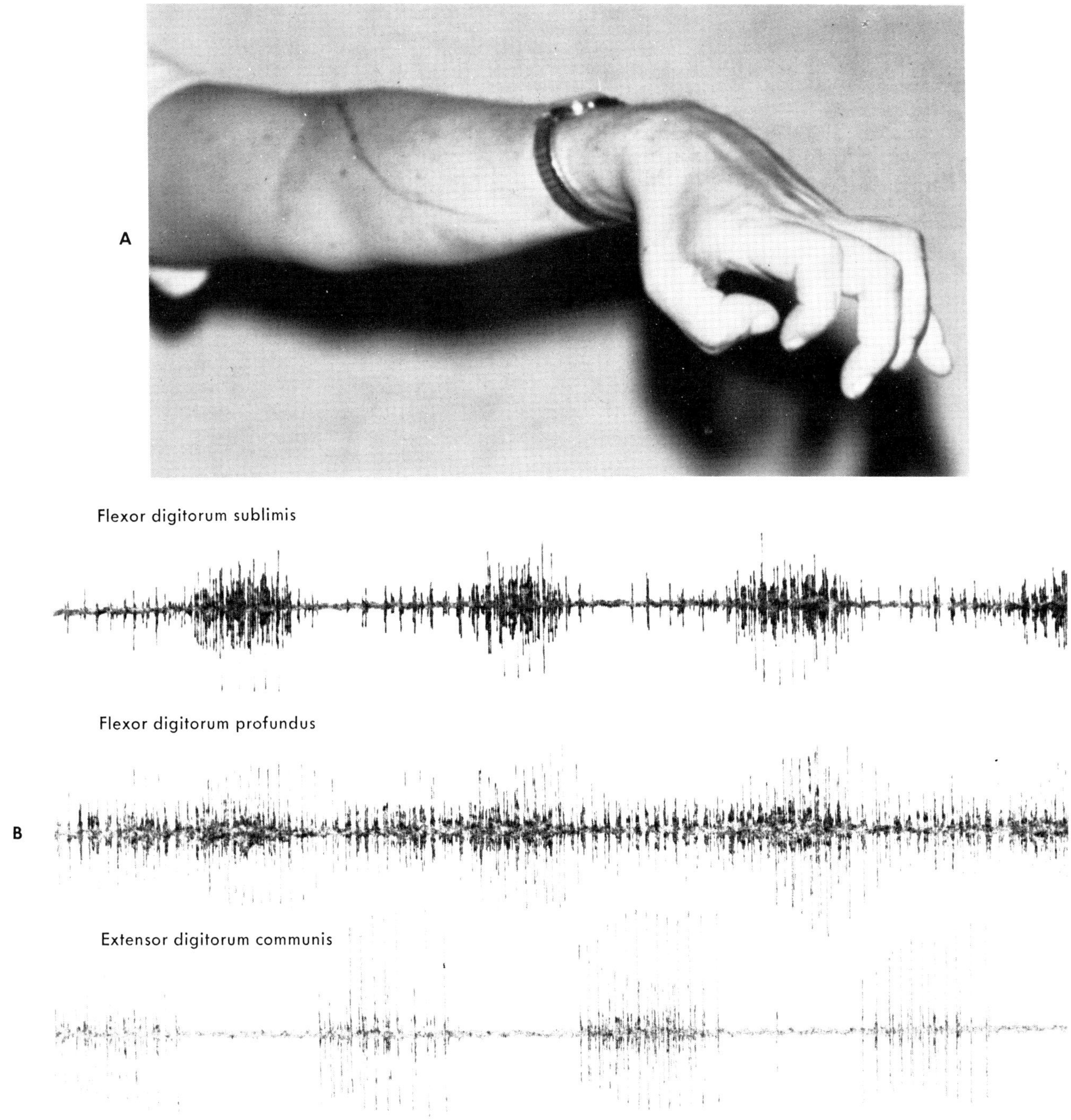

Fig. 15-5. A, Limited extension of interphalangeal joints in thumb and fingers. **B,** Electromyograms demonstrated abnormal firing of profundus tendon during finger extension. Sublimis tendon showed normal activity in flexion only. Extensor digitorum longus is normally active during extension. **C,** Improved extension was achieved following release of profundus tendons and lengthening of sublimis tendons, as well as lengthening of wrist flexor tendons. Full flexion was preserved postoperatively.

Chapter 16

Classification, evaluation, and indications for upper limb surgery in tetraplegia*

Erik Moberg

Until recently, surgical improvement of the upper limb in tetraplegia has been discouraged for fear that well-intentioned procedures would hamper rather than enhance residual function. If, however, one designs procedures that are reversible,[12] the risk becomes acceptable. For example, a contemplated arthrodesis can be pretested by simple wire fixation, and a local anesthetic block can determine the value of nerve section to control spasticity.

Today's literature abounds with surgical procedures to improve hand grip, but so far they are rarely used.† The various results obtained have been difficult to compare because very few authors have indicated the preoperative function. Most papers have classified their patients according to the level of cervical cord involvement, which does not provide enough detailed information about hand function. Some authors have used residual motor ability for operative criteria, which is an improvement, but still inadequate.‡ The status of the *afferent* impulse is of paramount importance to functional grip and must be considered in planning therapy and evaluating results.[12] Many quadriplegics have differing residuals in each arm. In a study of over 200 patients this difference was sufficient to require individualized treatment plans in opposite limbs of 50% of the patients.[14] Also the sensibility and motor function in any given limb do not necessarily correspond. We have seen as much as a four-segment difference in one patient.[12] These differences may occur because the medulla is subject to as much anatomic variation as is the peripheral nerve distribution, or because of asymmetry in the root, or because of plexus involvement.

* This work was made possible through the collaboration of several services in Scandinavia and extensive stays as Visiting Professor at the University of California, Irvine, Rancho Los Amigos Hospital, Downey, and the Veterans Administration Hospital, Long Beach, California.

† References 1, 1a, 2a, 3, 5-9, 10a, 12, 14-18.

‡ References 2a, 3, 6, 7, 16, 17.

CLASSIFICATION

I have developed a classification that considers all the above variations as a basis for surgical planning and that can also be used for multiple series comparisons.[12]

In order to have a truly useful voluntary grip one must be able to respond to different impulses (feedback). Thus our classification begins with an afferent evaluation—ocular and cutaneous.[4,11,13] The only useful test of cutaneous sensibility is two-point discrimination (see Chapter 4). Discrimination of 10 mm or better in the thumb pulp is the minimum cutaneous function required to lead a key grip.[12,14] This same test is fortuitously useful in determining proprioceptive ability.[13] Both sensibility and proprioception can therefore be quantitated and recorded numerically in each phalanx. Proprioceptive evaluation is an important but frequently neglected aspect of quadriplegia care. For example, marked muscle imbalance produces far less severe contracture if proprioception is present. If proprioception is absent, the resultant contractures can later destroy an initially promising surgical result.

My classification ignores the level of cord injury in favor of analysis of each individual limb. The two main divisions based on afferent abilities are group O, ocular afferents only, and group OCu, both ocular and functional cutaneous sensibility. The pres-

Table 3. Examined arms evaluated in Scandinavia and the United States and grouped according to Moberg classification*

Groups	*Percent of total number*	*Percent of triceps force of 3 or better*
O:0	12	0
O:1	24	3
O:2, O:3, OCu:0	6	(20? too few)
OCu:1	16	8
OCu:2	27	32
OCu:3	8	100
OCu:4-8	7	100

*Two thirds of all cases belong to groups O:1, OCu:1, and OCu:2. Less than one third have useful triceps muscle function.

ence of grade 4 muscles is then accounted for in the following scheme:

Group O (ocular afferents only)

O:0 No grade 4 muscles available
O:1 Brachioradialis (grade 4) available
O:2 O:1 plus radial carpal extensors
O:3 O:2 plus pronator
O:4 O:3 plus flexor carpi radialis
O:5 O:4 plus extensor digitorum communis
O:6 O:5 plus extensor pollicis longus
O:7 O:6 plus some of the long digital flexors
O:8 O:7 plus intrinsic hand muscles

Only grade 4 muscles are considered for transfer, as anything less usually functions poorly. Posttraumatic paraplegia patients rarely achieve above O:3, but this higher combination can be seen in other conditions.

An identical scale is created for OCu (i.e., OCu:0, OCu:1, etc.). In those patients whose limbs show fewer defects or near-normal function, direct description of the loss is usually preferable.

The classification can then be augmented by adding Tr− or Tr+ (for triceps) or the triceps can be listed by grade (i.e., Tr 3).

I have used this classification for 4 years on over 400 limbs and found it easily understood and practical. Table 3 shows the grouping of arms according to our classification.

Case selection

This classification is used as a basis for selecting appropriate procedures properly timed and in logical order. A candidate for reconstruction must be a wheelchair sitter. Pressure sores are a contraindication and indeed should be treated on an independent schedule so as not to interfere with the timing of the limb surgery.

The dominant hand should always be operated on first,[12] and the patient should not be permitted to influence this decision. If only ocular afferents are present, then only one hand should be provided with grip. If both limbs are fairly similar in their sensory and motor resources, then the preinjury dominant hand will persist. If the difference between limbs is greater than one step on the scale, then the better limb should be considered as dominant despite the preinjury status or even the preoperative preference.

If elbow extension requires restoration,[1,1a,10a,14] then this should be done first. This avoids the frustration of depriving the patient of his newly reconstructed hand function for the 3-month recovery period following elbow surgery. Even more importantly, functional elbow extension facilitates learning to use a newly transferred brachioradialis. It is very difficult to isolate brachioradialis function from the other elbow flexors in the absence of an antagonist elbow extensor.

Patients with high-order function may benefit from complex reconstructions. Those in the O:1 to O:3 range cannot expect more than key pinch sometimes accompanied by weak pronation.[12] The same is true of OCu:1 and probably also OCu:2 and OCu:3. In a few cases some finger flexion may possibly be added[6,8,17] especially if the extensor carpi radialis brevis is strong. In general, a tenodesed thumb has a stronger key pinch than when flexion is restored by tendon transfer.

In the occasional patient (7% of all patients) who has an OCu:4 limb, thumb adduction can be reconstructed, and finger flexion is optimistic. Patients with even less disability must be carefully evaluated to determine what, if any, individualized procedure would be of benefit.

One must not let the patient's impatience shorten the time between procedures or convince the surgeon to do two procedures at once. If the elbow and hand are done at one sitting, the patient is left helpless, and adequate retraining is delayed and impaired. The hand should not be done until the elbow recovers 90 degrees of flexion and full extension. Ideally each stage should await full recovery and retraining of the previous procedure. Impaired afferent impulses compounded by generally decreased endurance tend to prolong reeducation in these patients.

There are patients in whom elbow extension should be reconstructed even if there is no potential for improving hand function. Driving, wheelchair propulsion, and bimanual tasks can be improved. It is paramount that each patient fully understand the narrow functional range in which improvement is possible. Frequently, previously treated patients can relate realistic expectations to the patient better than the surgeon can, and they should be encouraged to do so.

CONTRAINDICATIONS

The following situations contraindicate surgical reconstruction:

1. *The bedridden patient.* The bedridden patient cannot be properly examined nor can postoperative reeducation be satisfactorily carried out. The patient must be wheelchair mobile.

2. *General inactivity.* Patients with major psychologic problems, especially when they lead to inactivity, make poor surgical candidates. The patient must eagerly seek the surgery. If he is at all hesitant, surgery should be postponed until the patient is convinced of its merit and limitations by discussion with others who have had the surgery. Unrealistic patients are difficult to deal with and will frequently discourage other candidates.

3. *Spasticity.* While it is generally a contraindication, spasticity in an occasional patient may be a useful adjunct to surgery.

4. *Abnormal muscle quality.* An occasionally seen phenomenon is slow "creeping" muscle activity. This peculiar quality is as yet unnamed and difficult to adequately test for. Even if they are under voluntary control, such muscles will not produce an acceptable transfer.

5. *Lack of proper rehabilitative facilities.* One must not lose sight of the total needs of the tetraplegic patient. Bowel care, urinary problems, and pressure sore prevention are even more difficult if the patient's arm is in plaster. Many general hospital wards lack the properly trained personnel and special facilities for such patients.

6. *Poor physician continuity.* The entire rehabilitative effort from surgery through reeducation must be in the hands of one surgeon with both the interest and the skill to manage the entire program. Fragmentation of care can be disastrous.

We have found that age per se and long-established tetraplegia are not contraindications to reconstruction (Table 4).

Table 4. Time between accident and reconstruction in a number of Scandinavian cases

Time elapsed (years)	*No. of cases*
<1	8
1-2	20
2-3	7
3-5	8
5-8	13
>8	14

SUMMARY

I have presented a classification for the tetraplegic upper extremity that emphasizes afferent sensory and proprioceptive impulses. The philosophy of patient selection for surgical reconstruction and the contraindications have been discussed. The reader is referred to previous references for details of the surgical procedure and reeducational program.[12-14]

REFERENCES

1. Bryan, R. S.: The Moberg deltoid-triceps replacement and key-pinch operation in quadriplegia: preliminary experiences, Hand **9:**207-214, 1977.
1a. DeBenedetti, M.: Restoration of elbow extension in the quadriplegic patient using the Moberg technique. Paper given at the annual meeting of the American Society for Surgery of the Hand in Dallas, 1978.
2. Freehafer, A. A.: Care of hands in cervical spinal cord injuries, Paraplegia **7:**118-129, 1969.
2a. Freehafer, A. A., and Mast, W. A.: Transfer of the brachioradialis to improve wrist extension in high spinal cord injury, J. Bone Joint Surg. [Am.] **49:**648-652, 1967.
3. Freehafer, A. A., von Hamm, E., and Allen, V.: Tendon transfers to improve grasp in cervical spinal cord injury patients, J. Bone Joint Surg. [Am.] **56:**951-959, 1974.
4. Granit, R.: The functional role of muscle spindles—facts and hypotheses, Brain **98:**531-556, 1975.
5. Lamb, D. W.: The management of upper limb in cervical cord injuries. In Proceedings of a Symposium held in the Royal College of Surgeons of Edinburgh, June 1963, London, 1963, Morrison and Gibbs Ltd.
6. Lamb, D. W., and Landry, R. M.: The hand in quadriplegia, Hand **3:**31-37, 1971.
7. Lamb, D. W., and Landry, R. M.: The hand in quadriplegia, Paraplegia **9:**204-212, 1972.
8. Lipscomb, P. R., Elkins, E. C., and Henderson, E. D.: Tendon transfers to restore function of hands in tetraplegia, especially after fracture-dislocation of the sixth cervical vertebra on the seventh, J. Bone Joint Surg. [Am.] **40:**1071-1080, 1958.
9. McDowell, C.: Tendon transfer to augment of wrist extension in the tetraplegic patient. In Proceedings of Veterans Administration Spinal Cord Injury Conference, **18:**78, 1971.
10. Moberg, E.: Criticism and study of methods for examining sensibility in the hand, Neurology (Minneap.) **12:**8-19, 1962.

10a. Moberg, E.: Editorial, Hand **9:**205-206, 1977.
11. Moberg, E.: Fingers were made before forks, Hand **4:**201-206, 1972.
12. Moberg, E.: Surgical treatment for absent single-hand grip and elbow extension in quadriplegia, J. Bone Joint Surg. [Am.] **57:**196-206, 1975.
13. Moberg, E.: Reconstructive hand surgery in tetraplegia, stroke and cerebral palsy: some basic concepts in physiology and neurology, J. Hand Surg. **1:**29-34, 1976.
14. Moberg, E.: The upper limb in tetraplegia. A new approach to surgical rehabilitation, Stuttgart, 1978, Thieme.
14a. Newman, J. H.: The use of the key-grip procedure for improving hand function in quadriplegia, Hand **9:**215-220, 1977.
15. Nickel, V. L., Perry, J., and Garrett, A. L.: Development of useful function in the severely paralyzed hand, J. Bone Joint Surg. [Am.] **45:**933-951, 1963.
16. Zancolli, E. A.: Structural and dynamic bases of hand surgery, Philadelphia, 1968, J. B. Lippincott Com- pany.
17. Zancolli, E. A.: Surgery for the quadriplegic hand with active, strong wrist extension preserved. A study of 97 cases, Clin. Orthop. **112:**101-113, 1975.
18. Zrubecky, G.: Operative und konservative Wiederherstellung einer Greifform von schlaff gelähmten Händen bei Halsmarkgeschädigten, Handchirurgie **4:**71-79, 1972.

Chapter 17

The upper extremity in cerebral palsy

M. Mark Hoffer

There are four factors to be considered in planning care for the upper limb in cerebral palsy. These are cognition, sensibility, placement, and control of the muscles of the hand.[3,4,9,11]

Cognition is often difficult to assess, especially when there is communication difficulty. Speech problems, difficulty in controlling facial musculature, and mood make intelligence testing for these children a considerable task.

Sensibility in cerebral palsy is never lost to sharp or dull discrimination. This is because gross sensation is thalamic and is rarely affected by cerebral palsy. It is the sophisticated cortical sensibility that is lost in these patients.[12] This sophisticated sensibility is best tested by texture, graphesthesia, or two-point discrimination. The specific test utilized depends on age and cognition of the child. Object identification is frequently used to test cortical sensibility, but it must be realized that motor control also affects this test.

Placement of the cerebral palsied hand is a combined problem of body, shoulder, and elbow action. The range of motion is limited by contracture or spasticity of these parts. The speed of placement is limited by motion disorders (dyskinesia, athetosis) which require that the arm make a circuitous pathway to an object. The precision of placement is limited by motion disorders (ataxia, tremors) which affect the end point of placement activities. It is convenient to document the speed and precision of placement of the studied hand on the opposite knee and the top of the head (Fig. 17-1).

Muscle control of the hand first depends on spasticity. Spasticity is defined as increased tone-to-stretch reflex. Minor degrees of spasticity may exist in limbs with good function. Severe spasticity, however, leads to secondary fixed contractures of muscle-tendon units and joints. These fixed contractures rarely develop in sophisticated upper limbs; when one sees these deformities, function is surely affected.

Retained perinatal reflexes are a second problem affecting muscle control in cerebral palsy hands. The posture of the head, neck, and body

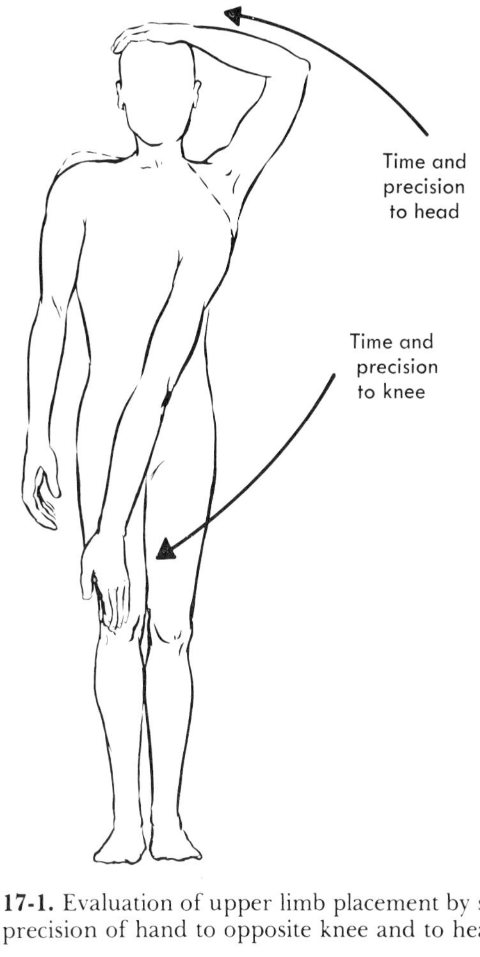

Fig. 17-1. Evaluation of upper limb placement by speed and precision of hand to opposite knee and to head.

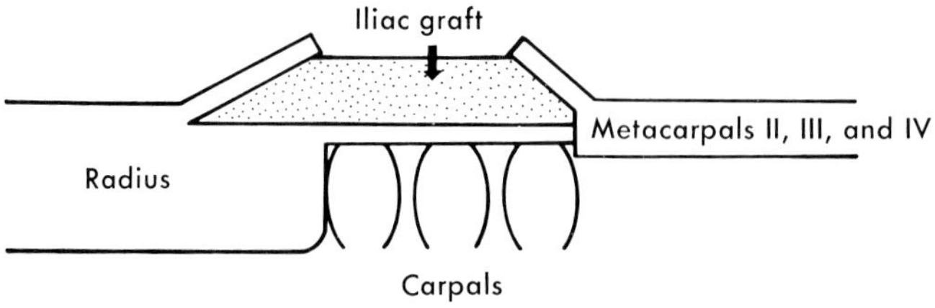

Fig. 17-2. Wrist fusion method using two cross pins, for hygiene or cosmetic reasons only.

may oblige a limb to go into mass flexion or extension when such reflexes exist. In the tonic neck reflexes the upper limb on the facial side of a rotated head goes into mass extension, while the occipital side goes into mass flexion (like a fencing posture). The tonic neck reflex also operates when the neck is flexed, obliging the upper limb to go into mass flexion, while when the neck is extended, the limb goes into mass extension. The upper limb can also be affected by primitive reflexes when the body is changed from prone to supine. Hands that are obligatory slaves to these primitive mass reflexes have poor functional potential.

A third problem affecting muscle control is that of synergistic tone patterns. Here the apparent strength of a muscle and its tone may be related to the position of adjacent joints, the activity of "agonists," and the activity of "antagonists." These synergistic muscle patterns make muscle testing very difficult. We feel that muscle tests for strength are valid only when patients have selective control of the muscle, free of dominance by the synergistic patterns. In studying synergistic patterns it is wise to study the muscle action in grasp, release, and pinch. Muscles that have uncontrolled tone throughout the patterns should be released or lengthened. When tendon transfers are planned, they should be made within the functional synergistic patterns. Here electromyograms may be helpful in making surgical plans.[8]

Realistic goals for hand use are based on the aforementioned four factors. An individual who has poor cognition, poor sensibility, poor hand placement, and no selective control of the muscles in the upper extremity has "all four strikes against him." A posture that permits hygiene is the only realistic goal for these hands. An individual who has good cognition and the other three strikes (poor sensibility, poor placement, and poor selective control) against him would be a candidate for creation of a hand that is cosmetically pleasing, and also facilitates hygiene. An individual with good cognition, sensibility, and placement but with some mus-

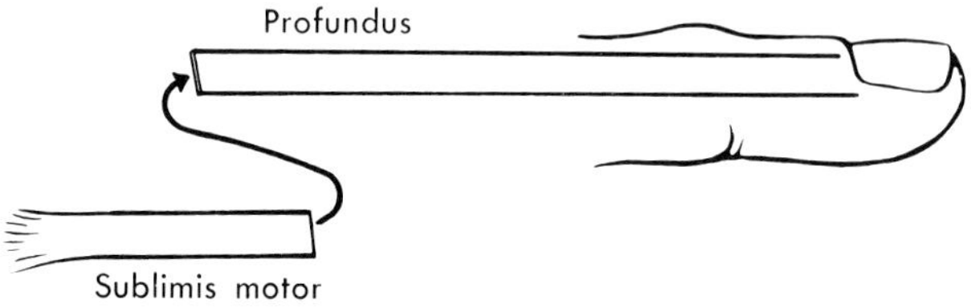

Fig. 17-3. Sublimis to profundus transfer of Braun for hygiene or cosmetic reasons only.

cle control problems would definitely benefit most from functional surgical procedures. An individual with all four factors working well obviously would have no real need for surgical intervention.

Hygiene and cosmetic operative procedures in patients with four or three strikes against them usually consist of correction of wrist flexion, thumb in palm, and finger flexion contractures. These individuals respond inconsistently to muscle transfers or simple lengthening procedures. Our policy for such hands is to perform radial-metacarpal wrist fusions with iliac bone graft and pin fixation. This decision is usually not arrived at till age 12 or 13 so that growth considerations are met (Fig. 17-2). At the same time we lengthen the muscle tendon units in the fingers by sublimis to profundus transfers[2] and perform tunnel and thumb releases (Fig. 17-3).

Functional procedures are performed on those individuals with good cognition, sensibility, and placement but with problems in muscle control. The problems in muscle control seem to revolve around the three main areas of pinch, grasp, and release (Fig. 17-4). When the thumb and palm deformity exists in these individuals, thumb-web release of the skin by Z-plasty (Fig. 17-5) and release of the adductor and first dorsal interosseus from the thumb metacarpal (Fig. 17-6) allow opening of the thumb from the palm.[7] In addition, it may be necessary to augment the thumb extensor by tendon transfer. Furthermore, there are times when one will see hyperextensibility of the thenar meta-

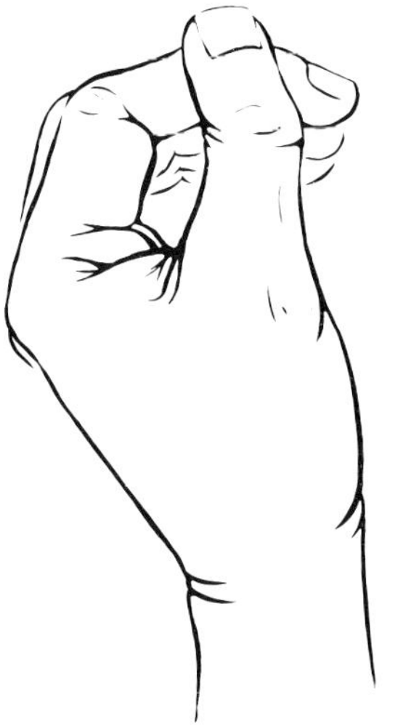

Fig. 17-4. Side pinch is goal in many cerebral palsied hands.

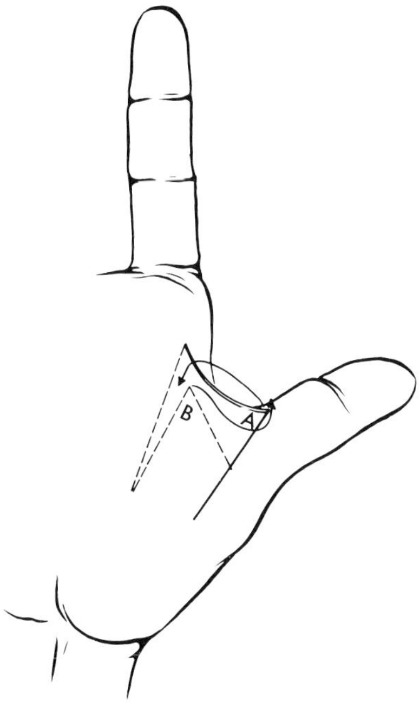

Fig. 17-5. Steps in Z-plasty of first cleft in cerebral palsy.

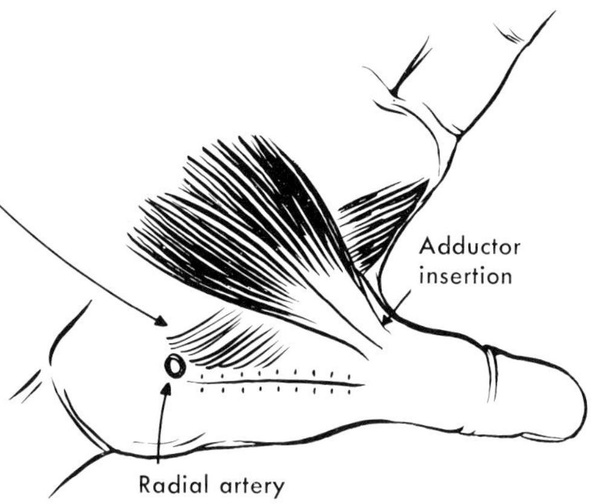

Fig. 17-6. Z-plasty is completed by intrinsic release of thumb.

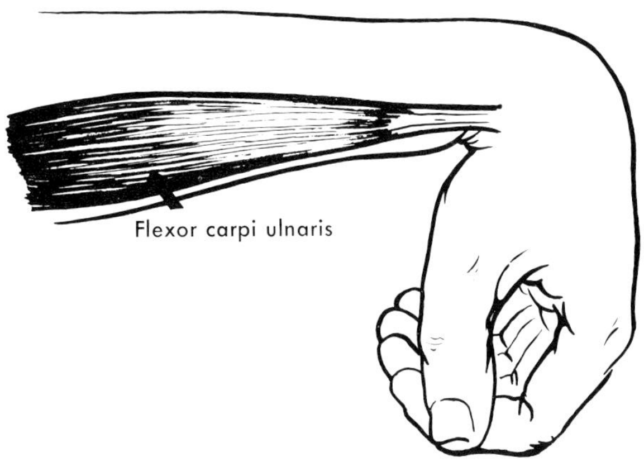

Fig. 17-7. Wrist-flexed grasp due to wrist flexor–finger flexor synergy.

carpophalangeal joint. For such loose joints, capsulodesis with temporary pin fixation of the joint is helpful.[2]

Patients with grasp problems are obliged to use wrist flexors at the time of finger flexion. This discoordinate action of wrist flexors and finger flexors weakens the effective power of the fingers (Fig. 17-7). Here a transfer of the wrist flexor to the wrist extensor would allow the patient to flex his fingers in vigorous grasp while his wrist is extended (Fig. 17-8). Before performing such a procedure, one should be sure that, with the wrist held in neutral, the fingers can be actively extended.[5] If they cannot, it is possible that one is dealing with a separate problem, that of release.

Those patients with problems of release have difficulty opening the fingers into extension with the wrist extended. They are obliged to flex their wrist to open the fingers. In this case there is often synergism between the finger extensors and the

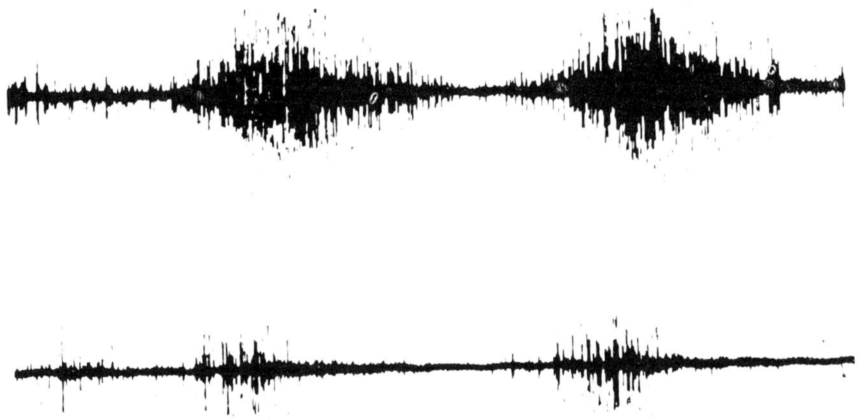

Fig. 17-8. An example of wire electromyogram used to help plan tendon transfer. Here a wrist-flexed grasp is seen clinically and postoperatively. By electromyogram, flexor carpi ulnaris and central wrist extensor are not active in grasp; thus transfer will be "phasic."

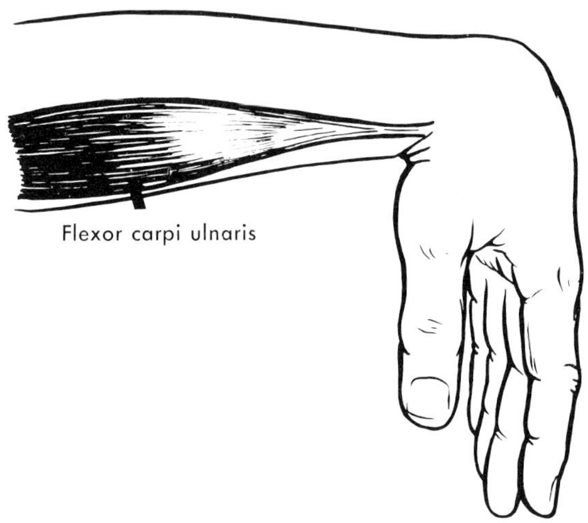

Fig. 17-9. Wrist-flexed release due to wrist flexor–finger extensor synergy.

wrist flexors (Fig. 17-9). This is reminiscent of the tenodesis action that one often sees in paralytics. However, in most cerebral palsy patients there is no fixed contracture, and it is a matter of synergistic release rather than tenodesis release. Again, the electromyograms can help define the pattern. When the flexed wrist–release combination is seen, transfer of wrist flexors to the finger extensors may be helpful (Fig. 17-10).

There are numerous other procedures that have been introduced for the care of these more sophisticated cerebral palsied hands. These include the sublimis tenodesis for the hyperextended proximal interphalangeal joint,[10] the use of the brachioradialis, which is an excellent muscle transfer,[4] and lengthening of the spastic and tight sublimis muscle at the musculotendinous junction. One should rarely perform flexor slides[6] in these more sophisticated

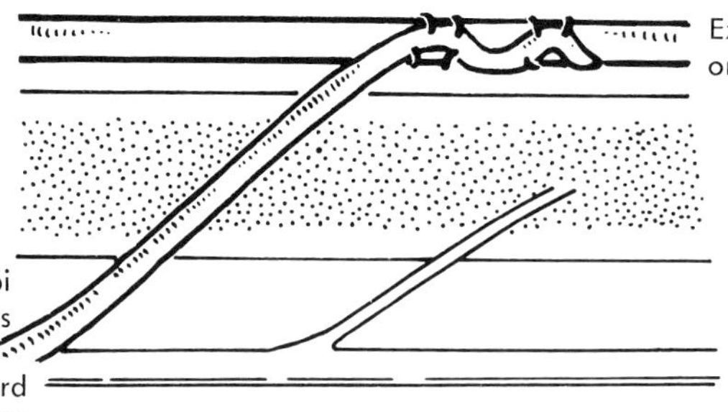

Fig. 17-10. Transfer of flexor carpi ulnaris. Tendon passed subcutaneously around ulnar aspect of forearm.

hands for fear that they will lose significant strength. Wrist fusions are poorly tolerated in functional cerebral palsied hands.

It must be admitted that making surgical plans for the cerebral palsied hand is very difficult. Each child seems different and unique. Intelligence, sensibility, placement, and muscle control are all difficult entities to test. Current experiments with functional orthoses and needle electromyograms promise to help us make more predictable and rational preoperative judgments in these complex children.

REFERENCES

1. Braun, R. M., and Vise, G. T.: Sublimis to profundis transfers in the hemiplegic upper extremity, J. Bone Joint Surg. [Am.] **55:**873, 1973.
2. Filler, B. C., and Stark, H. H.: Capsulodesis of the thumb MCP joint in cerebral palsy children, J. Bone Joint Surg. [Am.] **56:**199, 1974.
3. Goldner, J. L.: Reconstructive surgery in the hand in cerebral palsy, J. Bone Joint Surg. [Am.] **37:**1141-1955.
4. Goldner, J. L.: The upper extremity in cerebral palsy. In Samilson, R., editor: Orthopedic aspects of cerebral palsy, Philadelphia, 1975, J. B. Lippincott Company.
5. Green, W. T., and Banks, H.: Flexor carpi ulnaris transplant, J. Bone Joint Surg. [Am.] **44:**1343-1352, 1962.
6. Inglis, A. E., and Copper, W.: Release of the flexor-pronator origin of the hand and wrist in spastic paralysis, J. Bone Joint Surg. [Am.] **48:**847, 1966.
7. Matev, I. B.: Surgical treatment of flexion adduction contracture of the thumbs in cerebral palsy, Acta Orthop. Scand. **41:**439-445, 1970.
8. Samilson, R. L., and Morris, J. M.: Surgical improvement of the cerebral palsied upper limbs, J. Bone Joint Surg. [Am.] **46:**1203-1218, 1964.
9. Samilson, R. L.: Principles of assessment of upper limbs in cerebral palsy, Clin Orthop. **47:**105-115, 1966.
10. Swanson, A. B.: Surgery of the hand in cerebral palsy, J. Bone Joint Surg. [Am.] **42:**951, 1960.
11. Swanson, A. B.: Surgery of the hand in cerebral palsy, Surg. Clin. North Am. **48:**1129, 1968.
12. Tachdjian, M. O., and Minear, W. L.: Sensory disturbances in the hands of children with cerebral palsy, J. Bone Joint Surg. [Am.] **40:**85, 1958.

Chapter 18

The surgical treatment of drooling

Garry S. Brody
Theodore F. Wilkie†

Drooling (sialozemia) is salivary incontinence due to a lack of control rather than an overproduction of saliva (sialorrhea). This may be intermittent and can be caused by neuromuscular disorders or damage to the oral structure from neoplasm or trauma. Simple overproduction of saliva is virtually never the cause of drooling, although excessive secretion may be found in such patients as a secondary compensatory phenomenon. The commonest cause of clinical drooling is neurologic, primarily cerebral palsy with or without profound mental retardation.

Significant drooling occurs in those cerebral palsy patients with major suprabulbar involvement, and it assumes considerable importance in the daily lives of those so afflicted. Many such patients are able to control food and saliva loss when they consciously concentrate on the use of all the accessory mechanisms (Fig. 18-1). The head-back posture, conscious lip closure, posterior positioning of food on insertion, and conscious tongue control, as well as a hand-held towel, aid in keeping the face and clothes dry. These measures require considerable concentration, and continence deteriorates when the child is distracted. One of the most distressing consequences of drooling is the soiling of tabletop activities, tools, papers, and so on while the child is concentrating on his work or television and thus is distracted from conscious efforts at control. The social stigma of a wet chin and sodden shirt is extremely distressing even to moderately retarded children, but most prefer this to bibs and towels (Fig. 18-2). Many continually clutch cloths or paper tissues, wear terry cloth wristlets, or use other ingenious catchment devices devised by resourceful mothers. We have seen multihandicapped patients who refuse any other corrective surgery except for drooling control, which they consider their worst affliction, possibly because they have spent much of their life being reminded of it by the looks of revulsion from strangers and the remonstrations of those close to them (Fig. 18-3).

PHYSIOLOGY AND PATHOPHYSIOLOGY OF SALIVARY CONTROL

Previously reported cineradiographic studies[16,17] show that patients drool because of lack of proper control of the muscles of the oral cavity that

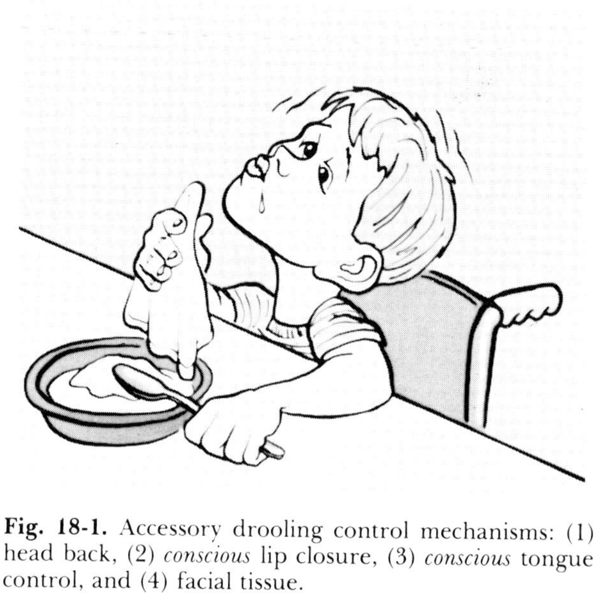

Fig. 18-1. Accessory drooling control mechanisms: (1) head back, (2) *conscious* lip closure, (3) *conscious* tongue control, and (4) facial tissue.

†Dr. Wilkie, to whom this volume is dedicated, passed away after participating in the final preparation of this chapter. To him belongs all the credit for the initial understanding of this problem and the basis of the operative solution.

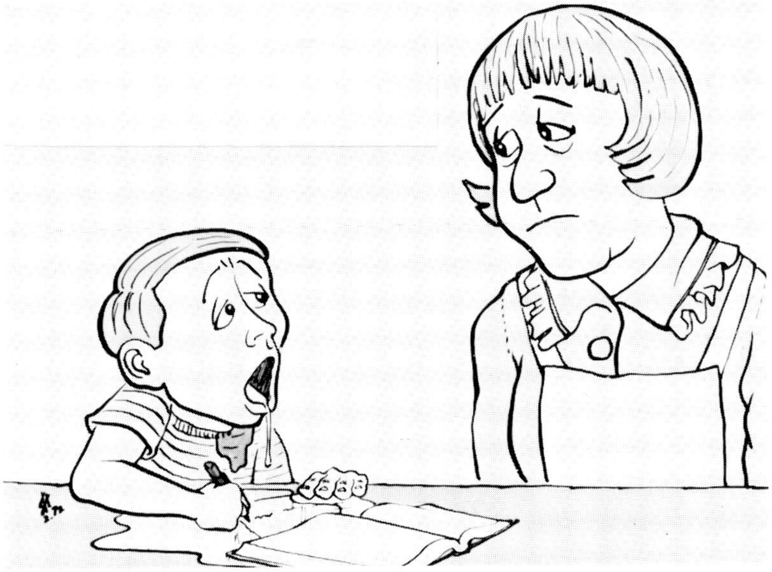

Fig. 18-2. "Social stigma" of a wet chin.

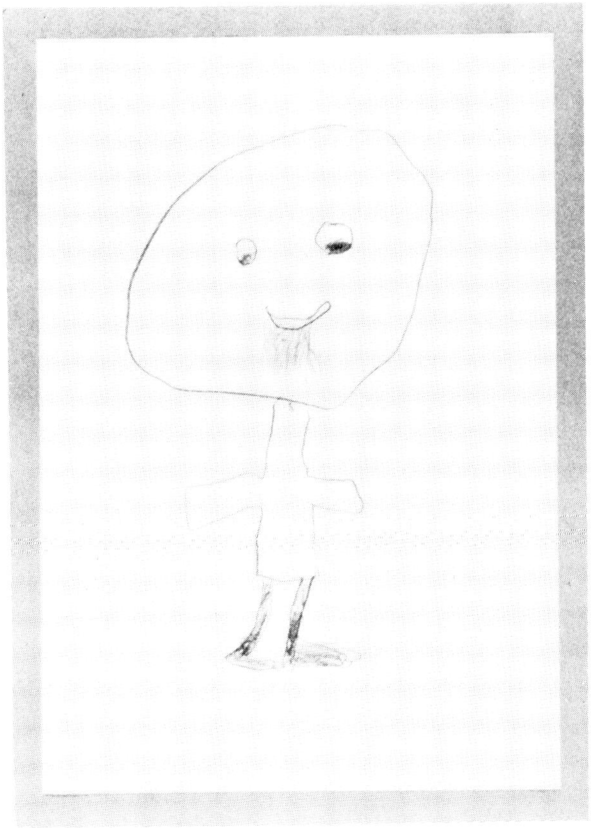

Fig. 18-3. Self-portrait of a child who drools. Child stated that scribbling under lips was "slobbering."

normally initiate swallowing (lips, cheeks, floor of the mouth, tongue, soft palate, and upper pharynx). A bolus of food or fluid (or saliva) is normally fed by the muscles of the cheek and floor of the mouth to the tongue. The tongue cups itself against the palate with an efficient seal, and the bolus is forced along the roof of the mouth to the oropharynx. Automatic swallowing reflexes take over as soon as the food has reached the lower pharynx and esophagus, propelling the bolus and closing and elevating the glottis. All patients studied were able to swallow normally once the bolus had reached the throat. It is therefore assumed that although the anterior (oral) phase can be severely abnormal, an abnormality of the posterior (or automatic) swallowing phase is probably not consistent with life, as death from aspiration would occur in infancy.

Virtually all patients who drool due to neuromuscular disorders have some problem with speech, which is not necessarily related to intellectual ability. (Two patients have been encountered who drool despite apparently normal speech, deglutition, and intelligence and whose drooling is therefore inexplicable. They both improved spontaneously by age 10 or 11.)

MANAGEMENT

Commonly this problem has been treated by encouraging resigned acceptance, due to ignorance, failure of other treatments, or the hope that neurologic maturation will permit the child to "grow out of it."

Drug therapy

Parasympatholytic drugs usually have not worked well. The drooling associated with parkinsonism may sometimes respond well to drugs such as amantadine and L-dopa.

Radiation therapy

Although control of drooling is perhaps a happy sequela of therapy for oral cancer, we have never encountered a cerebral palsy patient who has received radiation to control drooling. Undoubtedly radiotherapists hesitate to prescribe the dosage required to destroy salivary secretion for nonmalignant disease, especially in children. The dry, painful oral mucitis, the destructive effect on growth, and the resultant malignancies are unjustifiable side effects.

Ligation of the parotid ducts

Parotid duct ligation has been practiced for years in ablative surgery, but refistulization and parotitis are common sequelae. It would also seem more physiologic to preserve the parotid secretions for whatever digestive and other physiologic roles they may play if this can be done without compromising drooling control.

Tympanic neurectomy[8,11,13]

Denervating procedures attacking the auriculotemporal and submandibular ganglion or the tympanic plexus and chorda tympani work temporarily, but drooling eventually recurs. It is alleged by some that taste sensation returns after sectioning the chorda tympani, but we believe it is cruel to risk the destruction of the only pleasurable sensation some of these severely involved patients may have.

Physiotherapy

The Mueller technique[1,2,10] of oral stimulation is effective when started in infancy, but the success rate drops if initiated beyond age 3 or 4.

Salivary gland surgery

Rationale. The parotid and submandibular glands produce 90% to 95% of saliva, with the volume distributed approximately equally. The remainder is secreted by sublingual glands and the oral mucosa itself. Normally approximately 1,000 to 1,500 ml of saliva is secreted per day.[14] Ablative surgery has taught us that two or more salivary glands can be removed without serious physiologic consequence. The submandibular glands can be removed with relative ease, but parotid resection is most complicated with considerable risk to the facial nerve.

Wilkie postulated that if the saliva could enter directly into the pharynx, then the need for coordinated tongue and cheek manipulation would be bypassed.[16,17] Eating would not be affected, but drooling should be controlled. Denis-Browne[5] demonstrated that a strip of epithelium buried subcutaneously to reconstruct a urethra would spontaneously tube itself. This principle was borrowed to devise a technique of lengthening the parotid duct so that it could be rerouted toward the tonsillar fossa. A strip of mucosa attached to the parotid orifice is elevated and slipped into a submucosal tunnel that is made to exit at the anterior pillar, as low as technically feasible. We have adequate evidence that this mucosal extension spontaneously tubes itself, forming a duct that opens far enough posteriorly to deposit the saliva where pharyngeal swallowing can handle it. It soon became apparent to Wilkie that ductal rerouting alone was not sufficient; all four major glands must be dealt with, and *submandibular gland resection is required for complete salivary control.* Fistulization of even one parotid transplant after submandibular ablation is enough to produce recurrent drooling almost as severe as preoperatively.

PREOPERATIVE EVALUATION

A history of significant drooling is required to justify surgery. Typically these patients will saturate two to three bibs or shirtfronts per day. A diary should be kept for 3 to 5 days if there is some uncertainty as to the severity of the problem.

The careful preoperative detailed measurement of salivary loss and cineradiographic studies by Wilkie[16,17] securely established the mechanism and rationale for this surgery. Clinically this detailed workup is not required for the average patient.

Initially, prior tonsillectomy was recommended before diversionary surgery. Currently this is only suggested if the tonsils are significantly enlarged or subject to recurrent infection. Severely retarded patients who exhibit extensive pica should be considered for surgery only guardedly, as oral hygiene may become extremely difficult and the pica more offensive. The only *specific* contraindication is restricted mandibular excursion great enough to limit surgical exposure.

Informed consent should include the following discussion:

1. No alteration of eating or speech patterns can be expected.

2. The spectrum of good results may include some small amount of residual froth that may dry on the lips.
3. The residual saliva may be thicker, requiring increased oral hygiene.
4. Occasionally, excess dryness on awakening and a change in dental health may be encountered.
5. The family should be advised of the marked postoperative edema seen in the cheeks, peaking at 48 hours, and the 3 to 4 days of discomfort.
6. The complications specific to this procedure such as ductal stenosis and recurrent drooling should be discussed.
7. Drooling may recur during periods of acute illness or stress or while antiepileptic medication is being adjusted.

THE SURGICAL PROCEDURE

All four glands are operated upon at one sitting, requiring 1 to 2 hours for an experienced surgeon. Transnasal endotracheal anesthesia is used. *It is important to avoid placing restraining straps across the legs, especially in nonambulatory patients whose long bones may be osteoporotic. Postanesthetic spasms can fracture a fragile femur secured against such restraints.* Straps across the torso are safe.

The operation consists of bilateral submandibular gland resection and posterior transplantation of the extended parotid ducts.

Submandibular gland resection is done through symmetric 2 to 3 cm incisions parallel to the mandibular margin at the lowest pole of the usually visible subtle bulge formed by the gland. If the incision is truly parallel to and 2 cm below the mandibular border, the marginal branch of the facial nerve will

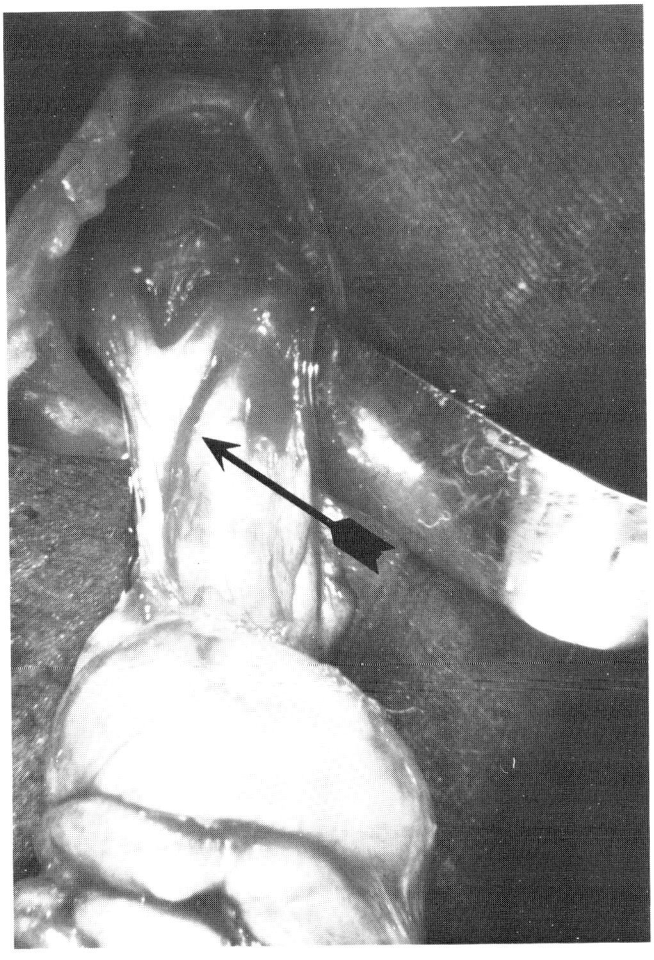

Fig. 18-4. Lingual nerve tented into wound by traction on parasympathetic fibers supplying submandibular ganglion.

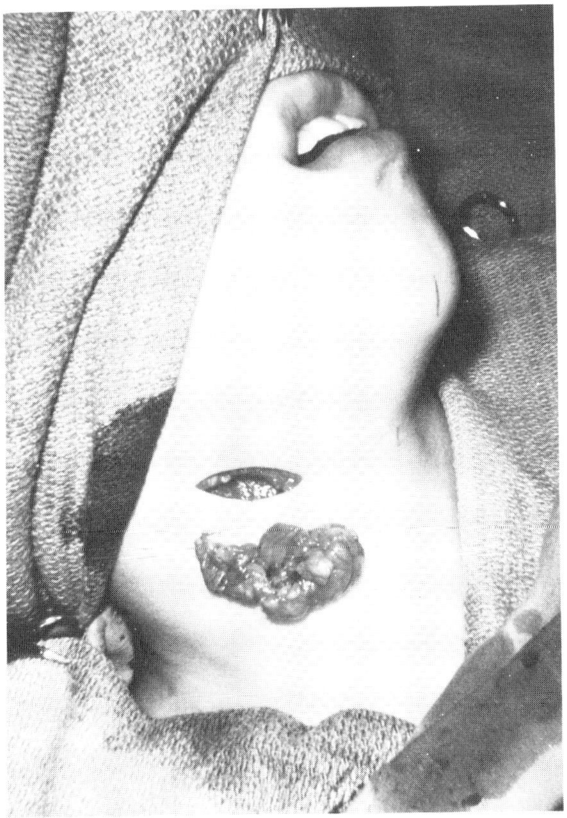

Fig. 18-5. Enlarged submandibular gland. (From Wilkie, T. F., and Brody, G. S.: Plast. Reconstr. Surg. **59:**791, 1977.)

be avoided. It is not necessary to be strictly in the skin creases if they conflict with this direction as scar hypertrophy has not been seen.

As the submandibular glands are not diseased or neoplastic the dissection should be subcapsular. This is an easy and constantly avascular plane on the superficial and deep aspects and inferior margins, and avoids the hypoglossal nerve, which will not be seen. The vascular arrangement on the anterior, posterior, and superior margins is highly variable. Radical excision of all glandular elements should be avoided as preservation of some sublingual glands is usually desired. (In some severely athetoid patients more aggressive removal of the sublingual

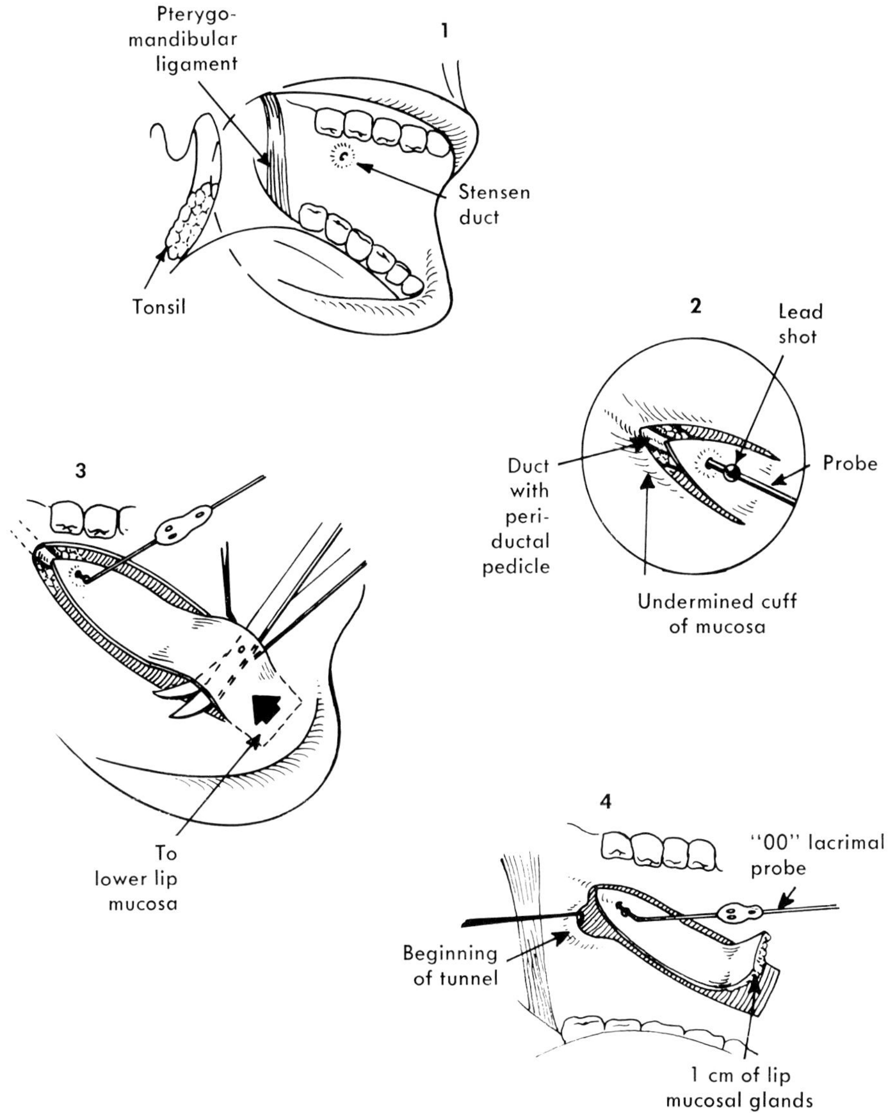

Fig. 18-6. Technique of parotid duct extension and translocation. *1,* Operative field is injected with lidocaine (Xylocaine) and epinephrine. *2,* A good cuff of mucosa must be undermined around duct to avoid kinking and to permit a watertight closure. *3,* Plane of dissection should be superficial to buccinator muscle. This flap is probably not totally vascularized, and distal portion therefore must survive as a free graft. Duct should not be skeletonized but should stay within leash of associated vessels and soft tissue. Cheek fat pad is seen at this point. Duct should be free enough to retropose into submucosal tunnel (see steps 6 and 8). *4,* Flap is raised obliquely anteriorly and caudad toward lower labial sulcus. If distal end of flap contains 1 cm of lip mucosal glands, it will be of sufficient length. *Short flaps produce stenosis.* Closure of cheek defect decreases redundancy and aids in control.

glands should be done as their thrashing tongues will whip the residual saliva into a stiff and offensive foam.) Meticulous care should be taken to avoid the lingual nerve, which frequently tents sharply into the operative field from traction on the specimen (Fig. 18-4). Pathologic examination of the resected gland has suggested glandular hypertrophy in a significant percentage but by no means all of the patients (Fig. 18-5). One could easily conjecture about the compensatory mechanisms that may cause this.

The modified technique of parotid duct extension and translocation currently used is diagramed in Fig. 18-6. The mucosa of patients on antiseizure

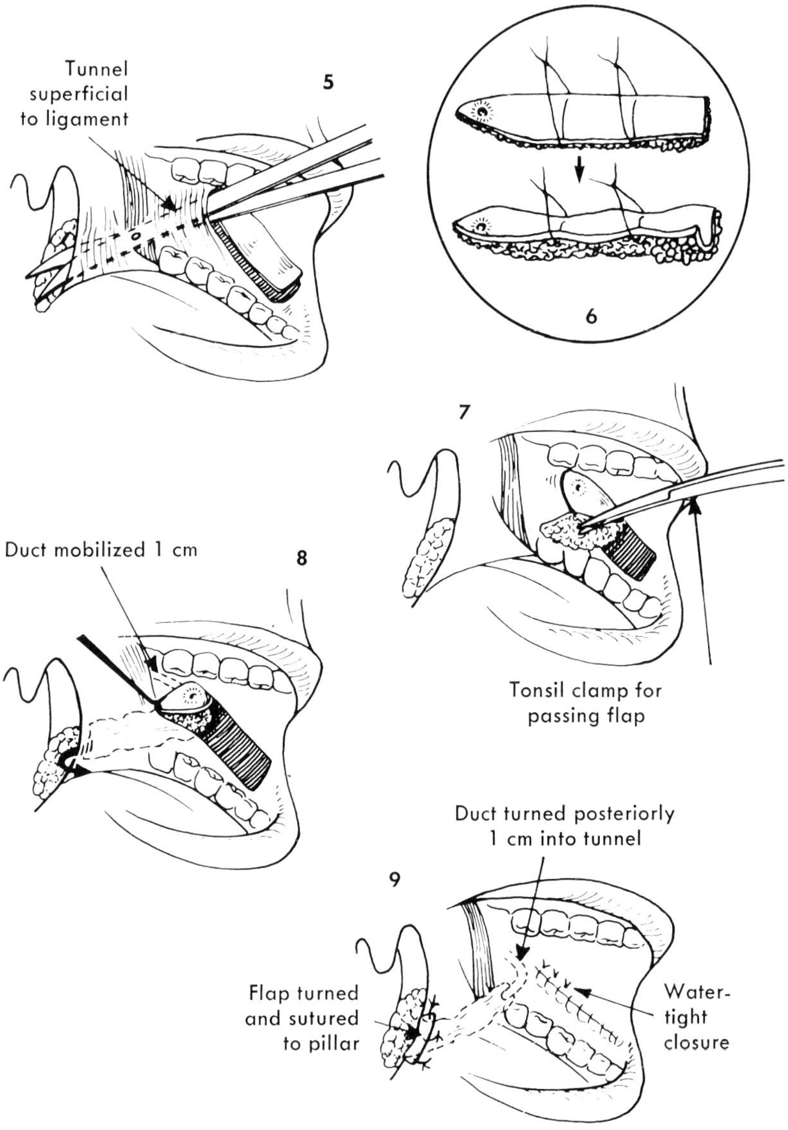

Fig. 18-6, cont'd. *5*, Mucosa just anterior to pterygomandibular ligament is thin, redundant, and difficult to dissect. Ligament may be sectioned if necessary. Perforation of mucosa leads to fistulas, which are difficult to correct. Tunnel exits at free edge of anterior pillar as low as possible. *6*, These two loosely tied sutures are of 6-0 catgut and catch only a tiny edge of mucosa. They prevent improper mucosal folding and ensure maximal raw surface contact for revascularization. *It is imperative to resist temptation to suture this strip into a tube.* Finger pressure along tunnel before suturing posterior tip will properly seat strip and ensure that it has not been pulled too tight. *7*, Tonsil clamp used to pass flap. *8*, Flap in submucosal tunnel. *9*, Completed procedure. (From Wilkie, T. F., and Brody, G. S.: Plast. Reconstr. Surg. **59:**795, 1977.)

medication is frequently thick, tough, and difficult to dissect but seems to heal readily and requires no special concern.

Postoperative course

These patients are most uncomfortable for 3 to 4 days and often develop rather dramatic facial edema, peaking in 48 hours (Figs. 18-7 and 18-8). This is probably due to saliva pouring into the cheek fat pads, as well as surgical trauma combined with poor lymphatic drainage from edema of the submandibular operative sites. Oral intake is poor in the first 3 to 4 days despite active encouragement of a liquid and then a pureed diet, so intravenous fluids are necessary. A nasogastric feeding tube inserted at the end of the procedure has been used recently to eliminate the need for intravenous feeding after the first day. Healing is usually complete, and drooling control manifested in 2 weeks, but hospitalization is rarely required beyond 5 to 7 days. Occasionally patients have had transient polyuria and minor changes in drinking and eating patterns. Nutrition is frequently improved.

Results

A combined series of 123 patients operated on over a 10-year period with a minimum follow-up of $1^1/_2$ years was reviewed. Tables 5 and 6 summarize our results. These were classified as the following:

1. Excellent: essentially normal salivary control
2. Good: slight loss of saliva frequently associated with dried froth on the lips
3. Fair: improved but with significant residual saliva loss, which can occasionally be a thick, offensive, brown, gummy froth
4. Poor: failure of significant control or overdryness

Complications

These complications represent the total series, and most are in the early cases. As the authors gained experience and the operation was modified and improved, the complication rate decreased.

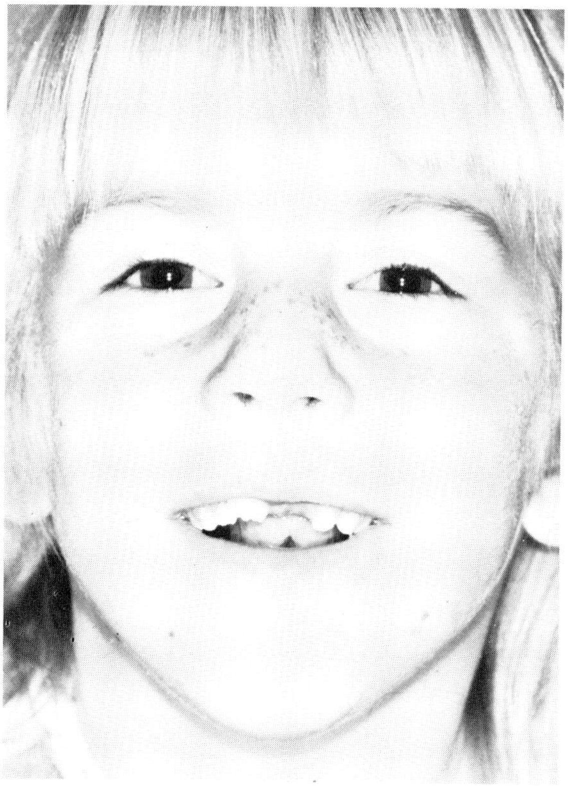

Fig. 18-7. Preoperative view. (From Wilkie, T. F., and Brody, G. S.: Plast. Reconstr. Surg. **59:**797, 1977.)

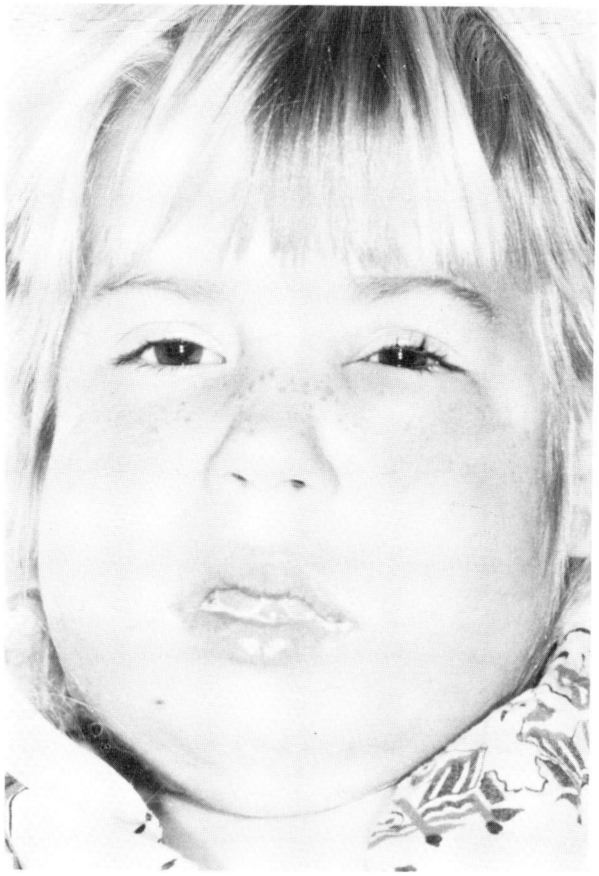

Fig. 18-8. View 48 hours postoperatively, showing marked edema. (From Wilkie, T. F., and Brody, G. S.: Plast. Reconstr. Surg. **59:**797, 1977.)

Table 5. Results of salivary gland surgery

	Wilkie	*Brody*	*Total*
Good to excellent saliva control	18	88	106
Fair to poor control	1	13	14
Overdrynness	0	2	2
Deaths (incidental)	0	1	1
TOTALS	19	104	123

Table 6. Complications of salivary gland surgery

	Wilkie	*Brody*	*Total*
Postoperative wound dehiscence	3	0	3
Stenosis manifested by cyst formation or recurrent drooling (fistula)	7	18	25
Corrected with second operation	6	14	20
Three or more procedures	1	3	4
Hygiene requirements increased	0	4	4
Dental or gingival deterioration	3	2	5
Transient parotid swelling	3	2	5
Septic parotitis	1	0	1

Cyst formation. Cyst formation can present intraorally (Fig. 18-9) or externally (Fig. 18-10) in the cheek. It is caused by total occlusion of the duct and responds well to simple opening posteriorly and orifice reconstruction if the duct has survived in its full length (Fig. 18-11).

Fistula formation (Figs. 18-12 and 18-13). Fistula formation is manifested by recurrent drooling and may occur up to 6 months postoperatively, presumably due to obstruction of the new orifice. It is rarely possible to examine these children satisfactorily in the office, and this is best done under general anesthesia, fully prepared to correct any defect encountered. The anesthesiologist should be requested to avoid atropinelike drugs so that saliva can be milked from the gland to help locate the orifice. When cyst or fistula formation accompanies incomplete survival of the mucosal extension, attempts at reconstruction have not always been successful, especially if the orifice is in the region of the pterygomandibular ligament. Almost every conceivable flap and graft have been used for secondary lengthening of the shortened duct, with only

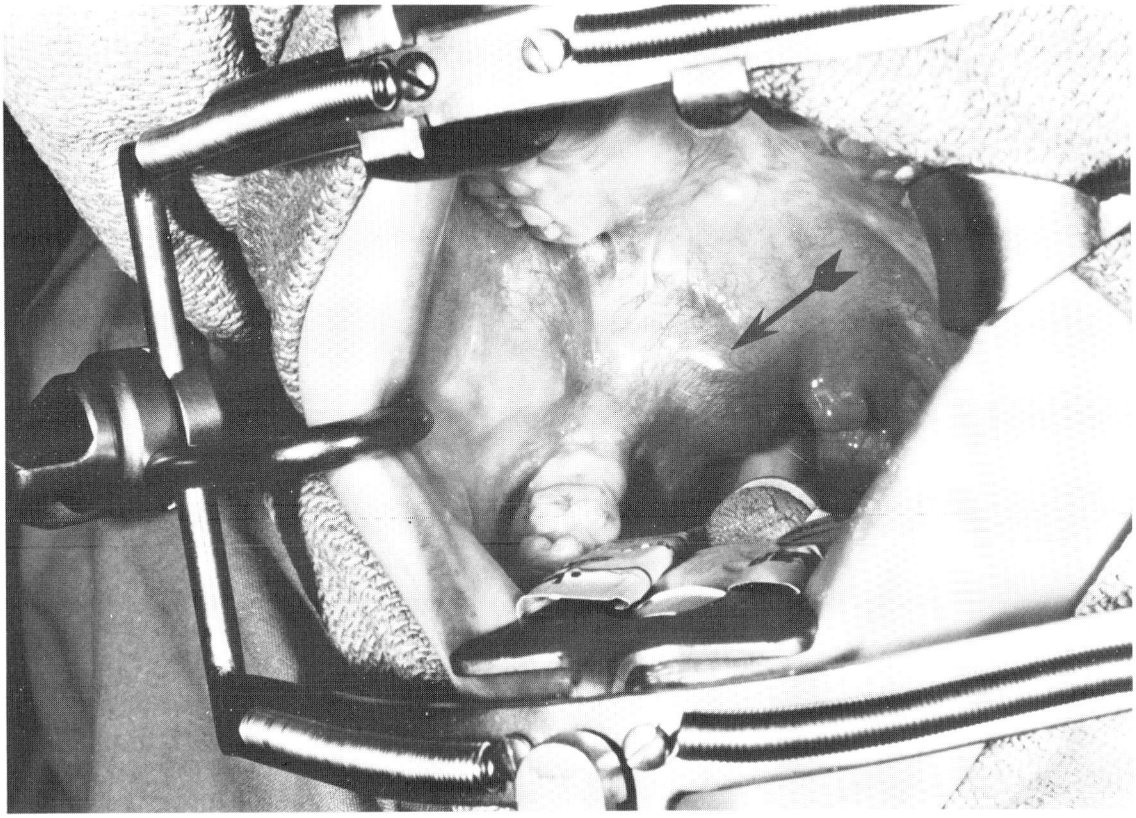

Fig. 18-9. Distended, obstructed, distal end of duct presenting intraorally. (From Wilkie, T. F., and Brody, G. S.: Plast. Reconstr. Surg. **59:**792, 1977.)

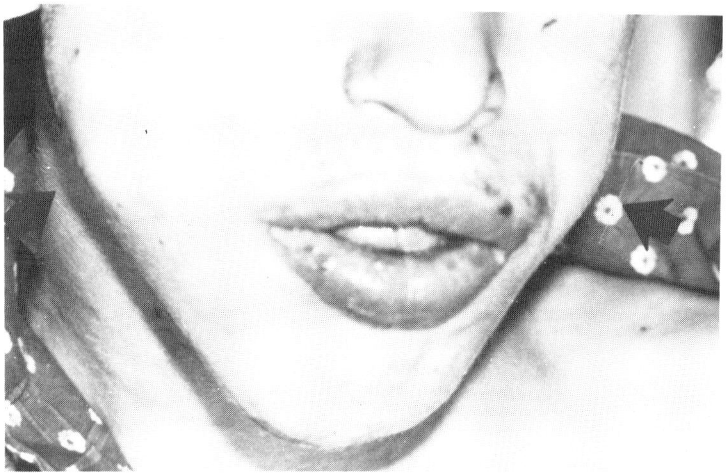

Fig. 18-10. Bilateral, distended ducts obstructed proximally, presenting extraorally. (From Wilkie, T. F., and Brody, G. S.: Plast. Reconstr. Surg. **59:**792, 1977.)

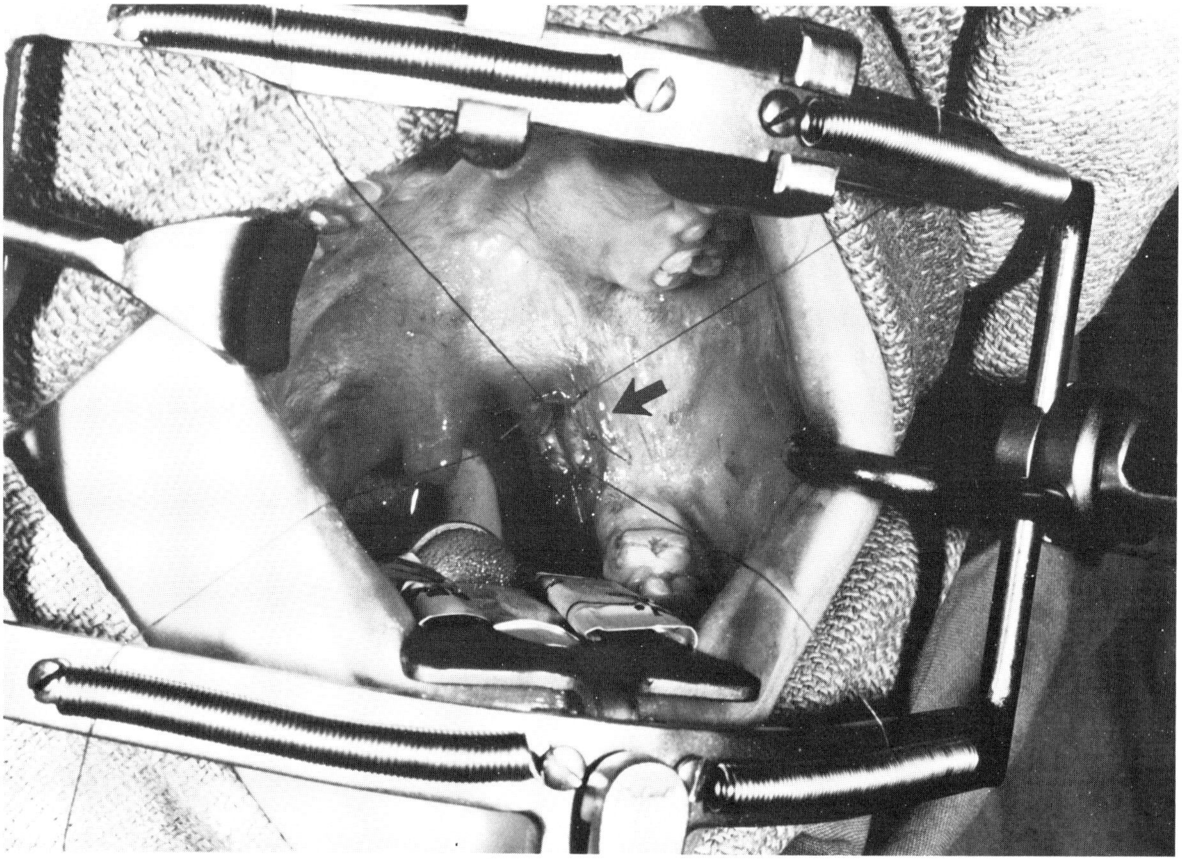

Fig. 18-11. Reconstructed posterior orifice. (From Wilkie, T. F., and Brody, G. S.: Plast. Reconstr. Surg. **59:**793, 1977.)

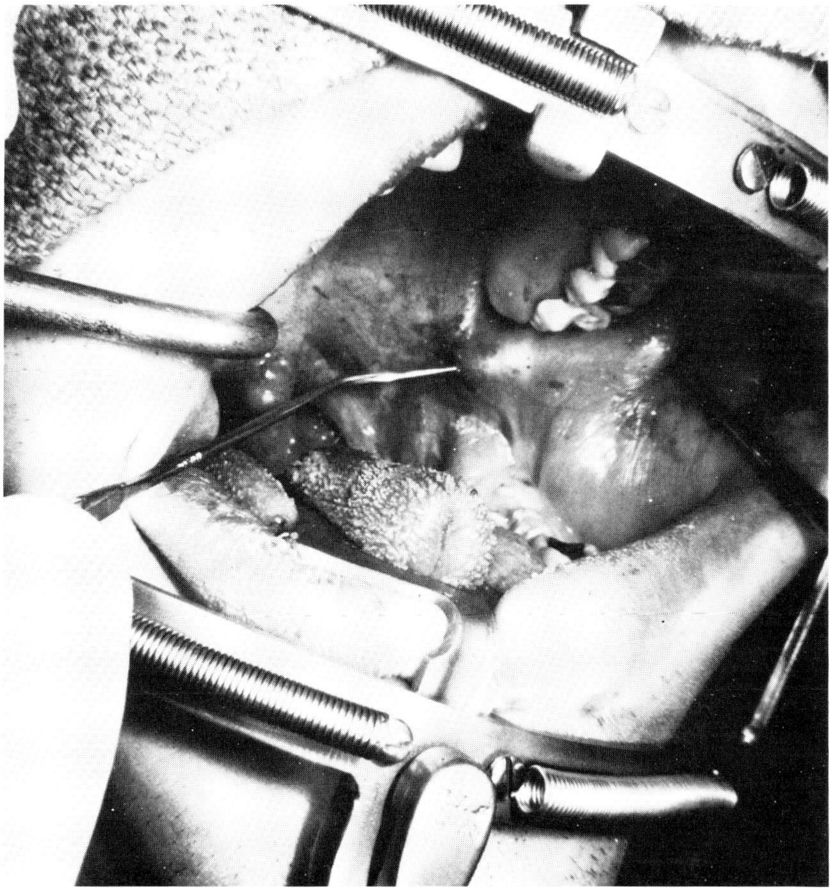

Fig. 18-12. Fistula at pterygomandibular ligament with posterior obstruction. (From Wilkie, T. F., and Brody, G. S.: Plast. Reconstr. Surg. **59:**793, 1977.)

partial success. If the orifice can be placed posterior to the watershed of the pterygomandibular ligament, this is usually sufficient for control. Attempts to suture in tubular splints have failed as the pharyngeal musculature usually milks these out within a few hours. In an occasional athetoid patient with persistent drooling, satisfactorily patent reconstructed ducts are found with no apparent fistula. Milking the submandibular ridges may produce some saliva. Resection and oversuturing of these ridges seem to control the residual saliva apparently produced by sublingual gland remnants or a small amount of gland left clinging to the submandibular duct stump. In one patient a ranula developed from this procedure.

Oral hygiene requirements are occasionally increased, especially in athetoid patients and those with gingival hypertrophy due to antiepileptic medications. The problems with pica have been discussed.

The role of saliva in dental and gingival health has never been clearly defined. While five patients in our series developed increased caries or gingival problems, it is hard to relate this to tampering with the salivary flow. The study by Ericson and associates[7] seems to support our contention that dental health is not affected.

Parotitis. One early patient developed acute unilateral parotitis immediately postoperatively, which was probably related to an infected tonsil. Transient parotid swelling was seen in five patients and was easily managed with antibiotics, tincture of belladonna in small doses, and avoidance of sour foods. Parotid swelling can be easily differentiated from the typical acute postoperative cheek edema by carefully relating the location of the swelling to the gland.

Discussion

Drooling surgery has a gratifyingly high success rate and rewards the surgeon with happy, grateful families and patients. It has been suggested by some

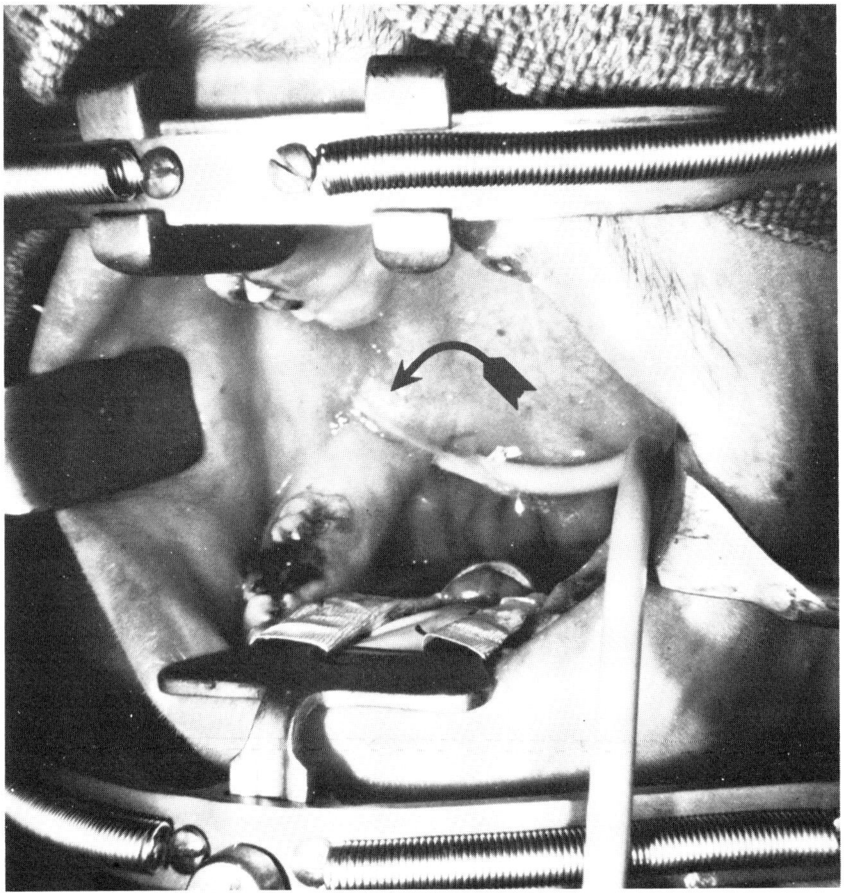

Fig. 18-13. Preligamentous fistula. Note saline stream *(arrow)*. Duct accepts no. 16 catheter with ease. (From Wilkie, T. F., and Brody, G. S.: Plast. Reconstr. Surg. **59:**793, 1977.)

that this is nothing more than a complicated parotid ligation and that control results from parotid atrophy. Radioactive technetium uptake studies have proven that there is continued parotid function, and observation during reexploration demonstrates the flow of clear saliva when the gland is milked. The minimal difficulty with parotitis suggests that the dissection technique preserves the competency of the sphincter at the orifice of Stensen duct.

Summary and conclusions

The surgical treatment of drooling as originally described by Wilkie has been reviewed. Collaboration between the authors has modified and improved the operative technique and clearly defined the indications, expectations, and results. A 10-year experience with 123 patients followed for at least $1^1/_2$ years has resulted in 86% good to excellent overall results. This procedure is indicated for drooling for any reason in a patient in whom nonoperative methods have failed and in whom general anesthesia is an acceptable risk. Severe intellectual impairment is not a contraindication as the increased ease of care justifies the procedure. In these patients a more relaxed criterion of success may be required.

Bilateral submandibular gland resection must be done on all patients and should be done at the same sitting.

Recurrent drooling or persistent cystic swelling constitute the two major complications that may arise; they imply stenosis of the transplanted duct. Many respond to a second operation.

REFERENCES

1. Bosley, E.: Teaching the cerebral palsied to chew, Cereb. Palsy J. **27:**8, 1966.
2. Bosley, E.: Development of sucking and swallowing, Cereb. Palsy J. **26:**14, 1965.
3. Buchner, A., and Sreebuy, L. M.: Enlargement of the salivary glands, Oral Surg. **34:**209, 1972.
4. Cohen, I. K., et al.: Parotid duct transplanation for correction of drooling in patients with cancer of the

head and neck, Surg. Gynecol. Obstet. **133:**633, 1971.

5. Denis-Browne: Operation for hypospadias, Proc. R. Soc. Med. **42:**466, 1949.
6. Enfors, B., Lind, M., and Soderborg, B.: Salivary gland scanning with 99m technetium, Acta Otolaryngol. (Stockh.) **67:**650, 1969.
7. Ericson, T., Nordblom, A., and Ekedahl, C.: Effect on caries susceptibility after surgical treatment of drooling in patients with neurological disorders, Acta Otolaryng. (Stockh.) **75:**71-74, 1972.
8. Goode, R. L., and Smith, R. A.: The surgical management of sialorrhea, Laryngoscope **80:**1078, 1970.
9. Morris, S. F.: Drooling: its assessment and treatment, National Disease Institute Newsletter, fall 1969.
10. Mueller, H. A.: Facilitating feeding and pre-speech. In Physical therapy services in the development disabilities, 1975, Springfield, Ill., Charles C Thomas, Publisher.
11. Ross, J.: Tympanic neurectomy for Frey's syndrome, Audio Digest—Otorhinolaryngolgy **3:**12, 1970.
12. Scholl, G. L., and DiChiro, G.: Clinical usefulness of salivary gland scanning, Semin. Nucl. Med. **2:**270, 1972.
13. Smith, R. A., and Goode, R. L.: Sialorrhea, N. Engl. J. Med. **283:**917, 1970.
14. Sreebny, L. M., and Meyer, J.: Salivary glands and their secretions, New York, 1964, Macmillan.
15. Townsend, G. L., Morimoto, A. M., and Kralemann, H.: Management of sialorrhea in mentally retarded patients by trans-tympanic neurectomy, Mayo Clin. Proc. **48:**776, 1973.
16. Wilkie, T. F.: The surgical treatment of drooling, Plast. Reconstr. Surg. **45:**549, 1970.
17. Wilkie, T. F.: The problem of drooling in cerebral palsy: a surgical approach, Can. J. Surg. **10:**60, 1967.

Chapter 19

Upper extremity deformities in Duchenne muscular dystrophy patients

John D. Hsu
David Taylor

Upper extremity deformities in Duchenne muscular dystrophy (DMD) patients are caused by muscle imbalance, muscle weakness, positioning of the extremities, and skeletal changes. A preventive program should be instituted at as early a time as possible to avoid further loss of function in an already severely disabled patient. Recognition of the potential problems that could occur if these deformities persist is important in a physician's overall management of the severely disabled child with Duchenne muscular dystrophy.

CLINICAL COURSE

Duchenne muscular dystrophy is a progressive disease affecting only male children. The inheritance is as an X-linked trait, but first generation spontaneous mutation occurs in approximately 40% of the cases. The clinical course varies slightly from patient to patient, but in general the following sequence of events occurs.[1,16]

Recognition of the disease is rarely made at birth or in very early childhood. The initial development of the child is normal. If there have been no previous encounters with the disease by the family, awareness is generally not made until age 3 or 4. Affected children are slightly slower than their peers at that time, they occasionally fall, and they have difficulty negotiating many flights of stairs quickly. Examination of their extremities reveals perhaps only a slight enlargement of the calves, thus the term "pseudohypertrophy." If enzyme studies are made, creatine phosphokinase (CPK), the most specific enzyme study for muscle disease, is highly elevated. Muscle biopsy is frequently made to confirm or clarify the diagnosis. Progression of the disease generally is manifested by weakness in the lower extremity, with the child's having difficulty getting up from the floor. These children need to push up and climb upon themselves, evoking Gower maneuver. Between 8 and 10 years of age there is more pronounced difficulty in walking due to lower extremity contractures in addition to the weakness. At this stage, maximum treatment effort is devoted to the lower extremity and maintenace of standing and walking. Various methods are available, including bracing and surgical procedures.[7,13]

Generally between 10 to 12 years of age, because of repeated falling, walking is no longer practical. Maximum effort is needed to stand, and despite bracing, the gait slows tremendously, thus eventually confining the child to a wheelchair.[3]

In the following years while the child is in the wheelchair, the muscle disease and wasting progress relentlessly. There is dependence on the arms and upper extremities to maintain independence. Arms and hands are needed for wheelchair propulsion, table-top activities, feeding, grooming, and self-care functions.

When the Duchenne muscular dystrophy patient reaches his early 20s, primary changes in the myocardium have become so far advanced that they cause heart failure. Wasting of the intercostal muscles make respirations shallow, eventually leading to respiratory failure. These patients finally die of cardiac or respiratory failure.

FUNCTIONAL EVALUATION

A functional ability method of testing the muscle disease patient was initiated by Swinyard and

Table 7. Muscle disease functional classification*

Level	*Activities*
1	Unlimited walking, unlimited self-care
2	Limited walking, unlimited self-care
3	Limited walking, limited self-care
4	Unlimited manual wheelchair propulsion (no walking), limited dressing, unlimited desk skills
5	Unlimited electric wheelchair propulsion or limited manual wheelchair propulsion, limited desk skills (moderate lifting)
6	Unlimited electric wheelchair propulsion or no manual wheelchair propulsion, limited desk skills (light lifting)
7	Unlimited electric wheelchair propulsion, no desk skills
8	No wheelchair propulsion, no desk skills

*Developed by Rancho Los Amigos Hospital, Muscle Disease Clinics, Occupational and Physical Therapy Departments.

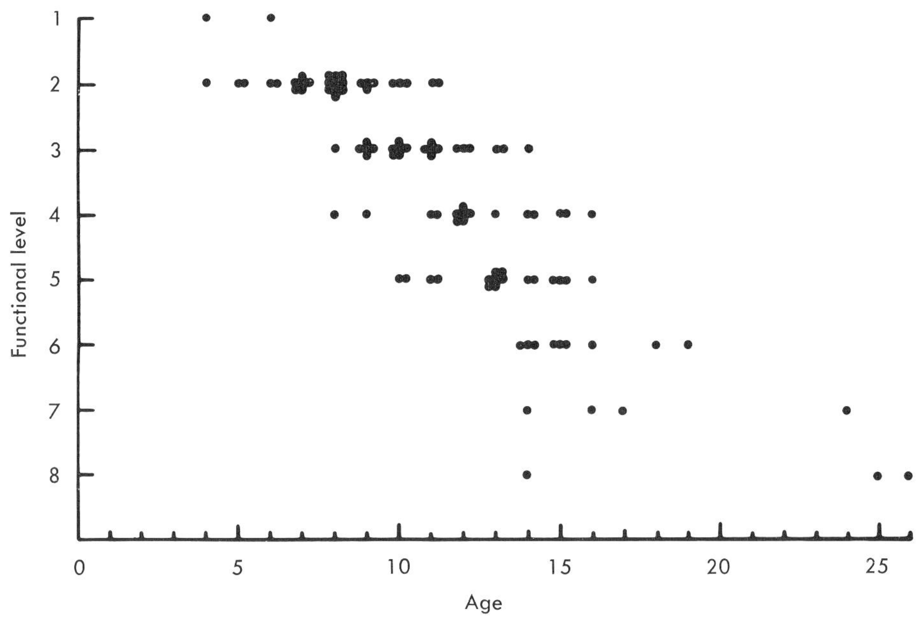

Fig. 19-1. One hundred four annual tests of Duchenne muscular dystrophy. Decreasing function is seen with increasing age.

associates,[14] later modified by Spencer and his colleagues,[15] Price,[11] and more recently at Rancho Los Amigos Hospital.[8, 9] An eight-step decreasing functional level scale, developed in the Muscle Disease Clinics, Rancho Los Amigos Hospital, specifically covers all activities of the Duchenne muscular dystrophy patient: standing, walking, wheelchair sitting, self-care, bulbar activities and those confined to bed. The scale is summarized in Table 7.

In assessing upper extremity function, special attention needs to be directed to levels 4 to 8. In level 4 the patient can propel his wheelchair and continue to be independent with upper extremity dressing, including the ability to pull his shirt over his head. Hygiene skills are retained. Level 5 represents significant loss of strength in the shoulder and upper extremity function. The child is now limited to tabletop activities and skills that require only limited lifting. He is able to feed himself, maintain his facial hygiene, and brush his teeth.

In level 6, the functional strength remaining is now in the wrist and hands. At level 7 the strongest muscles are the intrinsics. The primary function in this group is the ability to independently operate an electric wheelchair. Fig. 19-1 represents a summary of 104 functional test studies in 44 individual patients, ages 4 to 25 years, over a 5-year period (1972 to 1977).

UPPER EXTREMITY: GUIDELINES FOR MANAGEMENT

The Duchenne muscular dystrophy patient in a wheelchair becomes extremely dependent on his upper extremities. Progressive weakness results in a decrease in the level of function. Currently available literature has paid little attention to this stage and there are very few published guidelines for management.

Head and neck control

In the sitting Duchenne muscular dystrophy patient the ability to control the head and neck is very important for upper extremity function. In the patient whose spine is straight but head control is weak because of wasting of the neck flexors or extensors, modifications of the patient's equipment are necessary. With extensor weakness an outrigger from the top part of the wheelchair or body jacket can very effectively help control the neck (Fig. 19-2). Weakness of the capital flexors can be helped by positioning the patient with slight posterior wheelchair tilting, and resting the neck in the headrest can overcome this problem, but the patient may have some difficulty in seeing straight ahead and in controlling his wheelchair.

Scoliosis causes lateral deviation and tilting of the head and neck and presents difficulties in positioning. When scoliosis is present, the elbows and forearms are needed to support the trunk on the wheelchair rests, and most of the patients' efforts are directed to sitting himself upright, thus limiting activities. Various head slings have been tried, but these create pressure on the jaw and may not be used for more than a very short time. Individually molded seats of fiberglass or of other foam material have proven to be extremely useful in helping control and position the head and neck so that the arms and hands are not encumbered.[6]

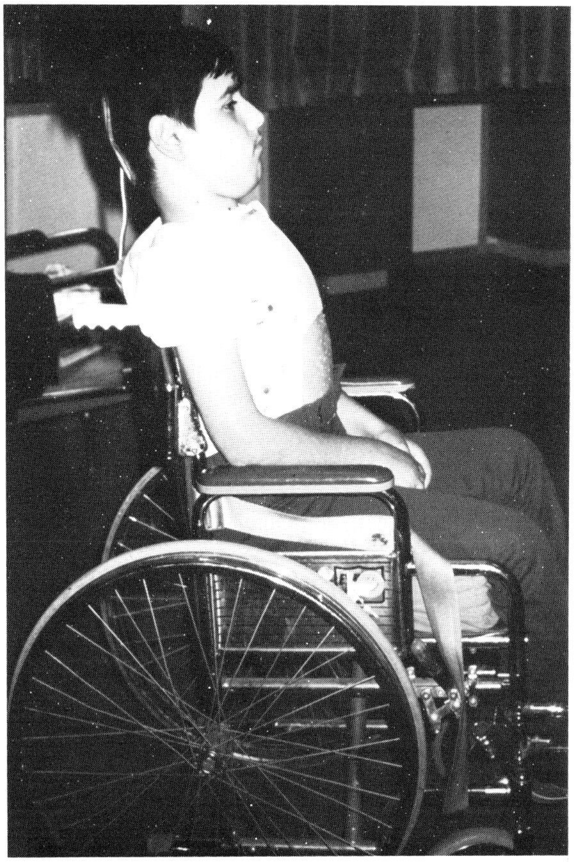

Fig. 19-2. Head support.

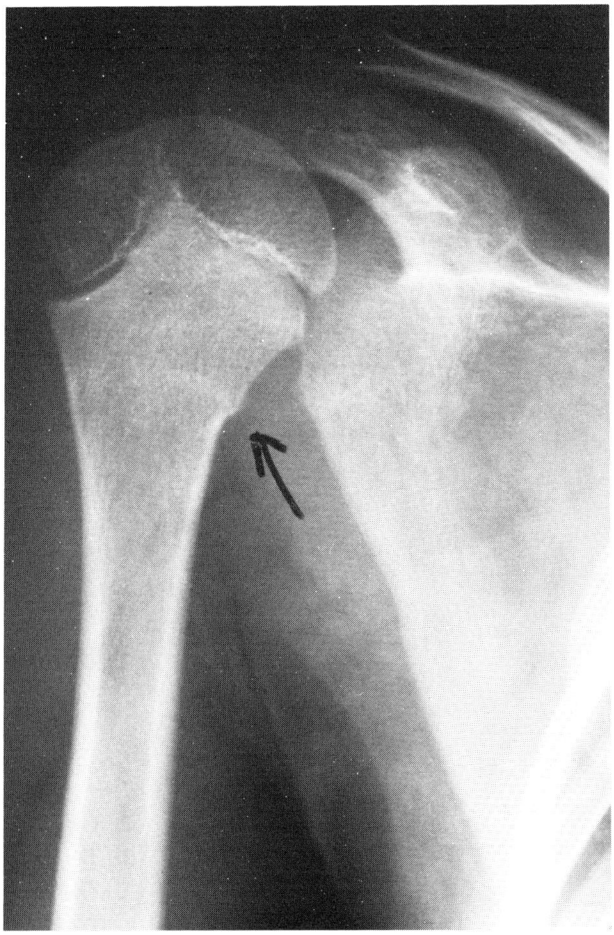

Fig. 19-3. Radiograph of right shoulder, showing undisplaced fracture.

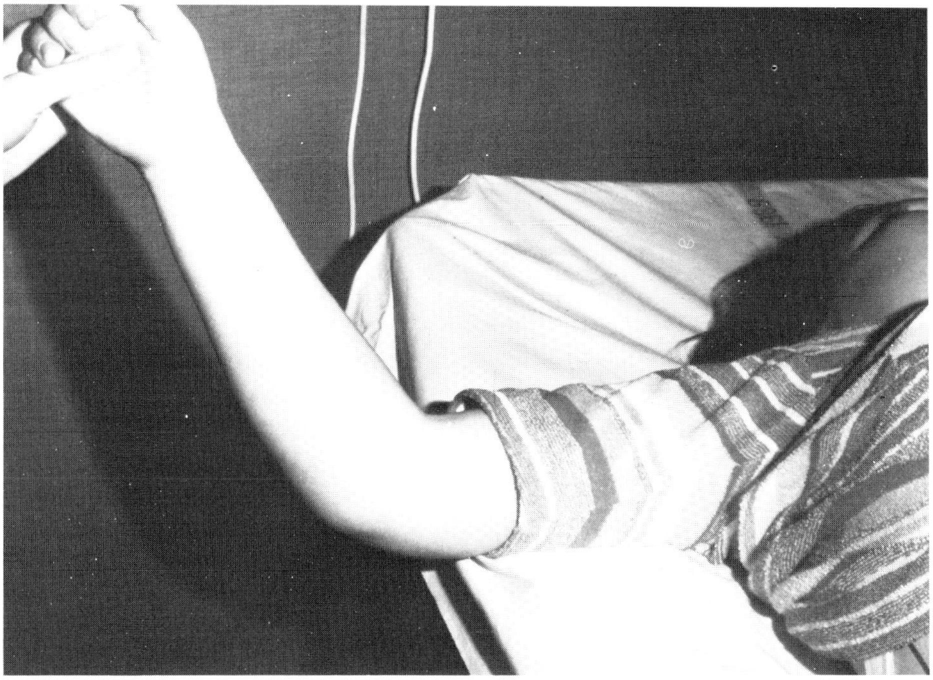

Fig. 19-4. Right elbow, showing elbow flexion contracture.

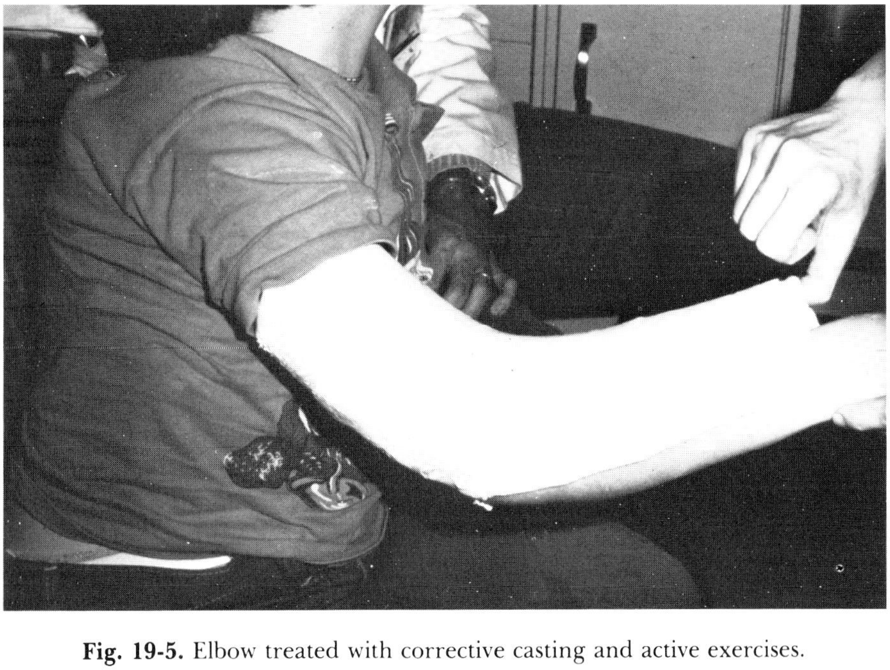

Fig. 19-5. Elbow treated with corrective casting and active exercises.

Shoulder

In the walking Duchenne muscular dystrophy patient there is generally very little limitation of shoulder range, but by age 12 to 13 there is approximately 90 degrees of active shoulder flexion and abduction left. In the sitting patient there is a natural tendency for the arms to form flexion contractures. However, the full range of motion can be maintained with passive ranging. With progressive wasting, further loss occurs. Contractures to 60 degrees are frequently seen in 13 to 14 year olds.

Because of disuse osteoporosis, the main danger in shoulder contracture is that in transferring and lifting patients, humeral fractures could easily occur[10] from forcefully abducting the contractural shoulder, coupled with the disuse osteoporosis. Fortunately, such fractures generally rarely displace and heal without difficulty (Fig. 19-3) with nothing more than immobilization of the affected arm in a sling. When the patient's arm becomes comfortable, ranging should be resumed. A Duchenne muscular dystrophy patient should be transferred by grasping him from behind, across the chest rather than under the armpits. Use of mechanical lifts and slings may be very useful in these patients as they alleviate the need for human exertion and uneven forces on fragile extremities.

Elbow

Elbow flexion contractures generally occur secondary to positioning in a wheelchair. In a study of 51 Duchene muscular dystrophy patients, range of motion in the elbow generally begins decreasing when the patients first go into a wheelchair. By age 17 this range diminishes to a still useful 90 degrees (30 degrees to 120 degrees), but by age 25 only 30 degrees of range remain. Flexion from 80 to 110 degrees is no longer useful. The elbows should be ranged gently to minimize contractures. Fixed contractures, past 30 degrees, can generally be improved by serial casts, followed by night splints and dropout splints as illustrated in Figs. 19-4 and 19-5. In the older patient, mobile arm supports help increase function.[2]

Forearm

Most tabletop activities are done with the forearm in pronation, and fortunately pronation is generally retained longer than supination. In the patients studied, loss of pronation to 60 degrees was not seen until the patients were 17 years of age. However, supination was lost much earlier, and very few patients had more than 60 degrees of supination by age 13 to 14.

Wrist

In the same series of patients, examination of the wrists of 15 patients whose functional level was 4 to 7[12,13] showed that ulnar deviation is present because the flexor carpi ulnaris muscle remains stronger than the other wrist muscles. Ulnar deviation, coupled with other contractures, weakens the hand and makes it difficult to pinch. In these pa-

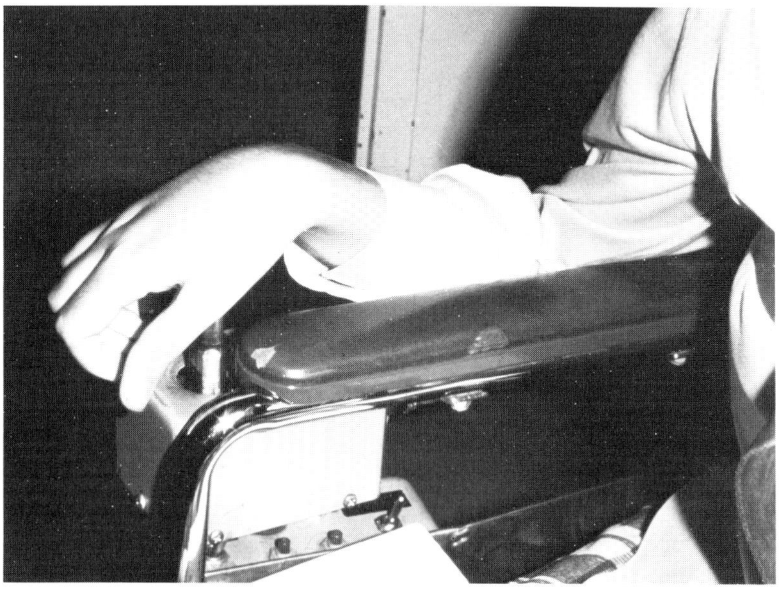

Fig. 19-6. Positioning of hand for driving electric wheelchair.

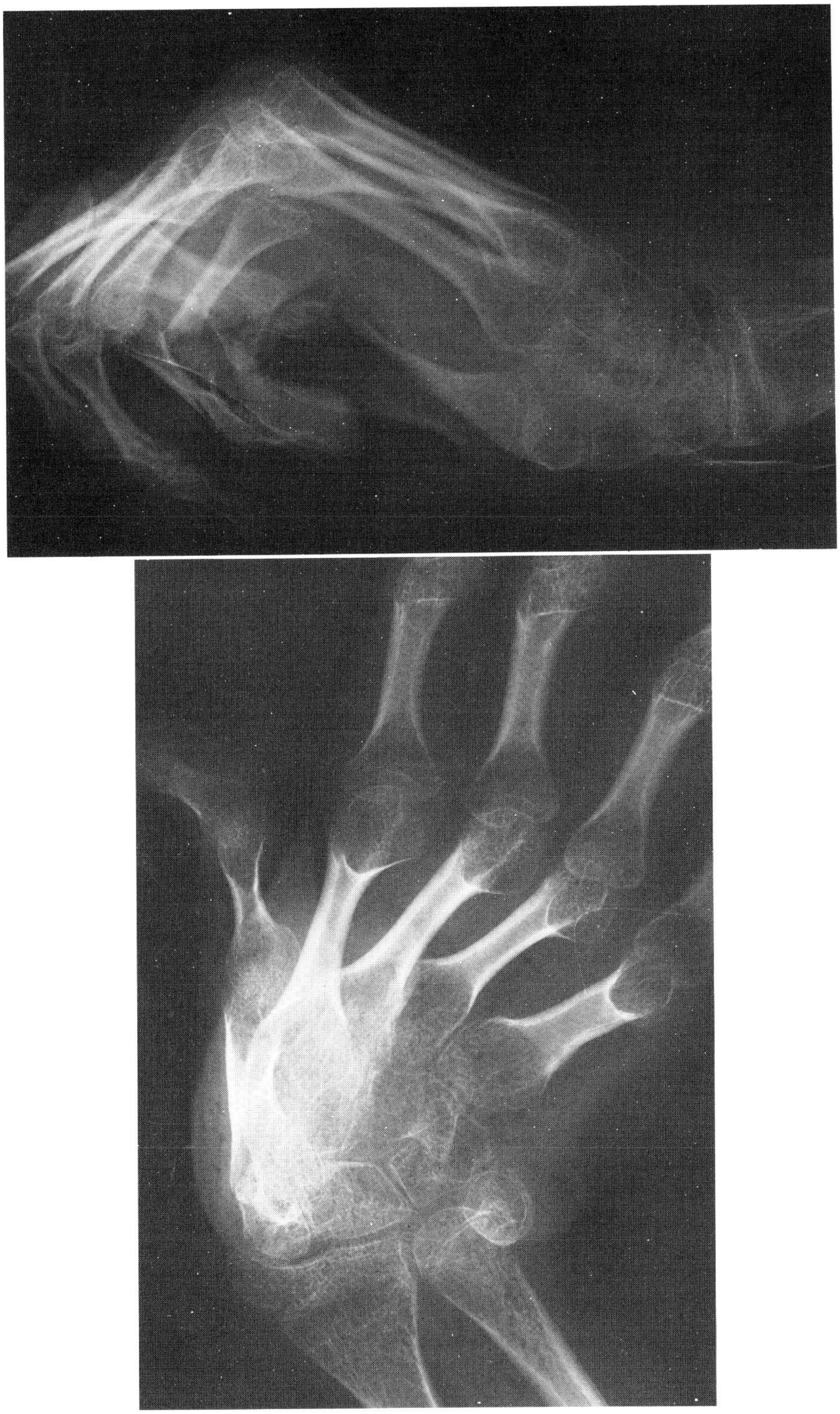

Fig. 19-7. Radiographs of hand, showing contractures and deformities.

tients transferring the flexor carpi ulnaris into the wrist as a dorsiflexor using the Green-Grice procedure gives more useful function.[5]

Hand and fingers

Thumb hyperextension at the interphalangeal joint secondary to a weak flexor pollicis longus muscle is seen in all patients. The opponens and adductor do retain some function, permitting side-to-side-pinch.

In the fingers, flexion contractures occur secondary to positioning in addition to the imbalance. Some of the most striking deformities that we have seen occur in right-handed patients with electric wheelchairs. These children use the right hand and fingers to drive the electric wheelchair resulting in the deformity illustrated in Fig. 19-6. Radiographs confirm fixed contractures (Fig. 19-7).

The nondriving hand is generally placed on the hand rest. If the wrist is allowed to dangle, marked wrist flexion contracture develops. If the distal hand is allowed to dangle, no appreciable wrist flexion contracture develops but there is a contracture at the metacarpophalangeal joint.

These contractures can be prevented by ranging, by better positioning, by using splints, and if necessary by better location of wheelchair control buttons or knobs.

SUMMARY

The need for maintenance of function in the upper extremities of the older Duchenne muscular dystrophy patient is discussed. Early recognition of the problems, use of protective splinting with the first occurrence of any muscle imbalance, and the necessity of faithful, aggressive, and persistent ranging of all upper extremity joints are important aspects in the management of the Duchenne muscular dystrophy child in order to retain maximum independence and function.

REFERENCES

1. Bonsett, C. A.: Studies of pseudohypertrophic muscular dystrophy, Springfield, Ill., 1969, Charles C Thomas, Publisher.
2. Chyatte, S. B., Long, C., II, and Vignos, P. J.: The balanced forearm orthosis in muscular dystrophy, Arch. Phys. Med. Rehabil. **46:**633, 1965.
3. Gibson, D. A., Albisser, A. M., and Koreska, J.: Role of the wheelchair in the management of the muscular dystrophy patient, Can. Med. Assoc. J., **113:**964, 1975.
4. Gonzales, V.: An occupational therapy intervention program for the individual with muscular dystrophy, Paper presented at A.C.T.A. Conference, San Francisco, Calif., Oct. 1976.
5. Green, W. T., and Banks, H. H.: Flexor carpi ulnaris transplant and its use in cerebral palsy, J. Bone Joint Surg. [Am.] **44:**1343, 1962.
6. Hospital for Sick Children: Manual for the construction of the hospital for sick children spinal support system, 1976.
7. Hsu, J. D.: Management of foot deformity in Duchenne's pseudohypertrophic muscular dystrophy, Orthop. Clin. North Am. **7:**979, 1976.
8. Hsu, J. D., Perry, R. E., Jr., Gonzales, V., Fracalosy, C., and Hash, D.: Functional abilities of the muscle disease patient, Dev. Med. Child Neurol. **17:**343, 1975.
9. Hsu, J. D., Perry, R. E., Jr., Gonzales, V., et al.: Functional abilities of the muscle disease patient, Exhibit presented at the A.A.O.S. Annual Meeting, San Francisco, Calif., 1975.
10. Marie, P., and Crouzon, V.: Un cas de fracture par atrophie osseuse de l'humerus chez un myopathique, Rev. Neurol. (Paris) **11:**239, 1903.
11. Price, A.: Repression of function in pseudohypertrophic muscular dystrophy, Milwaukee, 1965, North Shore Publishing Co.
12. Roy, L., and Gibson, D. A.: Pseudohypertrophic muscular dystrophy and its surgical management: review of 30 patients, Can. J. Surg. **13:**13, 1970.
13. Spencer, G. E., Jr.: Orthopaedic considerations in the management of muscular dystrophy, Curr. Pract. Orthop. Surg. **5:**279, 1973.
14. Swinyard, C. A., Deaver, G. G., and Greenspan, L.: Gradients of functional ability of importance in rehabilitation of patients with progressive muscular and neuromuscular disease, Arch. Phys. Med. Rehabil. **38:**574, 1953.
15. Vignos, P. J., Jr., Spencer, G. E., Jr., and Archibald, K. C.: Management of progressive muscular dystrophy of childhood, J.A.M.A. **184:**89, 1963.
16. Ziter, F. A., and Allsop, K. G.: The diagnosis and management of childhood muscular dystrophy, Clin. Pediatr. (Phila.) **15:**540, 1976.

Chapter 20

The hand in severe arthrogryposis

M. Mark Hoffer
Susan Swank
Valerie Gonzales

Arthrogryposis multiplex congenita is a nonhereditary syndrome, present at birth, consisting of multiple joint contractures and muscle weakness.[1,2] The management of such patient's lower extremities has been relatively well defined,[3-9] but upper extremity care has received less attention.[4,10,11] Our experience has been limited to the severely involved individual.

Twenty-one severely involved patients (ages 5 to 20), each observed by the authors for more than 5 years, were reviewed with respect to hand function (Table 8). None of these severely involved children had better than fair muscle grades in any of the hand musculature. All children had normal intelligence. All of them, even the children with severely paralyzed hands, had normal sensibility by sharp-dull, object identification, graphesthesia, proprioception, and two-point discrimination tests.[8]

Typical hand deformities included pronated forearms, flexed and ulnar-deviated wrists, digits rigid in a position of slight flexion, and thumbs in palm. Many patients exhibited an unusual type of index-to-small-finger pinch over the dorsum of the long and ring fingers (Fig. 20-1). Most used cross-wrist locking for grasp (Fig. 20-2).

None of these upper extremities could be used for crutch support. The prerequisites for crutch use are good grasp, good triceps or fully extended elbows, and good shoulder depressors (pectoralis major, teres major, and latissimus dorsi). Only

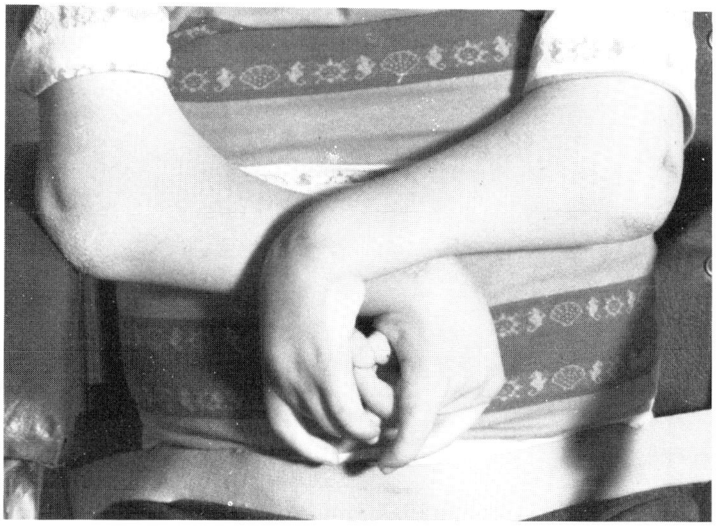

Fig. 20-1. Cross-arm grip.

Table 8. Hand function in 21 patients with arthrogryposis multiplex congenita

Patient	*Age*	*Ambulatory status*	*Surgery*	*Orthotic devices*
1	18	None		Mobile arm support discarded, electric wheelchair
2	12	None	Elbow release	Mobile arm support and myoelectric device discarded, electric wheelchair
3	7	With AFO*		
4	6	None	Forearm osteotomy, thumb release	Mobile arm support discarded, electric wheelchair
5	17	None	Wrist fusion, thumb release†	Myoelectric hand device, electric wheelchair
6	18	None	Elbow release†	Mobile arm support, electric wheelchair
7	18	Independent	Thumb release	Mobile arm support discarded
8	15	Independent	Pectoralis transfer†	
9	16	With AFO*		
10	20	Independent	Bilateral elbow release	
11	6	Independent	Bilateral elbow releases, wrist release†	
12	8	With AFO*		
13	17	None		Mobile arm support discarded, electric wheelchair
14	14	Independent	Elbow release, triceps transfer	
15	8	None		Mobile arm support discarded, electric wheelchair
16	18	With AFO*		Electric wheelchair
17	16	Independent	Bilateral thumb release	
18	6	None		Mobile arm support
19	15	Independent		
20	6	Independent	Wrist release, thumb release†	
21	17	Independent		

* AFO: ankle-foot orthosis (short leg brace).
† Improved function.

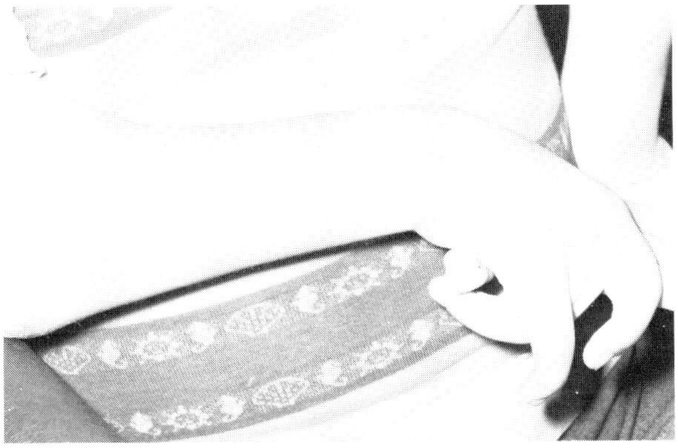

Fig. 20-2. Index-to-small-finger pinch.

those children with good or better key motors (hip extensors, quadriceps, and triceps surae) could accomplish free ambulation (13 of the 21 patients). Ankle-foot orthosis did aid ambulation in some. More elaborate above-knee orthoses did not help.

Bioengineering and orthotic measures were attempted in all of these patients. Positioning braces and plasters prevented progressive deformities but did not decrease those already present. Mobile arm supports (Fig. 20-3) were helpful teaching and classroom devices in eight children but were used after 5 years in only two. Two myoelectric control braces were fabricated, and one was well utilized after 5 years. Eight children used electric wheelchairs with upper extremity control devices specifically designed for them (Fig. 20-4). These children continue to use the electric wheelchairs after the 5-year observation period. The independence in mobility permitted by these chairs has been the most significant mechanical aid in their lives.

Twenty surgical procedures were performed on 11 of these patients. These included seven elbow releases, two tendon transfers for elbow flexion, two wrist releases, one wrist fusion, one forearm osteotomy, six thumb releases, and one sublimis release.

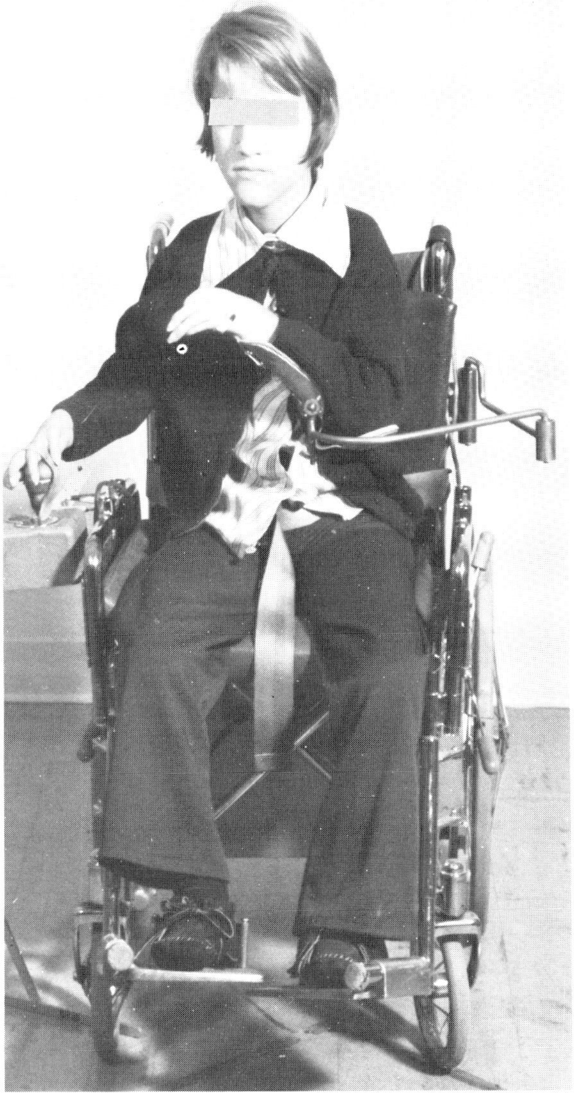

Fig. 20-3. Mobile arm support.

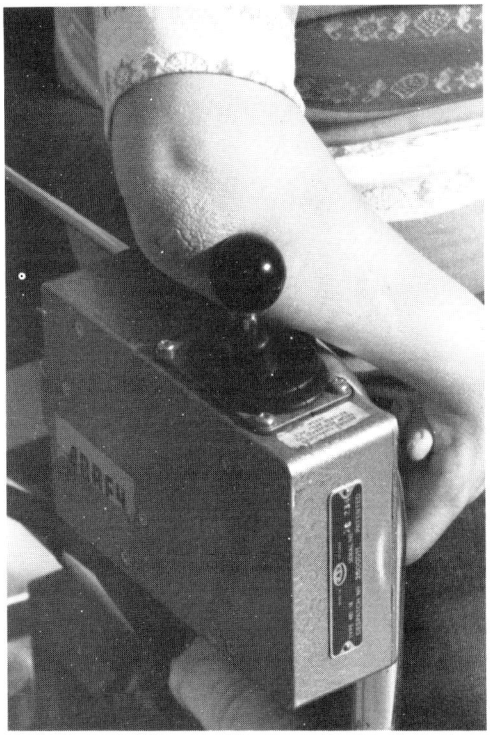

Fig. 20-4. Electric wheelchair control.

After surgery five patients had resultant improvement in function. Patients 8, 11, and 20 had fair hand muscles; the muscle transfers and releases helped them improve their function. Patients 5 and 6 had muscles graded poor or worse; their operative procedures permitted improved use of effective orthotic devices. Unfortunately, patients 2, 4, 7, 10, 14, and 17 had both poor muscles in the hand and poor orthotic function despite operative procedures. More sophisticated orthotic devices rather than more surgery would be helpful in these failure cases.

Our experience suggests that all arthrogryposis patients develop normal sensibility despite their lack of upper extremity function and therapy; complicated orthotic and bioengineering devices may be helpful teaching tools but are not functional in these children with the exception of the electric wheelchair; most children develop substitution hand use by the mouth or cross-wrist grip, and these probably should be encouraged.

REFERENCES

1. Adams, R. D.: Diseases of muscle, ed. 3, New York, 1975, Harper & Row, Publishers, p. 238.
2. Bharucha, E. P., Pandya, S. S., and Dastur, D. K.: Arthrogryposis multiplex congenita. J. Neurol. Neurosurg. Psychiatry **35:**425-434, 1972.
3. Drummond, D. S., Siller, T. N., and Cruess, R. L.: Management of arthrogryposis multiplex congenita. In American Academy of Orthopaedic Surgeons Instructional Course Lectures, Vol. xxiii, St. Louis, 1974, The C. V. Mosby Co., p. 79.
4. Friedlander, H. L., Westin, G. W., and Wood, W. L.: Arthrogryposis multiplex congenita, J. Bone Joint Surg. [Am.] **50:**89-112, 1968.
5. Gibson, D. A., and Urs, N. D.: Arthrogryposis multiplex congenita, J. Bone Joint Surg. [Br.] **52:**483-493, 1970.
6. Lloyd-Roberts, G. C., and Lettin, A. W. F.: Arthrogryposis multiplex congenita, J. Bone Joint Surg. [Br.] **52:**494-508, 1970.
7. Mead, N. G., Lithgow, W. C., and Sweeney, H. J.: Arthrogryphosis multiplex congenita, J. Bone Joint Surg. [Am.] **40:**1285-1309, 1958.
8. Moberg, E.: Objective methods for determining the functional value of sensibilty in the hand, J. Bone Joint Surg. [Br.] **40:**454-476, 1958.
9. Shariff, F. K., Horoupian, D., and Greenlaw, R. K.: Arthrogryposis multiplex congenita, Clin. Orthop. **94:**263-267, 1973.
10. Weeks, P. M.: Surgical correction of upper extremity deformities in arthrogryposis, Plast. Reconstr. Surg. **36:**459-465, 1965.
11. Williams, P. F.: The elbow in arthrogryposis, J. Bone Joint Surg. [Br.] **55:**834-840, 1973.

Chapter 21

The myelo-spino-dysrhaphic diseases: neurosurgical considerations

Thomas B. Ducker
Walker L. Robinson

Myeloschisis, myelocele, meningomyelocele, meningocele, cystic dermal sinus, diastematomyelia, and spina bifida occulta—a spectrum of disorders of developmental nervous system abnormalities that are referred to as the dorsal rachischisis diseases—remain a major problem in pediatric medicine. Meningomyelocele alone occurs from 0.2 per 1,000 live births in Japan to 4.2 per 1,000 live births in Ireland.[1,13,18] The exact incidence of these dysrhaphic states in the United States is not known, but clinically it appears to be occurring less often. Generally these children are born to parents who are very young and poor, and it is these people who are now having fewer children.

The exact cause or initiating event within the ontogenesis of the baby is not known. Etiologic agents, such as genetic translation,[16] metabolic disease,[17] chemical poisoning,[23] infection,[8] and irradiation[22] have all been implicated. Regardless of the initiating events, it is known that at approximately 4 weeks' gestation, when the embryo is 10 to 20 mm in crown-rump length, the lateral neural plates join anteriorly, then complete their closure posteriorly to form the embryonic neural tube. Failure of adequate closure, bleb formation within the closure, or splitting of the closure readily occurs in many embryonic specimens.[20] Any change within the cerebral spinal fluid dynamics can either deform or negate the cleft closure problem. Depending on the cephalad or caudal location along the neural axis and depending on the extent and the position of the bleb or closure defect, the various abnormalities are manifested in the newborn child. The exact importance of either increased or abnormal flow patterns of cerebral spinal fluid is not known, but this fluid certainly becomes part of the pathophysiologic process within the first trimester.[7] The defects in the bone are secondary to the developmental abnormalities of the nervous system tissue.[5]

CLINICAL CONDITIONS

The clinical conditions can be divided into four basic categories. First, the open myeloschises are part of the division of developmental abnormalities referred to as spina bifida aperta, described by Padget.[20] Second, the meningomyeloceles and meningoceles are referred to as the spina bifida cystica syndromes. Third, the conditions where there is a dermal sinus, an intradural lipoma or epidermoid, or simply splitting of the posterior bony arches are in the group referred to as spina bifida occulta. Fourth and finally, there can be abnormalities in the anterior neural plate, and such a defect will give rise to diastematomyelia and anterior meningoceles. Within each of the four categories there are at least two major disease processes, leading to at least eight separate clinical syndromes.

Craniospinal encephalocele

Encephaloceles occur at the upper end of the neural axis and are basically the same congenital problem that develops along the midline of the brain or the cranial-cervical junction. When they are located anteriorly with a small defect compatible with life, the child does not have a large or extensive neurologic deficit or abnormality. When the defects occur posteriorly, they can be compatible with life, but with considerable brain damage so that they are associated with mental retardation. The development of the encephaloschisis can be quite large so that certain children are born and do live with what appears as an outgrown, developmental, abnormal mass nearly as big as their head. The tissue within the myeloschisis sac contains few neurons and mostly undifferentiated embryonic neural tissue and glial scar. There is no functioning brain tissue within the sac. Consequently, amputation of the sac will not further damage the functioning neurons in the child. When the problem occurs at the cranial-cervical junction, it is associated with considerable scarring and kinking of the brain stem centers so that even early successful repair is fraught with a progressive neurologic deficit in the growing child, even in the face of adequate closure.

Myeloschisis

The myeloschisis abnormalities, where there is little to no dorsal covering of the neural tissue, typically occur along the thoracic spine. The neural plate literally is separated widely with no fusion of any of the elements posteriorly. With such wide separation of the neural plates, there is no inner neuronal functioning tissue. Neither do the astrocytic tissues mature normally. All developmental axons across the area are not protected by any pia mater or blood-brain barrier. Consequently, the neurologic loss at the lesion is complete and irreversible at the time of birth and diagnosis. This lesion most likely occurs early in embryonic maturation and is associated with marked deformity, not only of the local bony tissue, but also of the cervical-medullary junction, in that the Arnold-Chiari malformation is present in nearly all these children. No neurosurgical procedure can restore the lost neurologic function of these lesions.

Meningomyeloceles

The meningomyeloceles typically occur at the conus medullaris. The point where the spinal cord ends and the typical nerve root configuration of the cauda equina begins is the most common site of this problem. In the majority of these lesions there are cord structures at the base of the cystic developmental defect. The cord may be of a near-normal configuration or show a definite myelodysplasia. On occasion the myelodysplasia may be so marked that the neural tube has ballooned posteriorly and the cord structures lie on the back of the sac. In other rare cases the neural cleft or bleb deformity enlarges so that the entire myelocele contains a cystic cavity wherein the abnormal cord lies within the walls of the cyst. The neurologic loss within this lesion is directly related to the degree of myelodysplasia of the cord itself. If the cord is of a near-normal anatomic position, then there may be functioning nerve roots below the lesion. Good surgical closure of the defect with nerve roots within a relaxed dural sac figuration may aid in the preservation of neurologic function. However, if the cord is markedly dysplastic, then the internuncial neurons and the blood-brain barrier have been so marred that all the functional tissue has been, in essence, destroyed.

Meningoceles

Meningoceles typically occur in the lower lumbar spine where there are only nerve roots. The cauda equina, if given the chance to develop properly, contains no cord tissue. Therefore the cystic outpouching will contain only nerve roots. Nerve roots, in the developmental stage, can stretch and lengthen considerably and still maintain good function. Clinically, nerve roots within a meningocele are found by direct stimulation at the time of repair. Certain meningoceles can occur within the spinal canal, and these abnormalities are without nerve roots in most cases. Generally it is these lesions where the neurologic function below the level of the defect may be maintained. These obviously carry the best prognosis. In turn, it is such lesions that demand the most meticulous care by the neurosurgeon.

Dermal sinuses

A variance of spina bifida occulta is fistula formation between the dura sac and the ectoderm of the skin. The failure of the mesodermal layer to completely close between the central nervous system tissue and the cutaneous ectoderm will produce a dermal sinus. With the abnormality in the ectoderm, hair and other ectodermal tissue may be caught within the fistulous tract or may actually lie within the spinal canal.

Ectodermal or fat tissue may be trapped within the spinal canal, in epidermoid or lipomatous tumors, or both. Dermal sinuses may be found as an isolated entity or in association with one of these tumors.

Spina bifida occulta

Spina bifida occulta, manifested simply by a failure of the lamina to fuse in the posterior plane, is indeed a common problem, but it is not usually of clinical significance. It does not cause a neurologic deficit or a defect on the skin that would require surgical correction itself. It is only important for the surgeon to be aware of this possibility in planning any type of surgery on the back. The bony abnormality can cause surgeons who do laminectomies to be involved in the wrong tissue planes. The danger is unknowingly damaging the central nervous system tissues. Therefore routine films of the back are mandatory in any planned surgery of the back.

Diastematomyelia

Diastematomyelia is one of the two disorders that represent an anterior neural plate abnormality. Failure of the neural plate to fuse posteriorly gives rise to the other six disorders discussed above. Splitting or closure abnormality on the anterior aspect of the neural plate can lead to bony or soft tissue abnormalities. Diastematomyelia represents one of these disorders. When the anterior neural segment adjacent to the notochord is divided, the cord may duplicate itself into two separate halves, and at the same time the dural and bony structures may also divide so that each neural plate acts as a separate cord. When this occurs, the vertebral body may form a bony spicule within the midline. While the nervous tissue initially develops properly, this bony spicule may lead to anchoring or scarring of the cord and cause a delayed traction injury to the adjacent nervous system tissue as the person develops.

Anterior meningoceles

Anterior meningoceles are defects involving the dura and bony structures. They most commonly occur at the most caudal aspect of the neural axis and are congenital lesions that present themselves anterior to the sacrum. They contain spinal fluid with the sac lying within the pelvis. There is a communication through the sacrum into the spinal subarachnoid space. In the majority of cases a neurologic deficit is not the manifestation of these lesions; instead they manifest themselves as pelvic masses producing chronic constipation and bladder abnormalities. The lesions can be corrected surgically without leading to a neurologic deficit. However, there is always a danger that the lower sacral nerve roots may be involved. If this is so, it can lead to certain degrees of denervation of the bowel and bladder.[2]

NEUROSURGICAL PROCEDURES

The attitude toward surgery for these dysrhaphic states has been altered markedly in the last 15 years. The major impetus toward active treatment of such children is related to the total care of the patient. With successful control of bowel and bladder abnormalities and with a few glowing reports of improved neurologic function, early closure was advocated and is now becoming more commonly utilized. These earlier reports were responsible for catalyzing the changes in therapy and have led to more active treatment of these children.

Currently all children referred to our neurosurgical service with one of the dysrhaphic conditions are considered to be surgical candidates unless there are multiple major congenital abnormalities. Very rarely defects so large that closure is considered impossible have also led to nonsurgical treatment. These are large defects high along the neural axis where we know there is considerable scarring about the cervical-medullary junction. Also, parental refusal for surgery is a definite consideration, in that the family has to be completely informed as to the child's future with operative repair. In the past, certain authors have felt that the presence of a permanent, severe neurologic deficit coupled with hydrocephalus was a contraindication to surgery.[3,9] The feeling in the past was that the neurologic deficit itself could only lead to a pathetic retarded child. Prolongation of life for such an infant seemed to be unwarranted. This becomes a matter of philosophy. With the informed consent of the parents, we still occasionally do not perform surgery on these children in our clinic. If the child is not a surgical candidate, he or she is managed by our pediatric service. There is considerable counseling by our geneticists so that the family is fully informed of their chances of having a second such child.

Children who are to undergo operative repair of the defect have the lesion covered by a povidone-iodine (Betadine)–soaked gauze immediately. A detailed examination is carried out to evaluate the function of the lower extremities, including the presence or absence of an anal wink. Radiographs are obtained along the entire vertebral axis to evaluate the presence of multiple skeletal abnormalities that may occur with this condition. Operative repair is planned as soon as possible within the first 24 hours of life.

Recently a new method of treatment has been devised. The newborn with a meningomyelocele is treated sterilely from the moment the diagnosis is made. The child is wrapped in sterile blankets, the defect is bathed only with sterile solutions with no antiseptics used, and all personnel wear sterile gowns and masks. The defect is closed as soon as possible, using the operating microscope, in an effort to preserve as much nervous tissue as possible.[12]

General anesthesia is preferred in most cases. A warming blanket is used with rolled towels beneath the shoulders, pelvis, and ankles. The anal area is excluded from the field, even though there should not be bacterial contamination from this source immediately after birth. The entire back is prepared as widely as possible so that the surrounding tissues may be mobilized extensively. The specific technique used to close the defect varies with the type and size of the lesion. The purpose of all procedures is to free all nervous tissue and replace nerve roots and spinal cord segments within the vertebral canal without increasing the neurologic deficit.

The operative procedure depends on the cephalad-caudal placement of the lesion on the vertebral axis and the exact degree of the dysplasia. Encephaloceles are closed primarily by amputation of the adjacent central nervous system tissue with the goal of achieving the best cosmetic result possible. An effort to preserve neural function of the tissue herniated from within the cranial cavity is no longer made. Myeloschisis repairs are done with the thought that the neurologic deficit is permanent, complete, and irreversible. Consequently, neural tissue may be removed at this time in order to achieve a satisfactory bony and soft tissue alignment. Meningomyloceles constitute the area where surgical judgment is the most important. The healthy-looking cord tissue must be preserved and all nerve roots dissected free. If on stimulation the nerve root functions at the time of operation, then it absolutely must be dissected free and allowed to assume a more normal position within a spinal canal. If the nerve root tissue comes from a markedly dysplastic cord and does not conduct at the time of operation, then the preservation of all this tissue is less important. Meningoceles contain only nerve roots, which must be meticulously dissected and returned to the neural canal. Dermal sinuses need to be excised so that there is no communication from outside the skin to the inside of the dural sac. Obviously this is a setting for meningitis. It is also a setting for the development of delayed epidermoid tumors. In the closure of dermal sinuses the presence of an intradural lesion must be ruled out. Finally, spinal bifida occulta requires no treatment initially. These patients may develop lipomas and epidermoids at a later date. Diastematomyelia and anterior meningoceles are treated once the diagnosis is made, but they are not usually a problem within the first year of life.

Unfortunately, successful closure of meningocele usually does not mark the end of neurosurgical care. The higher or more cephalad the lesion and the more severe the dysrhaphic condition, the greater the likelihood that hydrocephalus will be present in the patient. In many cases the hydrocephalus is present at the time of the initial diagnosis.[11] At other times the hydrocephalus is clinically manifest immediately upon the closure of the defect, at which time there is no easy exit for the circulating spinal fluid. Ninety-five percent of children with these caudal defects have other abnormalities within the central nervous system. For example, Arnold-Chiari malformation of the cervical-medullary junction occurs in 70% to 90% of the patients.[22] There is a defect in the posterior arch of C-1 in more than 70% of the patients.[6] Various degrees of hydromyelia or cystic spinal fluid accumulation within the cord opposed to the brain occur in more than one third of the children. Syringomyelia, diplomyelia, and other abnormalities of nervous system tissue can occur. Other bony abnormalities associated with the disorders include the Klippel-Feil syndrome, platobasia, basilar impression, cervical malformations and asymmetry, and cervical ribs. In addition, these same children are more prone to have teratomas, lipomas, and sacrococcygeal dermoids.

Of all these lesions, hydrocephalus is initially the most important. In many cases it is difficult to determine whether to first treat the hydrocephalus or the meningomyelocele disorder. While there are obviously advocates for both sides, currently we tend to first close the posterior dural defect. This primary closure is followed within a day or so with a ventricular shunt operation if there is overt hydrocephalus initially or if the hydrocephalus manifests itself. It is not clear whether the hydrocephalus abnormality is related to the Arnold-Chiari malformation and posterior fossa circulatory abnormalities or is due to failure of proper development of the normal absorption channels along the superior sagittal sinus. However, the majority of the children treated in our clinic do have a ventricular shunt operation performed during the initial hospitalization. The exception obviously is the very low meningocele and the very high encephalocele, for these patients often do not require a shunt.

Both ventriculoatrial and ventriculoperitoneal shunts are suitable procedures, and both techniques have their proponents.[1,4,19] The advantages of a ventriculoatrial shunt are that it can be performed easily and that it does not require extensive tubing. When infection occurs with a ventriculoatrial shunt, it is usually a readily controllable septicemia due to a blood contamination. It seems that ventriculoatrial shunts are more commonly infected but usually do not lead to serious ventriculitis when infection occurs. The procedure should be avoided in the face of any active infection. Patients with increased cerebrospinal fluid protein and patients with congenital cardiac or cardiopulmonary abnormalities usually have a shunt to the peritoneum. Complications of the ventriculoatrial shunt readily occur when the child grows and the tubing becomes shortened from the atrium up into the superior vena cava.

On the other hand, ventriculoperitoneal shunts tend to work longer if the peritoneal catheter initially is made long in order to allow for axial growth. However, even though the shunts tend to work longer, require less replacement, and are associated with less obstruction, when an infection occurs, it is usually more serious and results in ventriculitis.[10,21] Exactly how the organisms of the peritoneal cavity, which may be gram-negative rods, are able to migrate as far as the head is poorly understood; however, it definitely does occur. Rarely, the ventriculoperitoneal shunt may be obstructed by omentum, bowel adhesions, or other pelvic structures. Regardless of the type of shunt diversion operation, there is no doubt as to the value of the procedure. In general, the current statistics indicate that the natural mortality in the condition can be readily halved, and the number of educable survivors can be doubled by such operative care.[14]

Other cerebrospinal fluid diversion procedures are available. These are not commonly used, but include ventriculopleural and ventriculoureteral shunts and ventriculostomies. All have varied degrees of success and failure. Since the advent of better tubing and valve systems, they have not commonly been used in the last 10 years.

The children after their initial care require long-term follow-up because of the patency failure of the shunts and because of the common occurrence of other congenital abnormalities along the cranial-vertebral axis. Delayed problems may occur, due to hydromyelia, syringomyelia, traction disorders, and so on. For example, children successfully treated for meningomyelocele in the dorsal region may readily develop difficulties with their cranial nerves due to traction and compression abnormalities at the cervical-medullary junction. In certain children the second dsyplastic area will cause a delayed death, in which the child's swallowing and breathing mechanisms fail. On occasion this can be corrected by a posterior decompression. In other cases the posterior decompression gives temporary relief, only for the problems to recur and the child to develop aspiration or respiratory failure.

The spectrum of abnormalities known as the dorsal rachischisis disorders is and will continue to be, a major problem in pediatric medicine. These disorders require cooperation among many medical and surgical disciplines in order to afford the best care. The child with one of these disorders has a constellation of lesions that present as he grows and develops. With newer medical and surgical therapies the length and quality of life for these patients are improving.

REFERENCES

1. Ames, R. H.: Ventriculo-peritoneal shunts in the management of hydrocephalus, J. Neurosurg. **27**:525, 1967.
2. Anderson, F. M., and Burke, L.: Anterior sacral meningocoele, J.A.M.A. **237**:39, 1977.
3. Bailey, P., et al.: Year book of neurology, Chicago, 1949, Year Book Medical Publishers.
4. Beucer, D., and Nulsen, F. E.: Control of hydrocephalus by valve-regulated venus shunt: avoidance of complications in prolonged shunt maintenance, Neurosurg. **283**:215, 1968.
5. Brucklehurst, G.: The pathogenesis of spina bifida: a story of the relationship between observations, hypothesis and surgical incentive, Dev. Med. Child Neurol. **13**:147, 1971.
6. DeLong, W. B., and Schneider, R. C.: Surgical management of congenital spinal lesions associated with abnormalities of the craniospinal junction, J. Neurol. Neurosurg. Psychiatry **29**:319, 1966.
7. Gardner, W. J.: The dysrhaphic states from syringomyelia to anencephaly, excerpta medica, New York, 1973, American Elsevier Publishing Co.
8. Johnson, R. T.: Viral infections and malformations of the nervous system, Birth Defects **7**:56, 1971.
9. Kahn, E. A., et al.: Correlative neurosurgery, 3, ed. Springfield, Ill., 1969, Charles C Thomas, Publisher.
10. Little, J. R., Rhoton, A. L., and Mellinger, J. F.: Comparison of ventriculoperitoneal and ventriculoarterial shunts for hydrocephalus in children, Mayo Clin. Proc. **47**:396, 1972.
11. Lorber, J.: Ventriculo-cardiac shunts in the first week of life, Dev. Med. Child Neurol. [Suppl.] **20**:13, 1969.
12. McLaine, W.: Personal communication, 1977.
13. Menkes, J.: Textbook of child neurology, Philadelphia, 1974, Lea & Febiger.
14. Milhorat, T. H.: Hydrocephalus and the cerebrospinal fluid, Baltimore, 1972, The Williams & Wilkins Company.
15. Naggan, L.: The recent decline in prevalence of anencephaly and spina bifida, Am. J. Epidemiol. **89**:154, 1969.
16. Nance, N. E.: Anencephalcy and spina bifida: an etiologic hypothesis, Birth Defects **7**:97, 1971.
17. Navarette, V. N., et al.: Subsequent diabetes in mothers delivered of a malformed infant, Lancet **2**:993, 1970.
18. Neel, J. V.: A study of major congenital defects in Japanese infants, Am. J. Hum. Genet. **10**:398, 1958.

19. Overton, M. C., III, and Snodgrass, S. R.: Ventriculo-venous shunts for infantile hydrocephalus: a review of five years experience, J. Neurosurg. **23:**517, 1965.
20. Padget, D. H.: Spina bifida and embryonic neuroschisis—a causal relationship, Johns Hopkins Med. J. **123:**233-252, 1968.
21. Rubin, R. C., et al.: Asymptomatic perforated incus and gram-negative ventriculitis as a complication of valve regulated ventriculoperitoneal shunts, J. Neurosurg. **37:**616, 1972.
22. Russell, L. B.: X-ray induced development abnormalities in the mouse and their use in the analysis of embroyological patterns, J. Exp. Zool. **114:**545, 1950.
23. Thiersch, J. B.: Therapeutic abortions with a folic acid antagonist, 4-aminonteroylglotamic acid (4-amino PGA), administered by oral route, Am. J. Obstet. Gynecol. **63:**1298, 1952.

Chapter 22

Meningomyelocele: plastic surgery considerations

Frank J. Gerow
Jonathan J. Dora

The plastic surgeon does not see the simple meningomyelocele closure. Primary closure of this defect is routinely carried out by the neurosurgeon after completion of the dural closure. Meningomyeloceles seen by the plastic surgeon will be those that the neurosurgeon recognizes to be difficult, either because of the complexity of the dural closure or because of the size of the skin defect. The plastic surgeon should encourage his neurosurgery colleague to consult with him prior to the anticipated surgery and then should plan to be present in the operating room from the beginning of the procedure. Initially, all epithelium on the wound edges should be preserved. In this regard the plastic surgeon will benefit from acting as the neurosurgeon's first assistant, retracting these wound edges for the neurosurgeon while the neurosurgeon proceeds with the neurosurgical aspects of the repair. Although the plastic surgeon may elect later to sacrifice some of this wound edge if the looseness of the tissue permits, there will be times when this tissue is critical. By his presence from the beginning of the procedure the plastic surgeon has an excellent opportunity to assess the difficulty encountered in acquiring a watertight closure of the dura mater.

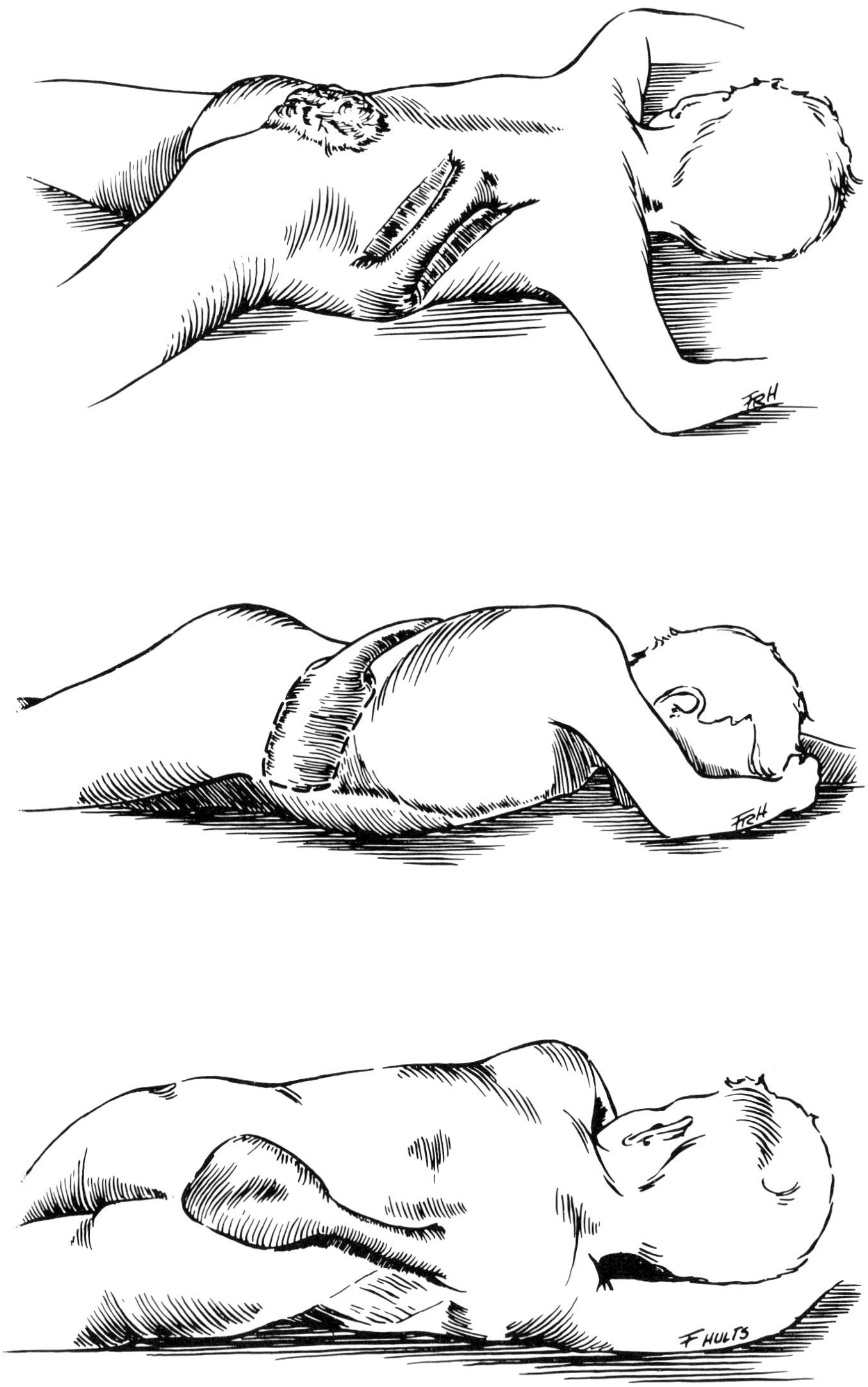

Fig. 22-1. Soderberg's multiple-stage bipedicle meningomyelocele closure. (From Soderberg, B. N., and Sutton, J. B.: U.S. Armed Forces Med. J. **7:**1214, 1956.)

HISTORY

A review of the literature reveals several landmarks in the management of meningomyelocele. Soderberg and Sutton[5] recommended a multiple-stage bipedicle closure that obviously precluded an early primary closure and increased the risk of intercurrent meningitis (Fig. 22-1). Edgerton[2] popularized the S-flap or the use of rotation flaps to close the meningomyelocele. This technique has some application in closure of lesions of limited size; however, the thinness of the flaps at the tips, the area in which the best closure is needed, makes this method somewhat risky (Fig. 22-2). Mustarde[4] has described a procedure involving a complex muscle-bone flap in which the laminae are fractured and the transverse processes and related musculature turned toward the midline to accomplish closure of the bony canal. The resulting defect is skin grafted (Fig. 22-3). DesPrez and associates[1] published a technique in which a double bucket-handle bipedicle advancement of a complex muscle-skin flap is created, involving flank incisions extending from the axilla to the groin with a dissection that results in the elevation and movement of the latissimus dorsi muscle with the overlying skin (Fig. 22-4).

The skin-subcutaneous defect enlarges in proportion to the infant's back once the neurosurgeon has accomplished the elevation of available dura and adjacent fascia and the precise closure so necessary to the success of any of these meningomyelocele procedures. If the dural closure is quite tight, with no leakage of cerebrospinal fluid, a wound closure may be considered that involves the local advancement of the wound edges and closure of the remaining central defect with a skin graft (Fig. 22-5). This type of closure is predicated on the ability of the dura to vascularize the overlying skin graft, which is most tenuous in the central area where closure is critical.

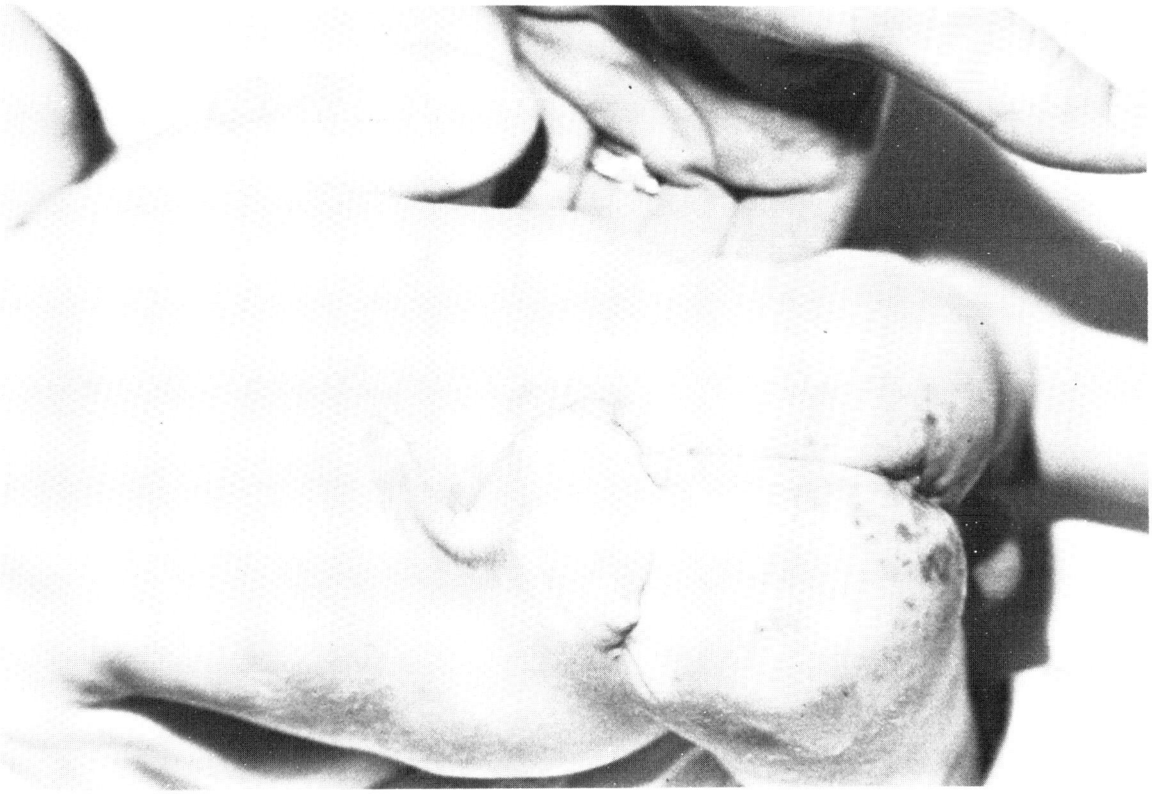

Fig. 22-2. S-flap meningomyelocele closure.

A

B

C

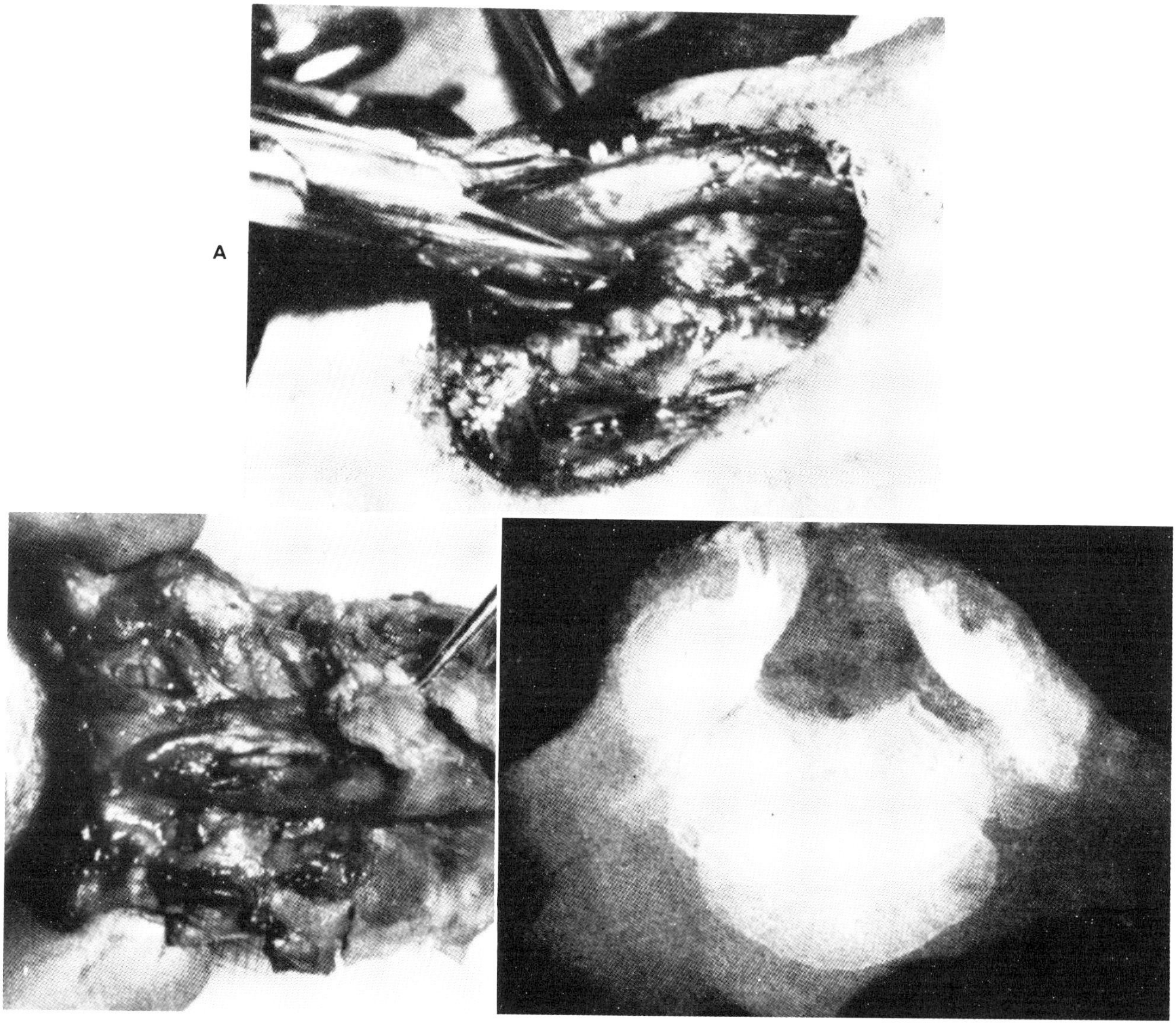

Fig. 22-3. Mustarde technique. **A,** Fracturing of spinous processes. **B,** Dissected specimen showing two spinous processes on one side fractured and brought over cord and meninges. **C,** X-ray film, showing fractured spinous processes brought over toward midline. (From Mustarde, J. C.: Br. J. Surg. **53:**36, 1966.)

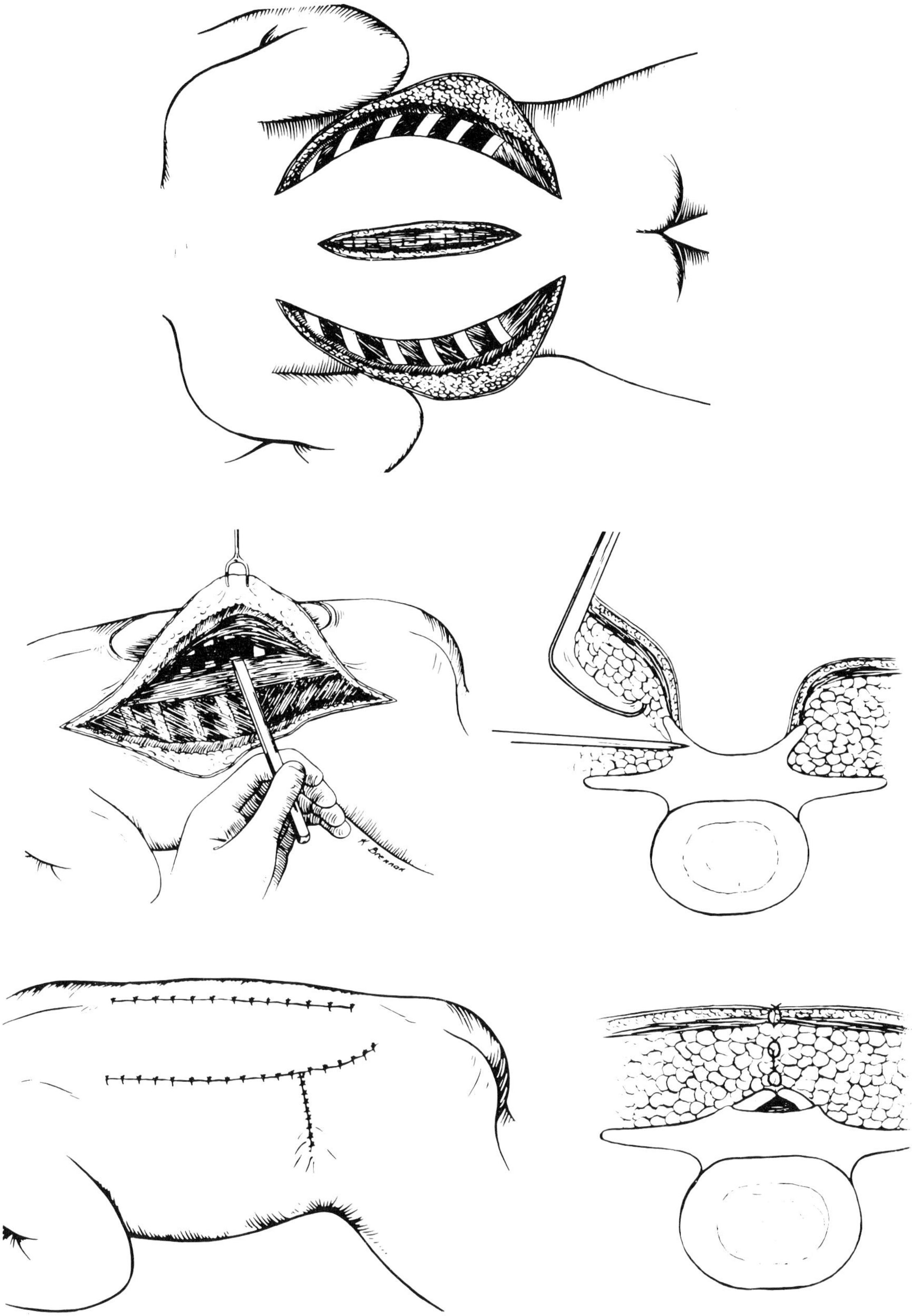

Fig. 22-4. Double bucket-handle bipedicle advancement of muscle-skin flap with flank incisions and elevation and movement of latissimus dorsi muscle with overlying skin. (From DesPrez, J. D., Kiehn, C. L., and Eckstein, W.: Plast. Reconstr. Surg. **47:**234, 1971. © 1971 The Williams & Wilkins Co., Baltimore.)

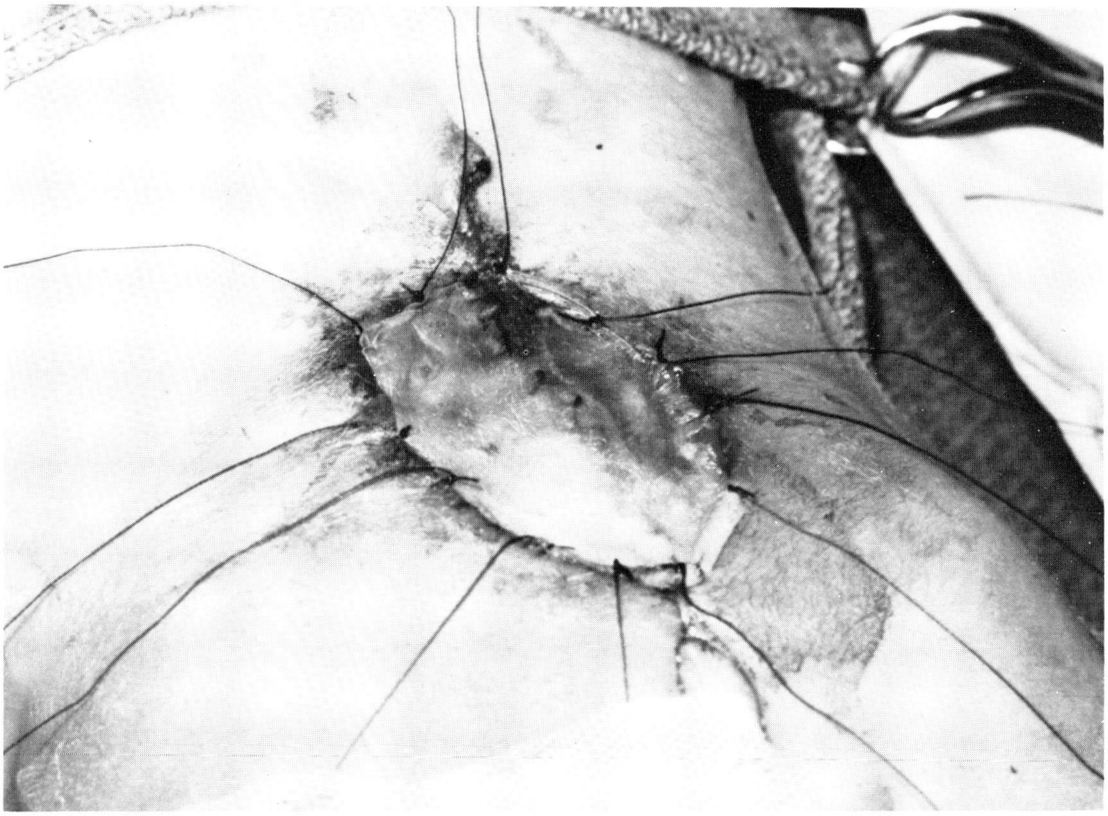

Fig. 22-5. Closure of central defect with skin graft.

SURGICAL METHOD: WOUND FLAP ADVANCEMENT TECHNIQUE

We favor the wound flap advancement technique. Following closure of the dura, the plastic surgeon begins the undermining of adjacent tissue immediately below the deep fascia and superficial to the muscle plane. Dissection at this level is easy and quite bloodless (Fig. 22-6). Diligent care should be taken to protect wound edges, and tension on the wound edges should be relieved during dissection to permit vascular recovery time. The use of rigid retractors in the wound should be avoided early in the dissection. A ribbon retractor may be necessary when the dissection has proceeded around the side of the trunk toward the anterior torso. It should be remembered that the rigidity of a retractor places an abnormal strain on the edges of the wound and that an electrocautery will ground out against a retractor if it is touched, damaging the flap.

Undermining is carried out widely with particular attention to the release of the fibrous tissue connections to the scapular spine, the dorsal spinous processes above and below the defect, the posterior iliac crest, and the sacrum (Fig. 22-7). Some bleeding will be encountered with the release of these fascial connections, and careful hemostasis is essential in these areas. These areas of bleeding do not, however, represent a blood supply critical to flap viability; this has been preserved by the subfascial dissection. The preservation of blood supply by this technique has been demonstrated by McCraw and associates.[3]

Along the midlateral line the lateral perforators will be encountered, and although the one or two perforators immediately opposite the somatic level of the meningomyelocele may have to be severed, the others frequently can be carefully dissected free and left as neurovascular connections between the musculature of the trunk and the overlying skin flap. Dissection is carried as far anteriorly as is necessary to mobilize the posterior wound edge to the midline; in the case illustrated (Fig. 22-8) the dissection was carried to the paraumbilical area. The wound edge may become slightly dusky but has proved to be viable in the 12 cases done with this technique.

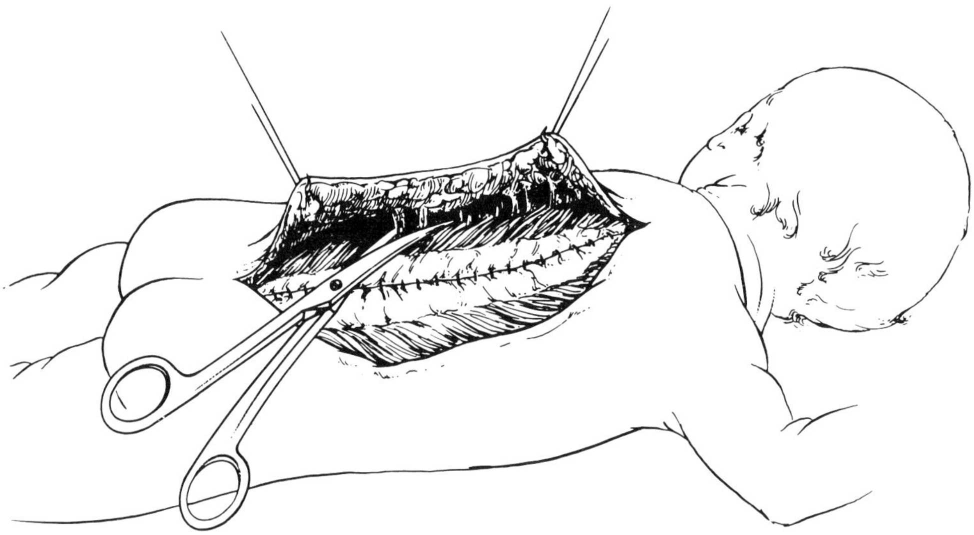

Fig. 22-6. Undermining immediately below deep fascia and superficial to muscle.

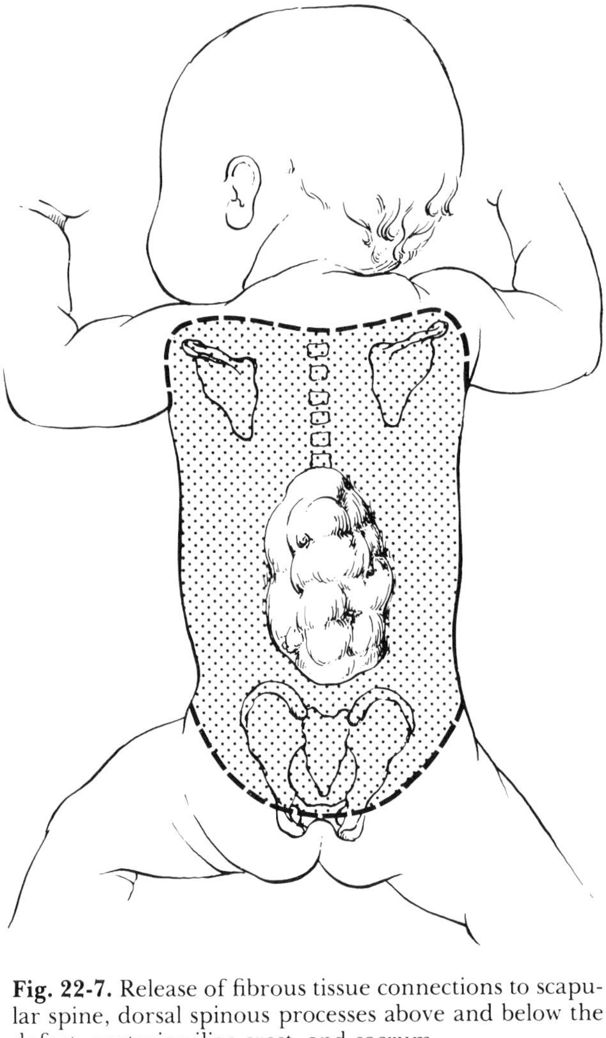

Fig. 22-7. Release of fibrous tissue connections to scapular spine, dorsal spinous processes above and below the defect, posterior iliac crest, and sacrum.

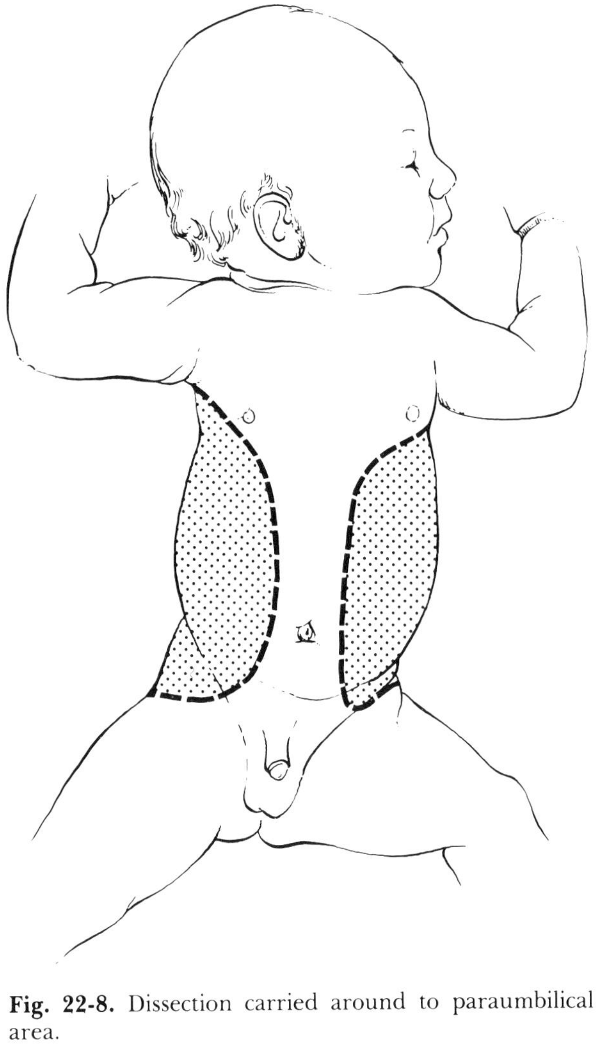

Fig. 22-8. Dissection carried around to paraumbilical area.

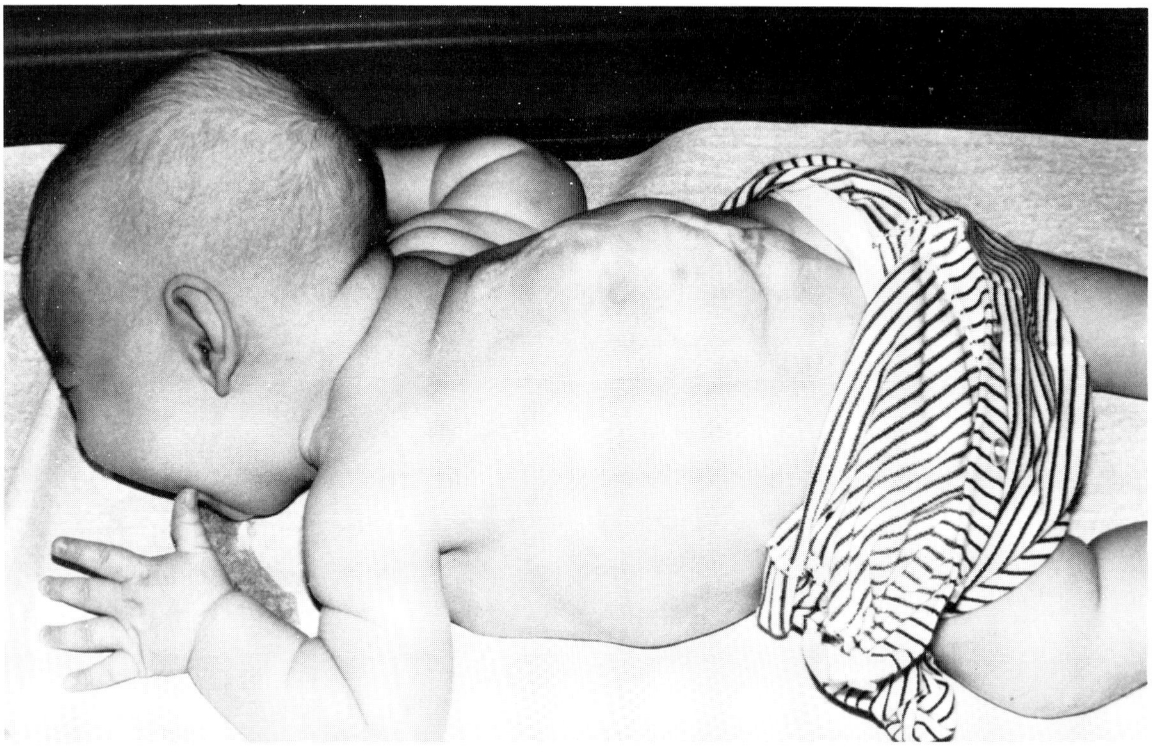

Fig. 22-9. Meningomyelocele closure over kyphosis.

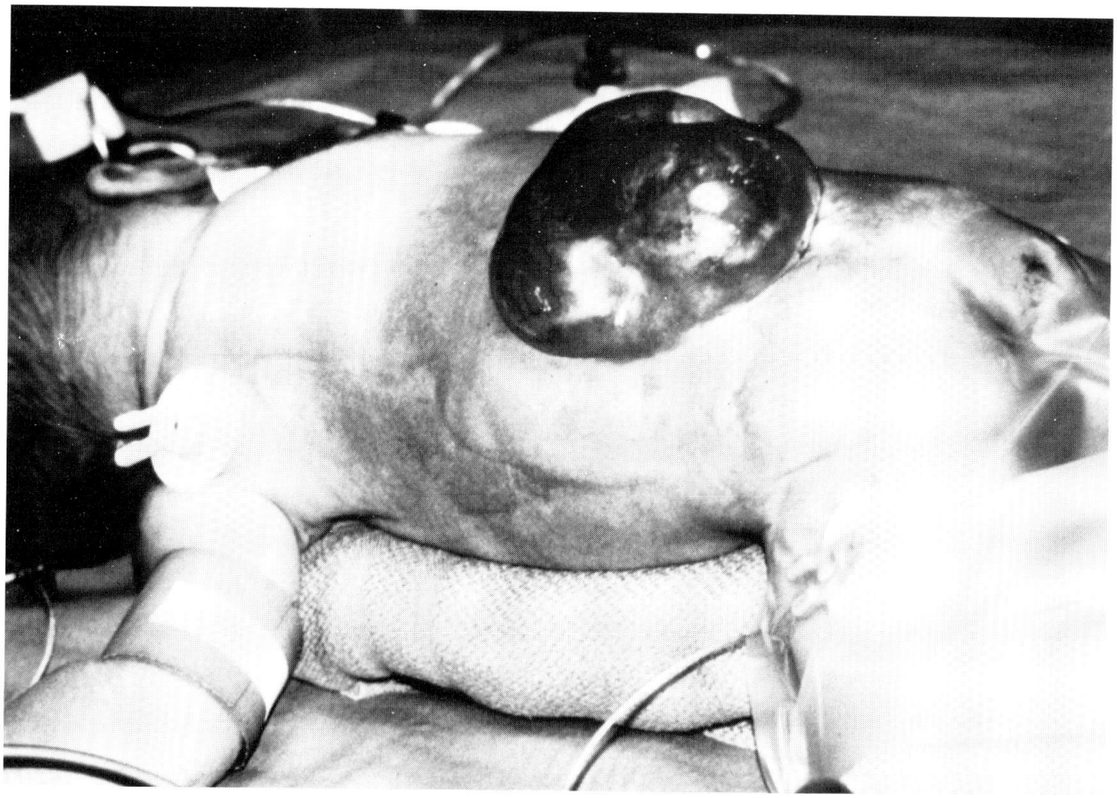

Fig. 22-10. "Dog-ear" effect following primary closure should not be revised until later date; tissues will often smooth out so that no revision is necessary.

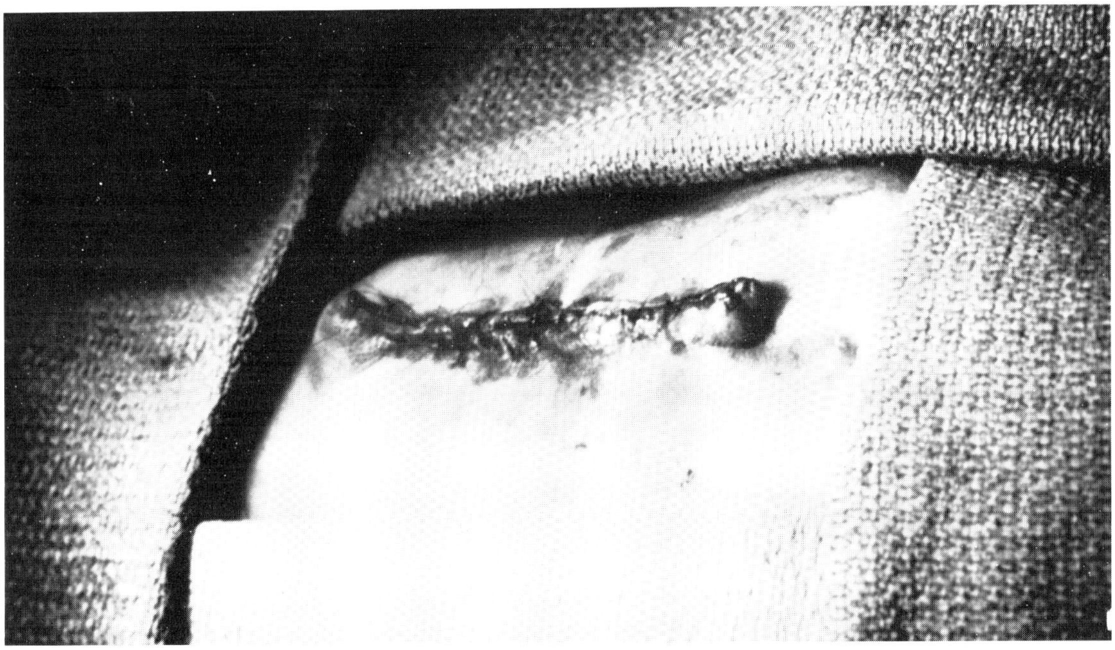

Fig. 22-10, cont'd. For legend see opposite page.

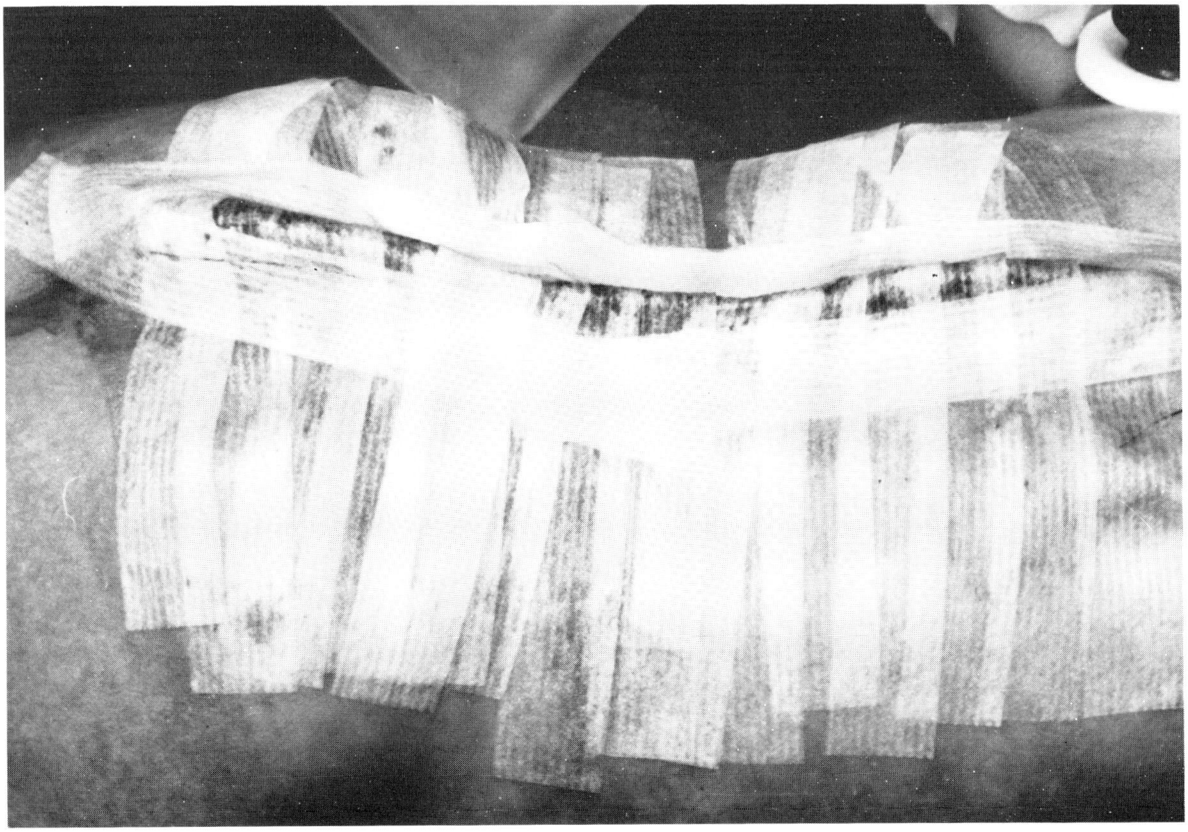

Fig. 22-11. Steri-Strip support of meningomyelocele closure.

The dissection will permit mobilization of these lateral wounds over a kyphotic deformity if such is present (Fig. 22-9). At the time of the primary closure, the "dog-ear" effect at each end of the wound is not disturbed; any trimming of this should be considered at a later date (Fig. 22-10). Generally the tissues smooth out enough that no revision is needed.

No drains are put in the wound. Deep closure is accomplished with a suture of individual choice; we prefer 3-0 plain catgut. A subcuticular closure of running nylon and interrupted nylon skin sutures completes the procedure. The interrupted nylon sutures are placed as half-buried vertical mattress sutures, alternating the sides on which the mattress effect is done to reduce the chances of wound necrosis from the external part of the suture. The wound closure is supported with Steri-Strips (Fig. 22-11) and dressed with fluffs and Elastoplast extending from the shoulder girdle to the thighs and flank to flank; the dressing thus restricts the spastic flexion motion characteristic of these infants.

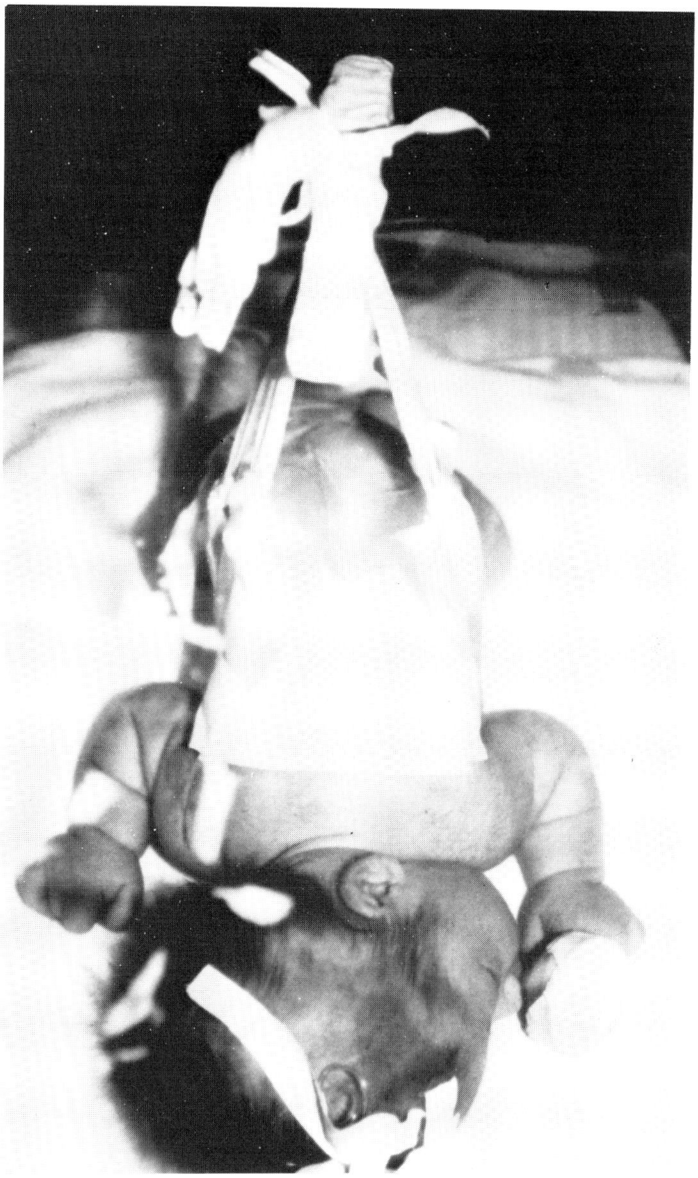

Fig. 22-12. Postoperative suspension system.

POSTOPERATIVE CARE

Postoperative management of a patient who has undergone this closure is quite important. The patient is suspended in the prone position from the top of the Isolette (Fig. 22-12) with Montgomery straps that have been carefully cut away to protect the skin over the prominence of the iliac crests (Fig. 22-13). The level of suspension just allows the infant's abdomen to clear the mattress and permits his knees and lower legs to touch the mattress. The patient is kept in this position approximately 5 days, monitored, and fed intravenously. Oral feeding can be started 2 to 3 days postoperatively, and if difficulty is encountered in feeding, the infant can be placed on one side long enough to accomplish the feeding and then returned to suspension.

The dressings are changed each day. Aspiration of fluid from beneath the flap is not undertaken unless the viability of the overlying wound is in jeopardy or the clinical picture suggests sepsis. If either of these occurs, aspiration is carried out in a sterile field through a percutaneous puncture located lateral to the wound and the dural reflection. If at 5 to 7 days postoperatively there is no fluid beneath the flaps and if the flaps are adhering to the underlying tissue, the patient may be removed from the suspension. The infant may be kept in the suspension system longer if necessary. Nursing personnel should be instructed to avoid the deliberate flexing of the patient's back at feeding time during the following week, and the patient is not permitted to lie on his back for at least 2 weeks postoperatively. Sutures are removed 10 to 14 days after the surgery.

RESULTS

Of the 12 patients treated in the manner described, only one experienced difficulty; this involved a wound infection with subsequent necrosis of part of the closure site. Conservative care and management of this problem later permitted skin grafting of the residual defect.

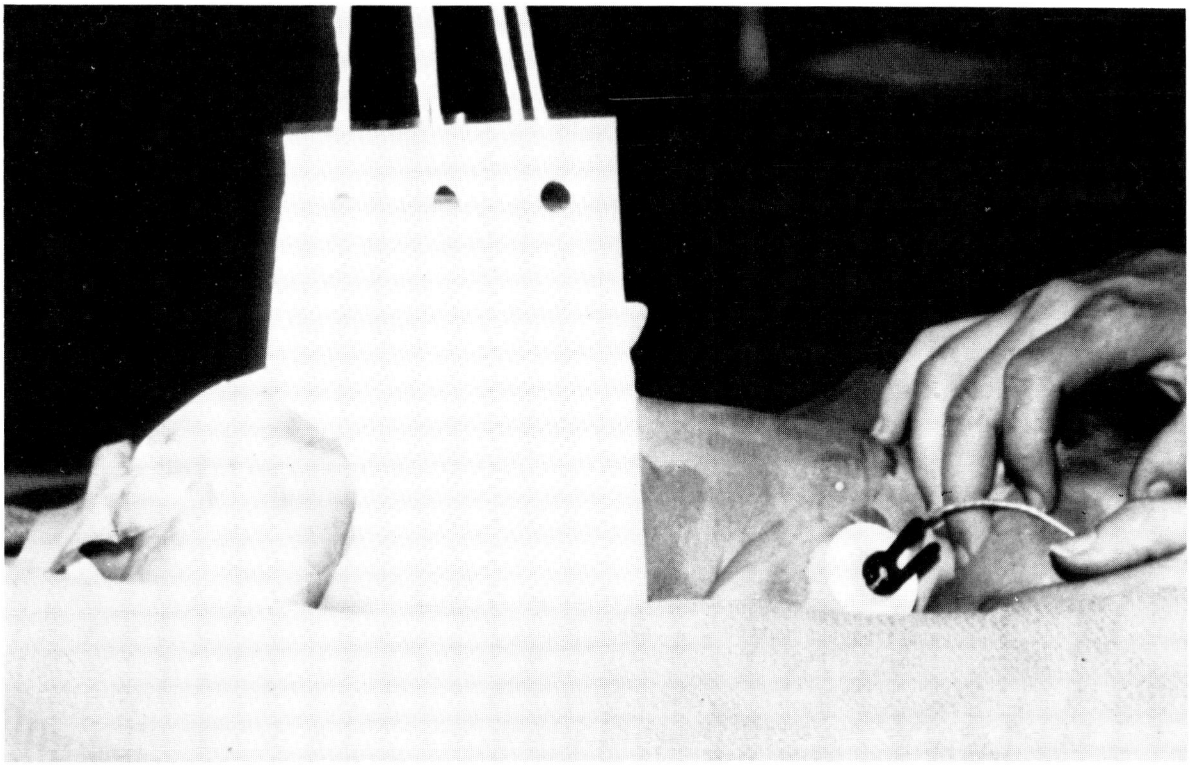

Fig. 22-13. Montgomery straps in suspension system are carefully cut away to protect skin over prominence of iliac crests.

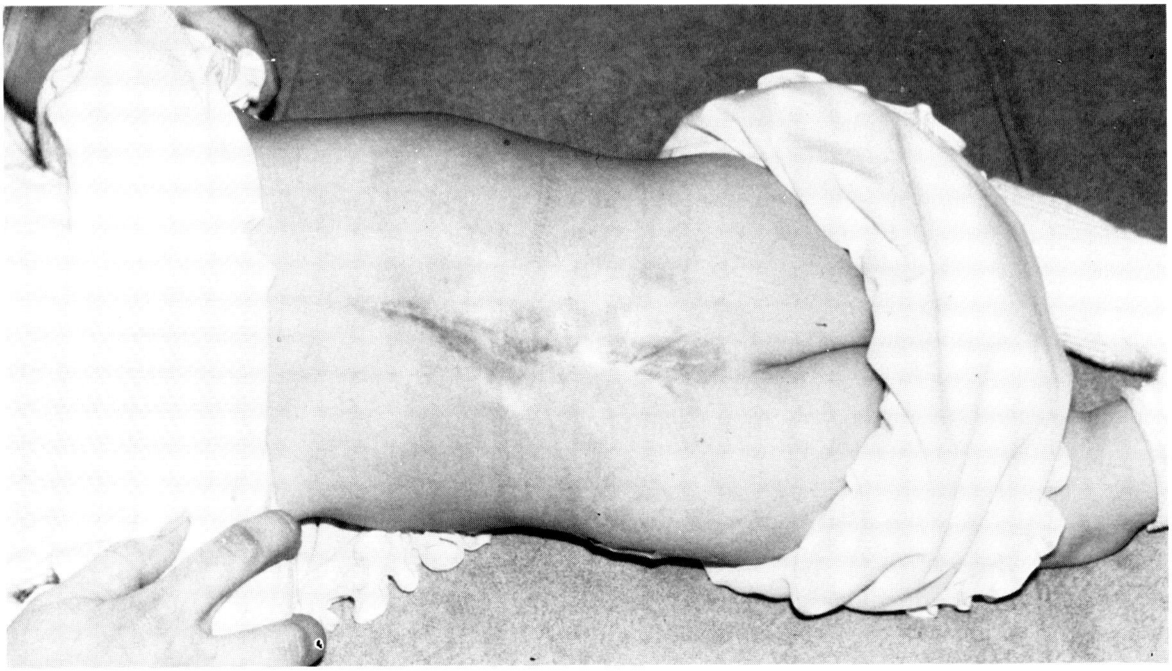

Fig. 22-14. Eighteen-month follow-up on patient treated with our wound flap advancement technique.

CONCLUSION

Fig. 22-14 represents an 18-month follow-up of a typical closure. This procedure of wound flap advancement is recommended for primary closure of the meningomyelocele. The technique involves extensive undermining of the skin and subcutaneous tissues of the torso at a subfascial level with advancement of the wound edges and primary closure. Emphasis is placed upon the method of suspending the patient in the Isolette after the surgery in such a way as to relieve tension on wound edges without applying compression to the lateral vasculature of the flaps. The results have been uniformly encouraging in the series presented.

REFERENCES

1. DesPrez, J. D., Kiehn, C. L., and Eckstein, W.: Closure of large meningomyelocele defects by composite skin-muscle flaps, Plast. Reconstr. Surg. **47:**234, 1971.
2. Edgerton, M. T.: Plastic repair of congenital defects associated with spina bifida and cranium bifidum, Surg. Clin. North Am. **32:**1327, 1952.
3. McCraw, J. B.: Personal communication, 1977.
4. Mustarde, J. C.: Meningomyelocele: the problem of skin cover, Br. J. Surg. **53:**36, 1966.
5. Soderberg, B. N., and Sutton, J. B.: Repair of meningomyelocele by plastic surgery, U.S. Armed Forces Med. J. **7:**1214, 1956.

Panel discussion on upper motor neuron disorders

SIMON FREDRICKS, Moderator
GARRY S. BRODY
THOMAS B. DUCKER
FRANK J. GEROW
M. MARK HOFFER
ERIK MOBERG
ROBERT L. WATERS

Question: Dr. Ducker, you discussed the embryologic origins of these spinal defects. Can these deformities also appear on the cranium?

Ducker: Yes, the entire spectrum from agenesis of the scalp to encephalomyeloskesis can occur along the midline. Nasofrontal encephaloceles will require dural repair as well as nasal and forehead reconstruction. Occasionally an infant will have an enormous lesion on the occiput which has no functioning neuronal components and can therefore be amputated and repaired.

Question: Dr. Waters, can you define spasticity for us?

Waters: Spasticity is a confusing term and should be replaced by muscle overactivity. For example, Mark Hoffer demonstrated how the tonic neck reflexes may be an important cause of overactivity in the so-called "spastic" patient. Just going from a supine to an upright posture may also stimulate overactivity. As a matter of fact, the upper extremity should always be examined with the patient upright. The recumbent patient has no labyrinthal input into his muscles. Merely sitting him up produces a sudden increase in flexor tone. The extensor patterning in the hemiplegic or cerebral palsied patient is another cause of overactivity. Other neurologic disorders, such as midbrain dysfunction, may produce rigidity. Thus spasticity has been an all-inclusive term and should be replaced by "muscle overactivity" further defined by an etiologic modifier.

Question: Dr. Hoffer, what late rehabilitative measures do you suggest for the walking myelodysplastic patient?

Hoffer: If a patient has no lower extremity muscle function and no sensation below the hips he does not ambulate. Patients with poorly controlled hydrocephalus don't ambulate. Many successfully walking children cease to do so after puberty because ambulation requires too great an energy expenditure for an adult. The child must develop ambulation himself, with our help, and lose it himself, again with our help and understanding. There is a very complex social interaction between the teenager, his parents, and the treatment team, and we mustn't cruelly encourage continued ambulation at great energy cost and at the expense of comfort.

Question: Would someone care to discuss the difference between congenital and acquired upper motor neuron lesions?

Hoffer: Generally the congenital or developmental upper lesion is purely motor while those due to trauma (at birth or later) will almost always have an associated sensory loss. Certainly the traumatic lesion is much more difficult to rehabilitate.

Question: How do you deal with established contractures in an upper motor neuron lesion?

Moberg: Not all contractures are bad, of course. I can recall one patient whose middle finger flexion contracture was essential for driving. But most contractures should be corrected. It is usually inadequate to just range the joints a few times per day, especially if proprioception is impaired. Dynamic splinting with elastic bands for counterpull can correct and control most contractures in preparation for definitive surgical correction.

Waters: In adults with acquired spasticity the contracture is usually myostatic and rarely periarticular. This can be tested with appropriate nerve blocks or during anesthesia when the patient is curarized. Thus your surgical procedure can be planned appropriately.

Ducker: Dr. Brody pointed out that drooling children can consciously control their salivary loss but resume drooling when distracted. Spasticity is similar. There is a tremendous unconscious system for rapid handling of proprioceptive information. The corticospinal system that controls conscious motion transmits signals at only 10 to 15 m per second. The spinocerebellar system in contrast is a servomechanism which is the fastest conducting part of the nervous system. Signals travel through three synapses at 120 m per second. Thus, this automatic system can make three circuits to set the muscle tone before you can think about moving your finger. The cerebellum has almost as many neurons as the entire cerebrum and is constantly setting and adjusting muscle tone with every activity and postural change day and night. When you lose fine control of muscle balance the stronger flexor muscles overpower the extensors, and the contracture is manifest.

Question: Dr. John McGraw is in the audience—would you care to comment on the method of closing meningomyeloceles?

McGraw: We feel that dividing the skin in a bipedicle flap is contraindicated. Recently we have been using a modification of John DesPrez's original latissimus procedure and lifting the muscle with the skin. The skin of the back is vascularized primarily through the latissimus muscle which in turn is supplied by the thoracodorsal artery and posteriorly by several perforators. The thoracodorsal fascia can be incised just lateral to the dural closure, and one can easily hand-dissect beneath the latissimus. By simply cutting the fascia anterior to the muscle one can easily close a 10 cm defect in a 6-pound baby. One gets both a muscle and skin closure in about 25 minutes with about 20 ml blood loss.

Question: One subject we have not addressed ourselves to is the neurologic deficits created by fibrous as opposed to neuromuscular contractures. Dr. Brody, how do you deal with congenital annular fibrous bands?

Brody: First, let me discuss the timing. If the band involves the superficial tissues only and shows no sign of peripheral edema or neuromuscular involvement, then one can wait until the infant is secure, using such guidelines as attainment of 10 pounds, 3 months, and so on. Again, if it is so severe that the peripheral part is almost autoamputated, then the procedure is also nonurgent and can be timed with the sociopsychologic readiness of the family to accept the final separation of the part. Those babies who demonstrate distal edema or neuromuscular deficit represent an urgent situation and should be done promptly. Surgically, the classic recommendations are to do a series of multiple Z-plasties in one or more stages. We have found this to be less than aesthetic as it is very difficult to avoid irregular surface bulges of the skin and subcutaneous tissues. Excellent results with smooth contours can be obtained by excising the band circumferentially and carefully dissecting out its deepest bands much like one would dissect a chordee or a Dupuytren band. The circumferential incisions should be serpentine and matched for fit proximally and distally. One should not try to save any of the skin in the trough, but rather excise to the limits of the depression where normal contour begins. Closure is not difficult, and the serpentine line prevents later scar contracture. By not attempting to salvage the circumferentially deficient skin in the trough with Z-plasties and flaps a much smoother contour is obtained.

Question: Dr. Gerow, do you feel that the carapace of contractured scar in a circumferential burn can produce a neurologic deficit?

Gerow: Yes. It is only recently that we have begun to appreciate that the swelling, fascial tightness, and subsequent scarring can produce subtle and sometimes severe neuromuscular deficits. We should now begin to think of decompressing these limbs for neuromuscular signs rather than waiting for vascular compromise.

Brody: I would like to elaborate on that a bit. The late, healed burn can present with classic signs of carpal tunnel or ulnar compression at the elbow. If the latter is present, there is often a history of prolonged elbow resting while grafts are healing.

Simple fascial release including the origins of the flexor carpi ulnaris is usually successful, and nerve transplants are rarely indicated. The problem is frequently one of diagnosis of these compression neuropathies in those limbs whose sensorium in grafted skin is already impaired. We are probably overlooking some but must rely more on the patient's symptomatology unless some motor deficits are apparent. Some patients complain of a burning type of hypersensitivity which is usually aggravated by compression garments. In these patients, nerve conduction studies may be helpful but are very difficult to do through the burn scar. The fact that every patient we have surgically released has been helped suggests to me that we are probably underdiagnosing the neurologic deficit.

Hoffer: We have seen three cases of ulnar nerve involvement in the heterotopic ossification about the elbow of burn patients. This can occur without any direct burn of the elbow itself or even of that limb. In these patients, transplant is mandatory.

Question: Dr. Waters, you have said that one should not release myostatic contractures excessively for fear of lengthening the musculotendinous unit beyond its range of effective action and thus weakening the grip. Do you find that after an optimum release further contracture occurs from continued muscular overreaction?

Waters: In cerebral palsy, those hands that have fixed musculotendinous contractures do not really work even after release. There are very few patients in whom a flexor slide on tendon elongations is justified. Occasionally a superficialis release may be beneficial, but if nonfunctional balance for cosmesis or hygiene is required, then we prefer the sublimis to profundus transfer described by Braun. Tendon transfers are usually more successful in cerebral palsy than are lengthening procedures. In adults with acquired spasticity and some residual function, again the effective available excursion is limited. We usually compromise by lengthening the motor unit by about one half of what it would take to get the hand to neutral. We have never lost function with this approach.

Question: Dr. Waters, is there a place for tendon transfers in the hemiplegic hand?

Waters: It depends on the cause. In the stroke patient probably not, but in the cerebral palsied child it can be quite useful. With head injuries, one must individualize the problem depending on the lesion, and electromyograms can be very helpful in deciding. Transferring of muscles that do not fire in their normal phase should not be done as they can be very unpredictable.

Fredricks: Thank you, gentlemen. Our discussion has perhaps gone afield from upper motor neuron disorders, but the term "contracture" can be used for muscle overactivity or cicatricial shortening. These two may be clinically difficult to separate, and thus I believe our discussion has been appropriate.

Part IV

Pressure ulcerations

Chapter 23

Pathomechanics of pressure ulceration

Paul W. Brand

The problem of pressure sores is complex. It involves questions of sensory denervation and of so-called trophic changes. It involves problems of paralysis and of the immobility of very sick and aged persons. Incontinence plays a part and is tied in with the effect of maceration of skin and of an infected environment. The factor of nursing care and hospital costs sometimes dominates the question and results in hot discussion of responsibility and of blame for failure to prevent a pressure sore.

In all this complexity, there is a central fact on which I want to concentrate today. It is the fact that every pressure sore results from the application of mechanical force. If we can understand exactly how skin reacts to force and under what mechanical circumstances it breaks down, then I believe we can minimize the significance of all the other factors. We should be able to modify and control the mechanical environment so that pressure sores are prevented.

This would have been clearly defined long ago but for the fact that most scientists have studied just one aspect of the problem and have not realized that there are at least four different ways in which

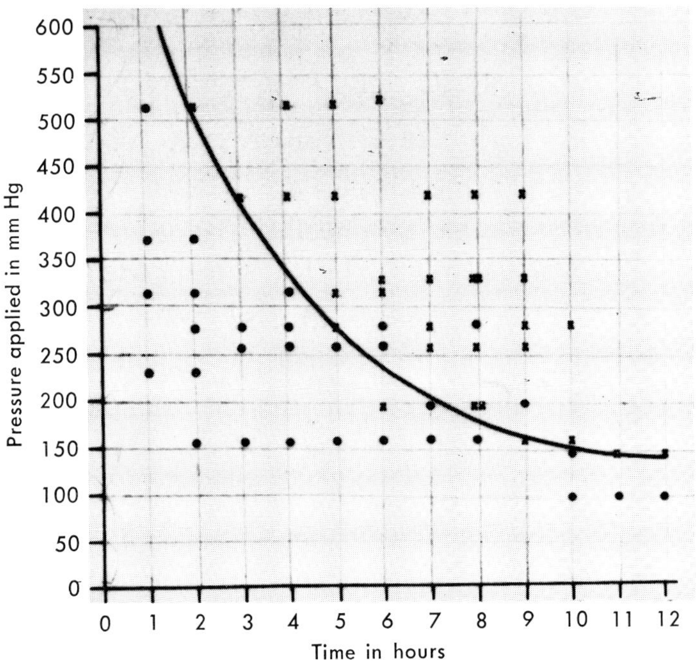

Fig. 23-1. Pressure-time relationship noted in 62 separate experiments on 16 dogs: x = ulceration; • = no ulceration. (From Kosiak, M.: Arch. Phys. Med. Rehabil. **40:**62-69, 1959.)

living skin and soft tissue can be destroyed by mechanical force and that these four ways are associated with widely different ranges of force and totally different factors in pathology.

The four ways to destroy tissues by mechanical force may be summarized as follows:

Forces	*Modifications*	*Results*
1. Low pressure: around 1 psi*	Continuous for several hours	Ischemic necrosis
2. High pressure: above 500 psi	With shear stress	Mechanical disruption
3. Moderate pressure: 20 to 100 psi	Thousands of repetitions	Inflammation, resulting in autolysis
4. Any localized pressure	On infected tissues	Spreading infection and osteomyelitis

LOW PRESSURE

The classic bedsore or decubitus ulcer is caused by ischemia. There may be other factors that make a patient susceptible to breakdown, but the central pathology is due to mechanical pressure sufficient to occlude the small blood vessels of the skin and subcutis. The pressure must be maintained for several hours if it is to cause real damage.

Kosiak[1] has shown that for ulceration to occur there is an inverse relationship between the level of pressure and the time it is maintained. The lower the pressure, the longer it must be maintained if it is to cause ischemic necrosis (Fig. 23-1).

The pathology of ischemic necrosis has been the most fully studied of the four types of tissue death, so I will not detail it here.

To prevent ischemic necrosis it is necessary to control either the pressure or the time or both. It is so difficult and expensive to provide total body support without exceeding the very small pressures that produce ischemia that I believe it is better to concentrate on control of the time factor. In bed this involves either frequent turning or alternation of body support areas by a method such as successive inflation and deflation of mattress segments. In a wheelchair it may mean training the patient to relieve the weight on his buttocks by lifting himself at regular intervals or by leaning forward frequently to transfer weight to his thighs for a change. In shoes it means that no new shoe should be worn for more than 2 hours at a time if the patient has insensitive feet. Even old shoes should be changed at noon and evening (about 4-hour intervals). It is worth noting that bandages may produce pressure and may trap a limb in ischemic status. Circumferential bandages cause pressure in inverse proportion to the radius of curvature of the limb. Thus a bandage around the foot will result in pressure sores at the lateral border where the radius of curvature is small rather than on the dorsum where the radius is large, even though the tension in the bandage is equal all round.

*1 psi is approximately 0.14 kg/sq cm.

HIGH PRESSURE

High pressure destroys tissue by direct mechanical disruption. It may be studied equally well in dead skin as in living. Yamada noted that human skin could resist stresses of 100 kg/sq cm. This is more than 1,000 times as great as the pressures that may damage by ischemia and more than ten times as great as the pressure ordinarily experienced on the sole of the foot when walking or running with a shoe on. It occurs when the body comes down on a very small area such as the point of a pin or an edge of broken glass or sharp stone. Shear stress is more likely to cause damage than is normal pressure or tension. Patients who are at risk because of loss of sensation will not suffer damage from this high level of mechanical force much more often than do normal people except when they apply force on their fingers to manipulate objects with very small hard handles. However, when they have damaged themselves, they may fail to take remedial action as a person would who felt pain. Anybody may step on a thumbtack, but a person without normal sensation may walk on it all day.

REPETITIVE MODERATE STRESS

The pathology of this type of tissue breakdown was quite unknown to me at the time that we started to study it about 8 years ago, although I had been treating ulcers caused by this type of stress for about 20 years. I had assumed, as I now find most doctors do, that a tissue breakdown was either due to ischemia or to direct mechanical damage. I now know that most "trophic" ulcers on the sole of the foot have had no continuous pressure to cause ischemia and no pressure high enough to damage the skin. They have a breakdown of tissue due to inflammation that has been caused by repetitive moderate stress and followed by more repetitive moderate stress until the tissues necrose.

We have subjected the footpads of many batches of rats to a wide range of carefully graded forces to match the forces experienced in walking. A machine was devised that would apply the stress repetitively many thousands of times to exactly the same part of the foot at exactly the same level of pressure.

Plate 1. Histology of repetitive stress. (Courtesy U.S. Department of Health, Education, and Welfare, U.S. Public Health Service Hospital.)

A B C

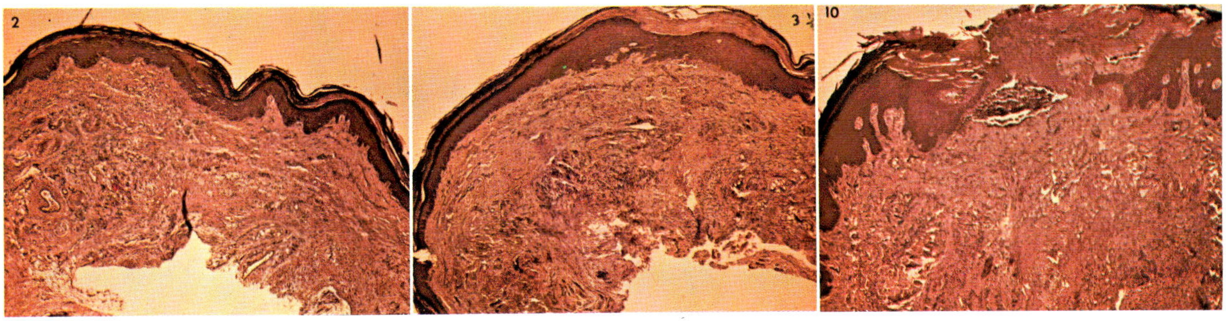

Experiment 1. All rats received 10,000 repetitions of stress each day for 10 days. For a human this is like a daily 7-mile walk at a fast pace on hard ground. Some rats were sacrificed each day for histology. **A,** Day 2. Some separation of epithelial cells. Some edema. A few inflammatory cells in subcutaneous tissue. **B,** Day 3. Epithelium shows some hypertrophy. Marked inflammation and some necrosis in deeper tissue. **C,** Day 10. Ulceration. Epithelium destroyed. Necrosis in deeper tissue. Epithelial hypertrophy on each side of destroyed tissue. This experiment shows how repetitive stress builds up an inflammatory state day by day until it finally causes ulceration.

A B C

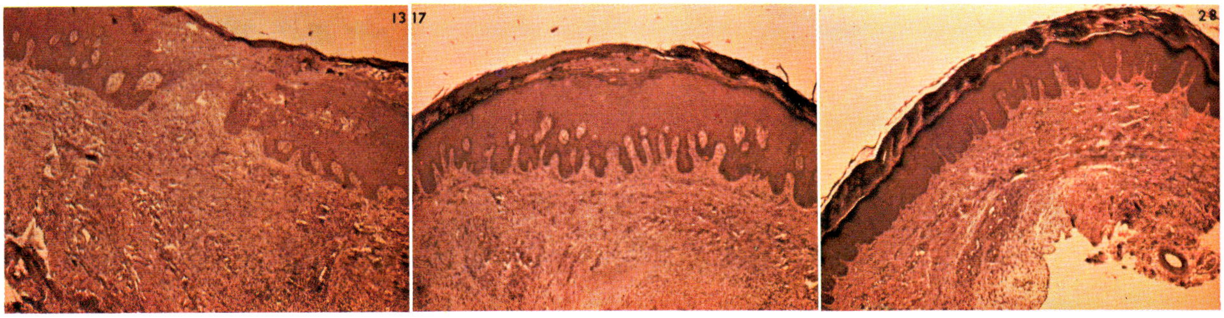

Experiment 2. Rats had the same stress as in Experiment 1 but only 8,000 repetitions per day, and only on 5 days per week. This experiment continued for 28 days. **A,** Day 13. Break in epithelium, which is hypertrophied on each side of the break. **B,** Day 17. Evidence of blister, which is absorbing. Very marked epithelial hypertrophy. **C,** Day 28. No sign of damage now. Marked hypertrophy of all epithelium. This experiment shows how same stress with 20% fewer daily repetitions and with rest at weekends allows feet to pass through inflammatory phase and move on to a hypertrophy, which protects foot from further damage.

The results of the tests at 20 psi at 10,000 repetitions per day are reproduced here because 20 psi is a pressure that is common for a human forefoot while walking and is quite painless and comfortable for several hundred repetitions on a normal sensitive foot (Plate 1).

For the first 2 or 3 days of these tests, the footpad that was being subjected to this program did not look very different from the other hind foot of the same rat, which was at rest. The foot under stress was a little swollen and was warmer than the other, but the skin looked normal. After about a week some of the rats had blisters, and by the tenth day there was frank ulceration and necrosis of the skin and subcutaneous tissue. Every day some of the rats were sacrificed for histologic study. Inflammatory changes in the footpad were present from the second day, and foci of necrosis by the third and fourth days. At this stage so many inflammatory cells and macrophages had invaded the area that the section looked totally different from normal footpad histology. Yet the skin was unbroken, and there was no evidence of infection.

The 10,000 applications of pressure on the tenth day were just the same as on the first day, but the skin, which had seemed to suffer no damage on the first day, broke down and ulcerated on the tenth day. What was the difference? From a mechanical point of view the tissue was more turgid and stiff on the tenth day, but the real difference was in the biologic and chemical responses of the changed cell population. We have not studied the enzymes in this system, but we know that inflammatory cells are rich in lysosomes, and they spill enzymes that are capable of digesting tissue. We suggest that the process we have observed could be called "autolysis" and that the cell change is a traumatic inflammation. The end point is a chemical or enzymatic necrosis (Plate 1, Experiment 1).

Noting that there was marked epithelial hyperplasia during the later stages of this experiment, we repeated it with modifications. We used the same pressure, 20 psi, but repeated it only 8,000 times per day and gave the rats the weekend off, so they had only 5 days of stress per week. On this program there was no ulceration. There was inflammation in the early stages and some local necrosis, but the footpads survived. By the end of 6 weeks on this program the inflammation had almost disappeared, the footpads were stronger and tougher than normal, and the histology showed hyperplasia of all elements of the epithelium (Plate 1, Experiment 2).

We repeated these experiments on denervated rat footpads and found a similar pattern except that the threshold for damage is lower in terms of the number of repetitions that can be tolerated at any given pressure. We have carried out extensive tests on the human foot to determine the range of pressures that are experienced in everyday activity. We have used transducers on the bare foot and in various forms of footwear. We find that normal feet experience up to 100 psi from time to time, but that pressures in shoes are usually less than 50 psi. If

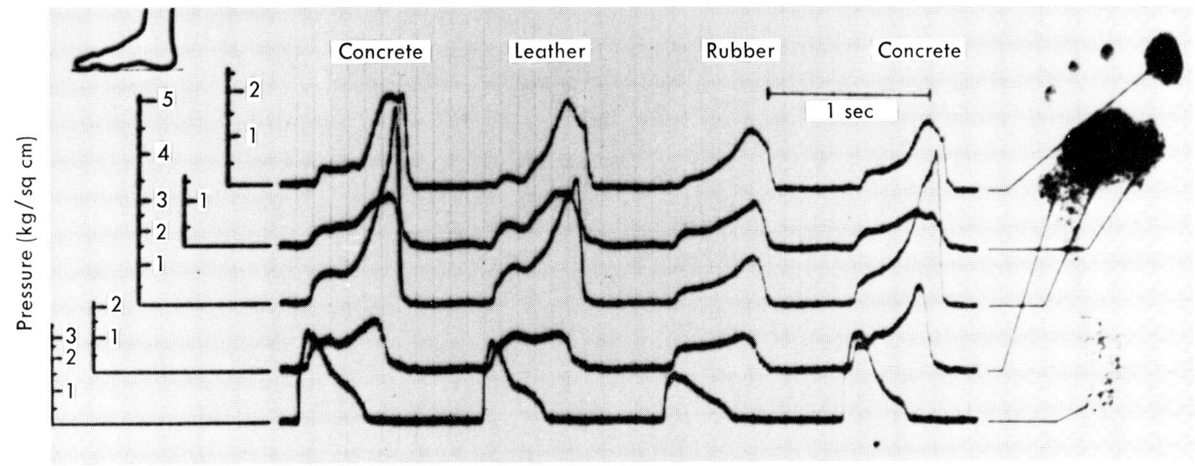

Fig. 23-2. Record of man with anesthetic foot walking barefoot. Successive steps were taken on polished concrete, 1.5 cm leather pad, 1.5 cm microcellular rubber pad, and polished concrete. Note that greatest benefit from microcellular rubber occurred at points of highest thrust and that most striking feature of step on rubber was that all areas tended to receive equal thrust. (From Brand, P. W.: J. Bone Joint Surg. [Br.] **45**(4):659, 1963.)

pressure can be kept down to 20 psi it is quite uncommon to get a breakdown, even in an insensitive foot (Fig. 23-2). Our clinical experience with humans parallels the rat footpad experiments. Long walking in hard shoes and on paved streets are the factors that produce ulceration. Each of these tends either to localize pressure and thus concentrate it to a few small areas or to cause repetition of the pressure until it produces inflammation and then until it breaks down. It is possible to prevent ulceration either by spreading the force more widely and thus reducing the pressure or by repeating the force less often.

In all these experiments we found that shear stress was much more damaging than normal (perpendicular) stress. For example, if the stress applicator were in the shape of a cylinder with a flat end, then we would get a circumferential bruise with no damage in the center. Even if the edges were rounded off, the maximum damage would be around the rim or even just outside the rim rather than in the area of maximum normal pressure in the center. This is the reason it is often unsafe to cut out a hollow in the sole of a shoe to relieve a high pressure point. The *edge* of the hollow may cause shear stresses that are worse than the original direct pressure. The same *edge effect* causes severe damage if a window is cut in a plaster cast to allow dressing of a wound. Shoes and casts should have *total contact* with elimination of *edge effects* and shear stresses as far as possible. For this reason we like Plastazote and similar heat-formed polyethylene foams that can be formed directly on the foot or on a model of the foot and that may then be inserted into an extra-depth shoe to equalize pressures on an insensitive foot.

From our studies of rats and humans we have learned that total protection and avoidance of all stress may not be good. Most living tissues and organs deteriorate and atrophy if they are not used. They hypertrophy if exposed to regular stress that is near the limit of tolerance. They break down if that tolerance is exceeded. The most valuable lesson we have learned is that the process of breakdown for feet is slow and gives time for evaluation and for change of direction. If the early stages of traumatic inflammation are recognized, then the patient may slow down a little or change the insoles of his shoes, and the foot may be saved.

The signs of inflammation are swelling and heat. We have found the thermograph and thermistor good for monitoring danger areas on feet and amputation stumps. The normal hand of a trained nurse or therapist can rapidly screen areas of potential danger and will quickly identify hot spots. These spots may then be measured by skin thermometry and checked at intervals until they return to normal.

The fourth type of damage from mechanical force is due to the spread of infection from an existing open wound or abscess. We are all so accustomed to the pain and tenderness associated with an infected hand or foot that we do not realize that without pain most infections would spread rather than heal. It is the immobility that is forced on us by pain that allows our own cells to localize the infection and deal with the invading organisms. In the absence of pain, an infected foot is walked on and an infected finger is used along with the normal fingers in full flexion and extension and participation in all the forces of grasp. Tissue fluids, loaded with organisms, are literally squeezed out into uninfected parts of the limb. Pus is forced out of the localizing inflammatory barrier and enters new areas. Uninfected joints and tendon sheaths and bones become infected, and whole segments of a limb are destroyed. Physicians, seeing a spreading cellulitis or osteomyelitis, usually try a new antibiotic. The old antibiotic would do, or even no antibiotic, if only the patient's own cells were given a chance by putting the tissues at rest and free from external force. When tissues are denervated and also infected, they should be protected from any outside force and from any movement. We advise a plaster of paris cast for every open wound or infection on the hand or foot of patients who lack normal levels of sensation. In a cast, the wounds of most such patients heal and their infections are dealt with in about the same time as for normal individuals with the same type of wound.

SUMMARY

There is no such thing as a single threshold between safety and danger in terms of mechanical force on the surface of the body. There are circumstances when 1 psi is dangerous, such as when it is maintained constantly until the tissue becomes necrotic from ischemia. There are times when 20 psi is dangerous, as when it is repeated frequently day after day or when it has a factor of friction and shear. There are times when 500 psi may be quite safe, as when it is perpendicular to the skin and is not sustained for a long time or repeated, and there are times when 5 psi may be very dangerous, if it occurs on an infected area when an adjacent uninfected area has no pressure.

However, if the pathology of breakdown of tissue from mechanical force is understood by the physician and by the patient, it is possible to modify the environment or to change the pattern and timing of the patient's interaction with the environment so that tissues are not damaged and may even become stronger as a result of mechanical stress. One of the safety precautions consists of awareness of the significance of local areas of high temperature and an alert response so that people without sensation may use hot spots, in the way others use pain, to serve as a warning that one of the complex interactions of pressure and time has reached a danger level, and the patient needs to give the affected tissue some relief.

REFERENCES

1. Kosiak, M.: Etiology and pathology of ischemic ulcers, Arch. Phys. Med. Rehabil. **40**:62-69, 1959.
2. Yamada, H.: Strength of biological materials, Baltimore, 1970, The Williams & Wilkins Company.

Chapter 24

Overall management of spinal cord injury

E. Shannon Stauffer

Patients with paralysis secondary to spinal cord injury have multiple medical problems that cross specialty boundaries. The plastic surgeon's participation in the rehabilitation program must be integrated with the overall goals and management plan for the patient's rehabilitation. An entire team must deal with the spinal cord–injured patient and his readaptation to a new life-style. The ultimate goal is to return this person to the highest functional level commensurate with his residual abilities. Emphasis should be on the functions that remain rather than on his disability. Consider, for example, a very high quadriplegic of a C-4 functional level. His muscle power may be minimal, but his residual abilities—mental and emotional, as well as physical—must be fully utilized for maximum potential. By contrast, a person with a low, partial paraplegia who is ambulatory with crutches may have little alteration in his preinjury life-style.

This discussion will deal with three concepts of the management of the spinal cord–injured person. The first is spinal stability, the second is prevention of medical complications, and the third is functional rehabilitation. When we are faced with a person with an acutely injured, unstable spine, our main task as physicians and surgeons is to restore protection to the spinal cord. This can be provided by immobilization of the spine in traction, rigid fixation by a halo body cast, or internal surgical stabilization. Recent advance in techniques of bone grafting and internal fixation provide the opportunity for early mobilization of the patient without continuous traction, thus preventing medical complications and permitting earlier and more thorough rehabilitation.

Treatment in traction still may be the most effective way of immobilizing certain types of fractures. The Gardner-Wells tongs have supplanted previous types of skull traction devices in most spinal injury units due to their ease of application. There are fewer parts to get lost and no need to drill holes or to use general anesthesia. The two sharp pins are placed through the skin into the scalp and cranium through wheals of local anesthesia. A spring-loaded pressure sensor indicates when the correct amount of torque has been applied to the pins (Fig. 24-1).

The halo may also be used for longitudinal traction (Fig. 24-2) to provide more control of the unstable spine and allow flexion, extension, tilt, and rotational forces to be applied to the spine. After the spinal fracture or dislocation has been reduced, the halo can be incorporated into a plaster or plastic body jacket, providing rigid immobilization, and the patient may then be mobilized out of traction and out of bed. If he is ambulatory, he may be discharged from the hospital with the halo jacket maintaining his spinal correction. If he is paralyzed, he may begin his rehabilitation program in a wheelchair.

Surgery may be used to reduce the dislocated spine and stabilize it with internal fixation to allow mobilization without external appliances. If the instability is posterior, as in facet dislocations, the most appropriate route is posterior reduction of the dislocation with interlaminar wiring. If the instability is anterior, as in the burst fractures of the midcervical vertebral bodies, the most dependable stability may be afforded by anterior removal of the comminuted vertebral body and replacement with a cortical strut graft from the fibula (Fig. 24-3). This provides rigid internal fixation and allows the patient to be out of bed in a light cervical brace to begin his rehabilitation. One of the most frequent complications that occurs after 6 to 8 weeks of bed rest is atrophy of the muscles under voluntary control.

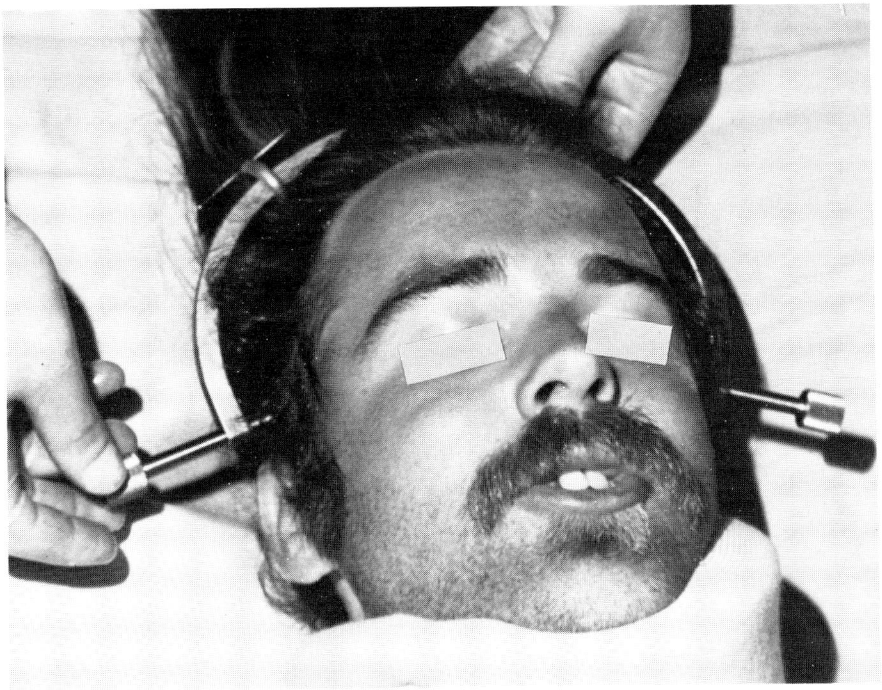

Fig. 24-1. Gardner-Wells traction tongs inserted with patient under local anesthesia.

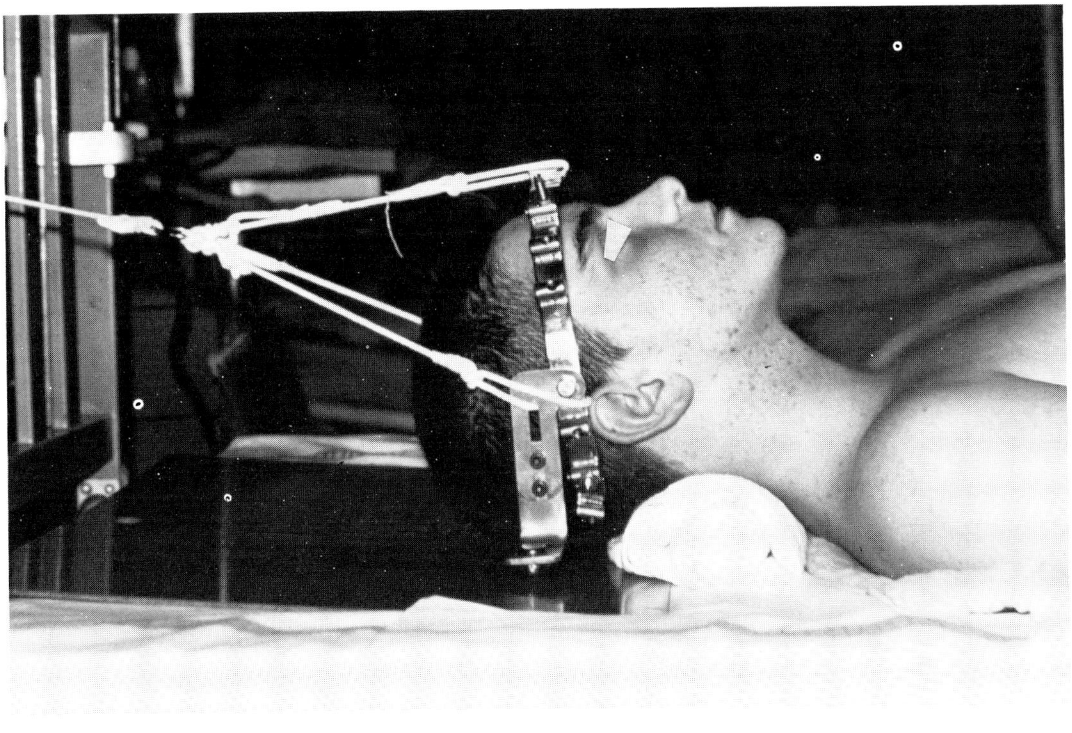

Fig. 24-2. Halo traction.

A

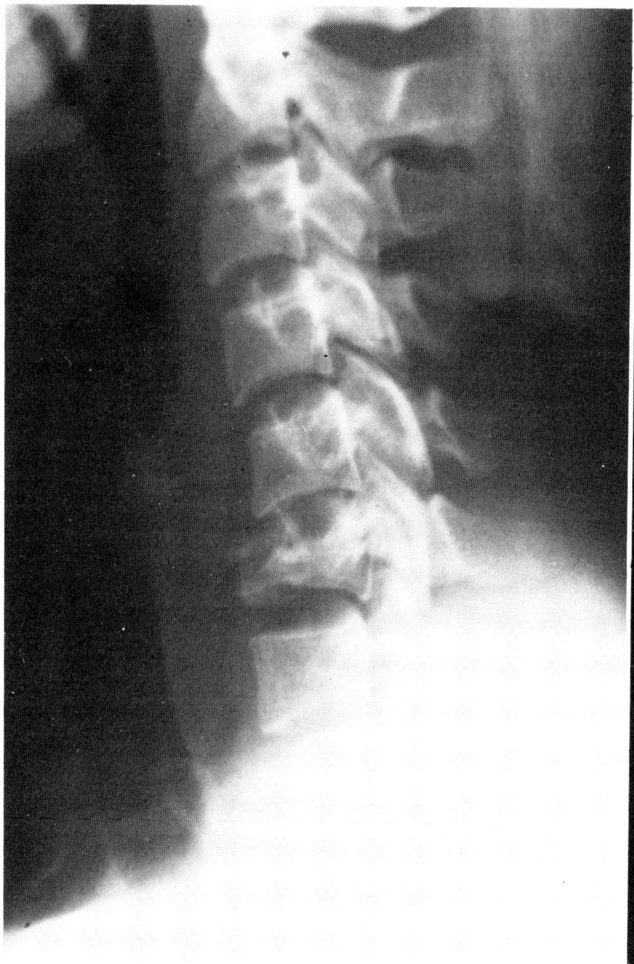

B

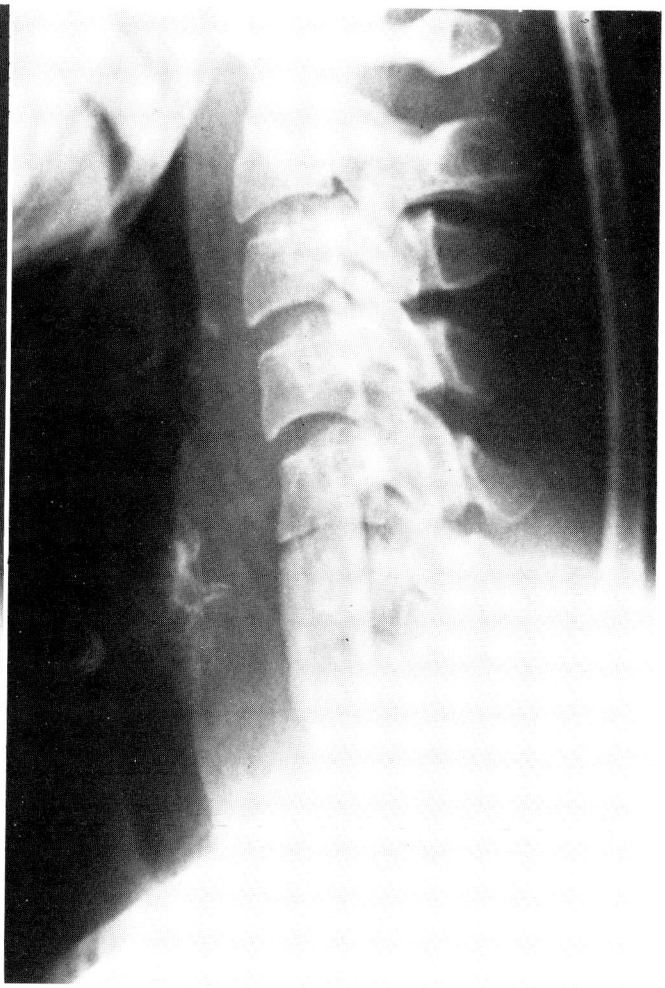

C

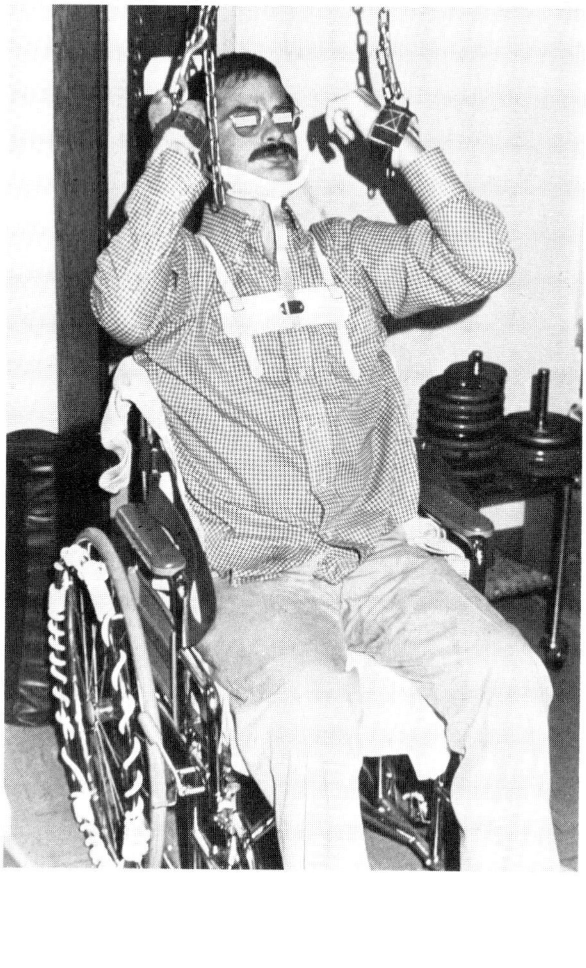

Fig. 24-3. A, Comminuted fracture of C-6 vertebral body. **B,** Fibular strut graft, providing immediate stability of fractured C-6 vertebral body. **C,** Early rehabilitation in wheelchair after fibular strut graft stabilization.

Early mobilization by wheelchair and an active exercise program decrease the patients' hospitalization time and the complication rate.

When dealing with fractures of the thoracolumbar spine, it is even more important to have a straight, stable spine. This is of particular interest to the plastic surgeon. The mild anterior angulation that frequently occurs with compression fractures of this area is not significantly disabling; however, lateral angulation producing a traumatic scoliosis results in a permanent pelvic obliquity if the fracture heals in the angulated position (Fig. 24-4). Thus sitting in a wheelchair with this pelvic obliquity produced uneven pressure distributed to the ischial tuberosities. The low side of the pelvis is in much greater jeopardy of breaking down with pressure sores of the insensitive skin over the ischial tuberosity and greater trochanter of the femur (Figs. 24-5 and 24-6). To the active, rehabilitated paraplegic, recurrent pressure sore formation may be a greater disabling condition than his muscle paralysis. The most common single factor that keeps an active paraplegic from participating in a normal life-style and being competitively employed is recurring pressure sores.

With the use of spinal instrumentation developed by Harrington[2] for the correction of scoliosis, we are able in many cases to reduce the thoracolumbar fractures and use the internal fixation devices to provide a straight, stable spine (Fig. 24-7). This allows the patient out of bed with a light plastic body jacket to begin his standing and rehabilitation program, thus decreasing total hospital time and lowering the complication rate. The patient is then

A

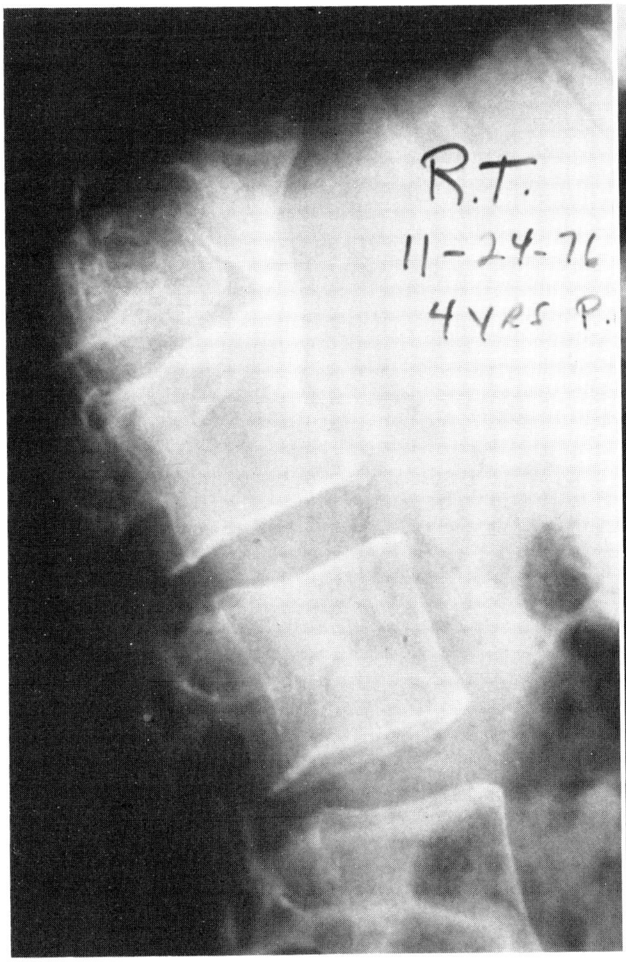

B

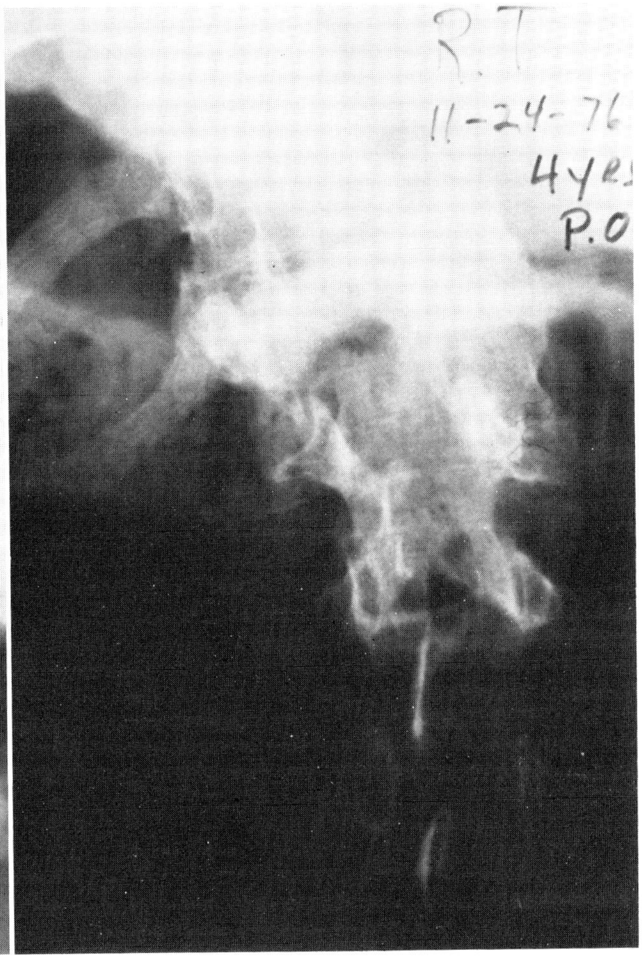

Fig. 24-4. A, Lateral roentgenogram of healed fracture T-12 on L-1 with residual kyphotic deformity. **B,** Anteroposterior roentgenogram of healed fracture T-12 on L-1 with residual scoliosis and pelvic obliquity.

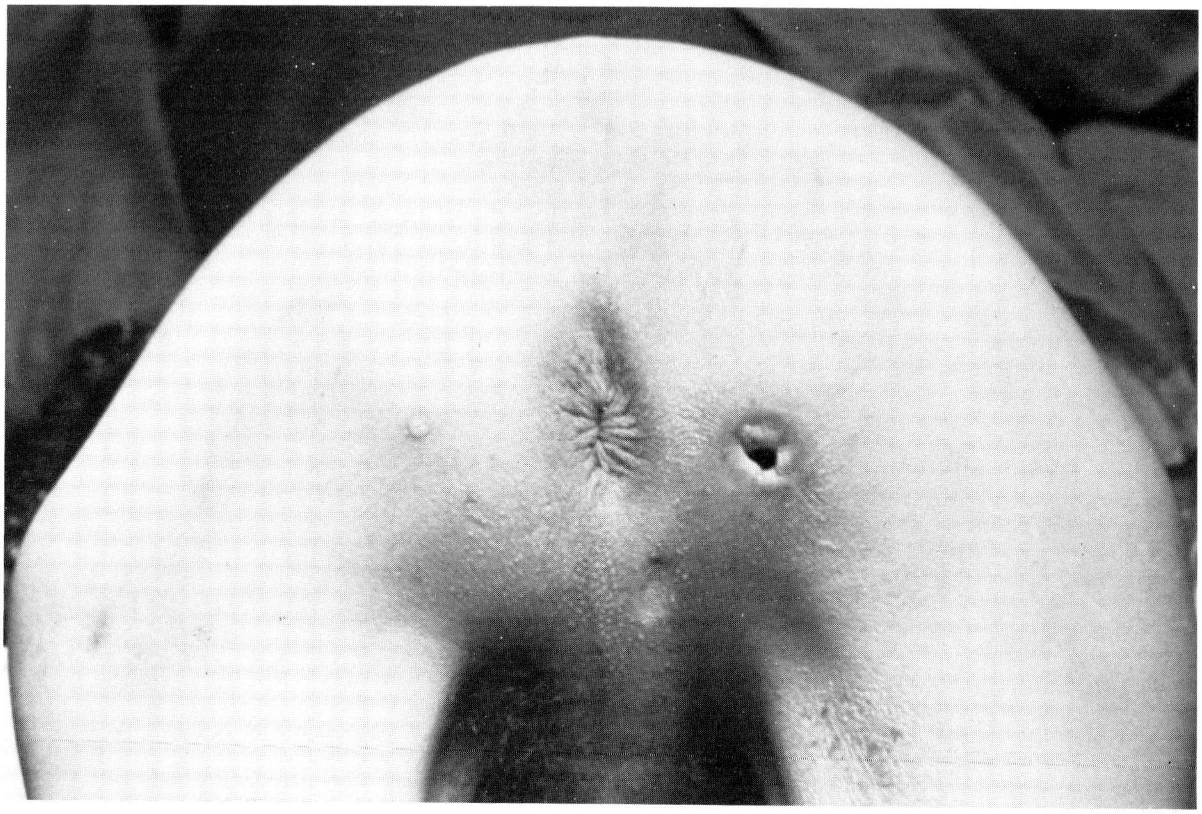

Fig. 24-5. Sitting pressure sore over low ischial tuberosity secondary to pelvic obliquity.

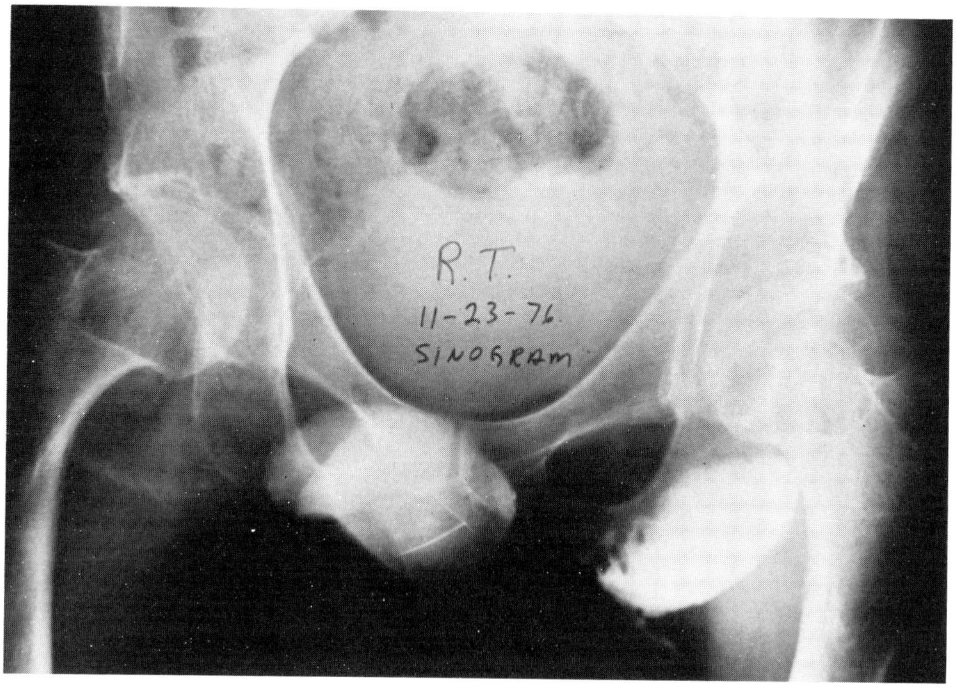

Fig. 24-6. Sinogram demonstrating extent of pressure sore and ischial bone involvement.

A

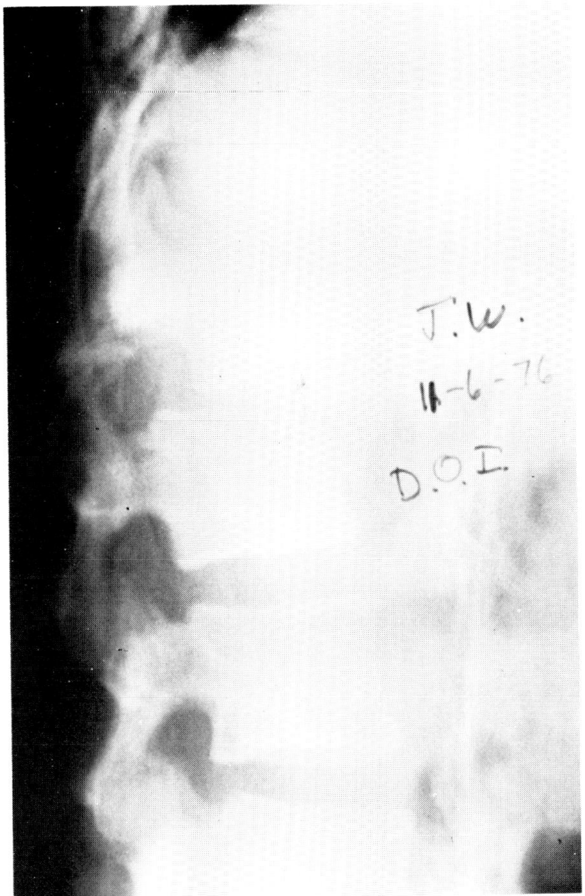

B

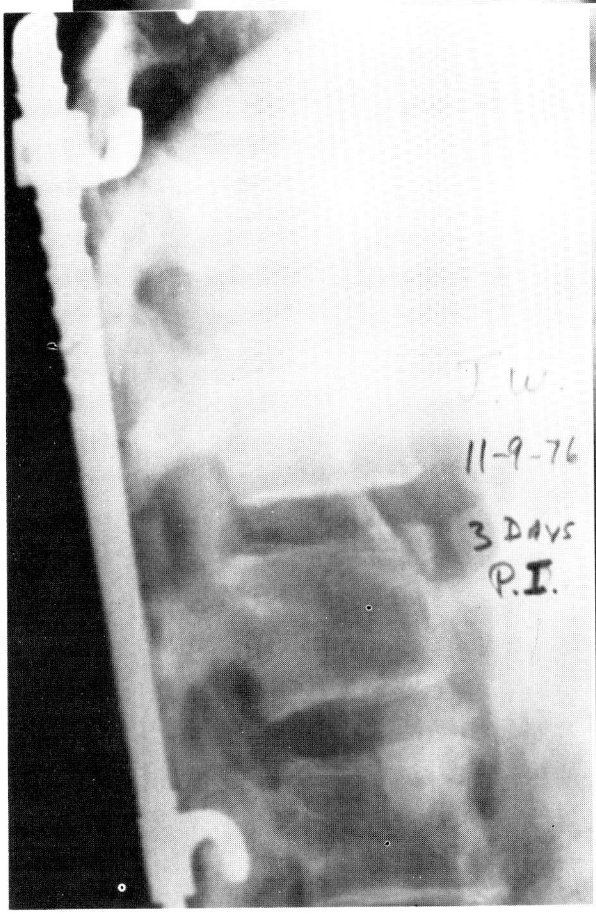

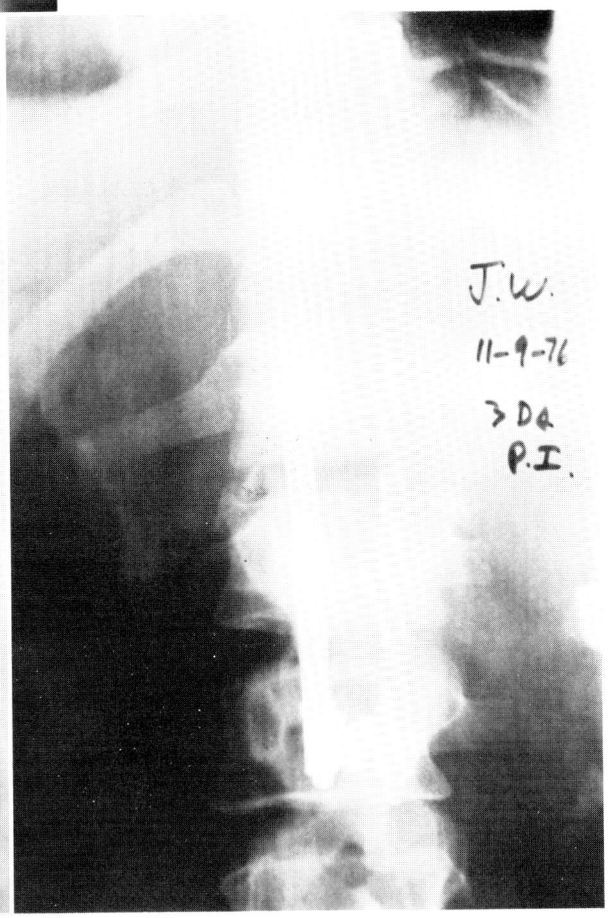

C

Fig. 24-7. A, Lateral roentgenogram of acute fracture-dislocation T-12 on L-1. **B,** Lateral roentgenogram showing postoperative open reduction and internal fixation with distraction rods. **C,** Anteroposterior postoperative roentgenogram, revealing no scoliosis or pelvic obliquity.

able to sit in a wheelchair with pressures evenly distributed over both ischial tuberosities. In treating patients with ischial pressure sores, it is therefore important to note the alignment of the spine as well as to measure the sitting pressures under the ischial tuberosities. Any element of pelvic obliquity must be considered when planning the surgical management of the pressure sore.

MEDICAL COMPLICATIONS

The many medical complications plaguing the spinal cord–injured patient involve most organ systems and are often preventable, if anticipated.

Pulmonary complications[1]

The respiratory complications of atelectasis and pneumonia are the most common causes of death in the early postinjury spinal cord–injured patient. The quadriplegic and the thoracic level–injured paraplegic are not able to voluntarily exhale and cough, as the only muscle of respiration under voluntary control is the diaphragm, which provides active inhalation but only passive exhalation. Therefore, the patient is at high risk of developing atelectasis from retained secretions, particularly if he is treated in the supine and prone positions in bed or on a Stryker frame. Ventilation therapy and active chest physical therapy must be instituted immediately in anticipation of this frequent complication. Nasotracheal suctioning and at times tracheostomy are necessary to remove retained secretions.

Renal complications

The greatest threat to life in the long-term management of the spinal cord–injured patient is renal infection and dysfunction. Spasticity of the bladder with overdistension leads to hydroureter, incompetent ureterovesical valves, and eventually hydronephrosis. With the presence of bacteria in the bladder, especially in the presence of an indwelling catheter, ascending pyelonephritis and destruction of kidney tissue occur. Current concepts of urologic care consisting of intermittent catheterization and judicious use of antibiotics have greatly decreased the complication of death from kidney dysfunction. Ongoing prospective studies indicate that kidney damage affects only 10% to 20% of well-managed patients during the first 8 to 10 years following injury.[9] Calculi in the bladder must be carefully sought, particularly as long as the patient has an indwelling catheter, and removed before they can cause permanent damage. With the decrease in the death rate from urinary tract infection the importance of adequate active rehabilitation has increased.

Fractures of long bones

Patients who have been paralyzed for over 1 year may suffer pathologic fractures of the femur or tibia secondary to osteoporosis.[4,8] These are usually long, spiral fractures, and treatment must consist of gentle immobilization of the fracture without causing excessive pressure on the skin over bony prominences or interfering with the patient's life-style. Most of the fractures can be satisfactorily handled by immobilization in a soft cotton "cast," a large pillow pinned around the leg, or a padded, removable knee-immobilizer splint. Circular plaster casts should not be used on anesthetic skin. This is overtreatment and frequently causes pressure sores that may progress to osteomyelitis and require amputation of the limb. These fractures which are characteristically in the supracondylar area of the femur or proximal tibia heal well with minimal immobilization that allows the patient to continue functioning in his wheelchair.

Amputation of lower extremity

Amputation of part or all of the lower extremity should be avoided if at all possible. Besides the irreparable damage to the patient's already distorted body self-image, amputation of a lower extremity distorts the pressure mechanics of wheelchair sitting. To properly distribute pressures over the soft tissues of the back of the thigh as well as the buttocks it is necessary to have the counterbalancing effect of the weight of the legs. Without this balance, flexion contractures of the hips may develop, and all of the weight is then concentrated on the ischial tuberosity. Sleeping in the prone or supine position becomes increasingly more difficult. Large areas of bone about the hip and proximal femur may be removed to treat pressure sores with satisfactory soft tissue closure without amputation of the entire extremity.

Cardiac arrest

One of the hazards of reconstructive surgery is intraoperative cardiac arrest. It has been long appreciated that spinal cord–injured patients have a higher incidence of cardiac arrest during surgery than do nonparalyzed patients. It has recently been shown that this is due to a hyperkalemia caused by sudden release of potassium from the motor endplates of the paralyzed muscles following administration of succinylcholine. This rapid hyperkalemia may cause cardiac arrest in systole but fortunately is transient, usually permitting resuscitation by the usual methods. This does not appear to be a problem during the first 5 to 7 days so that the initial emergency operation is usually uncomplicated.

However, risk of this hyperkalemia occurs from 2 weeks to 12 months after injury. Thus succinylcholine should not be used in these patients for tracheal intubation, but curare is safe as it does not have the same effect.

Tracheal suctioning of the patient in bed on the spinal injury unit may also cause a sudden cardiac arrest secondary to a vagovagal reflex. The nursing staff must be aware of this and monitor the pulse during suctioning to detect any arrhythmias that may occur, signaling impending arrest.

Intraabdominal pathology

One must remember that the spinal cord–injured patient does not have protective pain sensibilities to warn him of occult pathology. Therefore conditions such as appendicitis, duodenal ulcer, and peritonitis may progress and become fatal without detection if the patient is not carefully examined when he complains of mild abdominal discomfort, nausea, or loss of appetite.

Autonomic dysreflexia

Increasing blood pressure elevation and a slowing pulse may occur in patients with lesions above the sympathetic outflow, that is, T-4. Any stimulus to the spinal cord secondary to cystitis, kidney stones, bowel impaction, or pressure sores may cause hyperactivity of the sympathetic nervous system, producing peripheral vasoconstriction. This cannot be reversed by parasympathetic balance. As the blood pressure rises the vagus slows the pulse. The patient develops a slow pounding headache with sweating and "gooseflesh." This condition constitutes an emergency on the spinal injury unit; uncontrolled, it may lead to a cerebral hemorrhage and death. The cause of the dysreflexia must be found and corrected. It usually is due to irritation in the urinary tract; therefore the catheter should be removed, a new catheter inserted, the bladder drained, and if necessary, 30 ml of 0.5% pontocaine instilled into the bladder to anesthetize it. If this is not successful, a gloved finger with Nupercainal Ointment should be introduced into the rectum to search for a fecal impaction. If the problem persists, intravenous antihypertensive medication may be administered to control the blood pressure.

REHABILITATION

At the present time there are no surgical or medical techniques to resuture or repair injured spinal cords. Rehabilitation deals with helping the patient prevent medical complications and readapt his life to the highest functional ability commensurate with his level of injury.[5]

Early goal setting

Early goal setting is the basis of rehabilitation philosophy. The patient is evaluated by each member of the team, that is, physician, therapist, nurse, social worker, and psychologist, who plan a treatment program and estimate the time it will take for completion. These goals of realistic functional expectations are set during the first week and are related to the type and level of paralysis as determined by physical examination. Completion may take 6 weeks or 6 months. The patient and his family are informed of these goals and the time estimate required to permit realistic planning at home as well as in the hospital. The patient, and especially the family, must understand that long-term rehabilitation does not mean "waiting to get well." Eventually discharge-planning goals are set by the team members and discussed with the family.

Rehabilitation is based on patient education. The patient must learn to live a new life-style consistent with his altered physiology. The first lesson begins with pressure sore prevention. Pressure sores, if allowed to develop, are destructive to the rehabilitation program and destructive to the patient's psyche as they confine him to bed. Obviously, during the first several weeks it is the nurse's responsibility to prevent pressure sores, but this responsibility must be transferred as rapidly as possible to members of the family and to the patient himself. Several hand-held mirrors are some of the first and most important pieces of equipment that the patient must get. The family and the patient must examine the skin on the back over the sacrum, ischia, and trochanters each time he returns to bed from the wheelchair and each time he is turned in bed. This must become a lifelong habit, with the patient responsible for his own skin care. The development of a pressure sore while in the hospital is unacceptable, and all members of the team, including therapists, nurses, family, and patient, must assume responsibility for prevention. Learning to live and sleep in a regular bed is encouraged. As soon as possible the patient should be treated on a regular hospital bed with normal pillows used for bridging so that when he goes home for overnight passes and is finally discharged he can sleep in his own regular bed with pillows positioned to bridge bony prominences. Learning to sleep in the prone position is difficult for many patients but must be mastered before the patient is allowed to go home. This helps to prevent flexion contractures of the knees and hips as well as protecting the sacrum and trochanters from pressure sores. Ranging of all joints as well as strengthening of muscles is accomplished not only in the physical therapy unit but also by the patient's daily activities on the ward. The nursing service provides this ranging during the bath and transfer activities from bed. Muscle strengthening exercises are incorporated into transfer activities, wheelchair propulsion, self-dressing, and feeding.

Activities of daily living

As soon as the patient is mobilized to a wheelchair and can go to the occupational therapy treatment area, he begins to learn self-feeding and personal hygiene such as shaving, face washing, hair combing, bathing, and dressing.[3] Specialized hand splints may be necessary for some of these activities for the quadriplegic who has no voluntary grasp. Success at accomplishing each of these activities much be carefully documented as a gain in the rehabilitation process by the staff and the patient. Emphasis is focused on the abilities and goals that are accomplished rather than on the disability or what the patient cannot do. The program should be progressive, leading toward the designated discharge date. Even though the patient is not "getting well" or improving neurologically, he must be convincing himself that he is improving functionally day by day, week by week. As most of our spinal cord–injured population is between 16 and 24 years of age, their body image, personal hygiene, and how they appear to the rest of the world is very important to them.

Hand surgery

Before tendon transfers, tenodesis, or arthrodesis of joints are considered to improve hand function, the surgeon must be thoroughly familiar with the life-style and daily activity of the spinal cord–injured patient. Above all, do not take anything away from his function. Transfer and wheelchair propulsion are of maximum importance in the daily activities of the patient. Most patients can develop a gross grasp based on the active voluntary power of the wrist extensors and the spastic involuntary contraction of the finger flexors associated with wrist extension. If adequate grasp is not possible tenodesis-type hand splints may be used for those functions requiring prehension. If surgical reconstruction is considered, reversible procedures such as those described by Dr. Moberg elsewhere in this symposium are to be recommended. Most quadriplegics have voluntary wrist extensor control and are able to transfer in and out of their wheelchair and automobile and to drive with hand controls.

Ambulation

Patients with complete spinal cord injuries above T-12 (the spinal cord ends at L-1) do not ambulate functionally.[10] They may be able to stand with braces and walk in parallel bars or with an accompanying physical therapist, but they are not able to independently get up and down out of a chair, and ambulating with crutches and braces uses too much energy. To be a functional ambulator, a person must have a functional level of at least L-1 or L-2 with voluntary innervation of some muscles across the hip into the leg. Unfortunately, ambulation is equated with successful rehabilitation by many patients and rehabilitation staffs. Many unsuccessful, futile hours are spent in ambulation training that can only end in failure and discouragement for the patient. The patient with a functional level above T-12 may be taught to stand in a standing device for daily exercise but should not be encouraged to have functional ambulation as one of his rehabilitation expectations.

Wheelchairs. Each nonambulatory patient must have an individually prescribed and fitted wheelchair. This is his most important piece of equipment. The wheelchair must be no wider than necessary to permit passage through narrow doors and must be sturdy enough to withstand the rigors of the patient's weight and life-style. It must be accurately checked out for leg length, cushion configuration, and so on by a knowledgeable therapist prior to issuance to the patient.

Psychology

The psychologic consequences of a sudden, traumatic permanent injury are different from those of other medical disabilities.[7] The patient is usually a healthy, outgoing, vigorous young man or woman who suddenly is paralyzed and is going to remain paralyzed for the rest of his or her life. During the first month to 6 weeks the psychologic defense mechanism of denial prevents the patient from accepting realistic goals and discussions. During this time he usually is a "good" patient.

However, after about 6 or 8 weeks when he is up in his wheelchair going to physical therapy, he begins to realize that he will not get well, and he enters the stage of mourning. He mourns his former self, that is, his lifelong friend with whom he skied, rode motorcycles, and so on, which he will no longer be able to do. He then may slip into a depression during which he becomes a "bad" patient. He begins to bargain and become manipulative with the staff, will not keep his appointments, becomes obnoxious to the nursing staff, disagreeable to the physical therapist, and angry at the world in general and the medical profession specifically for not curing him of his illness. Unfortunately this period of depression frequently lasts about 6 months. About this time he has reached his rehabilitation goals and is discharged from the hospital. With all the rest of his problems he feels the staff has then given up on him and thrown him out of the hospital. He sits at home without the encouragement of the rehabilitation team and either stays depressed or begins to cope with the disability. It takes about 1 year for most patients to begin to cope with their disability, and at this point vocational retraining and counseling are effective. Notice we do not use the term "acceptance." Many years go by before a patient accepts the fact of permanent disability, and most patients never truly come to grips with it. They cope with life as it comes along.

Sexual counseling

Sexual counseling has become an important part of the rehabilitation program in the last decade, specifically as it relates to sexual options and parenthood among the handicapped. Even though only about 2% of the men can father children, it must be clearly pointed out to the women that their procreation system has not been disrupted and that they can conceive, tolerate pregnancy, and bear children with little difficulty.

SUMMARY

The overall management of the spinal cord–injured patient can only be accomplished by an informed team of medical and allied health specialists. The patient must be an active participating member of the team and must assume the responsibility of completing his rehabilitation and preventing medical complications. It is our function as health professionals to see that adequate care, education, and rehabilitation, as well as emergency medical services are available to all who are left with residual paralysis secondary to spinal cord injuries.

REFERENCES

1. Bellamy, R., Pitts, F. W., and Stauffer, E. S.: Respiratory complications in traumatic quadriplegia: analysis of 20 years' experience, J. Neurosurg. **39**(5):596-600, 1973.
2. Dickson, J. H., Harrington, P. R., and Erwin, W. D.: Harrington instrumentation in the fractured unstable thoracic and lumbar spine, Tex. Med. **69:**91-98, 1973.
3. Ford, J. R., and Duckworth, B.: Physical management for the quadriplegic patient, Phildelphia, 1974, F. A. Davis Company.
4. Freehafer, A. A., and Mast, W. A.: Lower extremity fractures in patients with spinal cord injuries, J. Bone Joint. Surg. [Am.] **47:**683, 1965.
5. Garrett, A.: Functional potential of patients with spinal cord injuries, Clin. Orthop. **112:**60-65, 1975.
6. Guttmann, L.: Spinal cord injuries, Oxford, England, 1973, Blackwell Scientific Publications Ltd.
7. Hohmann, G.: Psychological aspects of treatment and rehabilitation of the spinal cord patient, Clin. Orthop. **112:**81-89, 1975.
8. McMaster, W. C., and Stauffer, E. S.: Management of long bone fractures in the spinal cord injured patient, Clin. Orthop. **112:**44-53, 1975.
9. Price, M., Kottke, F. J., and Olson, M. E.: Renal function in patients with spinal cord injuries: the eighth year of a ten-year continuing study, Arch. Phys. Med. Rehabil. **56:**76-79, 1975.
10. Stauffer, E. S.: Ambulation in paraplegia, J. Bone Joint Surg. [Am.] **54:**1336, 1972.
11. Tobey, R. E.: Paraplegia, succinylcholine and cardiac arrest, Anesthesiology **32:**359-364, 1970.

Chapter 25

Pressure sores: preoperative considerations

Libby F. Wilson-Mackby
William W. Fish
Patti Harder

A pressure ulceration is one of the most disastrous complications that can occur in a spinal cord–injured patient. The lesion is always debilitating and frequently life threatening. The course of treatment is generally long and frustrating and frequently associated with loss of function. The cost of treatment is exorbitant. An aggressive approach combining the skills of many members of the health care team is usually necessary to minimize unfavorable results.

Prevention of recurrence is the most important component in pressure ulceration management. Recurrence may be preventable if the single cause or combination of factors producing the lesion can be established.

ETIOLOGY

At least 50% of individuals seen with pressure sores will be able to identify a personal crisis that occurred just prior to appearance of the lesion. When seen initially, these patients relate the onset of the ulceration to an overwhelming infection, for example, flu, pneumonia, or loss of services of their attendant. For this group of patients, carefully planned reconstruction of the area of tissue breakdown, judicious resumption of activities postoperatively, and possibly, assistance in locating a new attendant will be sufficient intervention to return them to their former level of function.

For the remaining 50% of patients with pressure ulcerations, the first phase of treatment should examine why the patient became ill. To establish the cause, we must first determine if the patient understands how ulcerations happen. Very frequently tissue breakdown occurs when the individual lacks an understanding of the mechanism of injury and his own responsibility for maintaining intact skin. He must be an active participant in his own care. During the first admission following injury the patient should be taught and must willing to practice (1) meticulous skin care techniques, (2) proper methods of transfer, (3) intermittent relief of pressure, and (4) self-detection of early signs of impending skin breakdown.

Physical deformities are the second important group of factors that contribute to tissue ulceration. The presence of axial skeletal deformities (such as kyphosis, scoliosis, or kyphoscoliosis), joint contractures, periarticular heterotopic ossification, or absent or underdeveloped lower extremities may lead to abnormal sitting postures, including pelvic obliquities, and frequently result in frank pressure sores.

Patient equipment can be identified as the third cause of tissue breakdown. Improperly fitted corsets, fatigued pressure cushions, wheelchairs with sagging upholstery that hammocks, or foot plates that are too high can produce elevated sitting pressures over susceptible bony prominences and precede the occurrence of tissue ulcerations.

These are some of the factors encountered when looking for the cause of pressure ulcerations in a given patient. The treatment of the lesion begins with elimination of the cause.

PRELIMINARY TREATMENT

Although for many patients the approach about to be outlined is merely preparation for surgery, for others it becomes the definitive treatment. In either case the average time spent in the hospital ranges from 8 to 10 weeks. Throughout this period of hospitalization, it is necessary to utilize the combined skills of a health care team consisting of surgeon, nurse, physical therapist, and social worker in order to achieve a successful outcome. Different institutions may include team members with other backgrounds, but one team member, the patient, remains constant. The first and most important step in any successful treatment program is obtaining complete patient cooperation. This cooperation is essential not only during the period of acute care but also over the long term if recurrence is to be prevented.

COMPREHENSIVE EVALUATION

On admission, patients are assessed by the various team members in these areas: (1) metabolism-nutrition, (2) hematology, (3) neuromuscular status, and (4) urology.

The overall status of the individual, including metabolic-nutritional status and hematologic status, is evaluated. It is generally accepted that patients with pressure areas are chronically debilitated. Their serum proteins, including hemoglobin, are depleted, and they are sometimes in electrolyte imbalance.

Neuromuscular function is determined to establish (1) level of injury (if not previously known), (2) level of function, (3) range of motion of both upper and lower extremities, and (4) degree of spasticity. Level of injury and level of function help to predict the patient's future independence in self-care and allow the team to prescribe an individual program of activities following healing.

Range of motion of both upper and lower extremities must allow the patient to lie prone and flat in bed during the preoperative and postoperative phases of his treatment. In order to sit normally the patient should have 90 degrees hip flexion bilaterally. If one or both hips cannot attain this range of motion, consideration must be given to methods of correcting the deficit or adapting equipment to accommodate the sitting pattern postoperatively.

Spasticity interferes with both preoperative and postoperative positioning. It can also lead to postoperative complications, that is, hematoma, failure of flap adherence, and possible development of new bursal cavities. Spasticity may also necessitate adjustment of adaptive equipment to permit sitting postoperatively.

Urologic complications, so common among spinal cord–injured individuals, not only further debilitate the patient, but can also be a potential reservoir for infection and the exciting focus of lower extremity spasms. Dysreflexia is a condition that should be recognized immediately by all team members.

SPECIFIC CONSIDERATIONS

Modification of the patient's condition begins with 24-hour-a-day prone positioning in bed. Conditions precluding this positioning should in most cases be corrected before surgical reconstruction is considered. This positioning program allows the ulceration to be completely pressure free. In order to prevent development of ulcerations at other sites due to the patient's remaining prone continuously, he should be "bridged" with pillows or placed on special mattresses, examples of which are the Poly-Float pad or the "mud-bed." Metabolic, hematologic, neuromuscular, and urologic abnormalities should be corrected.

The wound itself requires evaluation for presence of necrotic tissue or infection of soft tissue and bone and extension of the process into adjacent structures. Surgical debridement is undertaken within 48 to 72 hours after admission. This, in combination with frequent daily dressing changes, is extremely important in mechanical removal of nonviable tissue and stimulation of perilesional epithelialization. In those ulcers affecting bony structures, judicious yet thorough debridement is utilized, together with broad-spectrum systemic antibiotic coverage.

Septic arthritis occurs by extension from adjacent infected soft tissue. The hip joint may become infected through the posterior capsule or via the proximal femur from a trochanteric sore. Although it is potentially lethal, this complication is frequently not suspected, even in the presence of daily high temperature elevations. At times a sinogram may be of assistance in making the diagnosis. However, negative study does not rule out joint sepsis. If pyarthrosis is determined during operative debridement, immediate resection of both joint surfaces and the involved bone should be accomplished. Local suction perfusion is desirable but cannot always be carried out because of wound configuration. Finally, one of the most important phases of prereconstructive preparation is control of spasms. Once the above requirements have been dealt with, surgical reconstruction may proceed with a reasonable expectation of success.

SUGGESTED READINGS

Enis, J. E., and Sarmiento, A.: The pathophysiology and management of pressure sores, Orthop. Rev. **2**:25, 1973.

Freehafer, A., et al.: Infection of the hip as a complication of advanced neurological disease. In Proceedings of the American Orthopedic Association, J. Bone Joint Surg. [Am.] **50:**1497-1498, 1968.

Ger, R., et al.: The management of chronic cavities in the region of the hip joint, J. Bone Joint Surg. [Am.] **55:**758-760, 1973.

Guttman, N. L.: The problem of treatment of pressure sores in spinal paraplegics, Br. J. Plast. Surg. **7:**196, 1955.

Kosiak, M.: Etiology and pathology of ischemic ulcers, Arch. Phys. Med. Rehabil. **40:**62-69, 1959.

Reichel, S. M.: Shearing force as a factor in decubitus ulcers in paraplegics, J.A.M.A. **166:**762, 1958.

Scherr, D. D., Dodd, T. A., and Buckingham, W. W., Jr.: Prophylactic use of topical antibiotic irrigation, J. Bone Joint Surg. [Am] **54:**634-640, 1972.

Smith, T. K., et al.: Complications associated with the use of the circular electrical turning frame, J. Bone Joint Surg. [Am.] **57:**711-713, 1975.

Chapter 26

Control of spasticity in the spinal-injured patient

E. Shannon Stauffer

Spasticity is defined as a hyperactive stretch reflex of the musculotendinous unit. The normal muscle reflex is mediated by an intact lower motor neuron afferent loop. The stretch reflex becomes hyperactive when the upper motor neuron carrying inhibitory influences as well as voluntary motor control is injured or destroyed. This condition occurs most frequently with injuries to the brain or to the spinal cord cranial to the segment of spinal cord mediating the reflex. A person with an injury to his spinal cord will have normal voluntary function and normal reflexes above the level of the lesion. If, however, the lower motor neuron arc is interrupted, either at the anterior horn cell or at the peripheral axon, the stretch reflex will be decreased, and there will be no spasticity. For example, if the injury is to the cerebrum or cerebellum there will be hyperactive reflexes (spasticity) in all voluntary muscles of the upper and lower extremities, as well as in the trunk. Areflexia and flaccid paralysis occur in thc muscles innervated by nerves emanating from the area of a cord lesion (lower motor neuron injury). No voluntary control but hyperactive reflexes (spastic paralysis) occur below the level of the lesion (Fig. 26-1).

Moderate spasticity in the paraplegic or quadriplegic patient is not without benefit. The intact muscle reflex causes frequent contraction of the muscle, preventing atrophy. This provides some added padding against the development of pressure sores over the bony prominences. Frequent involuntary muscle contractions also maintain bone strength by preventing the severe osteoporosis seen in flaccid paralysis, thus minimizing the risk of pathologic fractures of the lower extremities. Many patients can incite useful spasticity to help in rolling

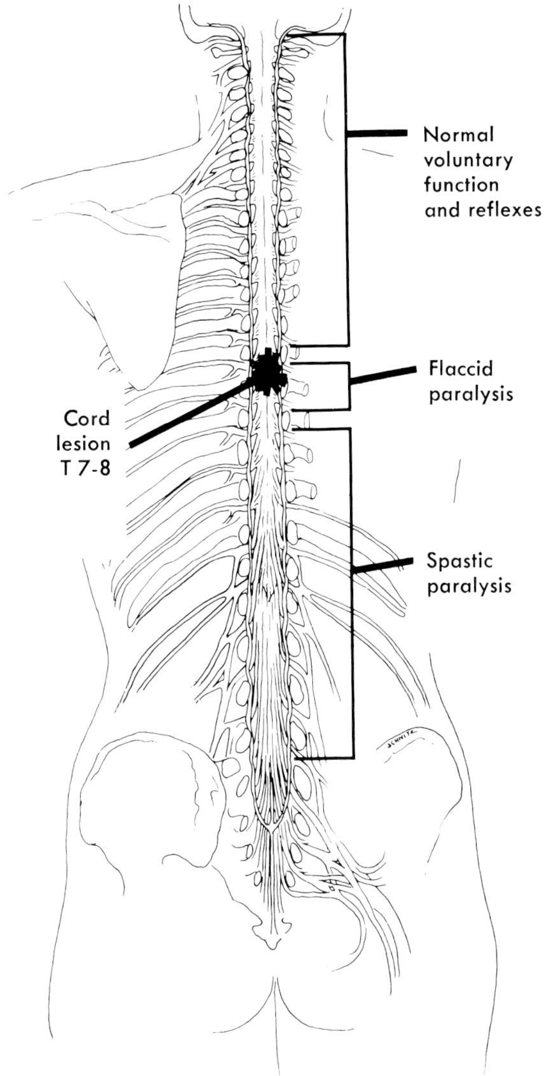

Fig. 26-1. Complete spinal cord injury (T7-8) produces flaccid paralysis of voluntary muscles innervated by injured area and spastic paralysis of muscles innervated below lesion.

over in bed, transferring from bed to wheelchair, and shifting position while sitting in the wheelchair. Intact bladder and bowel reflexes are necessary to develop automatic reflex emptying of the bowel and bladder without the need for catheterization. Maintenance of tone, bulk, and normal contour of the lower extremities are important cosmetically to a wheelchair-bound person.

Excess spasticity, however, is destructive. Continued, repetitive, unrelenting rhythmic contractions of the legs and trunk are painful and fatiguing to the paraplegic with retained sensation. The constant jumping of feet and knees is cosmetically undesirable. Positioning of the patient in the prone position for sleeping and resting may be impossible. Constant motion of the lower extremities may cause irritation to the bony prominences, such as the femoral trochanters or medial condyles, and produce pressure sores. The patient's rehabilitation may be impaired and his function decreased by excessive spasticity.

Immediately following a severe injury to the spinal cord the portion distal to the level of injury may become temporarily areflexic. Complete areflexia may last from several hours to several days and is termed "spinal shock." The first reflex that can be clinically demonstrated to return is the bulbocavernosus reflex. A positive bulbocavernosus reflex is demonstrated by a brisk anal sphincter contraction felt on the gloved finger inserted in the rectum and elicited by squeezing the glans penis. This refex is mediated through the sacral segments of the spinal cord, and when it is elicited, spinal shock is considered to be over.

During the first 3 to 6 weeks following injury the peripheral musculotendinous reflexes, such as the knee and ankle jerk, return. From 6 weeks to 6 months after injury these reflexes become hyperactive, and even minimal stimuli such as clothing contact, a breeze blowing across the skin, tapping the limb, or shaking the bed may cause involuntary contraction of the muscles. The flexor muscles are affected first, with hip and knee flexion and plantar flexion of the ankles the most common early signs of spasticity. In 6 months to 12 months the spasticity plateaus at about a year and maintains a constant level or begins to decrease. Surgical procedures should be delayed if possible until the spasticity has plateaued. Table 9 illustrates the time interval between onset of paralysis and the first operative procedure for spasticity in a group of 55 surgically treated patients.

Table 9. Time interval between injury and first operative procedure

Interval	*No. of patients*	
	Complete paralysis	*Incomplete paralysis*
6 months	4	2
6 months-1 year	5	3
1-2 years	3	6
2-5 years	4	8
5 years	5	15
TOTALS	21	34

CONTROL OF EXCESSIVE SPASTICITY

An essential part of the rehabilitation of the spinal-injured patient is early attention to prevention of joint flexion contractures. These are caused by spasticity, inadequate range of motion therapy, and improper positioning of the patient in bed. The patient must have a full passive range of motion of each joint every day. Specifically his hip flexors and adductors, hamstrings, and gastrosoleus muscles must be stretched. If these are allowed to develop myostatic contractures, the spasticity is accentuated. When in bed the patient should be positioned prone with hips abducted, knees extended, and shoulders abducted and externally rotated. Positioning of the legs with the hips in flexion and the knee extended maintains normal length of the hamstring muscles. This appears to be the most effective method of preventing contractures. If full range of motion cannot be obtained or the patient cannot be positioned in bed to maintain his range and spasticity increases despite therapy, then drugs are indicated. Double-blind studies have demonstrated that diazepam (Valium) and dantrolene sodium (Dantrium) are more effective than placebos and sedatives in decreasing spasticity and frequently do not have a concomitant somnolent effect.[2] At the present time the drug of choice is diazepam, as we have more experience with it and are more aware of its side effects. If diazepam is not effective, then dantrolene sodium may be substituted or added.

SURGICAL PROCEDURES

Surgical procedures to decrease the hyperactive stretch reflex should be considered if the patient has disabling or noxious excessive spasticity requiring chronic drug treatment 12 to 18 months after injury. The surgical procedures are all based on decreasing the hyperactive stretch reflex. This can be approached by weakening the muscles,[7] damaging the peripheral nerve externally[9] or in the spinal canal at the level of the cauda equina,[1,3-5,8] or destroying the spinal cord[6] tissue below the level of paralysis.

The muscle is weakened by lengthening the tendon or by division of the muscle belly. The peripheral reflex can be weakened by injuring the peripheral nerve by crushing,[7] injecting phenol, or transection.

Central measures to weaken the reflex include introduction of phenol[1,9] or alcohol[8] into the subarachnoid fluid at the level of the cauda equina, open section of the dorsal (sensory)[4] or ventral (motor)[3] nerve roots, or resection of the distal spinal cord.[6]

I prefer to do stepwise, peripheral procedures. The specific troublesome muscle must be first identified by repeated observation and examination of the patient. The most common musculotendinous unit that incites spasticity is the gastrocnemius-soleus group, followed by the hamstrings, the hip adductors, and the hip flexors. Frequently it will be found that rapid dorsiflexion of the foot causes ankle clonus that rapidly spreads to flexion of the knees and flexion and adduction of the hips. This could be caused by simply rolling the wheelchair over a door piece or over an uneven spot in the pavement. It is important to emphasize that one must not do too much to decrease spasticity at one operation, or previously masked spasticity in the opposite direction (extension) may occur and be more difficult to manage than the original problem.

Stepwise surgical procedures to decrease spasticity

If ankle clonus is the initiating factor for seeking treatment, a percutaneous three-level hemisection and stretching of the Achilles tendon (Fig. 26-2, *C*) may be performed. This can usually be done on an outpatient basis without anesthesia. This effectively weakens the musculotendinous unit and frequently decreases spasticity sufficiently without interfering with muscle bulk around the hip and thighs. If this is not sufficient, the patient is admitted to the hospital where the proximal spastic muscles are dealt with. It has been our experience that a single operation consisting of an intrapelvic iliopsoas myotomy and obturator neurectomy (Fig. 26-2, *A*) to decrease the hip flexor and adductor spasticity and a hamstring release at the knees, both medial and lateral (Fig. 26-2, *B*), to decrease the knee flexor spasticity is sufficient to allow most patients to be comfortable in the wheelchair without objectionable spasticity. The intrapelvic iliopsoas myotomy is preferred to the extrapelvic release of the iliopsoas tendon in the groin, as it is more predictable, affects the capsular insertion of the iliac muscle as well as the insertion of the psoas of the lesser trochanter, and simultaneously divides the nerve supply to the

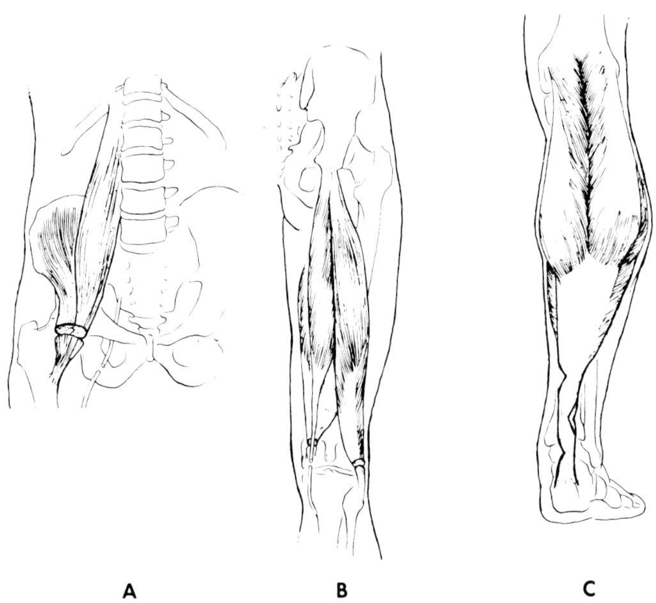

Fig. 26-2. Peripheral procedures to reduce excessive spasticity. **A,** Iliopsoas release and obturator neurectomy. **B,** Hamstring release. **C,** Three-level, percutaneous, heel cord tenotomy.

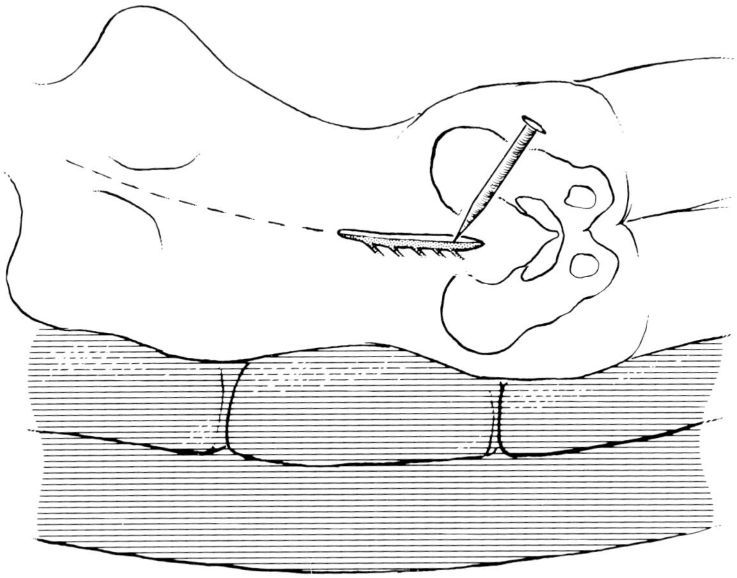

Fig. 26-3. Pooling of hyperbaric 5% phenol unilaterally in lumbar nerve root sleeves to decrease lower limb spasticity without affecting bowel and bladder arc.

distal part of the muscle. After the muscle heals, the proximal iliopsoas muscle may again be spastic, but the flaccid distal portion of the muscle will stretch. One must avoid injury to the femoral nerve during this procedure, as the extensor power of the quadriceps helps prevent knee flexion contracture.

Central (intradural) procedures such as rhizotomy and introduction of intrathecal absolute alcohol are major procedures and rarely indicated. Instability of the spine may ensue, and profound atrophy follows the complete destruction of the motor nerve roots.

Injection of 1 ml of a dilute (5%) solution of phenol in glycerin provides a hyperbaric solution that can be pooled in the lumbar nerve root sheaths (Fig. 26-3). With the patient lying on his side, the lumbar nerve roots are partially damaged, decreasing the spasticity of the leg muscles without interfering with the sacral nerve roots supplying the bowel and bladder. Only one side at a time can be done.

Intrathecal dilute phenol, however, is a temporary measure, and usually the spasticity will have returned in 6 to 12 months. This measure is of value for the patient with a complex problem of spasticity compounded by multiple joint contractures and pressure sores and who is not an optimal candidate for peripheral neurectomies, tenotomies, myotomies, or pressure sore closures.

In summary, the scheme consists then of subcutaneous lengthening of the Achilles tendon as an outpatient, followed by admission to the hospital for an obturator neurectomy, iliopsoas myotomy, and hamstring release. Intrathecal phenol, 5%, is reserved for those patients with complex problems, and intrathecal alcohol is used only for those patients who have severe pressure sores and must have their spasticity decreased completely and permanently as a lifesaving measure. Intrathecal alcohol, it must be remembered, produces complete flaccidity and condemns a person to (1) a permanent indwelling catheter in a bladder incapable of reflex emptying, (2) altered bowel reflex emptying, and (3) loss of erections.

Occasionally a person insidiously develops increased spasticity several years following his injury, and one must consider the possibility of occult, increasing, noxious stimuli introduced into the spinal cord setting as the cause. The two most common triggers for this are incipient pressure sores and renal calculi. Therefore, a careful examination of the pressure areas and an evaluation of the patient's kidneys, ureters, and bladder for stones must be undertaken. All possible areas of irritation must be considered and ruled out prior to a direct surgical attack on the spastic muscle unit.

If lower extremity spasticity remains a problem in spite of myotomies, tenotomies, and minor motor neurectomies, major neurectomies can be performed. A high femoral and sciatic neurectomy will produce a permanently flaccid lower extremity without interference of bowel and bladder reflex.

Table 10. Surgical procedures performed for spasticity

Procedure	*No.*
Tenotomies about the knee and ankle	40
Iliopsoas myotomy and obturator neurectomy about the hip	36
Miscellaneous tenotomies in the upper extremities	12
Intrathecal phenol injections	7
TOTAL	95

Fortunately this is rarely indicated. Table 10 lists the various procedures performed on 55 surgically treated patients. Amputation of spastic contracted lower extremities for easier transfer in and out of wheelchairs and easier wheelchair propulsion has been advocated in the past. I have found that paralyzed patients who have amputations of lower extremities are much more disabled and are less able to sit in a wheelchair. The weight of the lower extremities is essential as a counterweight to maintain proper balance in the wheelchair. Proper positioning distributes weight to the posterior thighs, minimizing excessive pressure over the ischial tuberosities.

Therefore a plea must be made to avoid amputation of the lower extremities. Rather pressure sore closures, bone resections, myotomies, and neurectomies should be done as necessary, thus maintaining the lower extremities for functional wheelchair-sitting balance.

REFERENCES

1. Cain, H. E.: Subarachnoid block in the treatment of pain and spasticity, Paraplegia **3:**152-160, 1965.
2. Corbett, M., Frankel, H. L., and Michaelis, L.: Valium, Amytal and placebo: trial on spastic paraplegics, Paraplegia **10:**19, 1972.
3. Freeman, L. W., and Heimburger, R. F.: The surgical release of spasticity in paraplegic patients. I. Anterior rhizotomy, J. Neurosurg. **4:**435-443, 1947.
4. Freeman, L. W., and Heimburger, R. F.: The surgical release of spasticity in paraplegic patients, II. Peripheral nerve section, posterior rhizotomy and other procedures, J. Neurosurg. **5:**556-561, 1948.
5. Kerr, S. A.: Anterior rhizotomy for the relief of spasticity, Paraplegia **4:**154-160, 1966.
6. McCarthy, C. S.: The treatment of spastic paraplegia by selective spinal cordotomy, J. Neurosurg. **11:**539-545, 1954.
7. Mechaelis, L.: Orthopaedic surgery in the limb of paraplegia, Berlin, 1965, Springer Verlag, pp. 8-12.
8. Sheldon, C. H., and Bors, E.: Subarachnoid alchohol block in paraplegia, J. Neurosurg. **5:**389-391, 1948.
9. Weiss, M., Rudnicki, S., Haftek, J., and Wirski, J.: Phenolisation of spinal roots and peripheral nerves in spastic paralysis, Paraplegia **4:**165, 1966.

Chapter 27

Surgery for pressure sores

Melvin Spira
Joseph Agris

The origins of many surgical procedures lie in antiquity, but the first description of surgical closure of decubitus ulcers by Lamon and Alexander[6] appeared in the literature in 1944. Interestingly, 6 years previously Davis[3] had recommended pedicle flap resurfacing of the scar epithelium of healed ulcers to provide satisfactory padding over bony prominences. Decubitus ulcers developing among the spinal cord–injured veterans of World War II stimulated many surgeons to develop techniques for the successful closure of pressure ulcers, as reported in a number of papers over the past three decades.

During the last 15 years at the Texas Institute for Rehabilitation and Research, we have personally closed or have supervised the surgical closure of over 200 decubitus ulcers. This chapter presents a distillation of the surgical experiences gathered from this period and describes our present operative approach and innovations in treatment of this physically, psychologically, and socioeconomically debilitating problem.

In an earlier work[11] we described in detail various causes of, and preventive methods for, decubitus ulcers. While paralysis, immobilization, anemia, spasticity, infection, skin trophic changes, age, and malnutrition have all been implicated in bedsore development, they are only predisposing factors. The precipitating cause invariably is pressure, and clinically, its result depends on duration rather than force. In our experience, utilization of a water-filled bed or cushion has extended the time period that skin over a bony prominence can tolerate continuous pressure without breakdown. The general basic preventive measures include the avoidance of excessive pressure over bony prominences, proper skin hygiene, adequate nutrition, and continuity of care.

Preoperative management involves both general body care and local wound treatment. Prior to surgery it is extremely important to establish the body positions the patient will be able to tolerate postoperatively so that undue pressure on the operated site and skin breakdown elsewhere can be avoided. In fact the ability of the patient to tolerate a specific position frequently will affect the proposed surgical plan.

A nutritional status conducive to wound healing must be obtained. Chronic infection, usually of ulcer or urinary tract origin, invites anemia, an important surgical consideration in paralyzed patients with cord lesions who tolerate poorly even minor changes in blood volume. A satisfactory blood volume with a hematocrit of 36 in a well-hydrated patient is desirable preoperatively. Maintenance of joint motion in preparation for the immobilization period necessitated by the surgery is important. Ideally spasms should be eliminated or markedly reduced, particularly if trochanteric or ischial ulcers are present; pedicle flap surgery in the presence of spasm invites postoperative complications.

Local wound care is directed toward the establishment of drainage, debridement of necrotic tissue, and development of granulation tissue in the ulcer bed. Saline-moistened coarse gauze dressings, changed frequently, and sharp debridement of the ulcer at bedside are mainstays of therapy. Salisbury and associates[9] have experimentally demonstrated the effectiveness of coarse gauze dressings over biologic dressings in microscopic debridement of a wound. Our routine, referred to as wet-to-dry

A

B

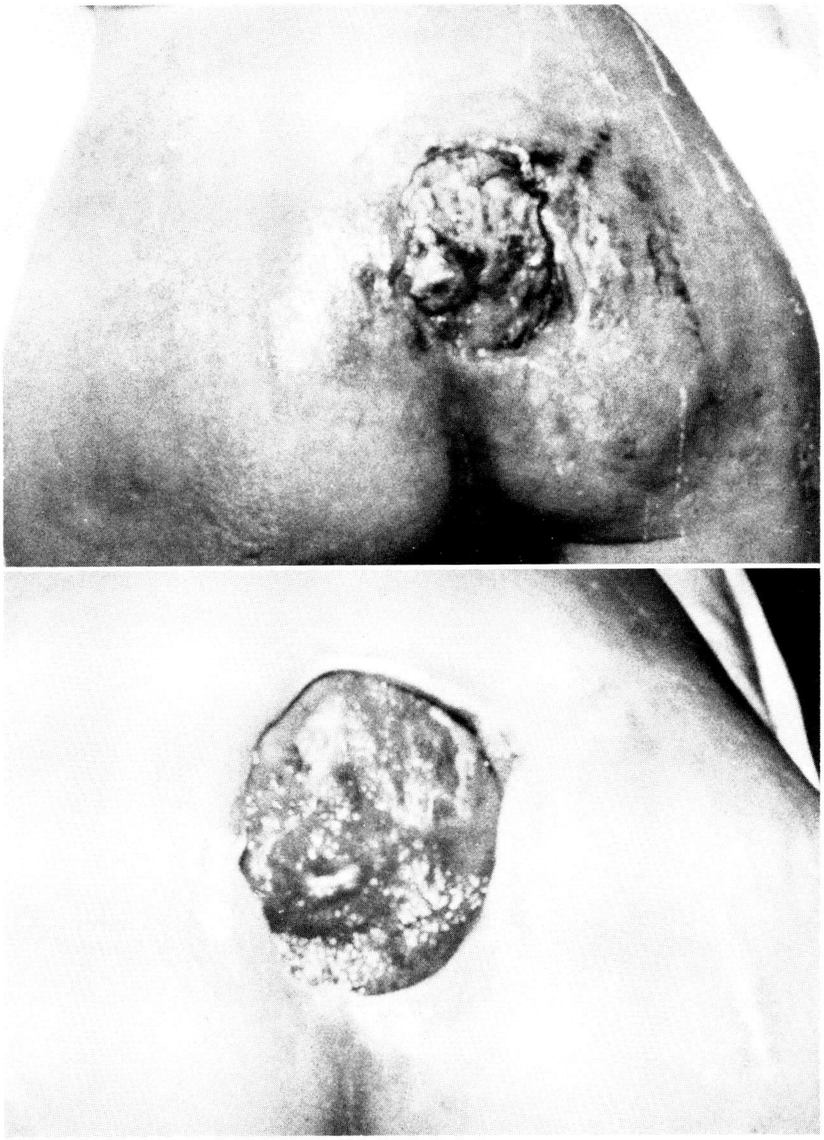

Fig. 27-1. A, Sacral ulcer prior to debridement with saline gauze dressings. **B,** Ten days later, wound is clean and epithelializing.

dressings, involves changing the dressing every 8 hours and wetting it every 4 hours, that is, between changes (Fig. 27-1). Such a dressing schedule poses no undue burden on any nursing staff and can be carried out at home. In our experience less conventional medications and techniques to accelerate the cleaning up of an ulcer prior to surgery are time consuming, expensive, and of unproven effectiveness. Occasionally, when an ulcer is very deep and undermined, a modification of Meleney's technique[7] is effective; equal parts of zinc peroxide, glycerin, and hydrogen peroxide impregnated in gauze and changed daily will accelerate wound debridement without incurring the risk of hemorrhage, a complication of sharp dissection of necrotic tissue.

Our goals in the preoperative preparation of decubitus ulcers are removal of necrotic tissue and reduction in the quantitative bacterial count, that is, a relatively clean wound. Peripheral epithelialization does occur concomitantly and serves as an excellent indication of a clean wound ready for skin graft or pedicle flap coverage; however, this scar-thin epithelium is usually sacrificed at surgery as such tissue will not serve as a satisfactory cover postoperatively.

A

B

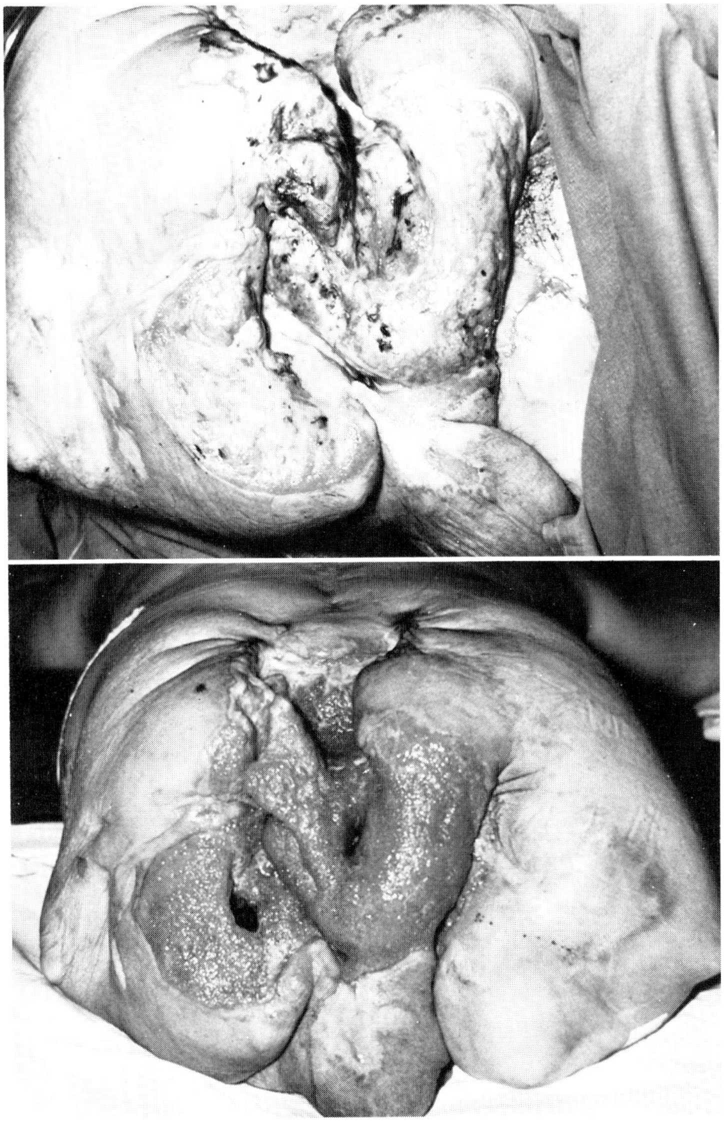

Fig. 27-2. A, Bilateral high thigh amputee with severe decubitus ulcers of stumps, buttock, and sacrum. **B,** Three weeks later on a program of saline and coarse gauze dressings (see text).

When the ulcer is located near the anus in the ischial or sacral areas, the patient is given a liquid diet 24 hours preoperatively and cleansing enemas the night prior to surgery. Paregoric, 10 ml every 8 hours to constipate, is begun, thus avoiding early fecal contamination. We have resurfaced the most extensive decubitus ulcers in these areas (Fig. 27-2) on this regimen without the need for a diversionary colostomy.

Most patients with paralytic spinal lesions undergo surgery under light premedication without a general anesthetic. It is imperative that a good intravenous passageway for fluid and blood replacement be established. In a patient with spotty sensation or in whom severe apprehension is a problem, general anesthesia with good airway control and tissue oxygen perfusion is superior to heavy doses of medications supplemented by local anesthesia.

The general surgical principles of decubitus ulcer surgery we have adhered to include the following:

1. Split-thickness skin grafts are utilized to close large multiple ducubitus ulcers in debilitated patients (Fig. 27-3).
2. Paraplegics may do well with skin grafts to sacral decubiti but may need flaps over the

C

D

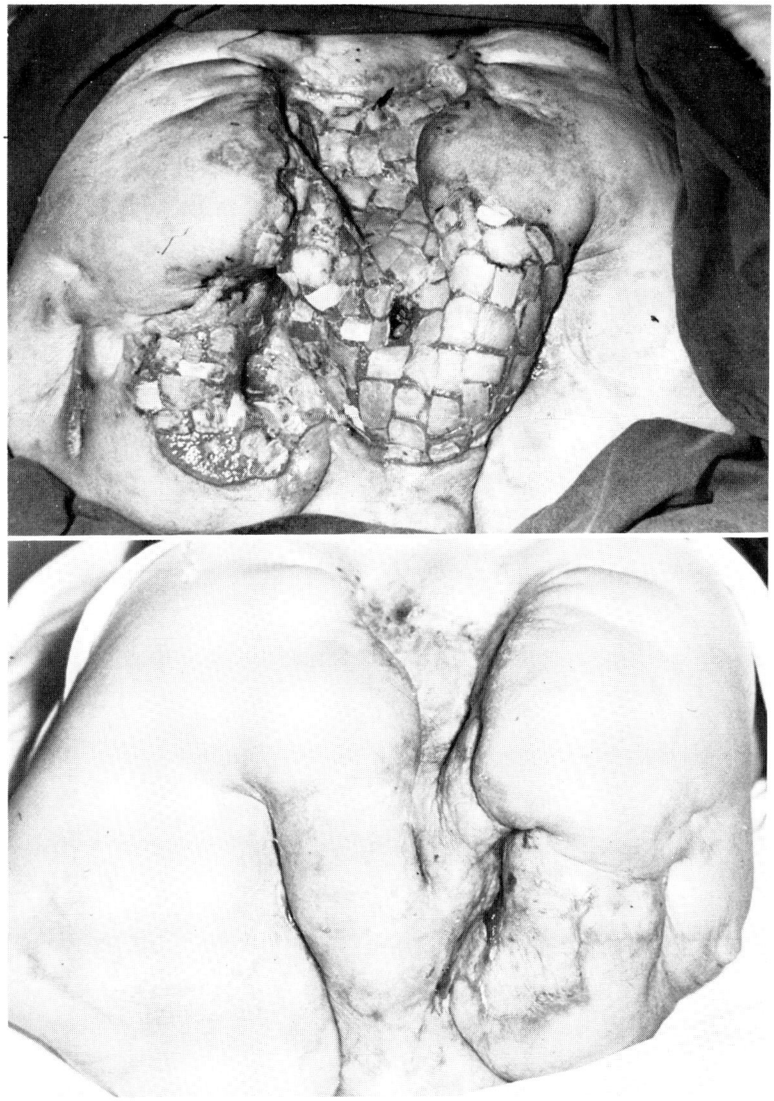

Fig. 27-2, cont'd. C, Following "postage stamp," split-thickness, skin grafting. **D,** Healing 1 month later.

ischial and trochanteric areas. Quadriplegics usually need flap coverage over the sacral area as well, with fewer problems seen at the ischial tuberosity sites.

3. Pedicle flap surgery in the presence of spasms carries a high rate of complications. Medical management of spasms with diazepam (Valium) or dantrolene sodium (Dantrium) is attempted initially, and, if this is unsuccessful, selective myotomies, intrathecal alcohol blocks, phenol blocks of peripheral nerves, or selective rhizotomies must be considered. Only a neophyte in the area of skin flap surgical treatment of decubiti would operate on a patient with severe spasms.
4. Postoperative body positioning must be planned preoperatively.
5. The ulcer wound and all adherent involved scar and remaining necrotic or partially viable tissue is excised.
6. Underlying bony prominences and heterotrophic bone are resected.
7. Good hemostasis must be obtained if hematoma and infection are to be avoided.
8. Where involved areas are small and adjacent

A 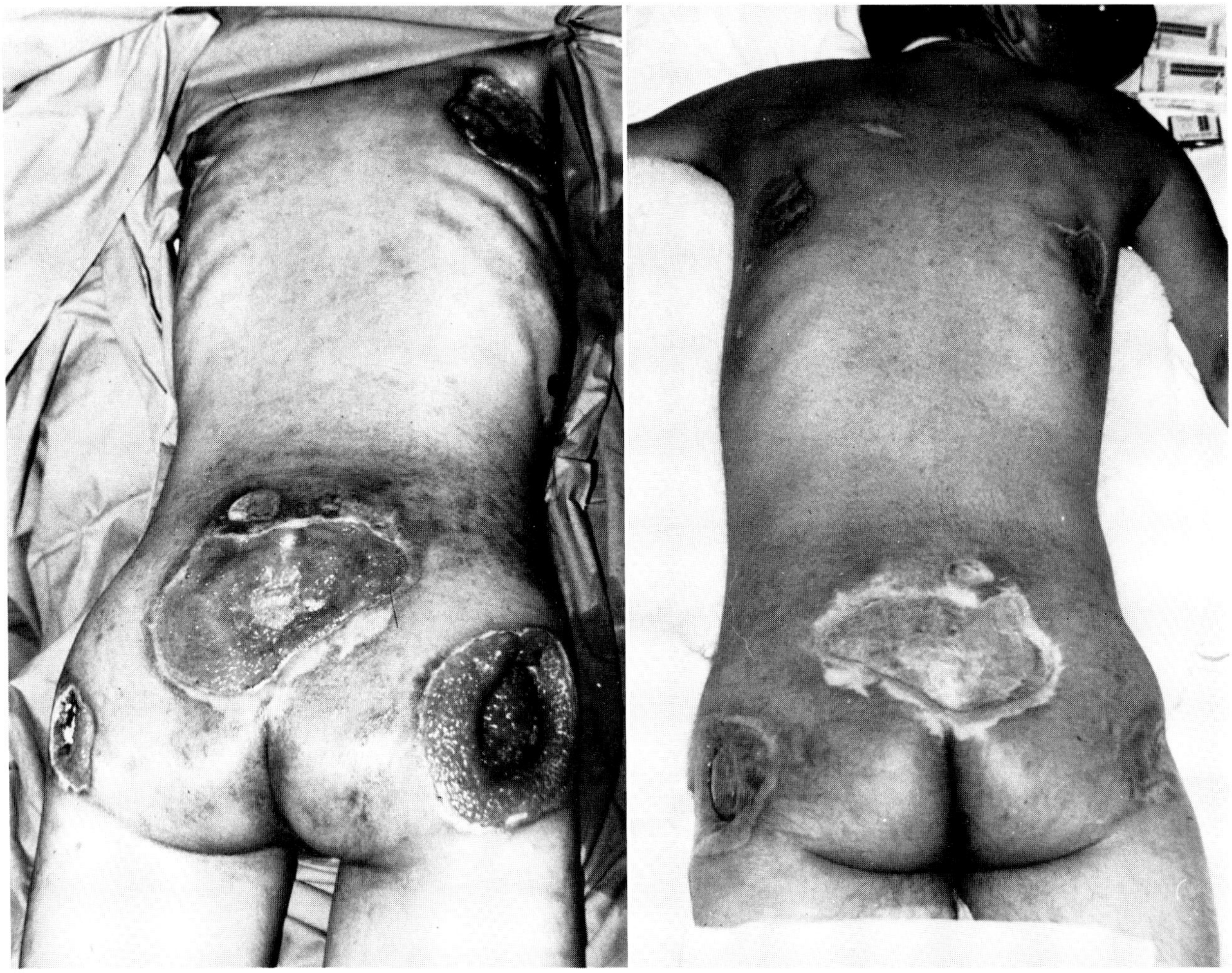 B

Fig. 27-3. A, Extensive decubitus ulcers over almost all bony prominences on debilitated quadriplegic. **B,** Healing after split-thickness skin grafting.

tissue loose, as in the ischial and trochanteric areas, direct closure without tension is preferable.

9. Larger ulcers should be resurfaced with a skin or skin-muscle flap wherever possible rather than with direct closure or split-thickness skin grafting.
   a. Small flaps that leave suture lines over pressure areas, predisposing the areas to repeated ulceration and to possible adverse reactions to future surgery, should be avoided.
   b. Underlying and adjacent musculature should be used to cover bare bone and fill voids where needed.
   c. Undue tension at the ulcer site can be avoided by using a split-thickness skin graft in the flap donor bed.
10. Proper wound drainage should be provided.
11. A bulky, light, but even pressure dressing is always applied.
12. Full weight bearing on operated ulcers is to be avoided for 12 to 21 days.

MANAGEMENT OF SPECIFIC SITES

Sacrum

In larger ulcers only the scar tissue adherent to the sacrum is excised, and the scar tissue that is not located on the pressure area is left in situ. Only the bone that is grossly protuberant, irregular, or sharp is resected; the entire sacral promontory is never resected; removal of this is accompanied by profuse and possibly uncontrollable bleeding. A wide variety of methods to resurface sacral ulcers has been proposed. These include direct closure, local advancement flaps, transposition flaps, bilobular pedicles, and larger rotational flaps. In many patients the skin above and lateral to the sacrum is thin and lacks the subcutaneous fat padding present over the buttock area. Therefore a large, superiorly based rotational flap, designed to include the upper portion of the buttock with extension into the loin area, is usually utilized (Fig. 27-4). With this technique, laxity of skin permits advancement of the rotated flap and frequently allows easy primary closure, obviating the need for a split-thickness skin graft (Fig. 27-5).

In larger ulcers, particularly in younger and

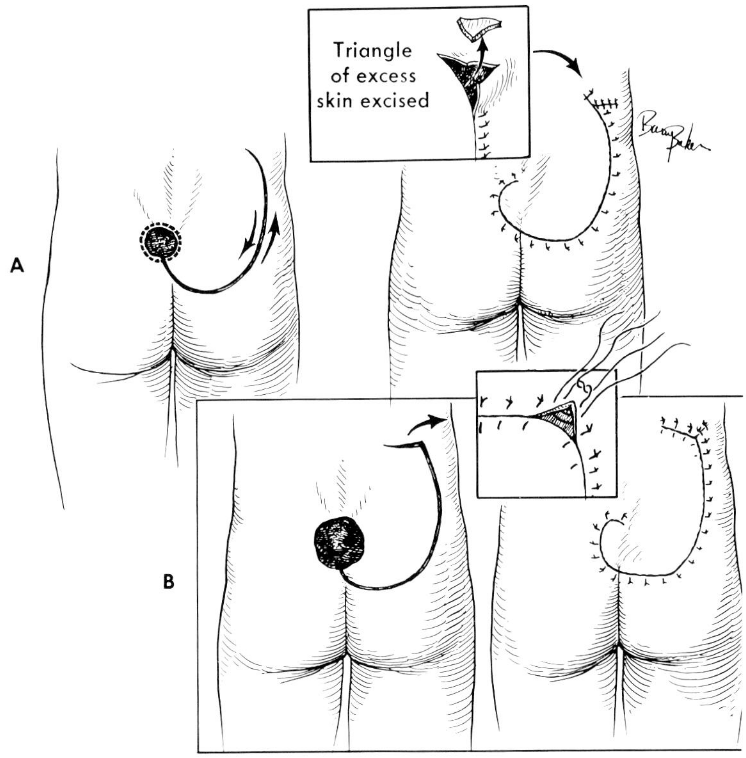

Fig. 27-4. Two variations of superiorly based pedicle flap for covering sacral ulcers.

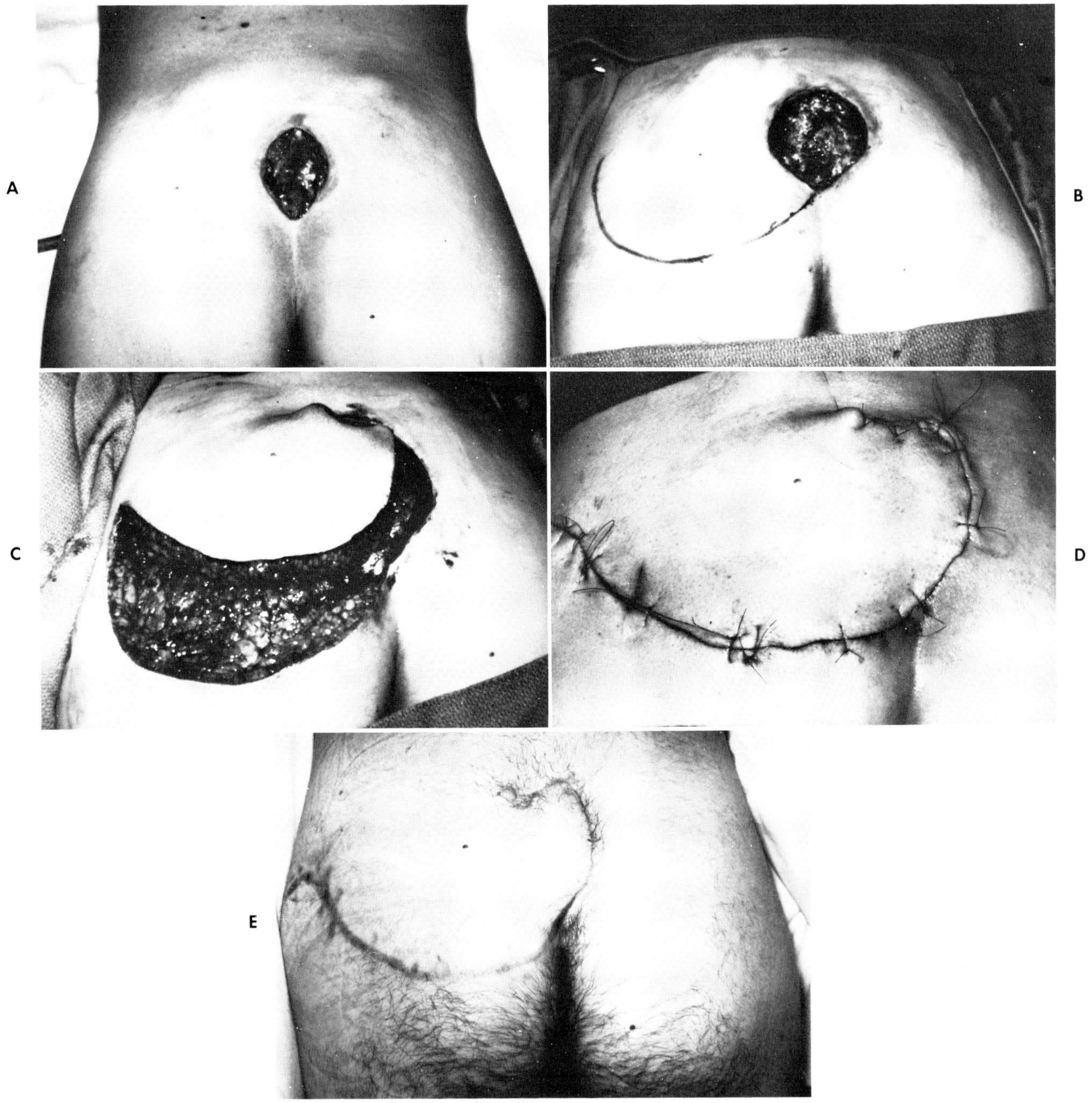

Fig. 27-5. A, Sacral ulcer prior to excision of peripheral scar. **B,** After excision, with flap outlined. **C,** Flap elevated with inferior margin well away from ischial pressure area, covering ulcer without tension. **D,** Subcutaneous and subcuticular closure. **E,** Three months later.

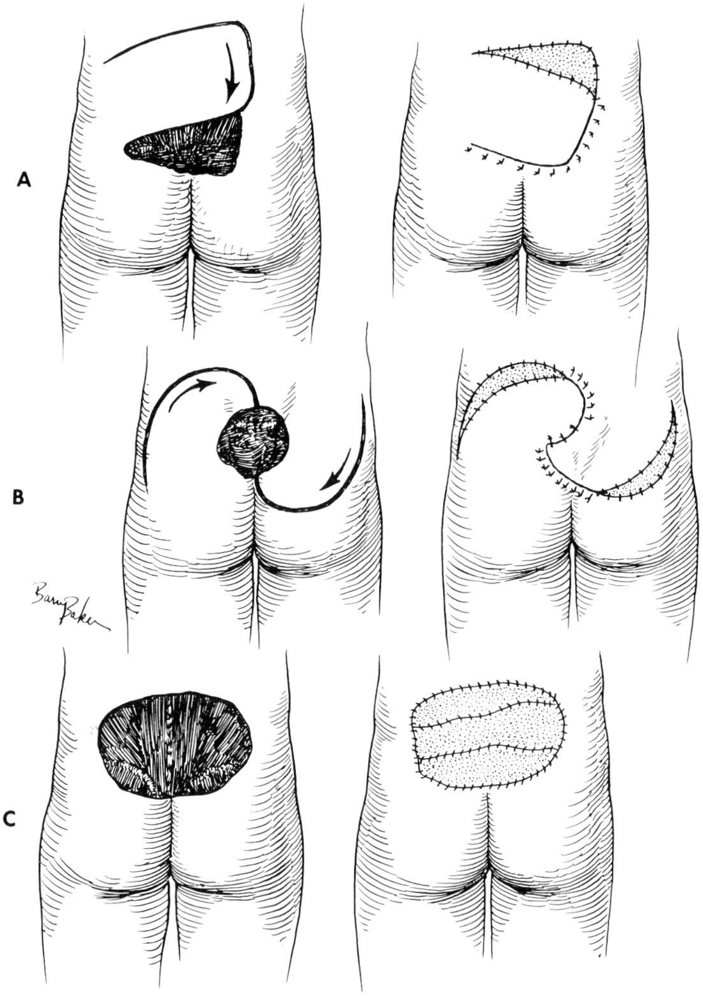

Fig. 27-6. Other methods of closing larger sacral ulcers. **A,** Large flap delayed at least once. **B,** Bilobular flaps used for larger defects. **C,** Split-thickness skin graft need not be sutured if patient is maintained prone.

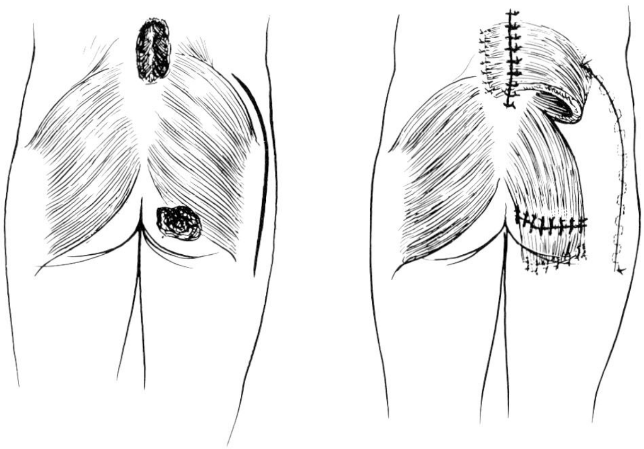

Fig. 27-7. "Turnover" gluteal muscle flap effectively provides additional padding and obliterates "dead space."

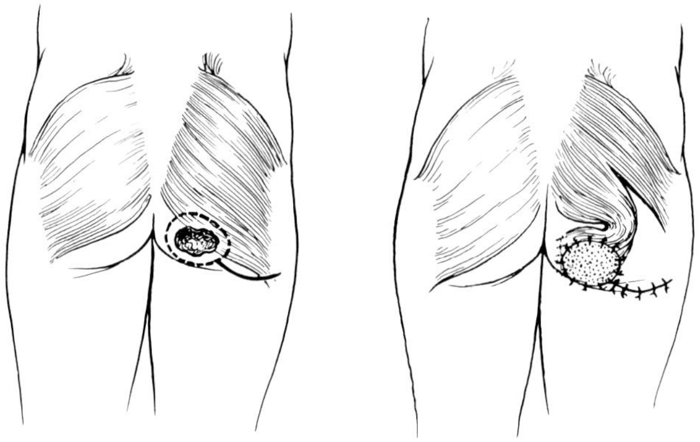

Fig. 27-8. Variation of muscle flap used with skin graft.

A

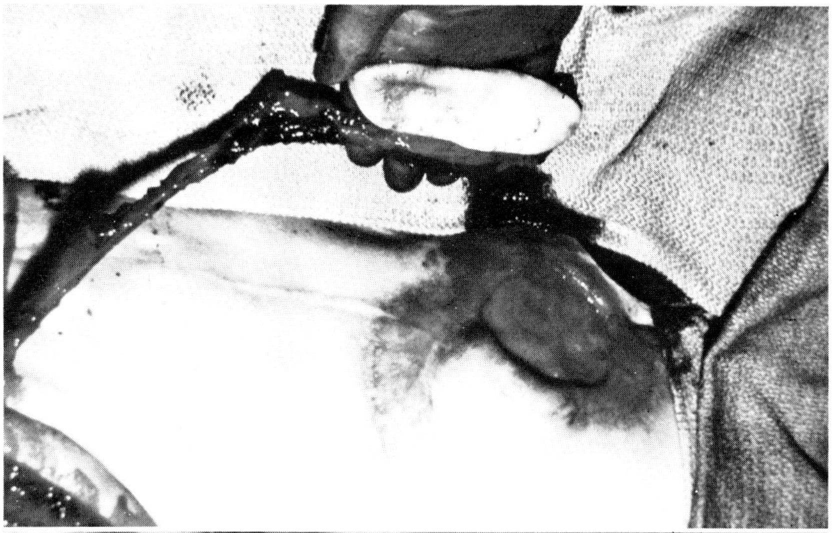

B

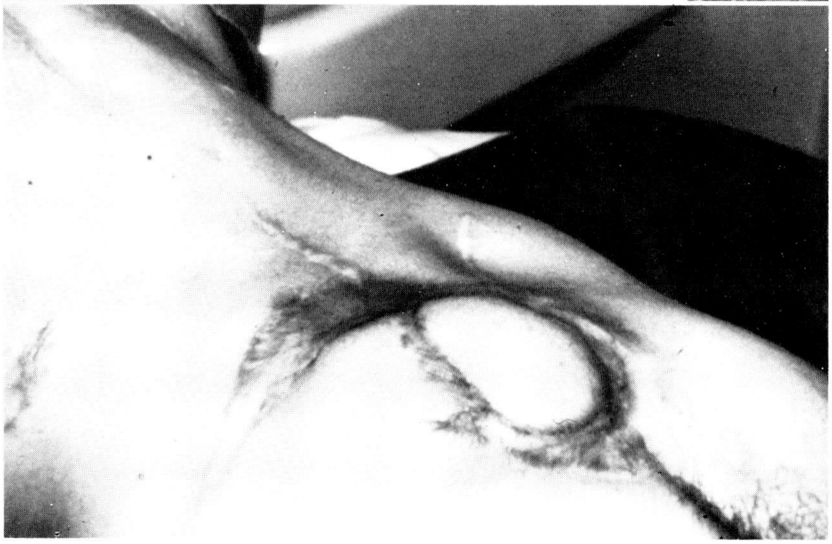

Fig. 27-9. A, Delayed intercostal neurovascular island flap being transposed to sacral defect. **B,** Healed flap has sensation. (Courtesy Dr. David G. Dibell.)

heavier patients, a back cut is needed to permit shifting of the flap without undue tension. The buttock *opposite* the side most involved by the ulcer is utilized, resulting in an off-center suture line, the midline being the site of usual recurrence. Occasionally we do employ an inferiorly based flap, grafting the donor site.

For larger ulcers, depending upon their shape and size, either a transposition flap, usually delayed, or a bilobular flap is utilized, using both sides of the loins (Fig. 27-6). In these instances split-thickness skin grafts are applied to the donor tissue sites where direct closure could endanger flap vascularity. In thin-skinned patients, additional padding can be provided by using a turnover gluteal muscle flap between the skin and the underlying bony prominence, as advocated by Ger and Levine.[5] This same flap can be effectively used as an adjunct to closure in patients who have had previous ulcers and closures at this site, as well as the ischial area where residual scarring may prohibit further utilization of local tissue (Fig. 27-7). The muscle flap can be sutured to the wound margins and a split-thickness skin graft placed directly on the muscle bed (Fig. 27-8).

A new technique has been developed by Dibell[4] and further advanced by Daniel and associates.[2] These innovative surgeons have employed a neurovascular island pedicle flap, based posteriorly on the eleventh or twelfth intercostal nerve and vascular bundle and brought down, either directly or in a staged delay procedure (Fig. 27-9) to resurface sacral decubitus ulcers, providing resurfacing, padding, and a degree of sensation that hopefully will prevent further pressure sores at this site.

Ischial tuberosity

Patients are always operated on in the hip-flexed position rather than with hips extended. Management of the tuberosity itself is controversial. We now advocate excision of the entire tuberosity and adjacent pubic and ischial rami. This radical approach, formerly reserved for recurrent ulcers rather than for management of primary pressure sores, is now utilized in almost all primary ulcer surgery at this site. Admittedly, total or near-total ischiectomy is laborious; bleeding is more difficult to control; and a deeper "dead space" must be dealt with. Mobilization of adjacent musculature to provide a "vest over pants" closure of this space or utili-

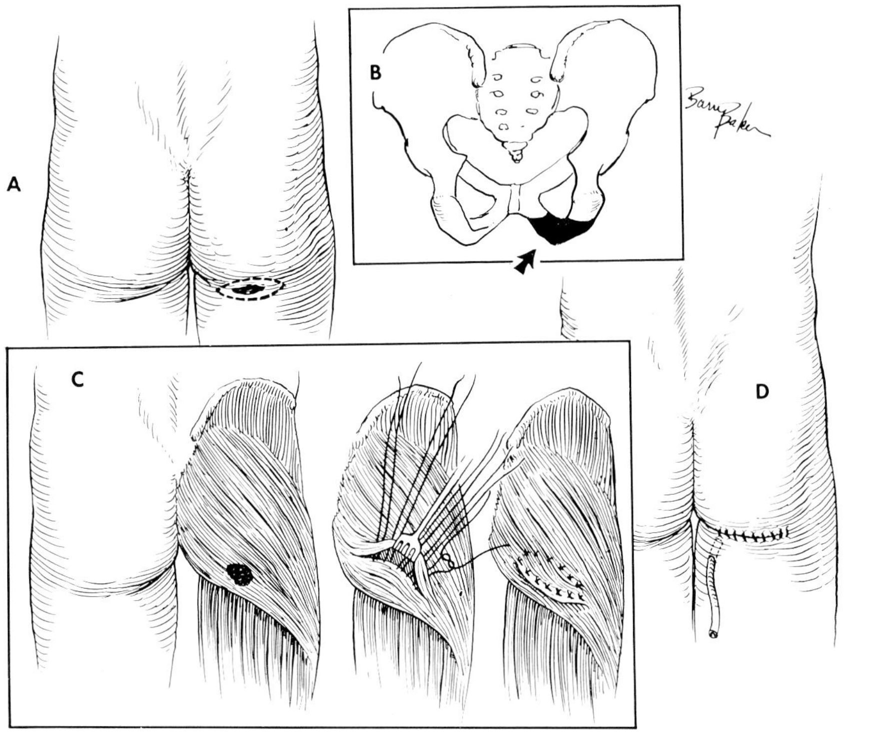

Fig. 27-10. Small but deep ischial ulcers are closed primarily, usually after extensive bony resection (blackened area in **B**).

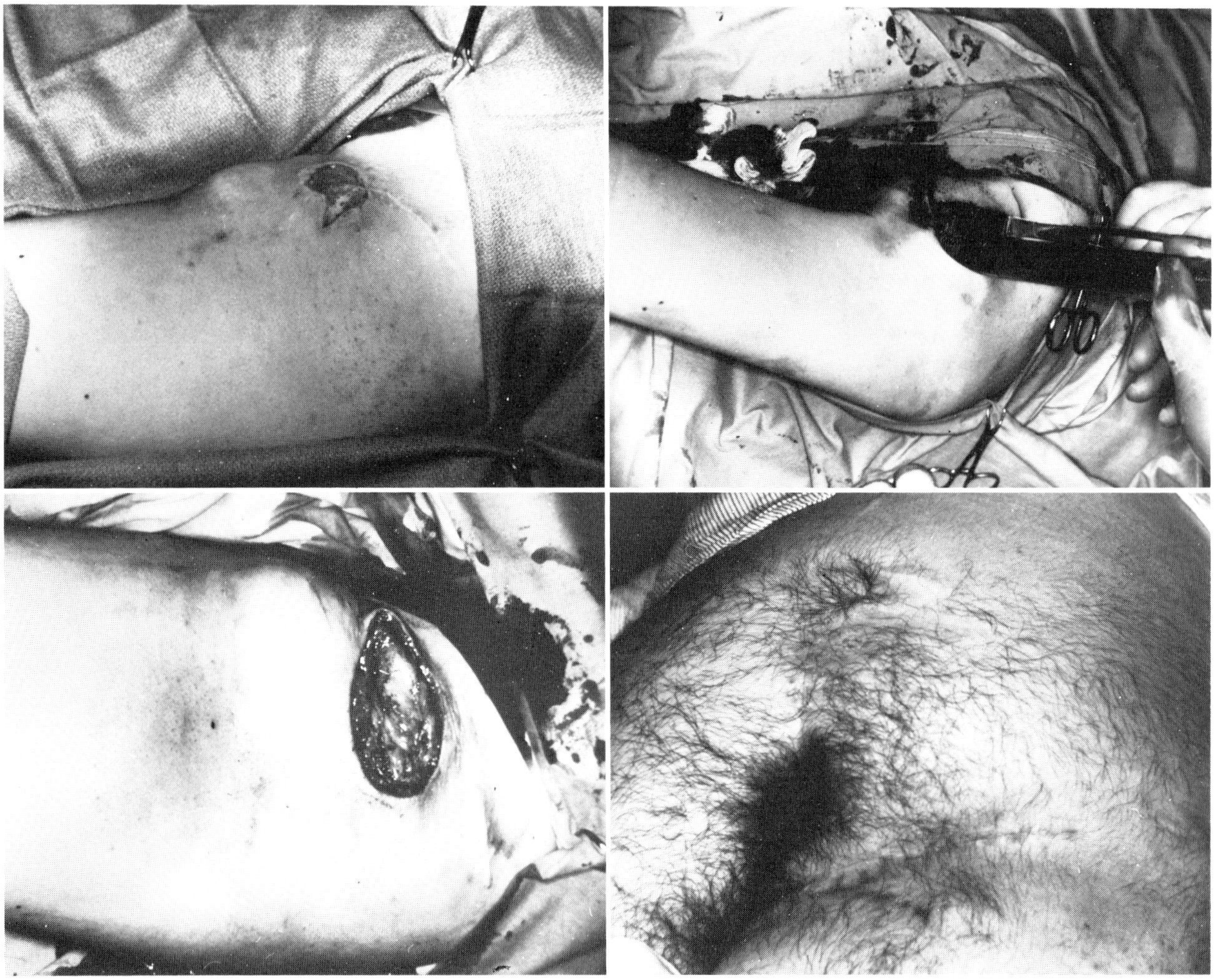

A B C D

Fig. 27-11. Recurrent ischial ulcer treated as illustrated in Fig. 27-10. **D,** Result 6 months after surgery.

zation of gluteal or hamstring muscles as a filler may be needed (Fig. 27-10). Removal of this large amount of bone is advantageous in that it usually permits a direct primary closure of the skin, obviating the need for the development of a pedicle flap (Fig. 27-11). When total ischiectomy is practiced, similar surgery to the contralateral ischial segment may be necessary to preclude future ulcer formation in that area and to promote an even, stable base on which the patient may sit.

Generally, a large, laterally based posterior skin flap is used to resurface the defect created by excision of ulcer and bone. The medial hamstring muscles, semimembranosus and semitendinosus, cut distally and rotated superiorly may be used to fill up any dead space, with care being taken not to injure the neurovascular bundle entering the muscles in their upper quarter (Fig. 27-12). The laxity of tissue of the upper inner thigh and perineum that adjoins this flap permits closure, obviating any defect here. We feel, however, that a split-thickness skin graft is needed inferiorly to permit inset of the flap into the ischial defect without tension (Fig. 27-13). We stress the importance of ischial ulcer closure with the patient in the prone position with hips flexed to simulate the sitting position. Excessive tissue tension at the repair site can be corrected at surgery. If the patient is lying prone during elevation and inset of the flap, when hip flexion as in sitting is resumed postoperatively, any tension in this area manifests as a spreading of the scar. Small transpositional flaps utilized in this area generally have been a disappointment. Such a flap, even if adequate initially, has associated scars that may preclude utilization of adjacent tissue at some future date. Again, we would employ the gluteus as a turnover muscle flap when dealing with an extensive ulcer in which repeated efforts to close it have failed (Figs. 27-7 and 27-8).

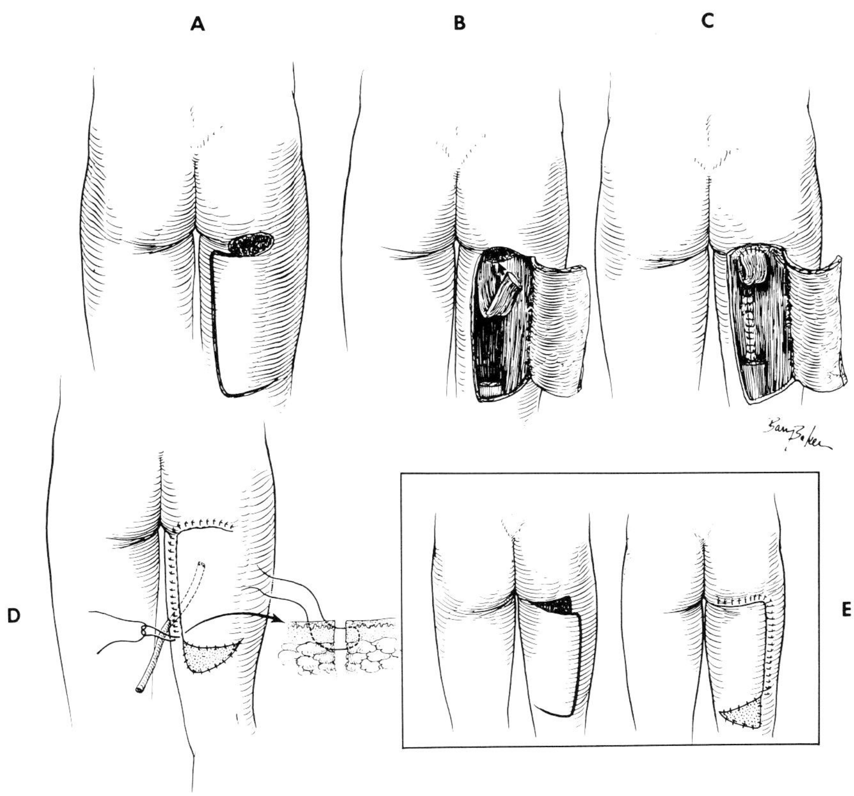

Fig. 27-12. Thigh flaps can be used to resurface larger ischial ulcers. **A,** Flap is designed to utilize upper three fourths of posterior thigh. **B** and **C,** Semitendinosus muscle used to obliterate "dead space." **D,** Illustrated closure using interrupted half-buried vertical mattress sutures. **E,** Alternate procedure.

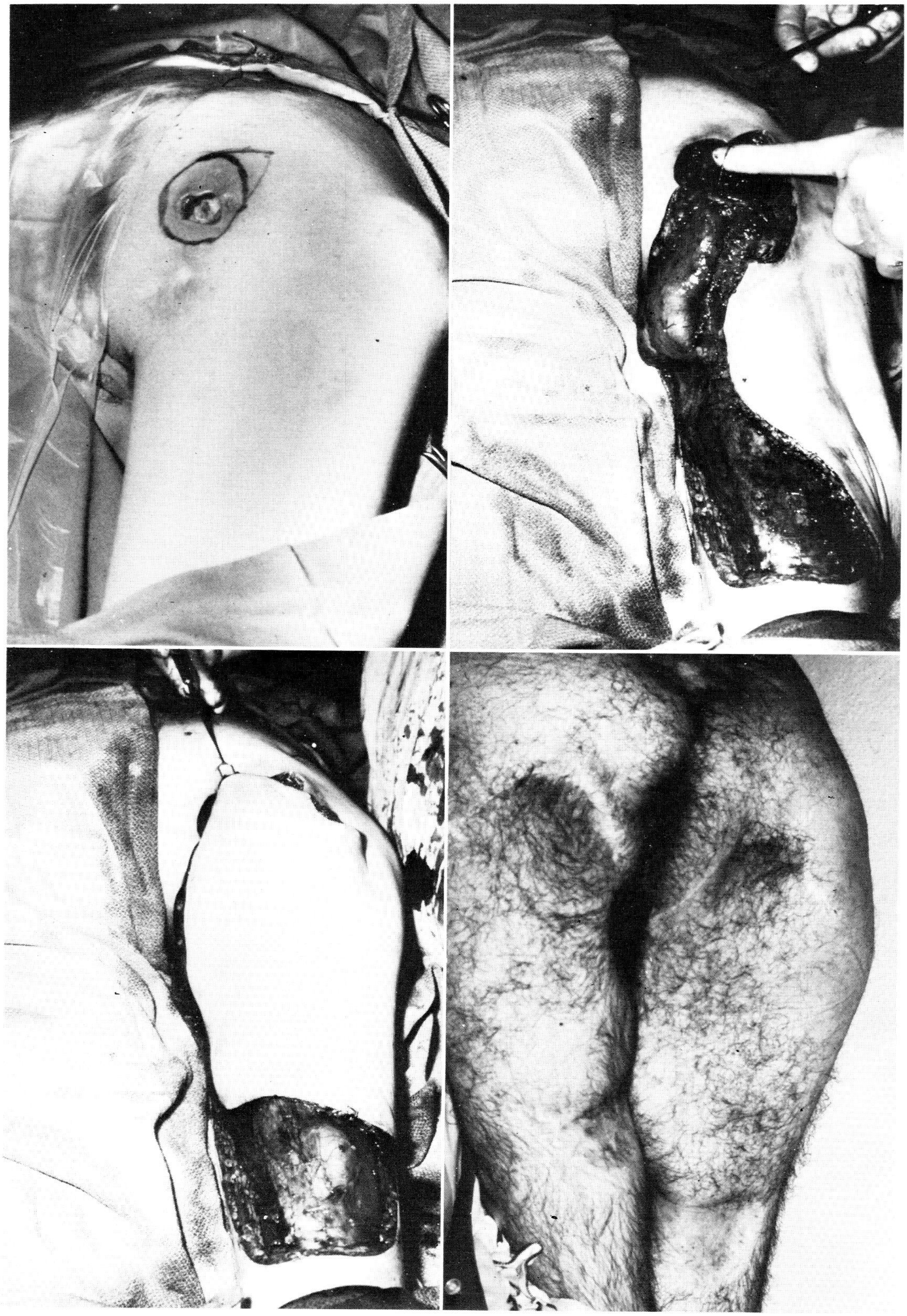

Fig. 27-13. Deeply scarred and undermined, this ulcer was completely excised with underlying ischium and resurfaced with pedicle flap, as illustrated in Fig. 27-12.

Trochanteric area

Excision of the head of the trochanter is mandatory. Ulcers here may be extensively undermined and must be excised, preferably in toto, together with the frequently present bursae. The flap donor site is dependent upon the size of the wound, direction of undermining, presence of scars, availability of local tissue, and the optimum postoperative position of the patient. In the larger ulcers, rotational advancement flaps are preferred to any type of transpositional coverage. To cover the usual resultant defect following excision of such an ulcer, a posteriorly based inferior flap is used and the inferior portion of the donor bed is skin grafted. The patient usually is maintained in the prone position postoperatively. When undermining is extensive, the elevated flap should include the roof of the ulcer. Any false or pseudomembranous lining should be sharply excised prior to inset. Following ostectomy of the greater trochanter, the raw bone is covered with a fascia muscle flap based below and anterior to the defect or with a vertical anteriorly based bipedicle flap (Fig. 27-14, *A*). A typical trochanteric ulcer covered with a long, posteriorly based thigh flap is illustrated in Fig. 27-15. Occasionally a combination of factors, including osteomyelitis resulting from extension of a necrotic ulcer into bone, severe heterotrophic bone formation, and hip fusion in extension, may necessitate resection of the head and adjacent proximal femur. If such bone removal is needed, it is best to go directly to resection of the entire proximal third of the femur. If the ulcer bed is deep, particularly when recurrence is the problem and the adjacent tissue is heavily scarred, the deep defect remaining is not covered with a flap but rather with stamp-sized split-thickness skin grafts or mesh grafts, usually applied to the wound as a delayed procedure.

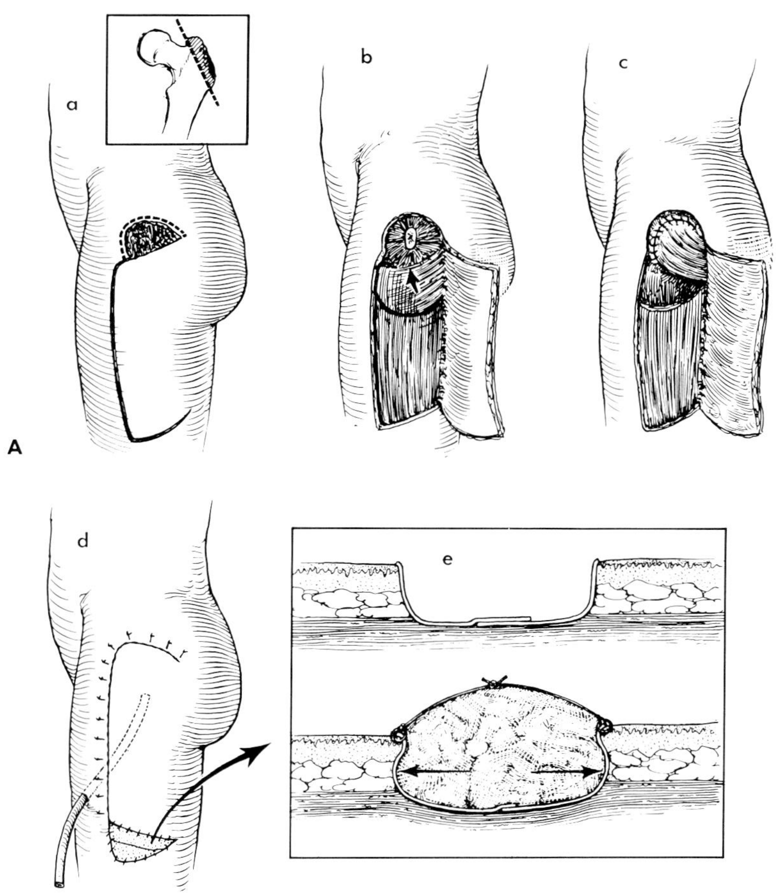

Fig. 27-14. A, Thigh flap used with local muscle flap to provide thick cover over resected trochanteric ulcer. Rapid method of overlaying split-thickness skin graft without sutures to cover donor defect is shown in *e*.

Continued.

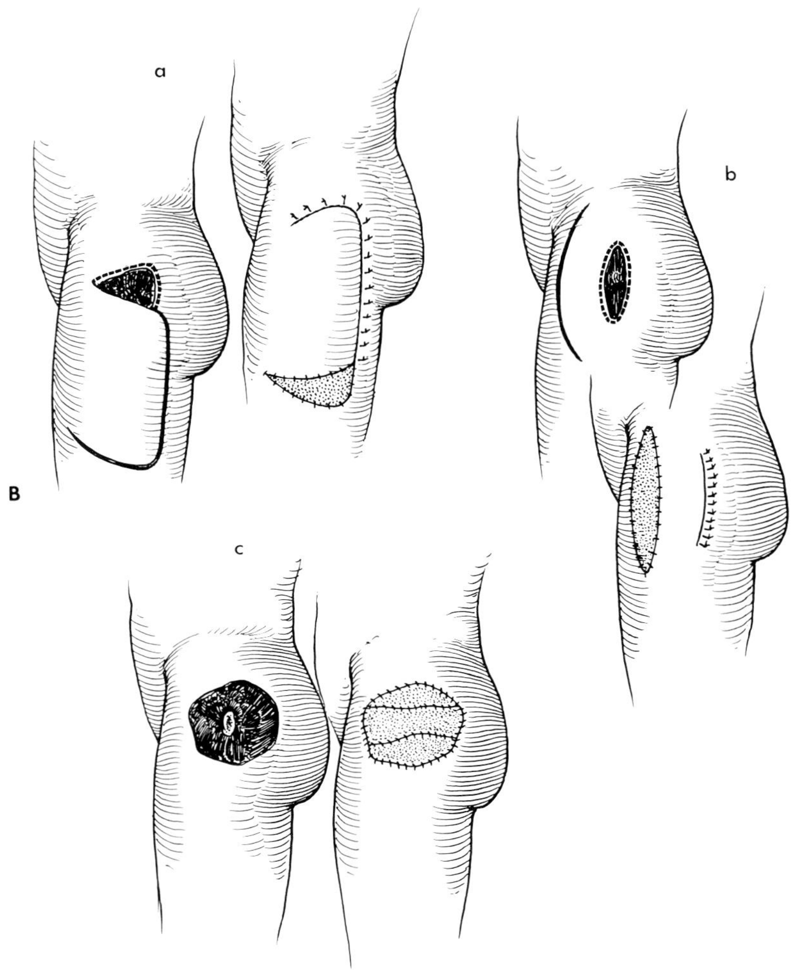

Fig. 27-14, cont'd. B, Variations of other methods useful in closure of trochanteric ulcer.

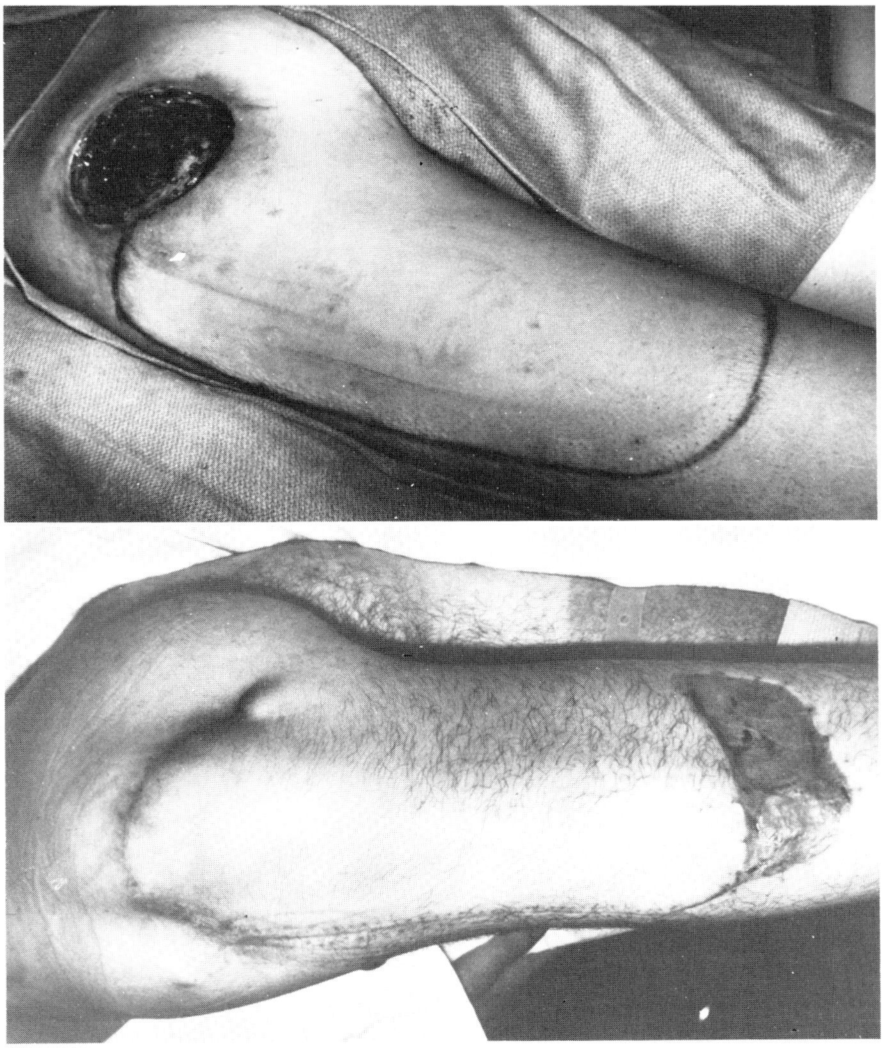

Fig. 27-15. Trochanteric ulcer closed by technique shown in Fig. 27-14.

Non-weight-bearing areas

Ulcers over normally non-weight-bearing areas are best managed by conservative method. The scapula, ischial crest, pretibial, and heel are common sites of ulceration in the immediate postinjury period and are not usually found after rehabilitation. Smaller ulcers are not debrided; the surgeon encourages peripheral epithelialization by keeping the area dry while avoiding prolonged pressure. It is an error to excise the eschar when it is elevated above the surface of the surrounding skin as this indicates less than full-thickness skin loss. Epithelialization from the deep dermal elements will heal the wound if a dry environment is promoted and infection prevented.

High thigh amputation

In selected cases a filleting procedure with utilization of a long thigh-leg flap to resurface multiple decubitus ulcers is the only available surgical procedure. A group of spinal cord–injured patients, fortunately few in number, will return time after time with a wide variety of decubitus ulcers in every conceivable pressure site, areas previously covered by skin flaps and grafts; their heavily scarred, ulcerated buttocks and thighs bear mute testimony to previous valiant efforts at surgical rehabilitation. For these patients the fillet procedure (Fig. 27-16) described by the senior author[10] and others, can be employed. Under tourniquet, the femur, patella, tibia, and fibula are removed supraperiosteally. The ulcers are excised, and the entire lower extremity is brought up, folded on itself, and employed to resurface ischial, trochanteric, and sacral areas as needed (Fig. 27-17). The same flap can be used to resurface pressure ulcers on the contralateral side. The operation is grossly deforming and unacceptable to many paralyzed patients, but as a "court of last resort" it has proven to be an effective rehabilitative measure in a few patients over the years. It certainly permits greater mobility, and when a hip disarticulation is not performed, the patient has a surprising degree of stability.

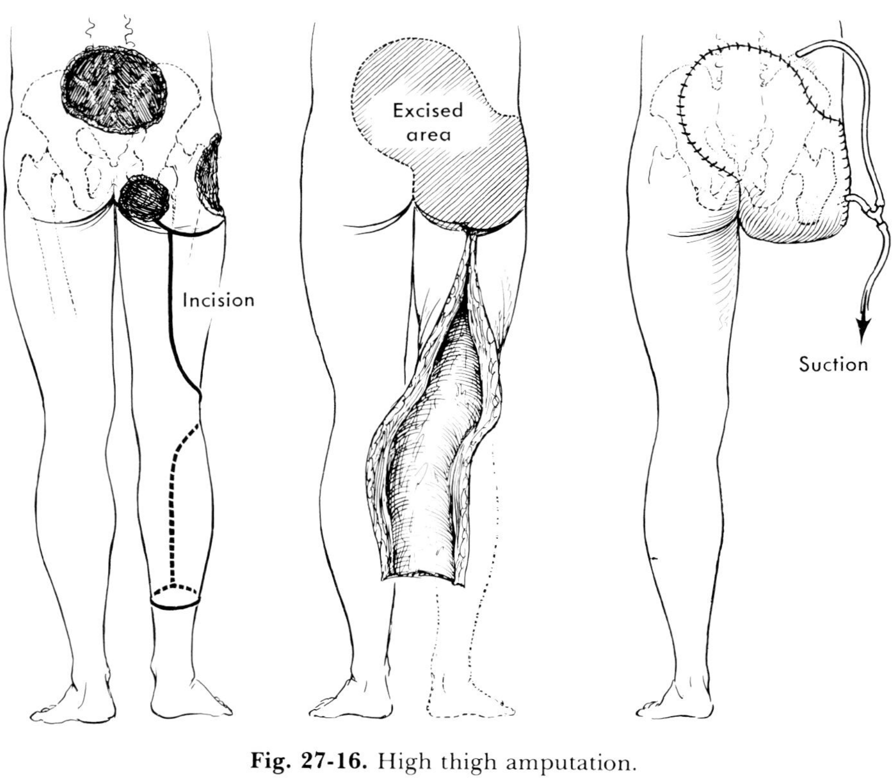

Fig. 27-16. High thigh amputation.

A B C D E F

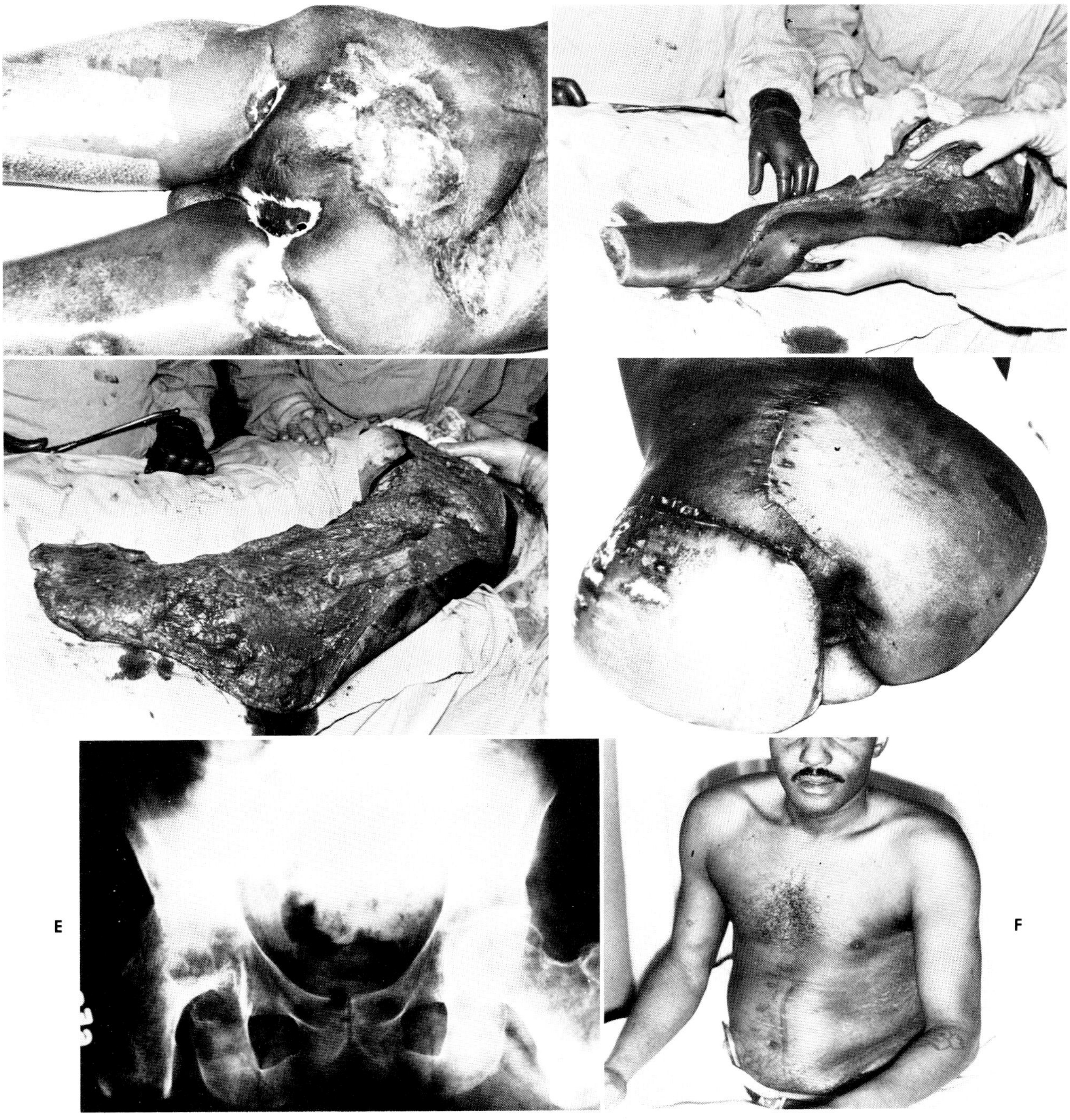

Fig. 27-17. A, Typical candidate for high thigh amputation. **B,** At surgery (see Fig. 27-16). **C,** Prior to completing bony resection. **D,** Closed ulcer healed. **E,** Postoperative roentgenogram. **F,** Patient demonstrating stability.

TECHNICAL DETAILS

If skin graft coverage is planned, the granulation tissue is lightly debrided to remove only the superficial layer with its high bacterial content; bleeding, which could preclude grafting, is avoided. Sheet grafts, while ideal for large flat surfaces, are generally not employed in the small deeper ulcers. Stamp grafts or mesh-type grafts are useful in that they adapt to convolutions and irregularities in the ulcer bed. Suturing is unnecessary. A moist-to-dry fluff gauze dressing over fine mesh gauze permits absorption of the wound exudate in the period immediately after grafting, when skin adherence is being established. Skin grafts are always checked and redressed within 48 hours of grafting. If the ulcer is to be covered by a flap, it is excised completely to remove all of the bed, including granulation tissue.

Hemostasis is expedited by electrocautery, and only the larger, arterial-type bleeders are tied with 3-0 catgut. All sponges are weighed, and blood loss, which is fequently underestimated, is replaced on a volume-for-volume basis. Thorough irrigation of the wound is carried out, using copious amounts of saline. *All* wounds are packed with warm, moist laparotomy packs, and steady pressure is maintained for about 10 minutes prior to beginning the repair.

A two-layer closure is performed, using a minimum of 3-0 catgut sutures in the subcutaneous layer and either a running subcuticular suture of 4-0 polyethylene or interrupted, half-buried vertical mattress sutures of 4-0 nylon. The running subcuticular suture, brought to the surface at 7.5 to 10 cm intervals, can remain in situ for 3 to 4 weeks without leaving suture marks, to minimize spread of the scar. Interrupted half-buried vertical mattress sutures secure good apposition at the wound margins and at the same time are not harmful to the epidermis of the flap. Simple interrupted sutures tend to impair vascularity of the pedicle margins, particularly in the distal segment, and are not employed except to "touch up" the suture line where a subcuticular suture has been utilized; they are removed early.

Prior to closure, drains are always inserted. With smaller flaps where undermining has not been extensive, the commercially available disposable suction apparatus is effective. When large flaps are involved, we prefer the placement of indwelling tubes (18-22 French) connected to a regular suction machine or wall vacuum.

If the original ulcer is large and infection has been a problem, especially if there is any question about obliteration of the dead space, we utilize a continuous through-and-through irrigation sump-

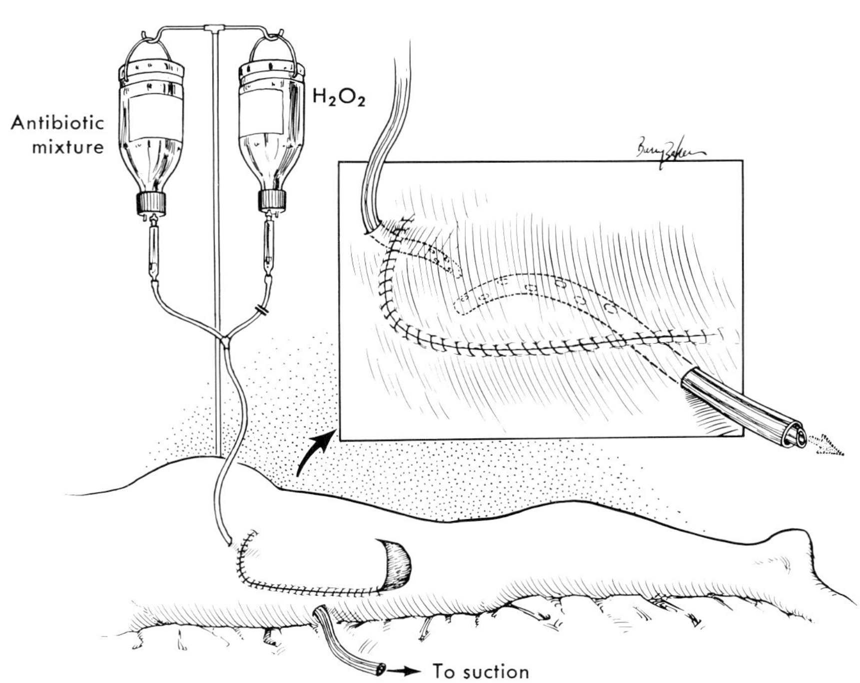

Fig. 27-18. Method of sump irrigation drainage described in text. Irrigant fluid can be varied.

type drainage, as advocated by Compere.[1] An antibiotic mixture of 1 g neomycin, 50,000 units bacitracin, and 50 g polymyxin in 1,000 ml saline drips slowly into the wound via a polyethylene catheter (Fig. 27-18) placed in the defect prior to closure of the flap. A bulky dressing is used, which is not applied in a wraparound fashion.

POSTOPERATIVE CARE

Close observation is mandatory for the first 24 hours after surgery. The routinely ordered postoperative hemoglobin test frequently is lower than anticipated. A hematocrit of 36 and hemoglobin of 12 are desirable; transfusion is considered when levels are below these figures. Symptoms of complications may be masked by the absence of sensation in the involved area, and the surgeon must rely on inspection of the wound. Therefore the flap tip is exposed on the first postoperative day with a complete dressing change every 2 or 3 days thereafter.

Positioning is so important that it becomes the personal responsibility of the surgeon to instruct the floor nurse and to make certain that appropriate padding is used. Most patients are kept in a position in which there is no pressure on the operative site for 14 to 21 days. We maintain our patients in the prone position (Fig. 27-19) for sacral and ischial procedures. For trochanteric ulcers the prone position is again preferred, but occasionally our patients are placed on a turning frame and early prone-supine-prone rotation is begun.

Drainage tubes are maintained for 2 to 3 days, longer if the flap is very large, debridement has been extensive, and drainage is greater than 50 ml a day. A solution of half to full strength hydrogen peroxide is occasionally used as an irrigant to maintain patency of the tube in the early postoperative period. With progressive decrease in exudate the tubes are eased out. We dislike leaving the drains in longer than 5 to 7 days except in certain instances (see below) for fear of the development of a permanent, pseudomembranous-lined sinus tract. If a constipation regimen has been begun preoperatively, it is usually maintained, with the patient on a clear liquid diet, until the drains are removed. Antibiotics are given the first week and then discontinued except for the usual urinary tract medication. Urine drainage is not modified from that which the attending surgeon had utilized and found effective prior to surgery.

Barring complications, the patient is returned to his previous activity regimen in slow stages, which rarely begin before the end of the second postoperative week. He may then lie on the opposite side for gradually increasing periods of time several times daily. If erythema develops, the activity routine is reduced. With maturation the resurfaced area will withstand reasonable periods of prolonged pressure. Taxing a single area with continuous pressure for more than 4 to 6 hours at a time is an invitation to skin breakdown. Various devices used to prolong this period of time are well-known and include the alternating air pressure mattress, silicone gel pad, sheepskin, sponge rubber, and air-or water-filled

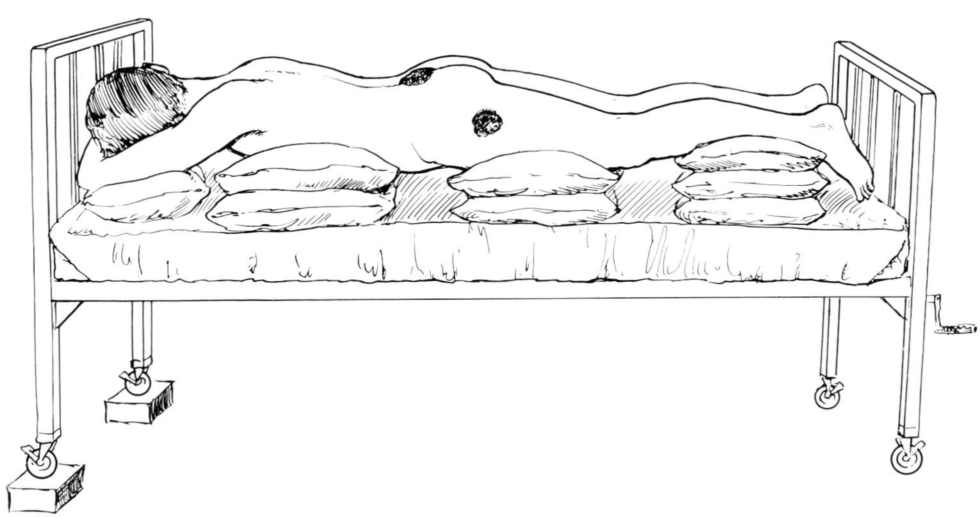

Fig. 27-19. Patient lying on pillows to maintain prone position without developing ulcers.

pad. Recently we have employed a commercially available "mud bed" to permit earlier pressure on the operated site.

COMPLICATIONS

The most serious early complication is embarrassed vascularity. When circulatory return is obviously delayed at the time of inset, serious consideration should be given to the return of the flap to its bed, especially if the signs of impaired circulation become progressively worse during surgery. Frequently the initial shock of cutting and elevating the pedicle will result in a pale distal segment that will gradually assume a more normal color. Injudicious clamping, especially of vessels at the pedicle base, may threaten flap viability. Gentle manipulation of the flap, using hooks instead of hands and clamps, is all that is needed to maneuver the flap.

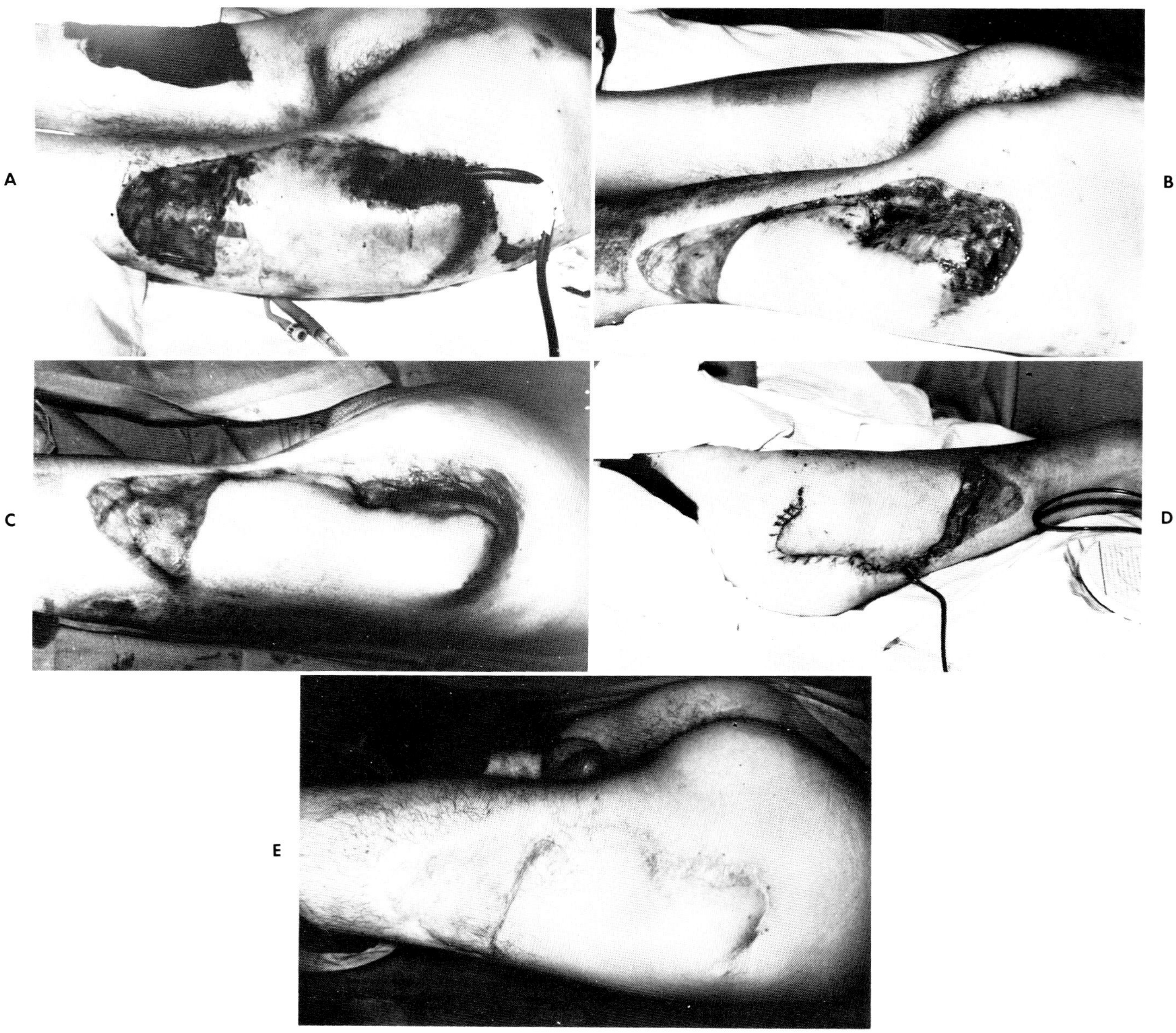

Fig. 27-20. A, Necrotic flap 5 days following inset. **B,** After debridement and "stamp" grafting. **C,** Wound healed and ready for revision. **D,** Flap reelevated and inset into defect left after excision of skin graft on bone. **E,** One year later.

If the flap is returned to its bed, the excised ulcer wound is wet-dressed and the surgical plan altered to fit the situation. If a healthy pedicle is inset, it is rare to discover 24 hours later that a variable amount of distal flap over the original ulcer site has become discolored or blistered. However, this may occur; possible causes include hematoma compromising venous return, too tight a dressing, and excessive pressure on the wound secondary to failure to maintain the desired position. Corrective measures are taken when possible. The percentage of survivability will become evident as necrosis develops a line of demarcation.

As noted above, full-thickness skin loss is evident by the formation of a thick, hard eschar, the margins of which are depressed below the adjacent tissue. Generally, sufficient subcutaneous tissue will survive to permit resurfacing of the site of complication with a split-thickness skin graft as a temporary covering. Rerotation of the original flap can be undertaken later, providing a large enough flap has been developed initially (Fig. 27-20).

Early wound separation may occur as a result of improper movement during patient positioning or spasms, while late wound separation usually results from infection or necrosis. Secondary suturing is notoriously unsuccessful with edema, induration, and infection working against the repair. Accepting the resultant defect is prudent. Moist dressings changed two to three times daily serve to achieve debridement quickly and to maintain a bed satisfactory for split-thickness skin grafting where necessary. The smaller defect will heal satisfactorily by peripheral epithelialization.

Despite drains, hematoma formation is an early complication, which if unrecognized and untreated may result in infection, flap necrosis, and later, wound separation. Larger hematomas in an ulcer bed under a flap often become infected because of contamination present at the time of surgery. Prompt evacuation is mandatory. If active bleeding persists, the flap must be opened in the operating room. Delay risks shock, especially in the weaker patients. To depend upon a pressure dressing in the face of arterial bleeding is poor surgical judgment. On the other hand, small hematomas in relatively clean wounds present no problem and are generally self-limiting.

An infected flap usually results from initially impaired vascularity with subsequent necrosis or hematoma formation. Treatment involves evacuation of pus and adequate drainage with appropriate local and systemic antibiotic therapy. A wound culture taken routinely at the time of surgery will be most helpful if this problem develops. We have been impressed by the use of a two-way irrigation drainage system utilizing an antibiotic solution slowly dripped through a 16-22 French catheter placed in the defect and siphoned off through an outlet of similar size connected to a low gastric suction machine.

When a large flap has been created and a split-thickness graft used in the donor bed, small partial losses in the grafted donor bed site are not uncommon. This area is well away from the pressure site, and even scar epithelium in the area is not subject to breakdown, hence the importance of a large flap in resurfacing. Some surgeons prefer delayed split-thickness skin grafting in an effort to secure a drier, firmer bed for the graft. If the presenting edge of the graft is sutured to the wound margins and adequate skin is used with overlapping (Fig. 27-8, *E*), obviating tenting, grafts generally do well.

LATE PROBLEMS

A recurrent decubitus ulcer is acutely disappointing to the patient, his family, paramedical personnel associated with his treatment, and the physician. The effect upon the surgeon of a patient returning with a decubitus ulcer directly in the center of a well-planned and executed flap is well-known. Reeducation of the patient and family must be included in the preoperative and postoperative treatment period. Maintenance of skin cleanliness and avoidance of prolonged pressure are the sine qua non of good home care. The patient must be on a hospital regimen that can be maintained following discharge. To send a patient home on a program impossible to carry out with the help available to him will negate the best surgical treatment and weeks of expensive hospitalization. We especially concentrate on "first offenders." This is particularly true if the patient develops his ulcers during the initial hospitalization for an acute injury. Efforts made with these patients are generally more rewarding than similar efforts with patients with multiple recurrent decubitus ulcers.

Early in the postoperative period the patient is instructed on the use of a mirror for daily personal observation of usual sites of ulcer formation (see Fig. 28-3). At the first sign of an ulcer, namely, erythema, all pressure is immediately removed from the area and a grease gauze dressing utilized. Local skin care primarily involves simple cleansing and avoiding undue pressure. Other adjuncts, including medications such as tincture of benzoin, infrared light, ultraviolet light, and ultrasound have not impressed us.

The paralyzed individual is encouraged to keep his normal weight, since excessive poundage limits mobility and makes nursing care more difficult. However, fat loss reduces the subcutaneous padding, diminishing protection over the usual pressure sites and predisposing to earlier breakdown. In the sitting position, foam rubber padding is helpful, and the gel pad is even more helpful. Weight shifting at regular intervals is especially beneficial in prophylaxis against pressure ulcers in paraplegics.

The importance of close follow-up cannot be overemphasized. The patient must be taught to return when a problem arises and not wait until a frank ulcer develops. Routine return visits are initially made weekly, later monthly, then quarterly. When a patient is unable to come in, the aid of a local Visiting Nurse Association is enlisted, and progress reports are secured by this organization.

FUTURE PROSPECTS

Certainly prevention is the goal of treatment as the cost of ulcers can be financially and physically demoralizing. What does the future hold? Establishing the patient in a weightless condition or environment would obviate all pressure and permit rapid healing; perhaps in the future we might be able to send some of our patients into outer space to facilitate healing of decubitus ulcers. Many efforts have been made to increase the size of the area of weight bearing as evidenced by the variety of cushions, pads, special beds, and floats that have become available over the past decade. The basic problem with all weight redistribution techniques is that pressure sufficient to ensure continuous patent capillaries and a good blood supply to the skin is always exceeded, that is, is over 30 mm Hg, in the area overlying a bony prominence. Air flotation beds that utilize compressed air are available to afford an even greater distribution of body weight than by more standard modalities. The removal of bony prominences as the surgical approach to weight redistribution is practiced by most surgeons dealing with decubitus ulcers. Decreasing the time an area is at risk is truly the only really practical method that can be employed almost universally. Rogers and Wilson[8] have shown that there is a time-pressure relationship and that no one can be maintained indefinitely in a particular position without incurring the risk of developing a decubitus ulcer. Restoring the body's alarm system by implantation of a thermometer to record temperature changes with prolonged pressure and an audible alarm or a mechanical device that would stimulate a viable nerve and refer the pain elsewhere, as well as the utilization in surgery of a neurovascular pedicle flap, described above, seems to hold promise. The ultimate answer to the problem of decubitus ulcers lies in the patient himself. He must be educated in the care of his own pressure ulcer–prone body. Personal mirror inspection at appropriate intervals, combined with the education necessary to avoid prolonged pressure and to keep these sites appropriately clean, will be rewarded by the avoidance of this debilitating and costly problem.

SUMMARY

We have described the operative treatment for various types of decubitus ulcers, including preoperative and postoperative care. The indications for, and the designs of, a variety of pedicle flaps for resurfacing these problem areas are discussed. Direct closure is used where feasible in smaller ulcers with large, widely based flaps employed for larger defects. Surgical complications are mentioned and their management discussed. Future possibilities in the prevention and treatment of decubitus ulcers are suggested.

REFERENCES

1. Compere, E. L.: Treatment of osteomyelitis and infected wounds by closed irrigation with a detergent-antibiotic solution, Acta Orthop. Scand. **32:**324, 1962.
2. Daniel, R. K., Terzis, J. K., and Cunningham, D. M.: Sensory skin flaps for coverage of pressure sores in paraplegic patients: a preliminary report, Plast. Reconstr. Surg. **58:**317, 1976.
3. Davis, J. S.: The operative treatment of scars forming bedsores, Surgery **3:**1, 1938.
4. Dibbell, D. G.: Use of a long island flap to bring sensation to the sacral area in young paraplegics, Plast. Reconstr. Surg. **54:**220, 1974.
5. Ger, R., and Levine, S. A.: Management of decubitus ulcers by muscle transposition, Plast. Reconstr. Surg. **58:**419, 1976.
6. Lamon, J. D., Jr., and Alexander, E., Jr.: Secondary closure of decubitus ulcers with aid of penicillin, J.A.M.A. **127:**396, 1945.
7. Meleney, F. L.: The prophylactic and active treatment of surgical infections With zinc peroxide, Surg. Gynecol. Obstet. **64:**387, 1937.
8. Rogers, J., and Wilson, L. F.: Preventing recurrent tissue breakdowns after "pressure sore" closures, Plast. Reconstr. Surg. **56:**419, 1975.
9. Salisbury, R., et al.: A comparison of coarse mesh gauze With biologic dressing on granulating wounds, Am. J. Surg. **131:**727, 1976.
10. Spira, M., and Hardy, S. B.: Our experiences With high thigh amputation in paraplegics, Plast. Reconstr. Surg. **31:**344, 1963.
11. Spira, M., Moore, J. L., Hardy, S. B., and Gerow, F. J.: Care of the decubitus ulcer patient, GP **39:**78, 1969.

Chapter 28

Patient management after surgery for pressure sores

Libby F. Wilson-Mackby
William W. Fish
Patti Harder

IMMEDIATE CARE

Following the reconstructive procedure for pressure sores the patient is again positioned prone 24 hours a day. He is maintained in this position, with his legs stabilized in abduction by a foam bolster, until wound maturation is sufficient to tolerate resumption of tissue stretching. If the postoperative course is uncomplicated, lower extremity range of motion is begun 6 weeks following surgery.

Large-bore suction catheters on continuous suction are used for 1 week postoperatively. These clear small amounts of drainage from the operative site and also promote flap adherence to the underlying bed. These catheters do not effectively drain true hematomas if they occur. Large postoperative collections require immediate return to the operating room for complete evacuation through the reopened wound. Delayed wound closure can be employed if oozing from wound margins is excessive at the close of the operative procedure. In order to allow for easy inspection of the wound, dressings are minimal. A single layer of a petrolatum-impregnated gauze directly over the suture line is sufficient.

Antibiotics, if used preoperatively, are continued through surgery and into the postoperative period. If osteomyelitis is present, low doses of the appropriate antibiotic agent are administered over a prolonged period of time—years if necessary to control deep-seated chronic pelvic involvement.

REHABILITATION

Frequent controlled joint ranging is begun 6 weeks after surgery. Range of motion continues until 90 degrees of hip flexion is achieved without producing excessive tension on the incision. The time required to achieve sitting range varies with the location and extent of the former ulceration and the preexisting status of the patient's joints. Individuals recovering from sacral pressure sores usually gain sitting range in 2 days. Those with trochanteric involvement require 3 days, and those with ischial lesions take 7 days.

The patient is then fitted with a 10 cm thick, high-density polyurethane foam cushion or other pressure-relieving material tailored to the specific length and width of the patient's own wheelchair to relieve pressure over sensitive weight-bearing areas (Fig. 28-1). These regions include the sacrococcygeal area, the ischial tuberosities, and the posterior trochanters. Pressure is redirected away from these areas and applied or loaded to high-tolerance regions by cutting out foam around susceptible areas and building up material at high-tolerance regions, for example, the distal thigh.

Objective measurement of external pressure generated under bony prominences is obtained with a pressure transducer. This apparatus consists of an inflatable plastic balloon containing a copper cross-grid, connected to a blood pressure manometer (Fig. 28-2). Unscarred skin over weight-bear-

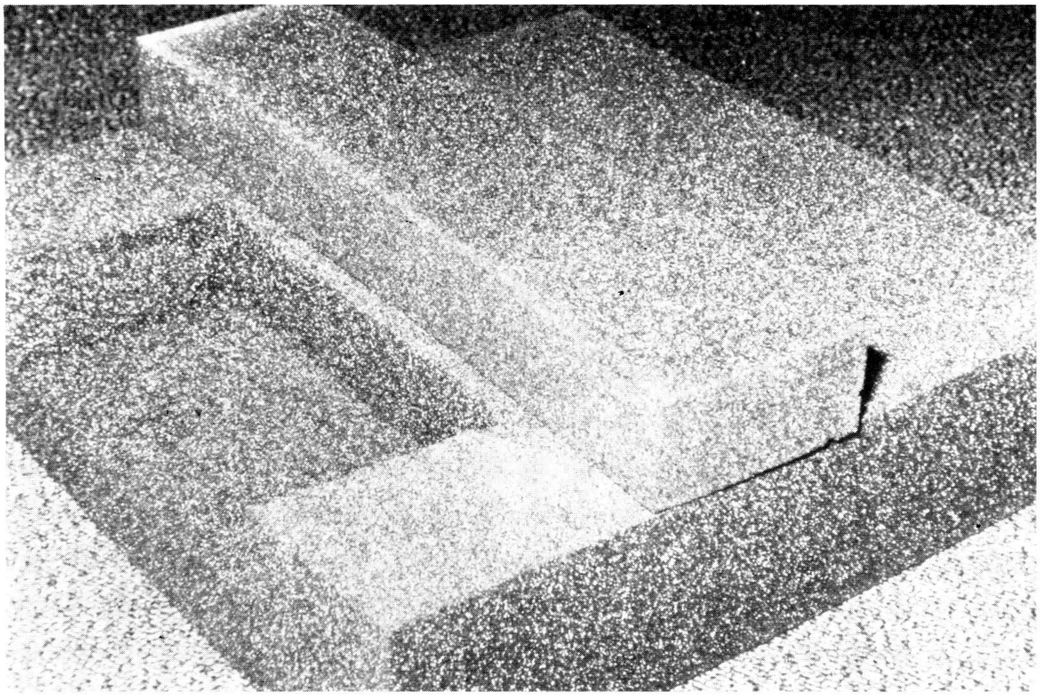

Fig. 28-1. Custom-fitted, foam wheelchair cushion cutout and femoral bar.

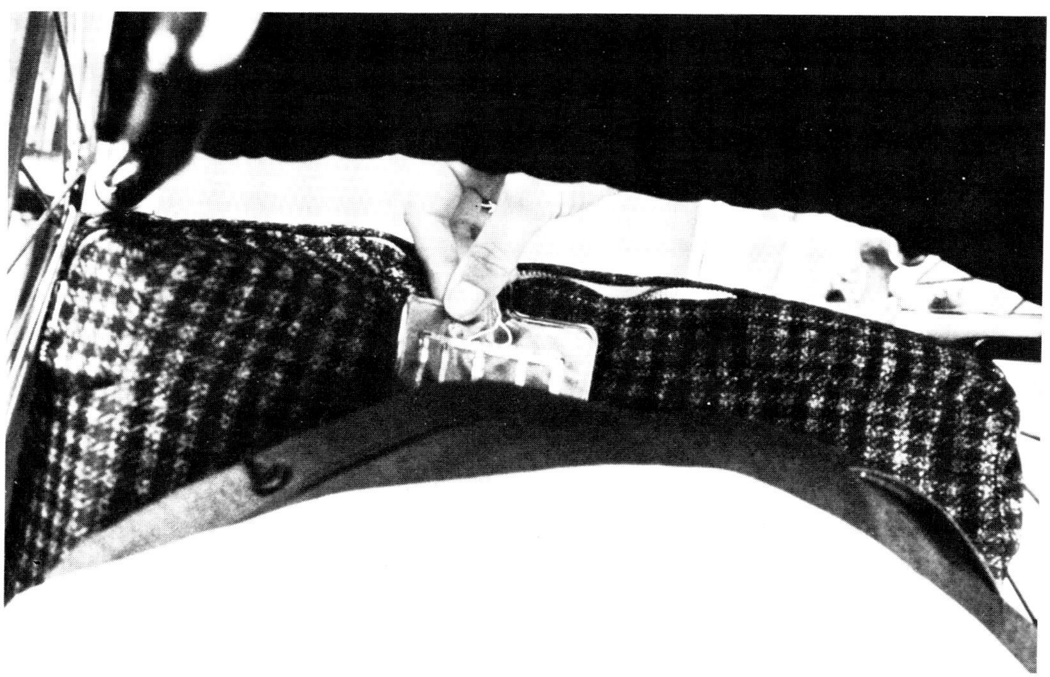

Fig. 28-2. Pressure transducer placed between patient and seat cushion to objectively measure pressures under bony prominence.

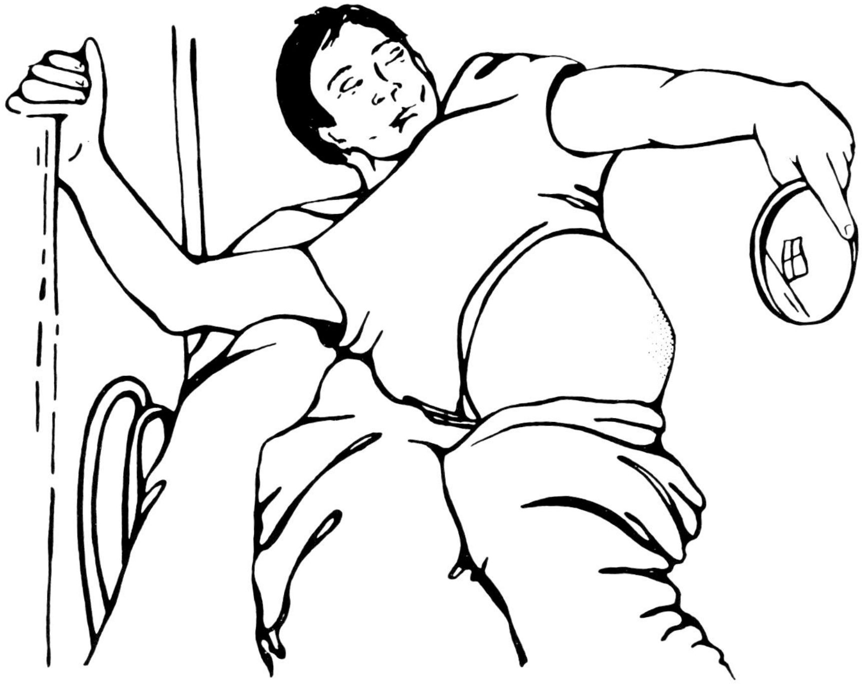

Fig. 28-3. Self-examination with mirror for early signs of excess pressure.

ing prominences has a varied pressure tolerance. The ischial tuberosities tolerate up to 40 mm Hg, while the sacrococcygeal area accepts only 15 mm Hg of pressure. Tissue that is scarred tolerates less pressure.

When cushion construction is complete, the patient begins on a sitting program to develop wheelchair tolerance of up to 6 hours. Time is generally increased at a rate of half an hour a day. The surgical site is checked before and after each wheelchair session and the program temporarily discontinued if wound appearance becomes unfavorable, that is, redness or blistering of the skin or scar (Fig. 28-3). Prior to discharge the patient will attain his preadmission activity level.

Throughout the postoperative course the educational principles of self-care are reviewed:

1. Meticulous skin care techniques
2. Proper methods of transfer from bed to wheelchair, and so on
3. Intermittent relief of pressure
4. Self-detection of early signs of impending skin breakdown

These are the responsibility of the patient.

Prior to discharge and in the follow-up visits the health care team must check for other factors that can contribute to formation of pressure ulceration. These include:

1. Abnormal sitting postures caused by axial deformities, joint contractures, heterotopic ossification, amputated or underdeveloped lower extremities
2. Faulty equipment: improperly fitting bracing devices or wheelchairs with sagging upholstery or improperly positioned foot plates

Pressure ulcerations are preventable.

Prevention is a team effort.

SUGGESTED READINGS

Enis, J. E., and Sarmiento, A.: The pathophysiology and management of pressure sores, Ortho. Rev. **2:**25, 1973.

Georgiade, N., Pickrell, K., and Maguire, C.: Total thigh flaps for extensive decubitus ulcers, Plast. Reconstr. Surg. **17:**220-225, 1956.

Guttman, N. L.: The problem of treatment of pressure sores in spinal paraplegics, Br. J. Plast. Surg. **7:**196, 1955.

McLeman, C. E., McLeman, M. T., and Landis, E. M.: Effect of external pressure on vascular volume of the forearm and its relation to capillary blood pressure and venous pressure, J. Clin. Invest. **21:**319, 1942.

Reswick, J. B., and Nickel, V. L.: A yearly report of progress at the Rehabiliation Engineering Center at Rancho Los Amigos Hospital, University of Southern California, 1972-73.

Reswick, J. B., and Rogers, J.: Experience at Rancho Los Amigos Hospital with devices and techniques to prevent pressure sores, Symposium, University of Stratchclyde, Glasgow, Scot., Aug. 1975.

Rogers, J., and Wilson, L.: Prevention of recurrence of tissue breakdown after pressure area reconstruction, Plast. Reconstr. Surg. **56:**419.

Smith, T. K., et al.: Complications associated with the use of the circular electrical turning frame, J. Bone Joint. Surg. [Am.] **57:**711-713, 1975.

Chapter 29

Pressure ulcerations in the insensitive foot

Vert Mooney
F. William Wagner, Jr.

Only 2% of patients with an ulcerated foot are those with the significant neurologic sensory deficits seen after sciatic nerve injury, with leprosy, or with various degenerative neurologic diseases. The patient most commonly seen with chronic foot ulceration is the diabetic. This paper presents our experience in the care of the dysvascular and insensitive foot. The principles for evaluation, prophylaxis, and treatment are based primarily on our experience with the diabetic foot, but are generally applicable to insensitive feet from any cause.

RATIONALE OF CARE

Three essentials are required in evaluation of the foot: (1) the ability to evaluate arterial blood supply in order to estimate adequate potential for healing, (2) the ability to control edema and permit tissue healing, and (3) the ability to control deformity so that the mechanical forces of ambulatory activity will not set the stage for destructive lesions that continue to threaten function.

For arteriovascular evaluation we have found the digital recording of peripheral pulses unrewarding. Success or failure of minor amputation in the presence or absence of pulses cannot be correlated.

Temperature of the skin has traditionally been used as a good clinical criterion for potential skin healing. Clinical experience has shown that cold skin will not heal. However, skin may be warm because of underlying inflammation and sluggish blood flow, giving a misleading impression of potential for healing success.

We must be aware that a significant number of diabetics, even with gangrenous changes and chronic infections, have sufficient arterial blood supply to achieve healing. There is no greater tendency toward occlusion of the small arteries in diabetics, even though it is coexistent with arteriosclerosis, than in nondiabetics.[8] In fact, Strandness and Priest[18] report that they found no specific disease of the small arteries and arterioles in the clinical and pathologic study of diabetics. It is now generally accepted that retarded healing in the diabetic is related, not to the absence of total blood supply, but to deficiencies of transfers across the pathologically thickened basement membranes of capillary and postcapillary venule beds.[17]

Aside from clinical judgment based on palpation of the skin itself with regard to temperature and turgor, a far more accurate method of evaluating arterial blood flow is the use of the ultrasonic probe. Using the Doppler principle, this system can monitor blood flow far more accurately than can physical examination. The presence or absence of arterial pulsation can be clearly identified, the character of blood flow noted (pulsatile or nonpulsatile), and the blood pressure at various levels in the lower limb can be accurately compared to the upper limb. By this peripheral vascular evaluation a more quantitative method of arterial blood flow evaluation can be achieved.[6,11,12,20]

The presence of edema also identifies vascular decompensation, thus enhancing tissue necrosis and allowing progressive inflammation. The nonsystemic factors that enhance edema formation are chronic dependency and inactivity. Moreover, in the diabetic, abnormalities of diffusion across the capillary membranes seem to enhance edema formation. Although venovalvular insufficiency and chronic thrombophlebitis have been traditionally considered the vascular culprits in local edema formation, we have been more impressed by the role of the lymphatics.

If we look at edema as increased interstitial fluid, the role of lymphatics becomes more apparent. The pressure of interstitial fluid at its physiologic level is zero or several millimeters of negative pressure.[10] Edema never forms until the interstitial fluid pressure rises above zero. A rise of only 1 or 2 mm Hg initiates an excess of interstitial fluid. The lymphatic system removes the larger molecules that are unable to return to the local circulation through the walls of the venous system. When the lymphatic system is inefficient, protein particles tend to accumulate, thus increasing the osmotic pressure. When the lymphatic system cannot draw the fluid and colloid material away from interstitial spaces, a vicious circle develops. Inflammation adds to this problem by creating an excess of protein, and this places extra stresses on the lymphatic system.

It has been our clinical impression that plaster casts worn by ambulatory subjects decrease edema fluid. This was confirmed by an experimental study in which ambulatory total-contact casts reduced the limb volume by 2.5% in normal subjects and by an average of 9% in edematous diabetic patients.[9] A more sophisticated method of evaluating the effect of rigid encapsulation (plaster cast) upon the muscle pump effect on lymphatic flow is the use of radioactive isotope studies. Technetium labeled sulfur colloid injected subcutaneously on the dorsum of the foot will arrive at the groin lymph node in 8 to 10 minutes. The same subject, however, can decrease the transit time by half when he exercises in a plaster cast.[1]

Therefore we feel that the most effective local mechanism to control edema is the total-contact plaster walking cast. In our experience this has been more effective than elastic devices because the muscle pump may be more effective and there is less opportunity for ill fit after plaster application. In contrast, elastic hose, bandages, and so on often become ill fitting, and areas become constricted in clinical use. Other benefits from the cast (the ultimate in well-fitting footwear) are the reduction of excessive mechanical activity at the local inflammatory site and protection from additional trauma that would further burden the demands for healing of the dysvascular limb.

In addition to the vascular problems reviewed, mechanical trauma as related to neurovascular foot problems must also be considered. In the obviously neurologically deficient individual, such as after peripheral nerve trauma, the effect of unnoted repeated mechanical trauma is more easily understood. Brand[4,5] has pointed out that in the relatively insensitive foot the destructive element rests in the summation of repeated minor trauma. Each tissue impact of itself may be considerably below destructive level, but it is the relentless repetition of these minor forces, unrelieved by normal minimal reflexive anatomic adjustments, that summates in a destructive lesion.

In the diabetic the role of neural deficiency is more subtle. In a consecutive series of 41 patients with minor foot lesions and a clinical diagnosis of diabetic neuropathy, Barrett[2,3] found relative anesthesia on the dorsum of the foot in 37 patients; only 4 had anesthesia on the plantar aspect. All patients could receive deep pain by standard pressure of the Achilles tendon but had decreased sensation at the areas of the lesions. Generalized sensory impairment was primarily in the distribution of the peroneal nerve and unrelated to the location of the ulcers. Clawson and Seddon[7] studied a number of patients with sciatic nerve palsy and found that in these patients the trophic lesions were at the location of deformity and high loading. Thus the trophic lesions of the neuropathic foot are related to pressure areas rather than anesthesia.

In summary the following points are pertinent: adequate arterial blood supply for healing must be available; edema must be controlled locally where possible; and trophic lesions are related to excessive or poorly appreciated force or both.

METHODS OF CARE

The greatest effort in caring for these patients must be focused on prophylaxis of additional lesions. Controlling edema and avoiding excessive tissue trauma are the primary goals. These will be successful only when there is adequate arterial blood supply to support healing in normal tissue repair.

Aside from clinical judgment based on skin temperature and the history of the duration of the lesions, the most precise method to evaluate potential for healing is the peripheral vascular evaluation, using the ultrasonic probe. This instrument, far more accurate than digital palpation, can identify the presence or absence of the femoral, popliteal, posterior tibial, and dorsalis pedis pulses and can characterize them as pulsatile or nonpulsatile. By occlusion of the arterial blood flow with a blood pressure cuff at the thigh and at the calf, a relationship between lower limb and upper limb blood pressure can be identified (normal ankle-to-arm pressure equals 1). On the basis of experience, minimal criteria for healing have been established. The ankle-to-arm ratio must be better than 0.45; one of the ankle pulses must demonstrate pulsatile flow; and in the diabetic, arterial pressures at the ankle should be above 70 mm Hg (in the nondiabetic it may be as low as 55 mm Hg). If the limb cannot meet these criteria, further attempts to salvage the part are unwarranted, and a local amputation will not heal.

If clinical evaluation and vascular studies suggest healing is possible, specific treatment programs are undertaken. First, the local lesion must be evaluated. The most minimal lesion would be a superficial ulceration that may have associated necrotic base or borders. In the treatment of dysvascular lesions we have not found surgical debridement to be of value as related to skin lesions. Incision into apparently viable tissue results in necrosis at the wound edge, as the insult of incision is too massive for this barely viable tissue to recover from. Control of edema is a necessity, and therefore these patients are placed in walking plaster casts.

It is inappropriate to start cast care, however, until all abscesses and deep necrotic tissue have been removed. Surgical debridement of all deep necrotic tissue is necessary, and wound drainage must be established. Therefore wide incision and drainage should be done to assure that all necrotic tissue is removed. Removal of necrotic bone will tend to decompress the severely stressed edematous tissues. Of course, if gangrene has developed, ablation of the necrotic area is necessary.

The total-contact plaster cast should be applied with the least amount of padding considered safe. Excessive padding rapidly packs down and converts the cast to an ill-fitting device with excess pressure points. If profuse drainage is still present, the use of a cast is inconvenient. Drainage should have slackened to the degree that the plaster will not be soaked and malodorous within a week. Because this device is to be a shoe substitute, the toes should be covered not only to avoid additional trauma but to stabilize temperature and avoid a potential pressure point on the dorsum of the toes. We have found lamb's wool or polyurethane foam to be a very resilient material between the digits and on the dorsum and plantar aspects of the toes (Figs. 29-1 and 29-2).

The long curing time of plaster of Paris (at least 1 day) until it has sufficient strength to allow full weight bearing is a disadvantage. If the patient cannot be trusted to be initially nonambulatory with crutches, a fiberglass cast should be used.

When healing has progressed through sufficient plaster cast applications until drainage is minimal, a "healing shoe" is used. It is made of closed cell polyethylene foam (Plastazote), a very resilient human interface material. Although it does not distribute the pressures as well as a total-contact plaster

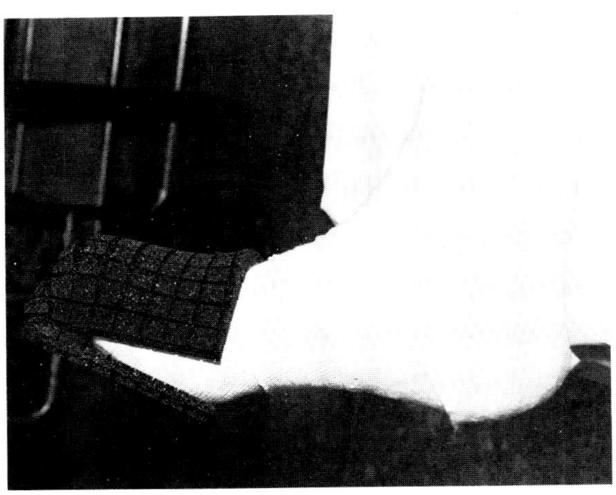

Fig. 29-1. Polyurethane foam being applied to toes in preparation for total-contact casting.

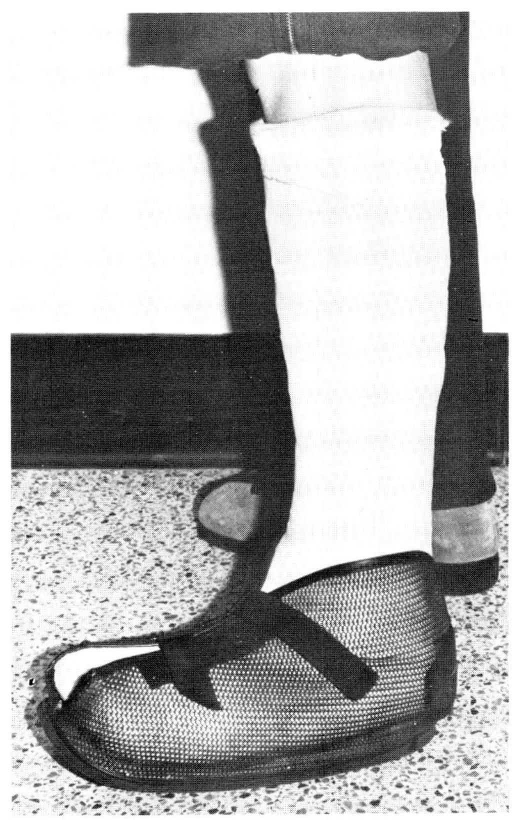

Fig. 29-2. Completed cast with cast shoe for ambulatory activity.

cast, the force distribution is better than standard footwear (Fig. 29-3). The Plastazote shoe must be considered a temporary step in the progression of footwear. It is constructed over casts built up to give extra room at the toe box and extra width in the heel; therefore it lacks wearing strength and aesthetic appeal. The patients wearing these shoes are advised that this is only a step in the process of healing. They are encouraged to use multiple white wool socks, which also serve as the wound dressings, rather than extra bandages about their lesions.

A more permanent shoe in which appropriate inserts have been molded to reduce potentially destructive mechanical forces to a minimum is the next step in providing rational footwear to the neurologically or vascularly embarrassed foot. The shoe must be an oxford type, therby guaranteeing adequate fit and avoiding fore-aft shift of the foot in the shoe. Poorly tolerated shear forces contribute a significant destructive force during ambulatory activity. Special inserts of Plastazote may be constructed to accommodate deformity and prominences. Body heat and functional forces will tend to mold the Plastazote along anatomic contours. If deformity is marked, molding can be accomplished at the initial fitting by heating the Plastazote sheets to their plastic state and having the patient stand on the sheet forming it according to the pressure loading. (Closed cell polyethylene foam is such a good insulator that the surface will cool sufficiently to be skin tolerable while the deeper parts of the plastic sheet will remain plastic and deform.) As the lighter grades tend to "bottom out" with use, the heavier grades should be used. The life of the insert can be lengthened by using a rubber or neoprene insert below the Plastazote insert. Thus appropriately fitted shoe inserts may be expected to last for 6 months to 1 year (Fig. 29-4).

A great deal of effort must be focused on the education of patients concerning local foot hygiene, the appropriateness of special footwear, and continual admonishment to avoid the "more stylish" shoes, which would be potentially destructive to their feet.

When lesions have healed under the influence of this progressive treatment, attention may be given to underlying deformities. In patients with persistent reactive changes, such as calluses and blisters, prophylactic surgical care should be

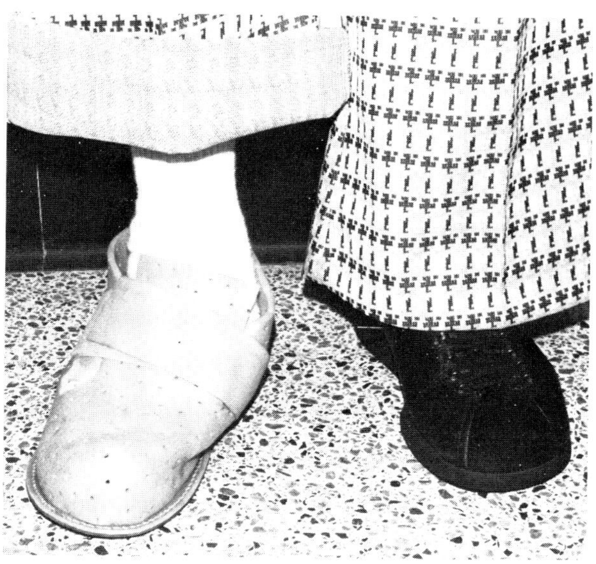

Fig. 29-3. "Healing shoe" made of Plastazote for lesions that are minimally draining or deformities inappropriate for surgical correction.

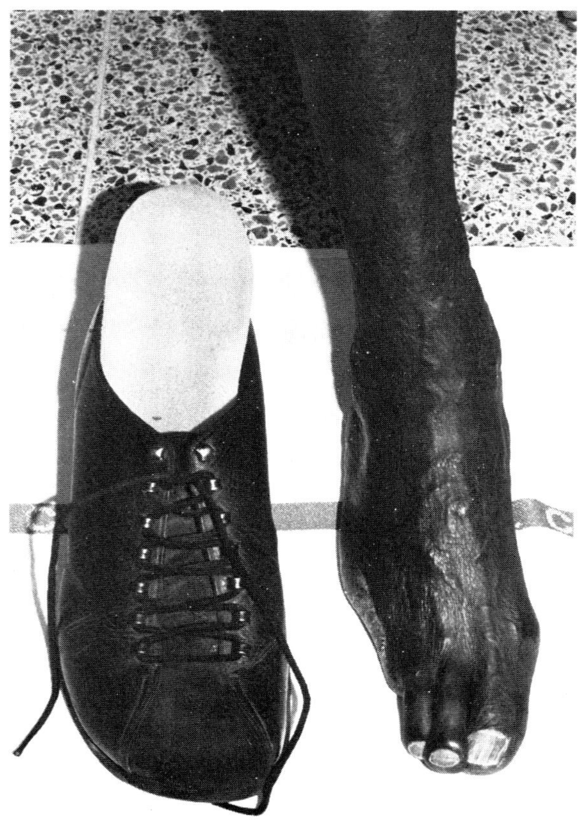

Fig. 29-4. Appropriate type of protective shoe with Plastazote insert and additional insert of neoprene rubber.

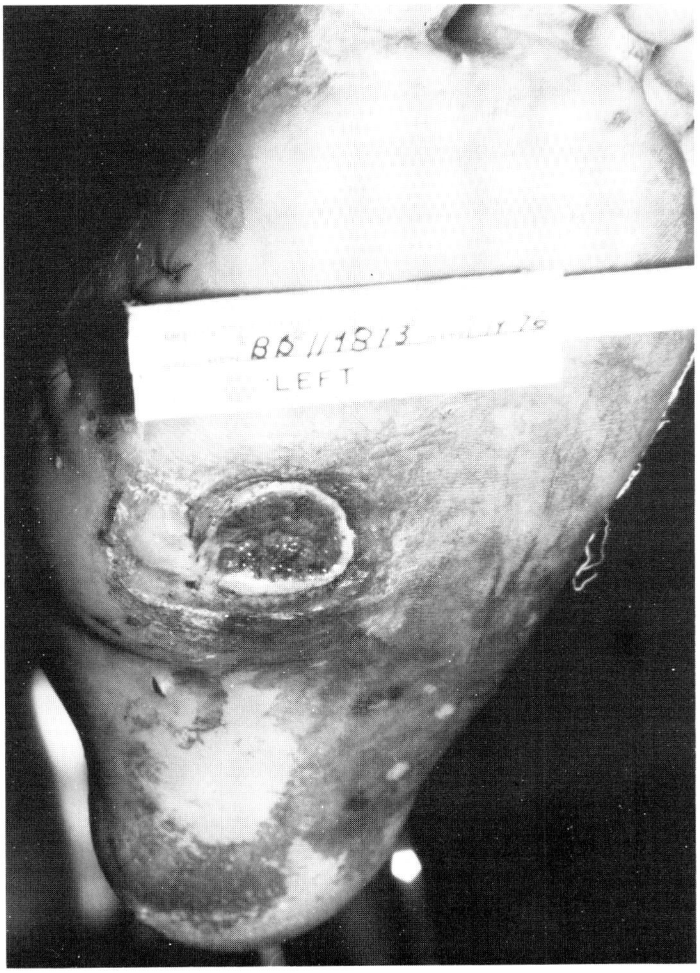

A

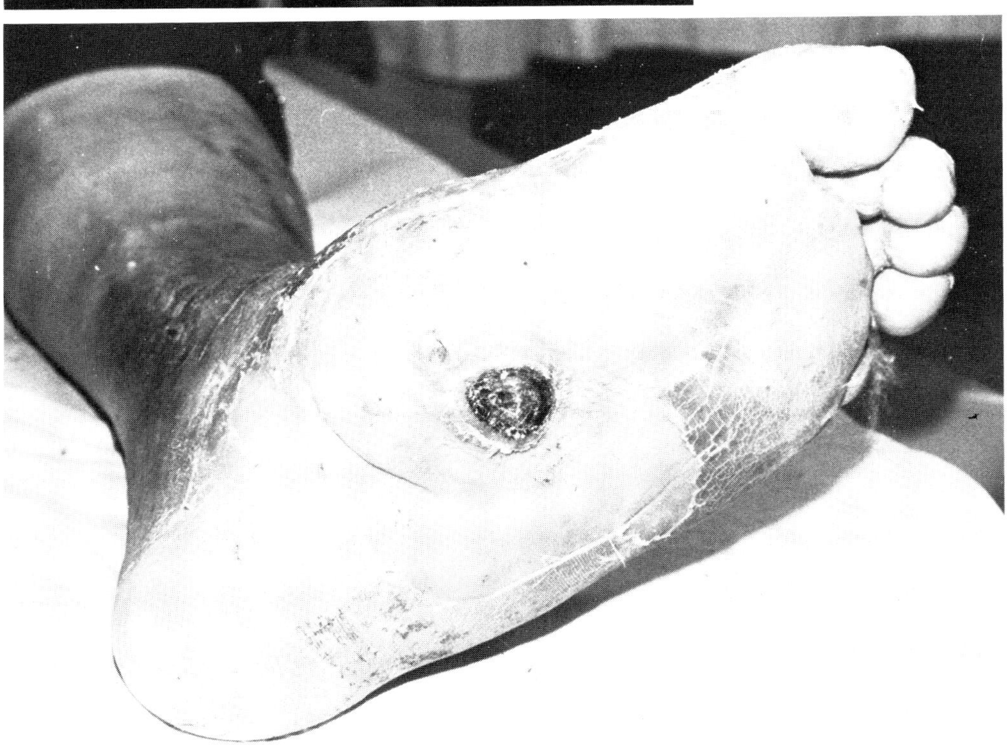

B

Fig. 29-5. A, Diabetic foot with chronic ulceration prior to surgical debridement and cast care, **B,** Diabetic foot after cast care, with healing lesions.

Table 11. Analysis of diabetic foot ulcers

		No. of feet	
		Preoperative	*Postoperative*
Grade 0	Foot deformity only	30	0
Grade 1	Superficial ulcer	28	4
Grade 2	Deep ulcer	25	5
Grade 3	Bone abscess	30	9
Grade 4	Gangrene	38	26
TOTALS		151	44

advised. Claw toes, bunions, ingrown toenails, and prominent metatarsals should be corrected in the dysvascular and neuropathic foot before tissue breakdown occurs. A small metatarsal neck osteotomy is a minimal procedure to avoid chronic plantar ulceration.

RESULTS

In an effort to formalize the concepts described above, a specialized foot care clinic has been developed. Currently this clinic cares for about 25 outpatients weekly, providing various types of specialized footwear from plaster casts through various types of shoes with appropriate inserts. Fig. 29-5 shows a typical example of a foot treated with progressive plaster casts. In this specific case, once the ulceration had eventually healed, the underlying skeletal deformity was corrected and appropriate specialized footwear prescribed thereafter.

A series of 151 consecutive diabetic admissions to the hospital were analyzed in 1972 (Table 11). In this group, 30 patients had prophylactic corrective surgery to resolve underlying foot deformities. All wounds healed in footwear that progressed through plaster casts and special shoes to standard shoes. Specialized footwear was no longer necessary for these patients because their feet now presented no unusual anatomic variations. In this series of patients the plaster cast method of primary and follow-up treatment was considered successful. Appropriate surgery was used in conjunction with plaster casting with progression into appropriate resilient footwear. Table 11 also describes the incidence of infection, necrosis, and need for higher revisions.

CONCLUSION

The rationale for care of the dysvascular neuropathic foot has been described. Prevention or correction of deformities is of primary importance in the insensitive, poorly healing foot. Control of edema is necessary to enhance the healing potential. Interest in defensive footwear, appreciation of interface forces, and the application of standard surgical techniques in this type of population can result in a significant improvement in patient care.

REFERENCES

1. Angel, J. C.: The mechanism of the healing cast, Orthopedic Seminars, University of Southern California, Department of Orthopedic Surgery, Rancho Los Amigos Hospital **4:**17, 1973-1974.
2. Barrett, J.: Neuropathy and diabetic pressure lesions, Orthopedic Seminars, University of Sothern California, Department of Orthopedic Surgery, Rancho Los Amigos Hospital **4:**5, 1971.
3. Barrett. J., and Mooney, V.: Neuropathy and diabetic pressure lesions, Orthop. Clin. North Am. **4:**43, 1973.
4. Brand, P. W., Bauman, J. H., and Girling, J. P.: Plantar pressures and trophic ulceration, J. Bone Joint Surg. [Br.] **45:**652, 1963.
5. Brand, P. W.: Pressure sores—the problem in tissue viability and clinical applications. In Kenedi, R. M. editor: Bed sore biomechanics, London, 1975, Macmillan International Ltd.
6. Carter, S. A.: The relationship of distal systolic pressures to healing of skin lesions in limbs with arterial occlusive disease with special reference to diabetes mellitus, Scand. J. Clin. Lab. Invest. **31**(suppl. 128):239, 1973.
7. Clawson, D. K., and Seddon, H. J.: The late consequences of sciatic nerve injury, J. Bone Joint Surg. [Br.] **42:**213, 1960.
8. Conrad, M. D.: Large and small artery occlusion in diabetics and non-diabetics with severe vascular disease, Gen. Circ. **36:**83-91, 1967.
9. Dorr, L. R.: Short-leg walking casts—pressure and volume studies, Orthopedic Seminars, University of Southern California, Department of Orthopedic Surgery, Rancho Los Amigos Hospital **3:**69, 1970.
10. Guyton, A. C.: A concept of negative interstitial fluid pressure based on pressures implanted in perforated capsules, Cir. Res. **12:**399, 1963.
11. Holstein, P.: Distal blood pressure as guidance in choice of amputation level, Scand. J. Clin. Lab. Invest. **31**(suppl. 128):245, 1973.
12. Lennihan, R., and Mackereth, M. A.: Ankle blood pressures as a practical aid in vascular practice. Angiology **26:**211, 1975.
13. Meggitt, B. F.: Orthopedic management of foot breakdown problems in the diabetic patient, Orthopedic Seminars, University of Southern California, Department of Orthopedic Surgery, Rancho Los Amigos Hospital **5:**311, 1972.
14. Mooney, V., and Nickel, V. L.: Rationale for amputee surgery in the diabetic—400 consecutive cases, Presented at Canadian Orthopedic Association, Jasper, Alberta, June 1971.
15. Morgan, N.: Walking cast treatment for diabetic foot lesion, Orthopedic Seminars, University of Southern

California, Department of Orthopedic Surgery, Rancho Los Amigos Hospital **4:**291, 1971.

16. Prietto, P. P.: Transmetatarsal amputation in diabetic patients, Orthopedic Seminars, University of Southern California, Department of Orthopedic Surgery, Rancho Los Amigos Hospital **3:**227, 1970.
17. Siperstein, M. D.: In Erasi, E., and Luft, R., editors: Pathogenesis of diabetes mellitus, New York, 1970, Macmillan Publishing Co. p. 81.
18. Strandness, E. E., Jr., and Priest, R. E.: Combined clinical and pathological study of diabetic and nondiabetic arterial disease, Diabetes **13:**366, 1964.
19. Wagner, F. W. W., Jr.: Classification and treatment outline for diabetic foot lesions. In American Academy of Orthopedic Surgeons Instructional Course Lectures, St. Louis, 1976, The C. V. Mosby Co.
20. Yao, J. S. T., and Bergan, J. J.: Application of ultrasound to arterial and venous diagnosis, Surg. Clin. North Am. **54:**23, 1974.

Chapter 30

The role of infection in chronic pressure ulcerations

Martin C. Robson
Thomas J. Krizek

In managing and rehabilitating the patient with a spinal cord injury, it is imperative that skin breakdown and ulcerations be prevented, or when present, corrected. The frequency of these ulcers in denervated areas and their geographic and temporal association with unrecognized or unrelieved pressure have made it axiomatic that pressure-ischemia and denervation are the major factors in the development of such sores. However, pressure-ischemia or denervation, singly or even in combination, does not always produce such ulcerations. Elaborate pressure-relieving beds, mattresses, and other devices, in concert with heroic nursing efforts, have failed to eliminate ulcerations as a clinical problem.

The initial clinical signs of impending ulceration are redness *(rubor)* accompanied by edema *(tumor)* and warmth *(calor)*. The denervation fails to allow the patient to appreciate pain *(dolor)* and has, in itself, produced a loss of function *(functio laesa)* that would enable him to move. These hallmark signs of inflammation may progressively increase in size and severity. The area then becomes fluctuant, and a small area of skin necrosis becomes obvious. Attended by systemic signs of sepsis, the process resolves itself either spontaneously or by surgical evacuation of the necrotic purulent contents. The resultant cavity is remarkably large relative to the surface loss of tissue.

It is clear that bacteria and local infection play an important role in the local management of these wounds, and the control of infection is paramount to spontaneous healing or successful surgical closure of these wounds. Local bacterial infection as a cause or at least a necessary adjunct in the development of these ulcers has not been completely investigated.

PRESENT EXPLANATION OF PATHOPHYSIOLOGY INCOMPLETE

Brown-Sequard noted that he could prevent the occurrence of skin ulcerations in guinea pigs and pigeons whose spinal cords had been sectioned by keeping the areas clean and free from pressure.[4] Since then there has been a continuing attempt to relate such ulcerations to the combination of neurotrophic factors, pressure, and metabolic factors. Of these, pressure has been the best documented. As pressure is incriminated, so is ischemia.[12] Numerous studies have shown that pressure obviously high enough to cause local ischemia can be generated over areas prone to these ulcerations.[13,15] If a pressure high enough to interfere with tissue circulation is present for a sufficient length of time, it will result in tissue breakdown. Yet one of the most baffling features of the problem is the variation in the susceptibility among patients to this effect of localized pressure. This variation should not be so marked if denervation alone, pressure alone, or the combination of denervation and pressure-ischemia were responsible for tissue breakdown.

Skin in normally innervated areas can be kept ischemic for 5 hours without irreversible damage. As short a time as 2 hours of ischemia in the quadriplegic patient can produce vesicle formation, which may progress to complete destruction of the skin even though the compressive effect is relieved. As pointed out by Peacock and Van Winkle, morbid anatomy of ulcers in denervated tissue is not similar to that observed when skin is rendered ischemic by simple obliteration of its blood flow.[18] Eschar formation is rare, and there appears to be a rapid sequence of events beginning with an erythemic reaction, progressing through vesicle formation and skin breakdown. The facts that eschar is not a prominent part of the pathologic process and that complete dissolution of the skin is so rapid suggest that an additional factor besides denervation and pressure is necessary to produce these ulcerations. One such factor might be localized infection.

EVIDENCE FOR ROLE OF INFECTION

The place of bacteria in these ulcers has been thought to be secondary. Certainly bacteria do play a late role. Robson and Heggers showed in 32 decubitus ulcers that only when the bacterial population was controlled does spontaneous healing occur.[21] Similarly they showed that definitive coverage of the ulcer could be performed only when the bacterial population was decreased. Bendy and associates found a similar relationship between the bacterial level in these ulcers and their rate of healing.[3] Besides this late effect in healing, it is postulated that bacteria play an early, possibly etiologic role. The marked pathology described by Peacock and Van Winkle is suggestive of bacterial invasion with dissolution of the skin by bacterial enzymes.[18]

In 1942, Groth showed that rabbits undergoing experiments of pressure necrosis reacted differently when infected than they did in their control state.[7] He showed that bacteria injected into the animals tended to be localized in the compressed areas; if the bacteria were pyogenic (staphylococci or streptococci), they produced liquefaction. In addition he showed that the localization could be prevented by pretreating the rabbits with antibiotics. Husain demonstrated that short periods of local pressure increased the susceptibility of tissue to local infection.[9] He injected streptococci intravenously and followed this by localized pressure to the leg. Samples of the tissue demonstrated the localization of streptococci in the area of the pressure.

The observations by Groth and Husain of localization of bacteria in areas of pressure can be explained in part by studies performed by Miles and associates. They showed that locally injected epinephrine temporarily diminished the flow of blood, thus decreasing the supply of phagocytes to the infected lesion.[17] Further demonstration of the effect of tissue ischemia on bacterial growth was made by these investigators. They showed the enhancement of staphylococcal and clostridial lesions in conditions of shock sufficient to lower the pressure in small arteries of the skin below a certain value with the degree of enhancement directly related to the amount of ischemia.[16]

Bacteria could play a role in several ways in a patient whose local area has been altered by denervation and pressure or ischemia. One mechanism could be "primary lodgment" through some breach in the epithelial surface, described by Miles. This breach could be mechanical, such as a wound, or a change in the chemical or physical character of the integument, caused by denervation or ischemia. An example of such a chemical change in the denervation skin is the occurrence of edema. Exton-Smith has documented the occurrence of edema in denervated tissue.[5] Edema fluid or plasma is known to neutralize the natural fatty acids of the skin lipids. Rickells and associates have demonstrated that these same fatty acids are streptococcicidal.[19] Therefore edematous denervated skin might be expected to allow streptococcal invasion and primary lodgment.

Another role of bacteria is their tendency to localize in an organ or area of the body with an altered local resistence. This idea of a locus minoris resistentiae has been suggested by Findlay to be due to the liberation of a histaminelike substance.[6] Any site of an inflammatory reaction releases histamine and allows the localization of bacteria.

To study the natural history of bacteria of the skin and bacterial infection in relation to denervation and ischemia, a review of normal flora is necessary. Kligman enumerates the common resident organisms: *Staphylococcus epidermidis, Micrococcus saccharolyticus, Sarcina,* streptococci, corynebacteria, *Herellea vaginicola,* and *Mima polymorpha.*[11] The more pathogenic organisms, such as *Staphylococcus aureus, E. coli, Klebsiella enterobacter,* and *Pseudomonas aeruginosa* are usually transients. The author points out how the balance between the transients and residents can be upset. Several of the mechanisms have been previously mentioned, that is, shock, ischemia, and breaks in the skin. He mentions the possibility of central nervous system dysfunction as a cause but cites no evidence.

The overwhelming weight of clinical evidence documents the inevitable presence of high levels of viable bacteria in the clinically evident pressure sore. The natural history, clinical appearance, and immediate findings at initial spontaneous or surgical drainage of these sores gives the inescapable picture of infection.

INFECTION CONTROL AND TREATMENT PRIOR TO ULCERATION

Since available evidence suggests that bacteria may play a significant role prior to ulceration, patients prone to develop ulcers need infection surveillance and, when appropriate, treatment. This may take several forms. The resident and transient skin bacteria are well established and normally exist at levels of 1,000 organisms per gram of tissue.[2] Clinical and experimental data have shown that a level of bacterial growth of greater than 100,000 organisms per gram of tissue is necessary in all species except beta-hemolytic *Streptococcus* for soft tissue infection and the potential for invasive sepsis to occur.[23] In our laboratories we have demonstrated experimentally that denervation alone or pressure alone can change the host resistance and allow primary lodgment to occur. Wounds created in denervated limbs and inoculated with known amounts of bacteria allowed greater soft tissue bacterial growth than identical wounds in normally innervated limbs. Similarly wounds created in controlled pressure areas allowed 100 times greater bacterial growth than wounds in nonpressure areas. If primary lodgment is the mechanism for infection in pressure-ischemic areas, a routine bacterial surveillance would predict a qualitative and quantitative change in the flora.

Bacterial surveillance of intact skin is more difficult than that of ulcerated wounds. Surface cultures are inaccurate and misleading. For instance, the dryness of the keratin layer is bactericidal against staphylococci. When the skin is intact clinically, biopsy techniques are not appropriate. However, Updegraff has described a plastic tape–stripping technique for the quantitative enumeration and cultivation of microorganisms.[26] This allows serial identification and counting of the bacteria in denervated and pressure-ischemic skin. Nonbacteriostatic tape is used to "strip off" the skin flora of a measured surface area. Colony counting provides a numerical value to present in a given area of the involved skin. This technique gives an internally consistent measure of bacterial growth and allows the areas of potential breakdown to be compared to other areas of the skin.

Another noninvasive technique to achieve routine qualitative and quantitative bacterial surveillance of intact skin is the use of RODAC contact plates. Once the keratin layer is removed by tape stripping, the contact plate gives a direct quantitative estimate of the bacterial population.

In addition to the qualitative and quantitative change of normal skin flora due to denervation, pressure, or ischemia, one must be concerned with altered host defenses due to edema. Soft tissue compressed between a firm surface and an underlying bony prominence becomes edematous. Since the edema fluid inactivates the body's defense mechanism against streptococci, the beta-hemolytic *Streptococcus* may well gain primary lodgment in this edematous tissue. Incipient areas of breakdown clinically appear to have cellulitis. They are red, warm, and swollen. We know that it takes fewer streptococci to cause soft tissue infection than other bacteria.[22] Therefore it seems appropriate to institute antistreptococcal measures in patients presenting with edematous inflamed areas prior to ulceration. These measures include repositioning to alleviate the edema and systemic penicillin or erythromycin.

Skin and soft tissue that has been injured by denervation or pressure-ischemia can become infected from endogenous sources by serving as a locus minoris resistentiae. Known sites of infection distant in the body may seed these locally resistance-depressed areas. The urinary tract is the prime source in the paraplegic patient. Therefore prevention and eradication of these infections is paramount if skin breakdown is to be avoided.

Between the incipient ulcer with intact skin and the classic ulcer, another type of wound may exist in which bacteria may play a role. The shearing-type abrasive injury is not a true pressure injury. However, this partial-thickness injury is bacteria prone, and if bacteria reach significant levels, this partial-thickness injury will convert to a full-thickness necrosis and resulting ulceration. Therefore these shearing injuries must be kept clean and the level of bacteria controlled. This can be done with a proper dressing or with topical antibacterials.

CONTROLLING BACTERIA IN ULCERATED WOUNDS

As opposed to the potentially contaminated incipient ulcer area, all wounds following breakdown and ulceration contain a tissue bacterial level. Although several techniques have been described to evaluate the true bacterial population of these wounds, the tissue biopsy method is the most accurate.[23] Following cleansing of the wound surface with isopropyl alcohol, a biopsy of the tissue is obtained and examined qualitatively and quantitatively for the presence of aerobic and anerobic bacteria. This allows one to know which of the several species that may be present on the surface of the wound have actually gained significant tissue levels. This is important when ulcers exist in close proximity to the rectum in patients who may be incontinent. Organisms thus overflowing into the ulcer may never gain lodgment and may be of no clinical significance as far as controlling the soft tissue infection.

The goal of bacterial control in the ulcerated wound is to decrease the bacterial level to 100,000 or fewer organisms per gram of tissue. Bendy and associates demonstrated that only when this occurred could the ulcer decrease in size and spontaneously heal by epithelialization.[3] Similarly Krizek and associates have shown that successful skin grafting is related to one's ability to decrease the bacteria in the wound to 100,000 or fewer bacteria per gram.[14] We have expanded this to all types of wound closure.[23]

The techniques of decreasing the bacterial load to acceptable levels are familiar to all of us. There remains no substitute for sharp debridement. The use of enzymatic debriding agents has not proved successful in these wounds and carries a risk of systemic sepsis. The pulsating jet lavage has proved to be an adjunct to sharp debridement. In the experimental animal it removes significantly more bacteria than the standard types of irrigation.[8]

Once the necrotic tissue is completely removed, the ulcer contains granulation tissue. This does not mean the bacterial level has been lowered to that consistent with successful wound closure. Granulation tissue does not occur in the absence of bacteria. It is not found beneath the surface of a successfully closed wound. Therefore the granulation tissue must be treated until the bacteria are numerically controlled, and there is an absence of streptococci. This can be done by cream-based topical antibacterials that penetrate the depths of the wounds and have a direct effect on bacterial growth. Systemic antibiotics do not reach adequate tissue levels in chronic granulation tissue and experimentally have been shown to have no effect on the bacterial level in granulating wounds.[20]

Since true bacterial control is only achieved by wound closure, the use of temporary biologic dressings for cleansing and temporary closure is both reasonable and of documented value. Porcine xenografts fail to establish biologic union with the underlying tissue and therefore are less effective than allograft skin or amniotic membranes.[24,25] However, the true control of infection in a granulating wound is closure of the wound with autogenous tissue.

The wound can be closed when the bacterial level is 100,000 or fewer organisms per gram of tissue if no streptococci are present. However, in the past this closure was jeopardized if any remote infection in the body had not been likewise controlled. Indeed the rate of infection at the time of closure has been reported to be threefold greater.[1] This has remained a problem in the closure of ulcers in the denervated patient with attendant urinary tract infections. However, recent data by Jennings and associates suggest that the closure may be protected with short-term high-level prophylactic antibiotic coverage.[10]

SUMMARY

Infection is an inevitable part of the clinical picture and a significant consideration in the therapy of ulcerations associated with pressure. There is an abundance of suggestive evidence that bacterial infection may be causative, or at least a necessary adjunctive factor in such ulceration. Pressure, denervation, edema, local ischemia, and alterations of tissue temperature are all part of the clinical picture. Each of these factors is known to reduce a patient's resistance to infection. All patients have a resident and transient skin flora of potentially pathogenic bacteria, the same bacteria found in ulcerations should they occur. Therefore attention to these bacteria is necessary at all time when treating patients prone to skin breakdown and ulceration. Real and practical approaches have been outlined to evaluate and control infection in these patients prior to and after the development of ulcerated wounds.

REFERENCES

1. Ad Hoc Committee of the Committee on Trauma, Division of Medical Sciences, National Research Council Report: Postoperative wound infections of ultraviolet irradiation of the operating room and the influence of various other factors, Ann. Surg. **160**(suppl.):1, 1964.
2. Artz, C. P., and Moncrief, J. A.: The treatment of burns, Philadelphia, 1969, W. B. Saunders Company.
3. Bendy, R. H., Nuccio, P. A., Wolfe, E., Collins, B., Tamburro, C., Glass, W., and Martin, C. M.: Relationship of quantitative wound bacterial counts to healing of decubiti: effect of topical gentamicin, Antimicrob. Agents Chemother. **4:**147, 1964.
4. Brown-Sequard, C. E.: Experimental researches applied to physiology and pathology, New York, 1853, H. Balliane.
5. Exton-Smith, A. N.: Nature of edema in paralysed limbs of hemiplegic patients, Br. Med. J. **2:**1280, 1957.
6. Findlay, G. M.: Histamine and infection, J. Pathol. **31**:633, 1928.
7. Groth, K. E.: Clinical observations and experimental studies of the pathogens of decubitus ulcers, Acta Chir. Scand. [Suppl.] **87**(76):207, 1942.

8. Hamer, M. L., Robson, M. C., Krizek, T. J., and Southwick, W. O.: Quantitative bacterial analysis of comparative wound irrigations, Ann. Surg. **181**:819, 1975.
9. Husain, T.: An experimental study of some pressure effects on tissues, with reference to the bed-sore problem, J. Pathol. **66**:347, 1953.
10. Jennings, S. A., Robson, M. C., and Jennings, M. M.: Preventing wound infection from distant endogenous sources in the rat, J. Surg. Res. **22**:16, 1977.
11. Kligman, A. M.: The bacteriology of normal skin. Maiback, H. I. and Hildick-Smith, G., editors: In Skin bacteria and their role in infection, New York, 1965, McGraw-Hill Book Company.
12. Kosiak, M.: Etiology and pathology of ischemic ulcers, Arch, Phys. Med. Rehabil. **40**:62, 1959.
13. Kosiak, M., Kubicek, W. G., Olson, M., Danz, J. N., and Kottke, F. J.: Evaluation of pressure as a factor in the production of ischial ulcers, Arch. Phys. Med. Rehabil. **39**:623, 1958.
14. Krizek, T. J., Robson, M. C., and Kho, E.: Bacterial growth and skin graft survival, Surg. Forum **18**:518, 1967.
15. Landis, E. M.: Microinjection studies of capillary blood pressure in human skin, Heart **15**:209, 1930.
16. Miles, A. A., and Niven, J. S. F.: The enchancement of infection during shock produced by bacterial toxins and other agents, Br. J. Exp. Pathol. **31**:73, 1950.
17. Miles, A. A.: Nonspecific defense reactions in bacterial infections, Ann. N.Y. Acad. Sci. **66**:356, 1956.
18. Peacock, E. E., and Van Winkle, W.: Repair of skin wounds. In Surgery and biology of wound repair, Philadelphia, 1970, W. B. Saunders Company.
19. Rickells, L. R., Squire, J. R., Topley, E., and Lilly, H. A.: Human skin lipids with particular reference to the self-sterilizing power of the skin, Clin. Sci. Mol. Med. **10**:89, 1951.
20. Robson, M. C., Edstrom, L. E., Krizek, T. J., and Groskin, M. G.: The efficacy of systemic antibiotics in the treatment of granulating wounds, J. Surg. Res. **16**:299, 1974.
21. Robson, M. C., and Heggers, J. P.: Bacterial quantification of open wounds, Milit. Med. **134**:19, 1969.
22. Robson, M. C., and Heggers, J. P.: Surgical infection. II. The beta-hemolytic streptococcus, J. Surg. Res. **9**:289, 1969.
23. Robson, M. C., Krizek, T. J., and Heggers, J. P.: Biology of surgical infection, Curr. Probl. Surg. March 1973.
24. Robson, M. C. Krizek, T. J., Koss, N., and Samburg, J. L.: Amniotic membranes as a temporary wound dressing, Surg. Gynecol. Obstet. **136**:787, 1973.
25. Robson, M. C., Samburg. J. L., and Krizek, T. J.: Quantitative comparison of biological dressings, J. Surg. Res. **14**:431, 1973.
26. Updegraff, D. M.: Methods for determining the distribution of bacteria in the skin, J. Am. Oil Chem. Soc. **44**:481, 1967.

Panel discussion on pressure ulcerations

LIBBY F. WILSON-MACKBY, Moderator

PAUL W. BRAND
VERT MOONEY
MARTIN C. ROBSON
MELVIN SPIRA

Question: Dr. Brand, would you care to begin by commenting on Dr. Robson's paper on the role of infection in pressure ulcerations?

Brand, P.: I feel that open wounds, whether innervated or not, are usually able to handle bacterial invasion if given optimal physical surroundings. Frequently, concentrating on the fear or presence of bacteria results in leaving the wound exposed and inadequately immobilized, which may do more harm than good. With good mechanical care one can frequently neglect the bacteriology. Let me describe our care of the foot ulcerations seen in the diabetic or leprosy patient. First, they are divided into acute and chronic. The acute ulcer is either fresh or shows signs of acute infection with fever, cellulitis, and so on. These patients are put on strict bed rest with elevation and antibiotics. When the acute inflammation subsides, the now-chronic wound is treated by cast immobilization, the antibiotics are discontinued, and the patient is permitted to ambulate. One word about culturing these ulcers. Dr. Garland reported on a series of legs amputated for infection and found that in over 50% of the cases, those surface bacteria available for culture bore no relationship to the deep infective organisms. Therefore, after treating many thousands of these patients, I've concluded that infrequently changed walking plaster casts without antibiotics are the treatment of choice of the chronic foot ulcer.

Spira: I agree with Dr. Robson that bacterial control is essential and would only disagree on the method. Historically we have gone through the eras of enzymatic debridement, 5% acetic acid, synthetic skin, porcine zoografts, and so on and now find that simple wet-to-dry saline dressings are as effective and certainly the least expensive method of wound care. I also believe that evidence of peripheral epithelialization about the ulcer is an excellent sign of bacterial suppression.

Robson: Well, both Drs. Brand and Spira have just agreed with me. Dr. Brand places the foot at rest and elevates it to get rid of the edema. We agree that edema is one of the causes of infection, and therefore his treatment increases the host resistance. Dr. Spira uses epithelialization as a sign of bacterial suppression, and our studies and those of Bendy show that epithelialization occurs only when the bacterial count is below 100,000.

Fredricks: We must be certain of the specifics of wound care and what the order "wet-to-dry" truly means. The uninformed nurse would lay a Topper (that terrible product of the purchasing agents' cost consciousness) and hold it on with some occlusive material. Disaster results. Proper care means a real gauze sponge carefully tucked into the depths and interstices of the wound to macerate the debris and suck it up with the bacteria into the material by capillary action. The moisture is permitted to evaporate through the top of the sponge, and the bacteria are desiccated. Once the wound is clean and bacterially depressed, then a mesh graft will hasten healing and permit continued wet dressing care. Once the wound is closed, then reconstructive flap rotation is more secure.

Robson: Perhaps the single most important modality is sharp debridement if there is any quantity of necrotic material. Only then can the residual debris be controlled by coarse mesh gauze. The interstices of fine mesh gauze are too quickly occluded by the wound coagulum. Antibiotics are the wrong material to be using topically. Antibacterials, however, such as zinc peroxide, are excellent at controlling wound streptococci and staphylococci.

Brand, P.: We do not hesitate to leave our leg plasters on a foot ulcer for a month at a time. We do less sharp debriding now as we feel that spontaneous separation occurs at a more accurate plane than we can do surgically. We use no other special dressings or drugs. The buttock ulcers, of course, do not lend themselves well to walking plasters, and here I do prefer wet dressings.

Mooney: One must make a distinction between a diabetic or arteriosclerotic ulcer and an ulcer due to pressure alone. When one debrides an ulcer due to intraarterial disease it must be immediately closed, directly or with a graft; otherwise, secondary eschar formation will undoubtedly result. These tissues cannot tolerate exposure with any kind of dressing short of biologic coverage.

Question: Dr. Brand, would you comment on the shear forces that would be generated by the square cutout cushions Dr. Wilson-Mackby described?

Brand, P.: Shear forces will be developed to some extent by any shape that is not a perfect contour fit. There are now many heat-moldable materials that can be used to obtain precise shaping. Cutouts are difficult to accurately locate and risk high shear forces on the edges. It is the same thing with shoes.

Spira: One can make a precisely contoured seat by filling a sturdy Mylar bag with glass beads, having the patient sit in it, and then sucking out the air. This will then become rigid and permanently hold its shape as long as the integrity of the vacuum is maintained.

Wilson-Mackby: With the relief built in, so to speak.

Spira: There was a recent study of the various commercially available cushions, and the price variations were extreme. There was very little difference in the pressure distribution seen with the Bye-Bye Decubiti at about $14 and the expensive Stryker Flotation Pad nearer $298.

Question: Dr. Robson, are there any other known alterations in wound healing in denervated tissue other than infection?

Robson: It is difficult to sort out which of the multifactorial processes, ischemia, denervation, pressure and temperature change, makes the difference. We have tried to create a model to isolate each factor, and we know that collagen synthesis is altered with denervation. There is difficulty in controlling temperature in any of the models, and thus far we have no real answer to that question.

Wilson-Mackby: Shannon Stauffer did some studies on wounds that crossed from innervated to denervated tissues. He could detect no difference in their tensile properties. We believe that the main reason that wounds in denervated tissues are subject to early disruption is that there is no protective pain reflex to prevent excess loading of the wound.

Brand, P.: In our rat studies we have shown that denervated foot pads break down more easily than normally to the same repetitive stimuli. The denervated foot becomes much more edematous, and this may mechanically increase the shear stress. Conversely, the denervated skin is the same as the unaltered tissue when subjected to a single large tearing force. I would like to emphasize that tissue can be overprotected. Skin and subcutaneous tissues respond to environmental forces in four different ways: atrophy, eutrophy, hypertrophy, and dystrophy. Over-protected tissues atrophy and become more fragile. Eutrophy implies normal activities with normal response. Hypertrophy occurs from overstressing within a tolerable range, and dystrophy (tissue breakdown) occurs when tolerances are exceeded. Perhaps we should go around our ward and slap our patients on the backside.

Spira: Frank Gerow and I attempted an experiment to see if gel implants would protect the tissues over bony prominences from excess pressures. After much difficulty we created a dog model and found that after an initial success they all eroded out.

Brand, P.: I hope that your comments will help to prevent someone else from trying what has failed so many times in the past. From time to time this idea surfaces, and people have the soles of their feet and other weight-bearing areas injected with silicone with disastrous results.

Wilson-Mackby: It is astonishing to see how frequently the wheel gets rediscovered.

Question: Dr. Spira, you have recommended amputation and filleting of the lower extremities for severe extensive pressure areas. Does the absence of the lower extremity not interfere with sitting balance?

Spira: Yes, there is no question that the lower extremity counterbalances, stabilizes, and helps to distribute forces when the patient is sitting. When we do a fillet amputation, the head of the femur and greater trochanter are left to extend the sitting base. If a hip disarticulation is required, then a specially molded seat must be fabricated.

Question: Also for Dr. Spira. You have recommended radical ischiectomy for ischial ulcers. Does this not transfer the forces elsewhere with subsequent erosions over the pubis and even through the urethra?

Spira: That is always a risk. However, our incidence of ischial recurrences is less. If done unilaterally then frequently the opposite side is placed at risk. The procedure offers no panacea against neglect.

Chapter 32

Nerve repair and crossover grafting in facial nerve palsy

Hans Anderl

Historically many variations of static and dynamic suspension operations have been developed to restore support and animation to the paralyzed face, and more recently, free muscle transplants have been used by Thompson,[10] Freilinger,[5] and others. All these operations have been, however, merely substitute procedures. True reconstruction can only be accomplished by successful restoration of direct facial nerve function. The recent advances in microneural surgery by Millesi and others have enlarged the scope of reinnervation and have considerably improved results. The modern operating microscope permits accurate atraumatic dissection of the nerve fascicles and precise repair with exceptionally fine suture material.

When a fresh nerve is sectioned following trauma or tumor ablation, primary direct repair of nerve ends is advisable, Secondary repair is complicated technically by the need to locate the tiny nerve endings in scar, and repair is therefore frequently less accurate. If primary repair is not feasible, the nerve endings should be tagged with colored sutures for ease of future location. Electric stimulation is often helpful in locating the distal branches when the nerve is freshly cut.

If there is a significant gap between the nerve ends, primary grafting can be done if the wound is clean. Each branch should have its own graft to minimize inappropriate movements resulting from axonic misalignment.

There are, however, situations in which reconstruction of the ipsilateral facial nerve is not possible even by bridging the defect from nerve roots in the cranial fossa as described by Dott, House, Fisch, and others. A spinocervical or hypoglossal nerve anastomosis may be employed to reinnervate the facial

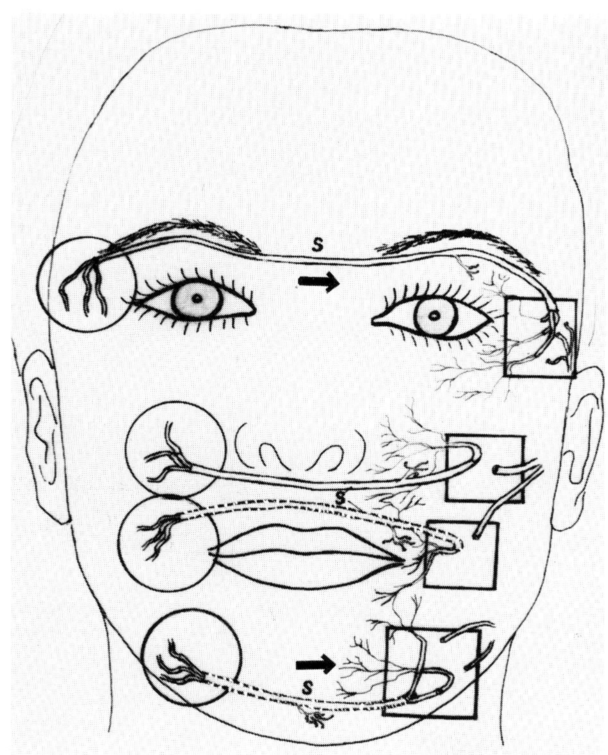

Fig. 32-1. Sural nerve grafts from right side of face (intact) to left side of face (paralyzed). Circles indicate anastomoses to healthy facial fascicles, squares indicate anastomoses of sural graft to corresponding main branches of facial nerve. Two grafts can be exchanged *(dotted line)*. (From Rubin, L.: Reanimation of the paralyzed face, St. Louis, 1977, The C. V. Mosby Co.)

muscles to produce symmetry in repose but grimacing and asymmetric mass function usually result during animated expression.

Because of the rich nerve supply of the muscles of expression, several filaments can be sacrificed without noticeable effect. When branches are injured due to trauma or even when entire rows of nerve ends are severed to treat spasm and twitching, little loss of function is noted. This fortuitous fact and the development of microneural surgery led to the idea of reinnervating the paralyzed face from the normal side via crossover grafts. Smith[9] and Scaramella[8] first described such a facio-facial anastomosis. We have independently conceived a method of specific nerve-muscle groupings for optimum reconstruction (Fig. 32-1). There are four main functional muscle groups, each innervated by its own branch:

Temporal	Ramus temporofrontalis
Orbital	Ramus zygomaticus
Buccal	Ramus buccales
Mental	Ramus marginalis

PROCEDURE

The operative procedure is in two stages. First, sural nerve grafts are positioned across the face and anastomosed to selected donor facial nerve fascicles on the normal side. Four to six months later when the axons have grown through the graft, the distal anastomosis is performed. Incisions (Fig. 32-2) are made on the normal side over the peripheral distribution of the various facial rami. After the skin and subcutaneous tissue have been dissected, three to four fascicles are selected from the peripheral plexus of the ramus zygomaticus under optical magnification of about 10. The appropriate selection of nerve fascicles is aided by initial use of a nerve stimulator and then blockade of those fascicles to be severed, with a drop of local anesthetic. If good function remains, then the fascicle can be cut. Six to eight fascicles from the buccal division and occasionally two to three fascicles from the marginal division are selected in the same manner (Fig. 32-3).

After the donor fascicles have been selected, sural nerve transplants are taken from both legs obtaining grafts up to 60 cm long. After the physician has bluntly tunneled across the face, the passage of the transplants may be facilitated by adding 1 cm incisions in mid tunnel. For orbicularis oculi function, a 15 to 17 cm graft is passed through the frontalis muscle and superior border of the orbicularis muscle with the distal end of the sural nerve oriented on the paralyzed side of the face. Thus axons growing out of the "cutaneous" branches of the graft can contribute to the reinnervation of the muscle.

For the lip and cheek musculature, two sural nerve transplants 13 to 15 cm long are passed through the upper lip. In the lower lip a 6 to 8 cm graft is implanted in the muscle of the chin. On the paralyzed side, all ends of the transplants are positioned posterior to the frontal border of the parotid gland, above and below the anatomic location of the facial nerve branches, thus eliminating additional scarring that could make their subsequent reloca-

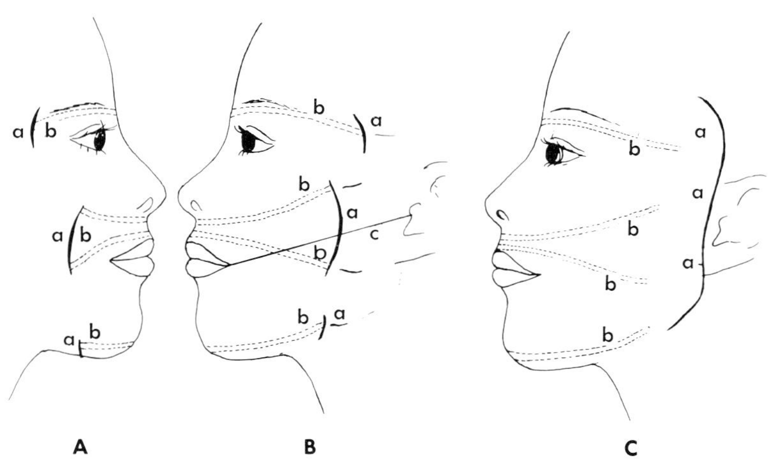

Fig. 32-2. A, Incision lines, *a,* on healthy side of face. **B,** Incision lines, *a,* on paralyzed side of face; *b,* sural grafts; *c,* imaginary line where Stensen duct can be located. **C,** Incision line, *a,* to perform a supplemental face-lift. (From Rubin, L.: Reanimation of the paralyzed face, St. Louis, 1977, The C. V. Mosby Co.)

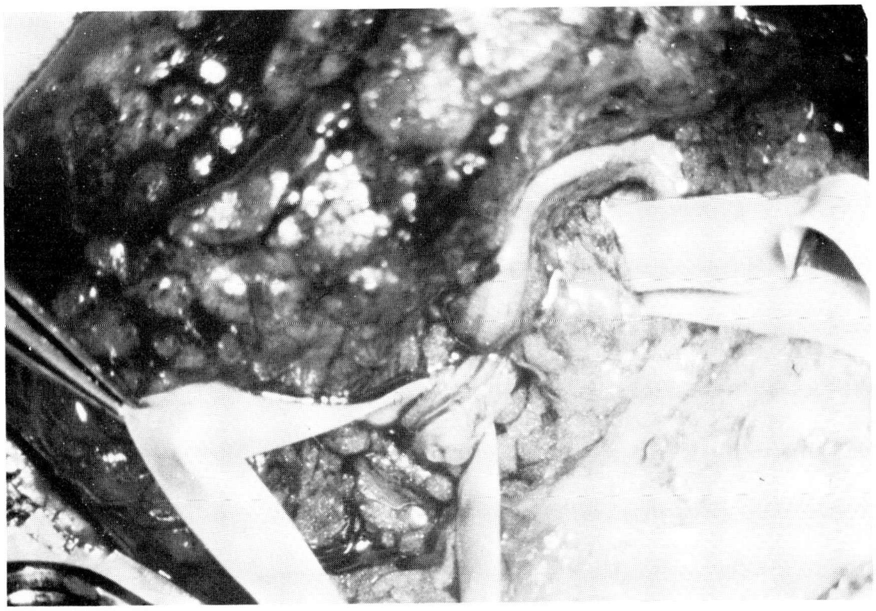

Fig. 32-3. Two large facial fascicles in the buccal area. (From Rubin, L.: Reanimation of the paralyzed face, St. Louis, 1977, The C. V. Mosby Co.)

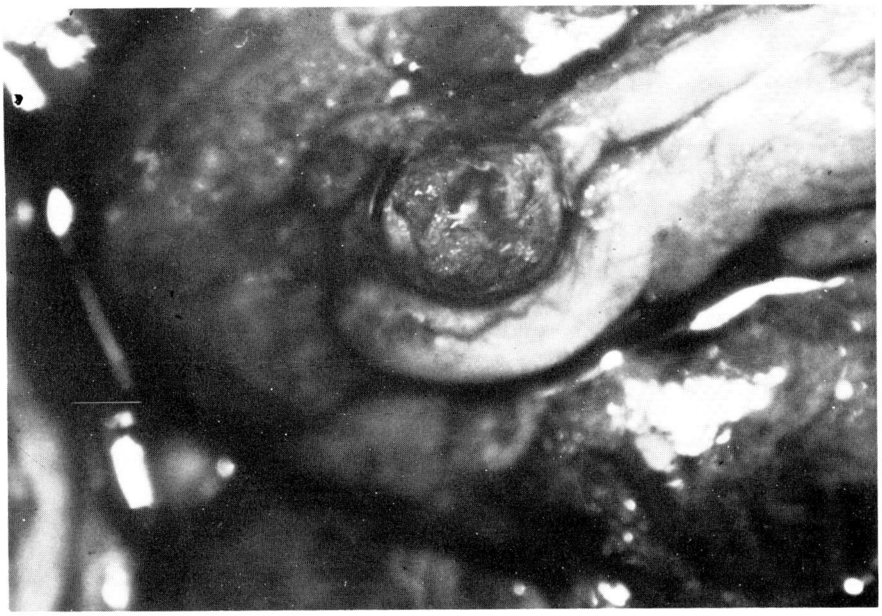

Fig. 32-4. Neuroma at end of a sural graft. (From Rubin, L.: Reanimation of the paralyzed face, St. Louis, 1977, The C. V. Mosby Co.)

tion more difficult. The ends are marked with colored suture brought out through the skin and cut close to the surface.

As a final step the microneural anastomosis is done using the technique described by Millesi and associates.[6] The fascicles of the sural nerve grafts are separated from each other for 1 to 2 cm and then brought into contact with the donor fascicles with enough slack to lie in a small tension-free loop. Only one suture of 10-0 silk is necessary. The suture lines are covered with a protective patch of subcutaneous fat, minidrains are inserted, and the wound is closed. Four to six months later the nerve grafts are anastomosed to the appropriate recipient branches on the paralyzed side through an incision over the zygomatic arch anterior to the parotid gland and over the mandible near the facial artery. All the major branches of the paralyzed facial nerve can be easily visualized through this incision, and they are severed 1 cm within the parotid gland. The distal segments are rotated to the end of the corresponding previously marked nerve grafts.

The thickening of the graft end represents an amputation neuroma and demonstrates the success of axon growth along the transplant (Fig. 32-4). This must be excised. After the ends of the sural grafts have been split into their individual fascicles, they are anastomosed to the previously prepared recipient facial nerve fascicles in the same fashion as on the donor side of the face (Fig. 32-5).

In some children or in the presence of excessive scarring the distal anastomoses on the paralyzed side may be impossible. If this occurs, a direct implantation of the nerve into the muscle may lead to some indirect neuromuscular innervation. We consider physiotherapy an important adjunct to facial nerve transplantation. Treatment should start at the onset of the paralysis and continue until the reinnervation is complete.

A successful clinical result can be verified by electromyography. Direct stimulation of the original paralyzed facial nerve stem with high-intensity current should produce no response. Stimulation of the facial nerve stem on the donor side should evoke a good response potential from the formerly paralyzed muscles. This method of cross-face nerve transplantation can be applied in all paralyses in which the muscles are still capable of regeneration.[1-4] Thus it is futile to use this technique if palsy was present for more than 1½ to 2 years. Electromyog-

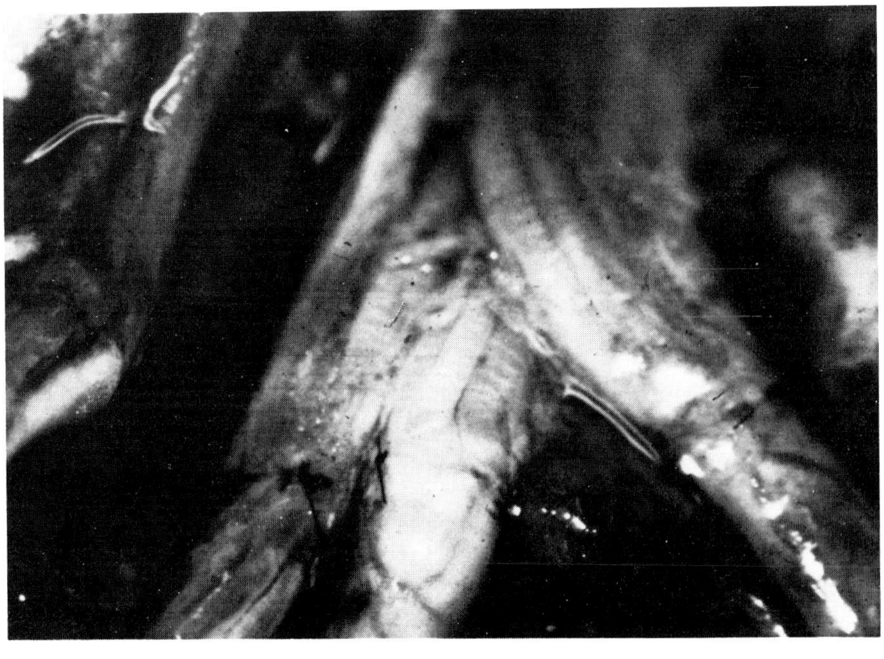

Fig. 32-5. Anastomoses of a sural graft to fascicles of a main facial branch on paralyzed side. (From Rubin, L.: Reanimation of the paralyzed face, St. Louis, 1977, The C. V. Mosby Co.)

raphy will help to determine muscle potential by evoking a fibrillation response. If the muscles are atrophied beyond salvage, the principle of cross-face nerve transplantation may be applied in conjunction with a free muscle graft implanted into the muscle or anastomosed to the nerve as Thompson[10] has described. Freilinger[5] has used such a combination to remotor a temporal muscle that was redirected to elevate the cheek and mouth. It is probably better to use a muscle that is already available, such as the temporal or masseter muscle, as free muscle transplants lose a considerable amount of fibers. We combine cross-face nerve transplantation with a Lexer-Rosenthal[7] procedure by direct suture of the transplant to that nerve segment which leads to the transposed half of the masseter. This idea was proposed together with Dr. Lalardrie.

In addition to these direct approaches to the facial nerve, we have also used temporary static and dynamic procedures to enable the patient to obtain eye closure while waiting for recovery. Lid springs in the upper lid (Morel-Fatio), lid magnets (Mühlbauer), or a Silastic membrane (Anderl)[1a] to support the lower lid was inserted in all patients on a temporary basis and could be removed after reinnervation. Since 1971, 18 patients, including two children aged 4 and 6, have been treated by this method. Six patients had good results (Figs. 32-6 and 32-7), five patients show satisfactory function, and three are still recovering. One patient has poor function, and three patients demonstrate essentially no recovery (Table 12).

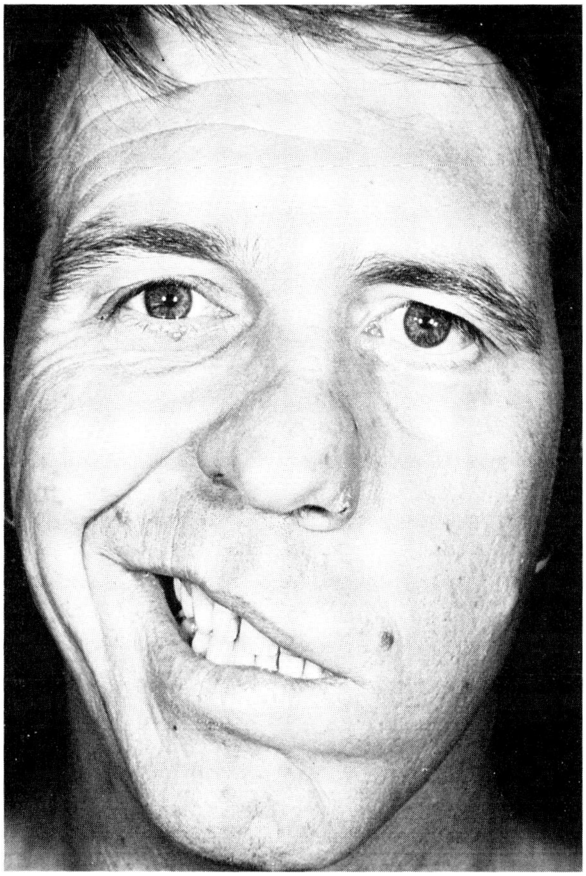

Fig. 32-6. Complete Bell palsy on left side of face (no spontaneous recovery after 12 months). (From Rubin, L.: Reanimation of the paralyzed face, St. Louis, 1977, The C. V. Mosby Co.)

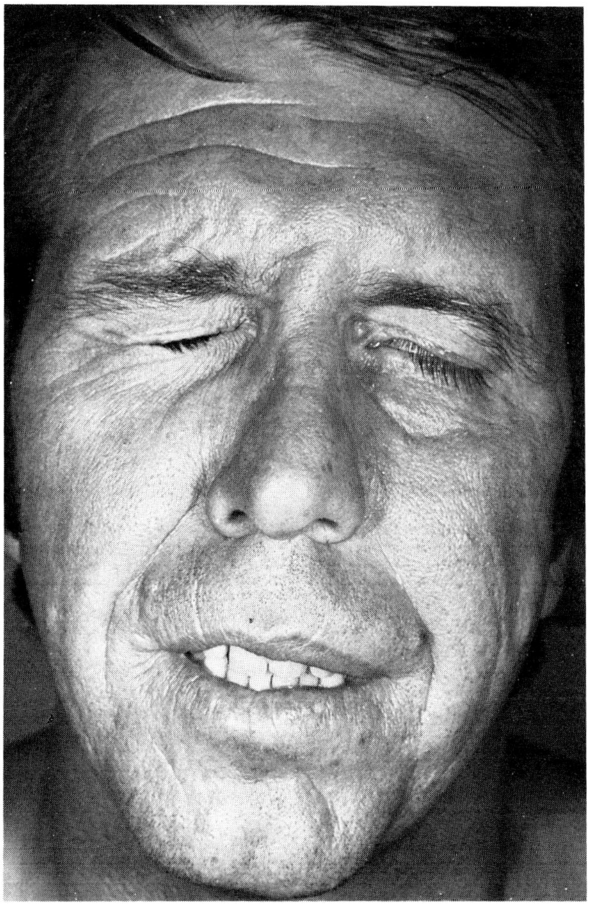

Fig. 32-7. Patient in Fig. 32-6, 5 years after cross-face nerve transplantation. (From Rubin, L.: Reanimation of the paralyzed face, St. Louis, 1977, The C. V. Mosby Co.)

Table 12. Results of facial nerve repair (crossover) from 1971 to 1976

No. of cases	*Diagnosis*	*Results* Good*	*Results* Satisfactory†	*Results* Bad‡	*In recovery*	*Follow-up (years)*
8	Cerebellar tumor	2	4	1	1	0.5-4.5
5	Basocranial fracture and decompression	3	1		1	1-3
2	Bell palsy	1			1	4.5
7	Parotid gland carcinoma; irradiation			1		1.5
2	Radical operation of the ear			2		4.5-5

*Symmetry, active lifting of angle of mouth and cheek, lid closure almost perfect.
†Fair symmetry, cheek tone and slight lifting, two-thirds lid closure.
‡Little or no symmetry, little muscle action, poor lid closure.

SUMMARY

1. A two-stage procedure for cross-face nerve transplantation using sural nerve grafts is described.
2. Temporary adjunctive procedures must be used to protect the paralyzed eye while reinnervation is incomplete.
3. The procedure is useful when all possibility of ipsilateral repair has been exhausted, and viable muscle remains on the paralyzed side.

REFERENCES

1. Anderl, H.: Nerventransplantation bei facial sparese. Jahrestagung der Schweiz, Ges. Plast. Wiederhorst. Chirurgie, 1972.

1a. Anderl, H.: A simple method for correcting ectropion, Plast. Reconstr. Surg. **49:**156-159, 1972.

2. Anderl, H.: Reconstruction of the face through cross-face-nerve transplantation in facial paralysis, Chir. Plast. **2:**17-46, 1973.

3. Anderl, H.: Cross-face-nerve transplantation in facial palsy. In Converse, J. M., editor: Reconstructive plastic surgery, Philadelphia, 1975, W. B. Saunders Company.

4. Anderl, H.: Cross-face-nerve transplantation in facial palsy (principles and further experience). In Marchae, D., and Hueston, J., editors: Transactions of the Sixth International Congress of Plastic and Reconstructive Surgery, Paris, 1976, Masson, pp. 332-340.

5. Freilinger, G.: A new technique to correct facial paralysis, Plast. Reconstr. Surg. **56:**44-48, 1975.

6. Millesi, H., Ganglberger, J., and Berger, A.: Erfahrungen mit der Mikrochirurgie peripherer Nerven, Chir. Plast. Reconstr. **3:**47, 1967.

7. Rosenthal, W.: Die bleibende Facialis parese und ihre Behandlung, Dtsch. Z. Chir. pp. 223-261, 1930.

8. Scaramella, L.: Lanastomosi tra i due nervi facciali, Arch. Otol. **82:**209-215, 1971.

9. Smith, J. W.: A new technique of facial animation. In Transactions of the Fifth International Congress of Plastic and Reconstructive Surgery, London, 1971, Butterworth, p. 83.

10. Thompson, N.: Autogenous free grafts of skeletal muscle, Plast. Reconstr. Surg. **48:**11-27, 1971.

Chapter 33

Management of facial paralysis associated with tumors of the parotid gland

John Conley

There have been two significant advances in the management of tumors of the parotid gland that have added a rationale to the treatment and to the facial paralysis resulting from the treatment. The classification of these tumors permitted their treatment to be correlated with their prognosis. This information established the surgical technique that was applicable for that particular problem. Excisional surgery in this region was a constant threat to the facial nerve, and in certain instances, all or part of the nerve was either destroyed or compromised by the tumor or removed in the radical excision, with a resultant partial or total facial paralysis. This paralysis should be rehabilitated when this is realistic, and the best time to do it is simultaneously with the ablative technique.

A

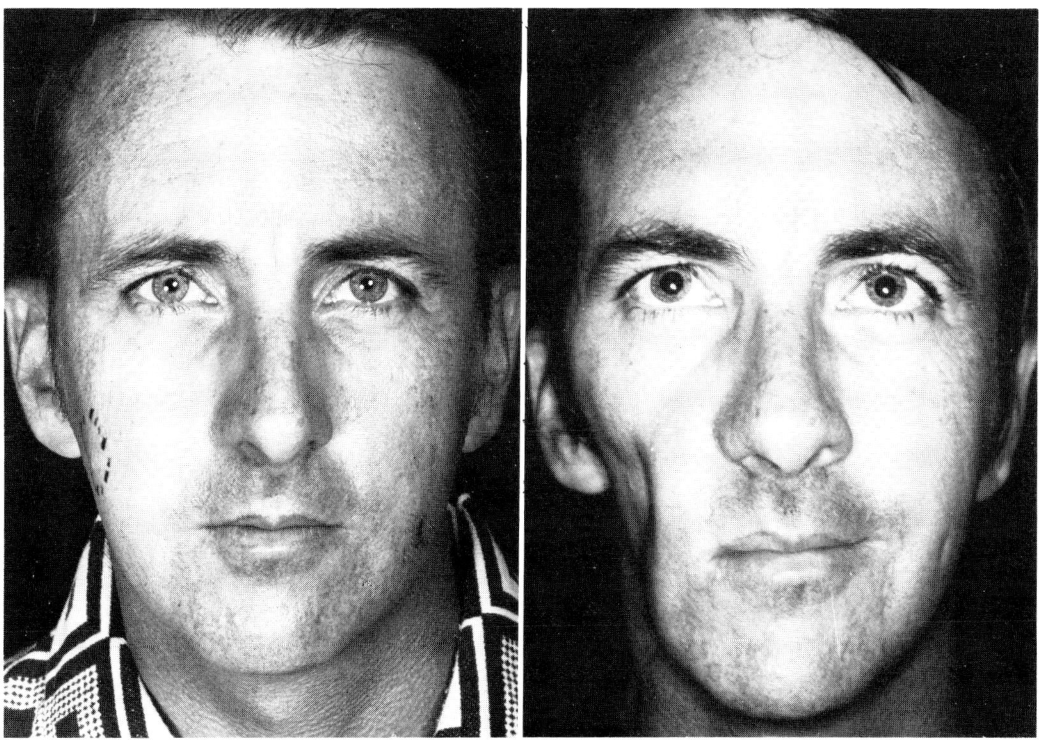

B

Fig. 33-1. A, High-grade mucoepidermoid carcinoma of pyramidal lobe. **B,** One year after radical resection and nerve graft with good movement about orbit and commissure.

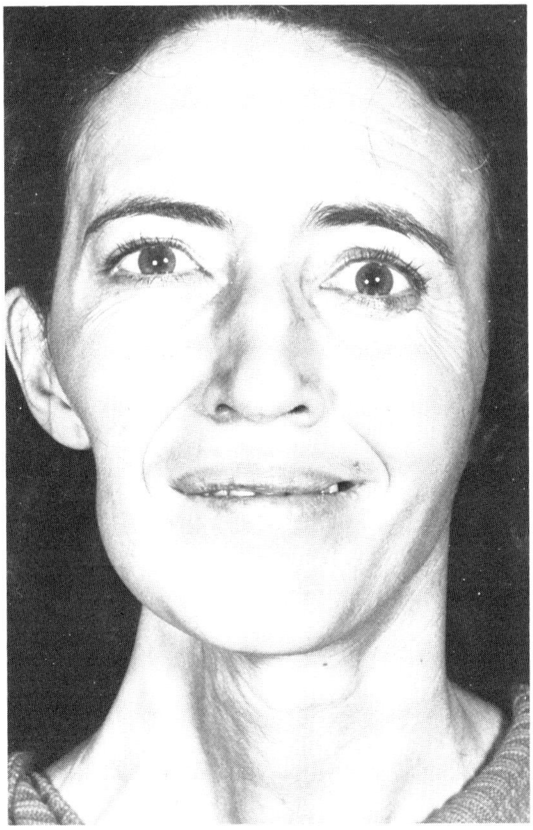

Fig. 33-2. Excellent return of movement about orbit, cheek, and commissure after radical resection for recurrent carcinoma following nerve graft.

Benign tumors and cysts rarely compromise the facial nerve, but their position, size, and intimate attachment may make the conservation operation extremely difficult. Large tumors at the deep lobe, confluent, multiple, recurrent benign tumors that have enmeshed the nerves, and nerves that are encased in scar tissue are at high risk of advertent or inadvertent resection.

Facial nerve paresis exists preoperatively in 17% of cases of malignant neoplasms in the parotid gland and in 40% of the primary neurilemomas of the facial nerve. In these instances the decision regarding nerve resection has already been made by the biologic process.

Of all malignant tumors in the parotid gland, 83% require a decision regarding resection of an intact facial nerve. This judgment is made at the time of the primary operation based on the information derived from frozen section or after the final diagnosis is established from the permanent sections. In a review of 278 malignant tumors of this gland, 68% underwent radical ablation.[1] The remaining 32% had some type of facial nerve conservation, with all or part of the nerve still intact at the end of the operation. None of these partial resections were grafted. Of those undergoing radical resection, 26% had a complete facial nerve graft. Forty-two percent were not grafted because the wound was too extensive or they were selected for hypoglossal crossover, muscle inter-

A

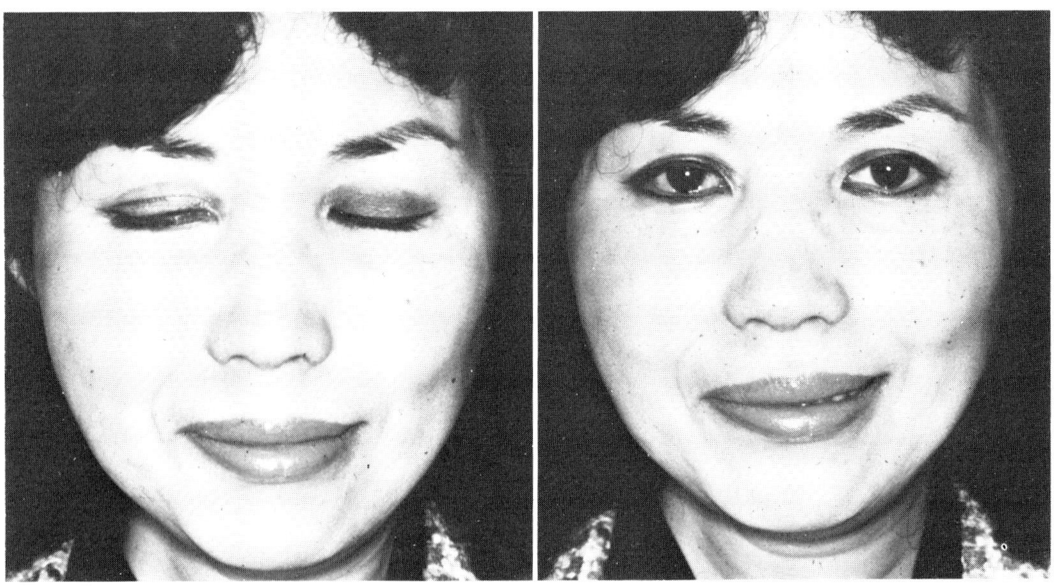

B

Fig. 33-3. A, Radical parotidectomy with interdigitation of masseter muscle into mimetic muscles. There was no nerve graft. **B,** Good return of movement about eye, cheek, and commissure.

digitation, or muscle transfer. Separate reports have covered 150 facial nerve grafts and 122 hypoglossal crossovers.[1]

There is little need to graft segmental or divisional resection of the facial nerve, as there is rarely more than a 10% to 15% deficit with excision of the main upper or lower division.

TOTAL FACIAL NERVE GRAFTS

Total facial nerve grafting is carried out immediately in radical parotidectomy when the condition of the wound and the patient permits it. There will never be a better anatomic presentation of the nerve elements in the wound. Reentry into the wound after heavy scarring, fibrosis, and nerve atrophy adds immeasurably to the technical difficulties. The usual donor areas are the sensory branches of the cervical plexus with a segment of nerve containing four or five branches. This graft is approximated to the proximal facial nerve stump with 8-0 atraumatic monofilament suture material. The peripheral branches are usually approximated with one suture. There is no question but that magnification with loupes or the dissecting microscope increases the precision of nerve approximation. Many of these grafts, however, have been placed without the aid of magnification with excellent return of function. The nerve graft is generous in length, thus eliminating any possibility of tension on the suture line. The suture line is encased in a soft nonconstrictive silicone tube, 1 cm long. All these wounds must be drained.

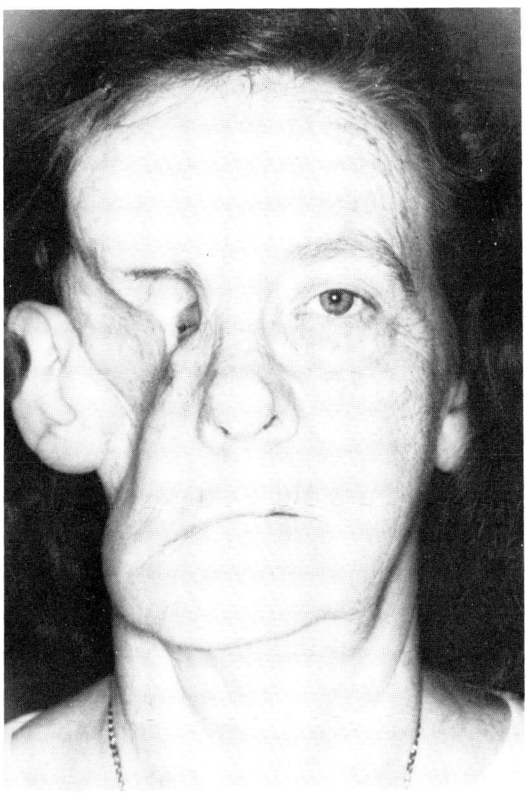

Fig. 33-4. Massive ablation for recurrent carcinoma, eliminating need for nerve grafting.

When the above criteria are applied, one can expect some degree of movement in the face in 95% of the cases. The first signs of return of movement appear in the cheek and about the commissure of the mouth. The interval of time is from 6 to 12 months, depending upon the length of the graft, the accuracy of the anastomosis, and the volume of regenerating axons. The tone of the face during this interval is better than one would expect in a paralyzed face, and many individuals do not require an elective tarsorrhaphy. The movement spreads from the middle third of the face into the cheek and about the orbit. The forehead and platysma movement usually do not return. Improvement in tone, movement, and coordination continues for another 2 years. The movement is always weaker than the normal side; it is basically mass movement in character; and it exhibits varying degrees of dyskinesia. The natural response to emotional expression on the paralyzed side of the face is markedly limited but can be improved by persistent training and awareness.

TRANSFACIAL NERVE GRAFTS

Transfacial nerve grafting may be considered in radical ablations in this area when the proximal segment of the facial nerve on the ipsilateral side is not available for grafting. It is axiomatic that when the proximal segment is available it offers the best opportunity for rehabilitation. Radical temporal bone resections, stroke, central neoplasms, neurilemomas of the central part of the facial nerve, severe Bell palsy, and degenerative disease may obliterate the possibility of using the proximal segment of the facial nerve. Although transfacial nerve grafting may be used in many of these instances, it has several deterrents: (1) it is a multistaged procedure; (2) a separate operation on the leg is required; (3) there is a protracted morbidity; and (4) a small volume of axons is produced. It is an illusion to think that a transfacial nerve graft will produce normal emotional expression, and, indeed, nothing will in a paralyzed face. The transfacial nerve graft unquestionably has a place in the rehabilitation of the paralyzed face, but I doubt whether criteria for its use have been established as yet.

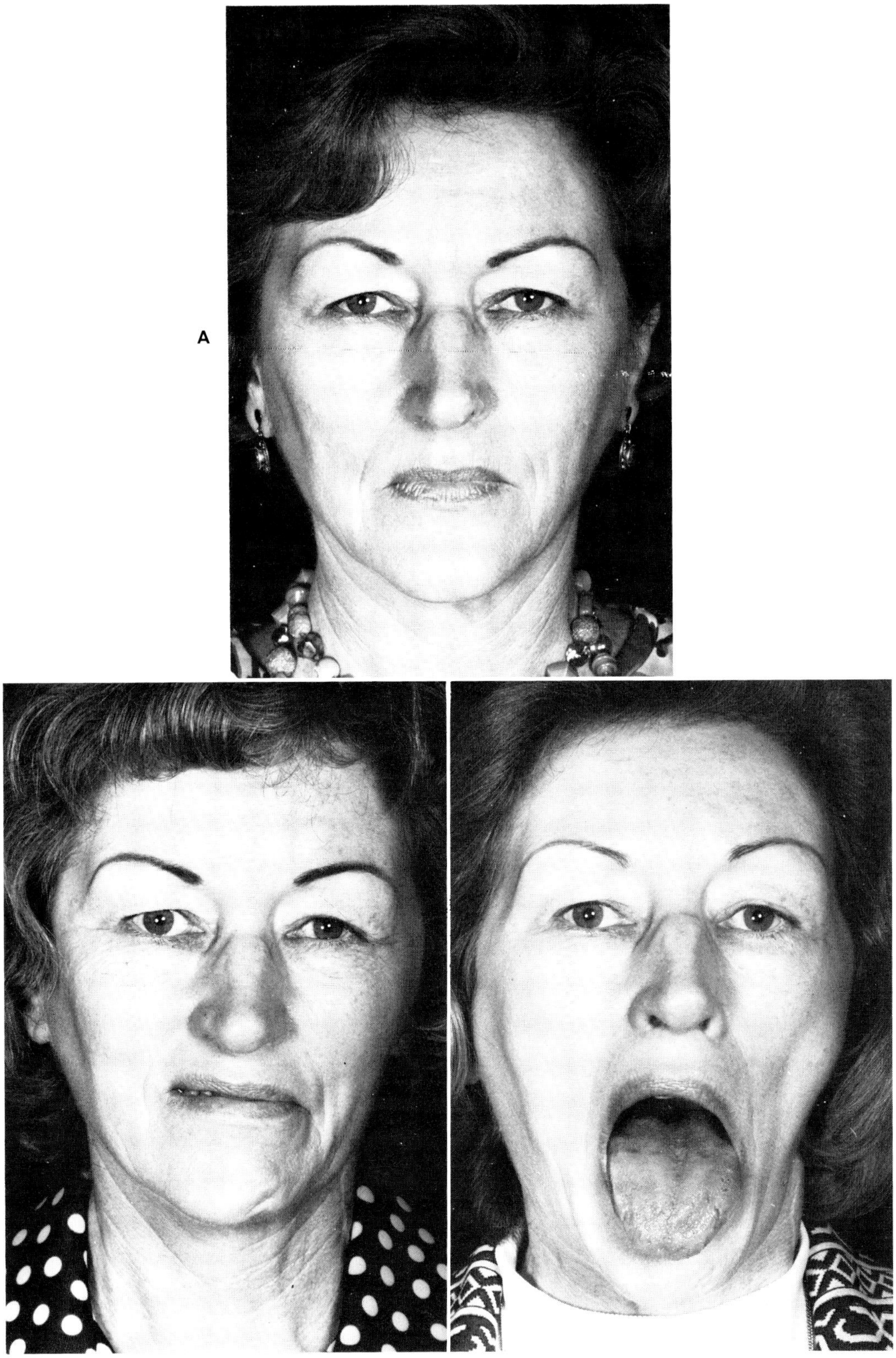

Fig. 33-5. A, Carcinoma of left parotid gland. **B,** Hypoglossal crossover 10 months following radical resection. **C,** Good movement and minimal atrophy of tongue.

HYPOGLOSSAL CROSSOVER

In many of the above situations, it is simpler to carry out a hypoglossal crossover. This concept has come under severe criticism from certain writers. This stems from the fact that this nerve has a high neural energy input and that its physiologic functions are associated with talking, chewing, and swallowing. This means that when an approximation is extremely accurate, when the peripheral facial nerve segment is in high quality of receptivity, and when a large volume of axons pass from the hypoglossal nerve into the facial muscles, there will be excessive movement of the face during the functions of talking, chewing, and swallowing. When it is an integral part of the radical operation for a malignant process, there are very few complaints because of the overriding emphasis placed on the treatment of the cancer. Individuals, however, who have had a facial paralysis for over 2 years have quite a different psychologic attitude. Dissatisfaction is considerably higher in this group. None of the patients in our series requested or were willing to revert to the status of facial paralysis. I therefore consider the hypoglossal crossover to be a very valuable technique in the rehabilitation of the face in individuals who have undergone radical ablation for malignant neoplasia. In all other cases I feel that the attitude of the surgeon and the patient must be critically analyzed before advocating this technique (Fig. 33-5).

MUSCLE INTERDIGITATION

In all cases where immediate nerve grafting is unrealistic, muscle interdigitation has become a routine part of the technique. The cut surface of the masseter, pterygoid, or temporalis muscle is spliced into the cut surface of the mimetic muscles. This interdigitation theoretically permits the axons of the masticatory muscles to grow directly into the axons of the mimetic muscles. This type of interdigitation places the axons in almost direct approximation with each other so that only a few millimeters of open-field transit are necessary. Movement is apparent within 3 months, appears first about the commissure, and then spreads around the middle third of the face. It also is basically mass movement and is produced essentially upon tightening the muscles of mastication.

CONCLUSION

There are more complex and more sophisticated methods of rehabilitating the paralyzed face resulting from radical resections for malignant neoplasia, but they are rarely carried out as part of the primary technique. As a delayed operation they may include combinations of muscle transfer, cross-facial-nerve grafting, and nerve switching. The results are never as satisfactory as when the rehabilitative process is carried out as part of the primary operation.

REFERENCE

1. Aitken, J. T.: Growth of nerve implants in voluntary muscle, J. Anat. **84:**38, 1950.

SUGGESTED READINGS

Anderl, H.: Reconstruction of the face through cross-face-nerve transplantation in facial paralysis, Chir. Plast. **2:**17, 1973.

Bunnell, S.: Surgical repair of facial nerve, Arch. Otol. **25:**235, 1937.

Conley, J.: Facial nerve grafting in treatment of the parotid gland tumors, Arch. Surg. **70:**359, 1955.

Conley, J.: Facial rehabilitation following radical parotid gland surgery, Arch. Otolaryngol. **66:**58, 1957.

Conley, J.: Facial nerve grafting, Arch. Otolaryngol. **73:**322, 1961.

Conley, J.: Salivary glands and the facial nerve, Stuttgart, W. Ger., 1975, Thieme.

Dott, N. M.: Facial paralysis; restitution by extra-petrous nerve graft, Proc. R. Soc. Med. **51:**900, 1958.

Erlacher, P.: Direct and muscular neurotization of paralyzed muscles. Experimental research, Am. J. Orthop. Surg. **13:**22, 1915.

Fisch, U. P.: Operations on the facial nerve in oto-neurosurgical operations. In Yasargil, M. G., editor: Microsurgery, Stuttgart W. Ger., 1969, Thieme, p. 208.

Freeman, B. S.: Facial palsy. In Converse, J. M., editor: Reconstructive plastic surgery, Philadelphia, 1964, W. B. Saunders Company, vol. III, p. 1124.

Freeman, B. S.: An immediate combined approach for rehabilitation of the patient with facial paralysis, Plast. Reconstr. Surg. **37:**341, 1966.

Gutman, E., and Young, Z.: The reinnervation of muscles after various periods of atrophy, J. Anat. **78:**15-43, 1944.

House, W. F., and Crabtree, J. A.: Surgical exposure of petrous portion of the seventh nerve, Arch. Otolaryngol. **81:**506, 1966.

James, A. B., Karlan, M., Kinsey, D. L., and Meagher, J. M.: Spontaneous regeneration of the seventh nerve, Arch. Surg. **81:**283, 1960.

Kettel, K.: Repair of the facial nerve in traumatic facial palsies. Results of decompression, nerve suture and nerve grafting in one hundred twenty-seven cases, Arch. Otolaryngol. vol. 66, 1957.

Lathrop, F. D.: Surgical repair of facial nerve: technique, Surg. Clin. North Am. **36:**583, 1956.

Martin, H.: Supplementary report on spontaneous return of function following surgical section or excision of the seventh cranial nerve in surgery of parotid tumors, Ann. Surg. **146:**715, 1957.

Maxwell, J. H.: Repair of the facial nerve after lacerations, Trans. Am. Acad. Opthalmol. Otolaryngol. **58:**733, 1954.

McCabe, B. F.: Facial nerve grafting, Plast. Reconstr. Surg. **45:**71, 1970.

Miehlke, A.: Die Chirurgie des Nervus facialis, Munich, 1960, Urban and Schwarzenberg.

Millesi, H., Berger, A., and Meissl, G.: Fascicular nerve grafting, using a microsurgical technique. In Transactions of the fifth International Congress of Plastic and Reconstructive Surgery, London, 1971, Butterworth, pp. 586-592.

Pulee, J. C.: Facial nerve grafting, Laryngoscope **79:**1562, 1969.

Scaramella, L.: L'anastomosi tra i due nervi facciali, Arch. Otol. **82:**209, 1971.

Smith, J. W.: A new technique of facial animation. In Transactions of the Fifth International Congress of Plastic and Reconstructive Surgery, London, 1971, Butterworth, p. 83.

Sunderland, S.: Funicular suture and funicular exclusion in the repair of severed nerves, Br. J. Surg. **40:**580, 1953.

Thompson, N.: Treatment of facial paralysis by free skeletal muscle grafts. In Transactions of the Fifth International Congress of Plastic and Reconstructive Surgery, London, 1971, Butterworth, pp. 66-82.

Thompson, N.: Autogenous free grafts of skeletal muscle, Plast. Reconstr. Surg. **48:**11, 1971.

Chapter 34

Intratemporal repair of the facial nerve

Melton J. Horwitz

Paralysis of the seventh cranial nerve produces a very obvious distortion and disfigurement of the face, which is unfortunately increased when the patient experiences an emotion, pleasurable or otherwise. The patient's mental status may also reflect depression due to this physically deforming condition. The facial nerve travels through a longer bony canal than any other nerve in the body. In the absence of traumatic injury or obvious disease of the facial nerve as it emerges from the temporal bone, abnormality leading to paralysis will lie within the intratemporal course of the nerve in 90% of the patients.[19] It is for this reason that intratemporal facial paralysis is considered to be an otologic disease requiring a thorough neurootologic evaluation.

ANATOMY

The facial nerve exits the pons in the posterior fossa together with the nerve of Wrisberg (nervus intermedius). They enter the porus acusticus of the internal auditory canal together with the cochlear and vestibular divisions of the eight cranial nerve. The facial nerve occupies the anterior superior quadrant in the internal auditory canal. At the fundus of the canal the seventh nerve exists between the cochlea anteriorly and the superior semicircular canal and its ampulla posteriorly. It enters its bony canal, the fallopian aqueduct, and travels in its labyrinthine course to the geniculate ganglion.

At the geniculate ganglion the greater superficial petrosal nerve leaves on an anterior course, passing medial to the middle meningeal artery, and enters the pterygoid canal. Secretory motor fibers to the lacrimal gland are carried in the greater superficial petrosal nerve for lacrimation. From the geniculate ganglion the facial nerve takes a posterior course, creating its first genu, and enters the middle ear medial to the ossicular chain. In its tympanic course the nerve passes superior and adjacent to the oval window niche and the stapes. The second genu or bend of the facial nerve occurs in the mastoid antrum where the nerve is just inferior and adjacent to the horizontal semicircular canal. At the genu or in the uppermost portion of the vertical course the branch to the stapedius muscle originates.

The facial nerve continues to descend in its vertical course where it gives off the chorda tympani nerve. The chorda tympani takes a retrograde course, passing through the middle ear lateral to the incus medial to the malleus, and exits via the petrotympanic fissure. It carries secretory motor fibers to the submaxillary and sublingual glands and sensory fibers for taste from the anterior two thirds of the tongue. The facial nerve continues its descent in its vertical course and exits the mastoid at the stylomastoid foramen. In its extratemporal course it gives off motor branches to the postauricular muscle and the posterior belly of the digastric, and then the main trunk passes forward into the parotid gland where it divides into an upper and lower division to innervate the facial musculature.

ETIOLOGY

The etiology of peripheral facial nerve paralysis can be classified under four major headings: trauma, infection, neoplasm, and idiopathic (Bell palsy). Trauma usually occurs in the form of a skull fracture or a penetrating missile. Fractures of the temporal bone are more often longitudinal than transverse. Longitudinal fractures may be associated with conductive hearing loss due to ossicular dislocation or tear of the tympanic membrane. The facial nerve is paralyzed in 10% to 18% of the cases of longitudinal temporal bone fracture; this paralysis is of delayed onset.[14] The site of involvement is usually the horizontal course of the facial nerve and is secondary to ischemia and compression. Transverse fractures run perpendicular to the long axis of the petrous portion of the temporal bone. They may cross the internal auditory canal and usually involve the cochlea, resulting in a sensorineural hearing loss. Facial paralysis occurs in 38% to 50% of transverse fractures and is usually immediate in onset and complete.[14] The facial nerve may be avulsed or severed at any point from the internal auditory canal to the horizontal portion.

Facial paralysis may be associated with acute inflammatory processes of the middle ear and mastoid. Treatment with antibiotics and a myringotomy will usually produce a resolution of the infection and paralysis. Involvement of the mastoid may require a mastoidectomy with or without a decompression. In chronic otitis media the middle ear and mastoid may be involved with granulation tissue or cholesteatoma or both. Facial paralysis occurring in a chronically draining ear is an indication for immediate surgical intervention. The sheath of the nerve is usually not opened in the presence of active inflammation. Herpes zoster oticus (Ramsey Hunt syndrome) frequently involves the facial nerve at the geniculate ganglion. A transmastoid and middle fossa approach is performed to decompress the nerve[5] if there is absence of lacrimation.

Neoplastic involvement of the facial nerve accounts for less than 5% of all cases of facial paralysis.[19] Involvement may be infiltrative and destructive but usually is secondary to compression of the nerve.[3] The paralysis most frequently is characterized by slow onset with progressive loss of function. Facial nerve neuromas may occur at any point along its course.[18] After removal of the neuromas a graft is usually performed to restore facial function.

Idiopathic paralysis of the facial nerve (Bell palsy) is a diagnosis made by exclusion. If the paralysis does not respond to medical therapy and electric excitability studies indicate degeneration, then decompression of the nerve is indicated. If there is a difference between the normal and the involved side of greater than 3.5 mA, degeneration of the facial nerve is occurring.[1,11] Total loss of electric excitability indicates severe degeneration of the facial nerve.

DIAGNOSTIC TESTS OF FACIAL NERVE FUNCTION

The site of the lesion or involvement of the facial nerve can be ascertained by testing the function of the various branches of the facial nerve. A lesion at or proximal to the geniculate ganglion will produce diminished or absent lacrimation. Lacrimation is tested by performing the Schirmer test (Fig. 34-1). Tearing is tested by placing a small strip of filter paper over the margin of the lower lid, and the amount of tearing of the eye on the normal side can be compared with the tearing from the eye on the paralyzed side.

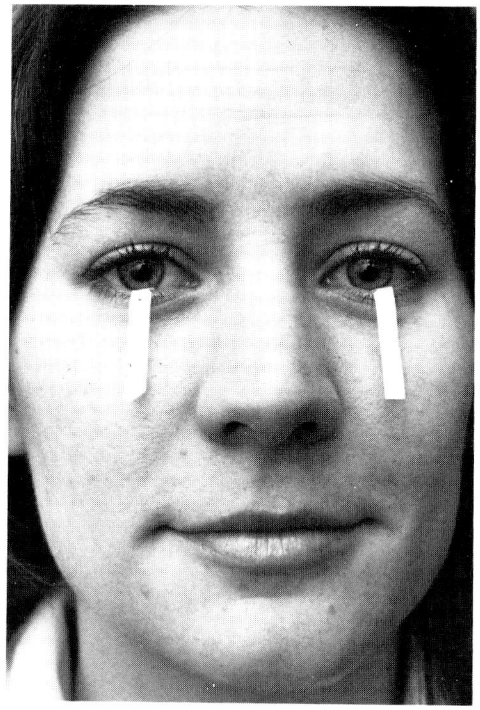

Fig. 34-1. Schirmer test is performed to test lacrimation function of greater superficial petrosal nerve. Normal and abnormal sides are compared. Normal lacrimation is 15 mm in 5 minutes.

A lesion in the horizontal or tympanic portion of the facial nerve will not interfere with lacrimal function; however, it will interfere with the ipsilateral stapedial reflex. In a normal ear the stapedius muscle will contract reflexively to a pure tone at a level of 85 decibels. The contraction will occur bilaterally and simultaneously.

A contraction of the stapedius muscle will stiffen the ossicular chain, resulting in an increase in the acoustic impedance of the sound transmission mechanism of the middle ear [2] (Fig. 34-2). Using an acoustic impedance probe, the physician can detect the change in the impedance. If the facial nerve is intact proximal to the motor branch to the stapedius muscle, the muscle will contract in response to the sound stimulus. If the function has been inter-

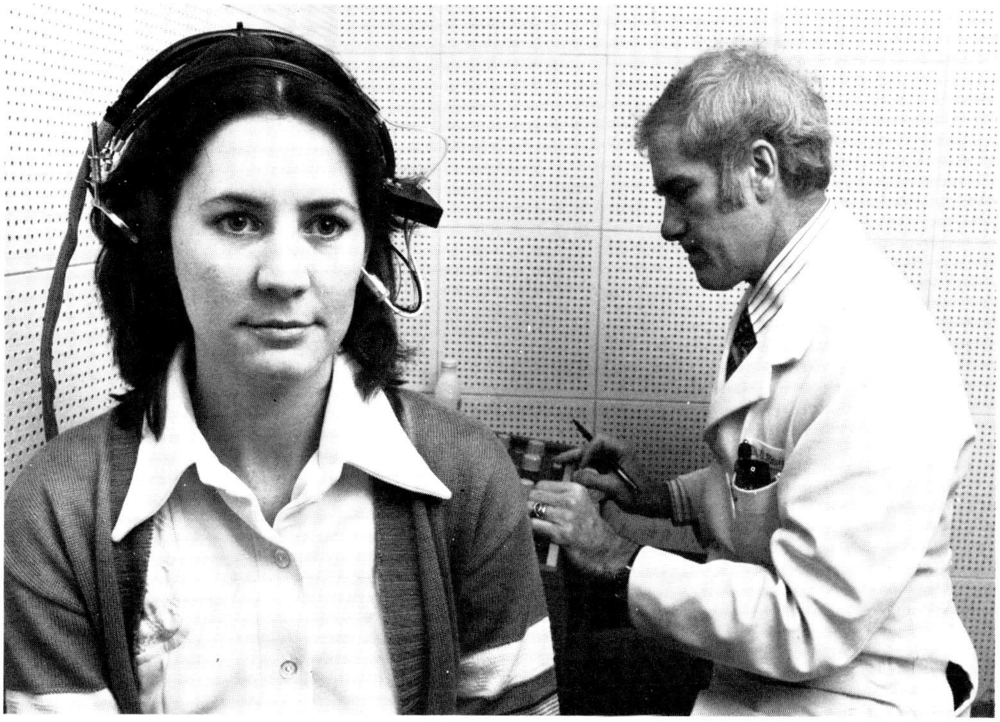

Fig. 34-2. Impedance audiometry is performed to test function of motor branch of facial nerve to stapedius muscle.

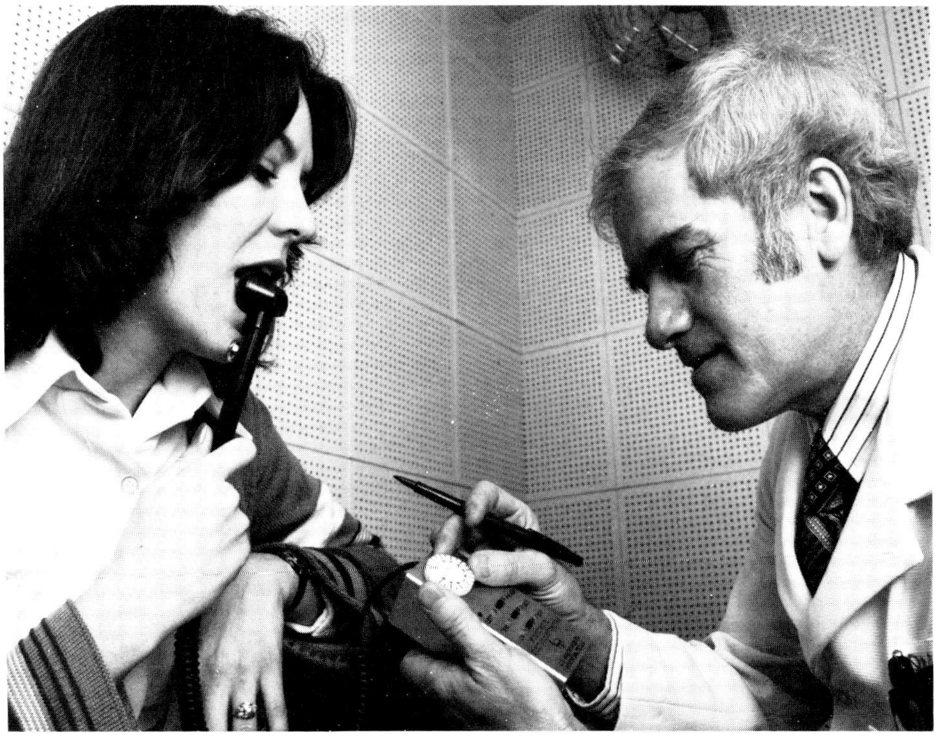

Fig. 34-3. Function of chorda tympani branch of facial nerve is tested with electrogustometry. Small positive current is delivered through gold-plated electrode held against anterior portion of tongue to elicit bitter or metallic taste.

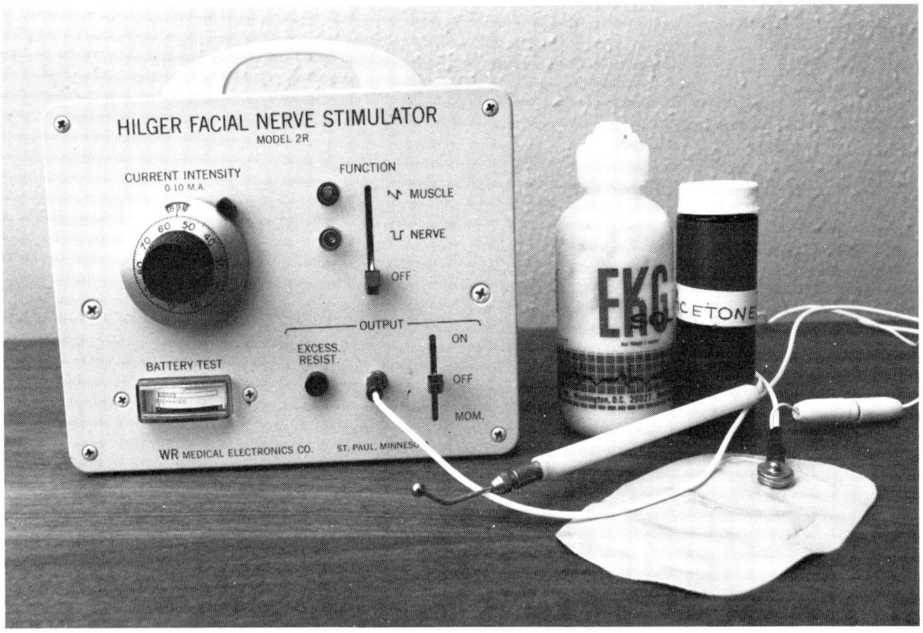

Fig. 34-4. Hilger facial nerve stimulator is used to test facial nerve electric excitability. Skin is initially cleansed of cosmetics, oil, or squamous debris with acetone, and then conductive electrode paste is applied.

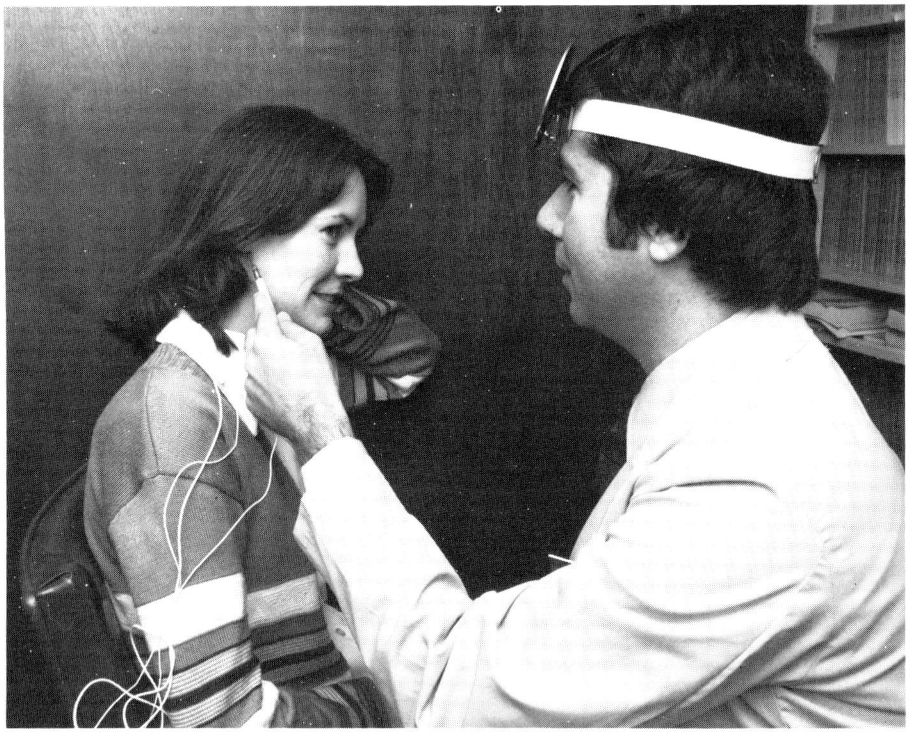

Fig. 34-5. Percutaneous facial nerve excitability is tested by applying current at angle of mandible until threshold contraction is observed. Normal and abnormal sides are compared; a difference of 3.5 mA or greater indicates degeneration.

rupted proximal to the stapedial branch, no change in the impedance will be detected.

A lesion in the vertical course of the nerve within the mastoid bone will reduce the taste function of the anterior two thirds of the tongue and diminish the salivary secretion from the submaxillary gland on the involved side. In this case the lacrimation and stapedial reflex will be intact and normal. The chorda tympani nerve function can be tested by electrogustometry (Fig. 34-3). By applying a small positive electric current to the tongue, a metallic or bitter taste is experienced by the patient. An absent or diminished response can be measured.

Facial nerve excitability testing is performed by applying a percutaneous electric current of low-intensity pulse of 1 msec or less at the angle of the jaw (Fig. 34-4). Both the paralyzed and the normal side are tested, and a comparison is made (Fig. 34-5). A difference of 3.5 mA or greater points to degeneration of the facial nerve.[11] It must be remembered that nerves undergoing degeneration will retain their ability to conduct a current for 72 hours. Therefore the nerve excitability must be carefully followed in a patient who has no evidence of voluntary contraction but does respond to electric stimulation. In addition to these diagnostic studies, a complete audiogram, electronystagmogram, and x-ray films of the petrous pyramids are obtained in the diagnostic workup of facial paralysis as indicated.

PRINCIPLES AND TECHNIQUE OF FACIAL NERVE SURGERY

The primary objective of facial nerve surgery is adequate exposure of the facial nerve at any point in its course without further injury to the nerve and with preservation of hearing and vestibular function. First and foremost, the surgeon must be familiar with the anatomy of the facial nerve throughout its entire intratemporal course. He must be able to use the operating microscope with ease, since brilliant illumination and magnification are of extreme importance. Experience in the use of various types of drills with both cutting and diamond burs is also important. The use of suction irrigation must also be mastered. Continuous suction irrigation keeps the field free of blood and bone dust. It also prevents possible damage to the facial nerve and adjacent structures by keeping the bone cool.

TRANSMASTOID APPROACH

The transmastoid approach allows for access to the facial nerve in its entire vertical course, horizontal course, and labyrinthine portion between the geniculate ganglion and the cochleariform process.[12] It is the usual procedure employed when there is serviceable hearing and normal vestibular function. Using the transmastoid approach preserves the normal anatomy and physiology of the outer, middle, and inner ear.

The patient is placed on the operating table in the supine position, and general anesthesia is used. A postauricular incision is made 1 cm posterior to the postauricular fold and carried down to the periosteum of the mastoid bone. The periosteum is then elevated superiorly along the superior temporal line and anteriorly until the cribriform area and spine of Henle are identified. The mastoid cortex is then drilled away initially along the superior temporal line and along a line tangential to the posterior bony external auditory canal. This exposure is then enlarged until the antrum of the mastoid is entered by identifying the horizontal semicircular canal and the perilabyrinthine cells. The mastoid is then further exposed to identify the tegmen of the mastoid covering the middle fossa dura, the sigmoid sinus and the sinodural angle, the mastoid tip, and the digastric ridge (Fig. 34-6). The fossa incudis and the ossicles are identified from their posterior aspect in the epitympanum. Having identified these important structures, the surgeon proceeds to thin the bone over the posterior bony canal wall. The facial nerve in its vertical course is then outlined by thinning the bone from the fossa incudis to the digastric ridge. The takeoff of the chorda tympani nerve is identified in order to delineate the facial recess, which is a triangular area of bone bordered by the fossa incudis superiorly, the vertical portion of the facial nerve medially, and the chorda tympani nerve laterally. The facial recess is then opened as widely as possible in order to visualize the pyramidal process, the stapes, incus, and horizontal portion of the facial nerve to the cochleariform process, in addition to the promontory and round window.

If the decompression is to be carried up to the geniculate ganglion, the bone above the body of the incus and malleus head is then removed, and the ampullated end of the superior semicircular canal is identified to avoid trauma to the labyrinth. Not infrequently it is necessary to disarticulate the incudostapedial joint to avoid a possible sensorineural hearing loss should the ossicular chain be touched by the high-speed drill. If the working area is limited, the incus may be removed until the decompression is completed and then replaced and secured in place with Gelfoam.

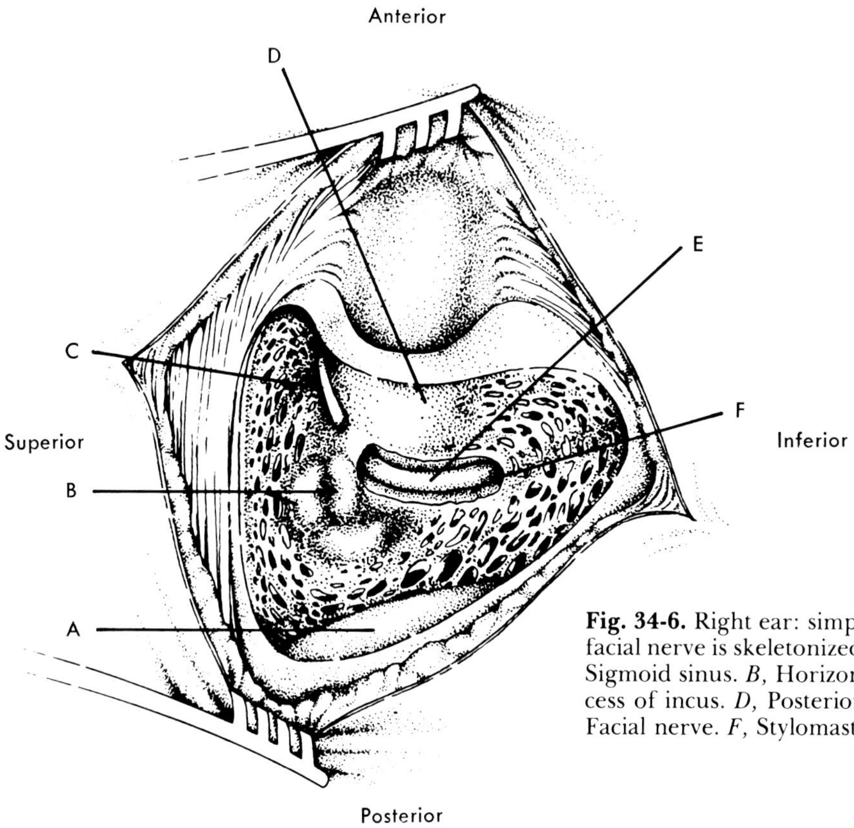

Fig. 34-6. Right ear: simple mastoidectomy is performed, and facial nerve is skeletonized in vertical and horizontal course. *A,* Sigmoid sinus. *B,* Horizontal semicircular canal. *C,* Short process of incus. *D,* Posterior wall of external auditory canal. *E,* Facial nerve. *F,* Stylomastoid foramen.

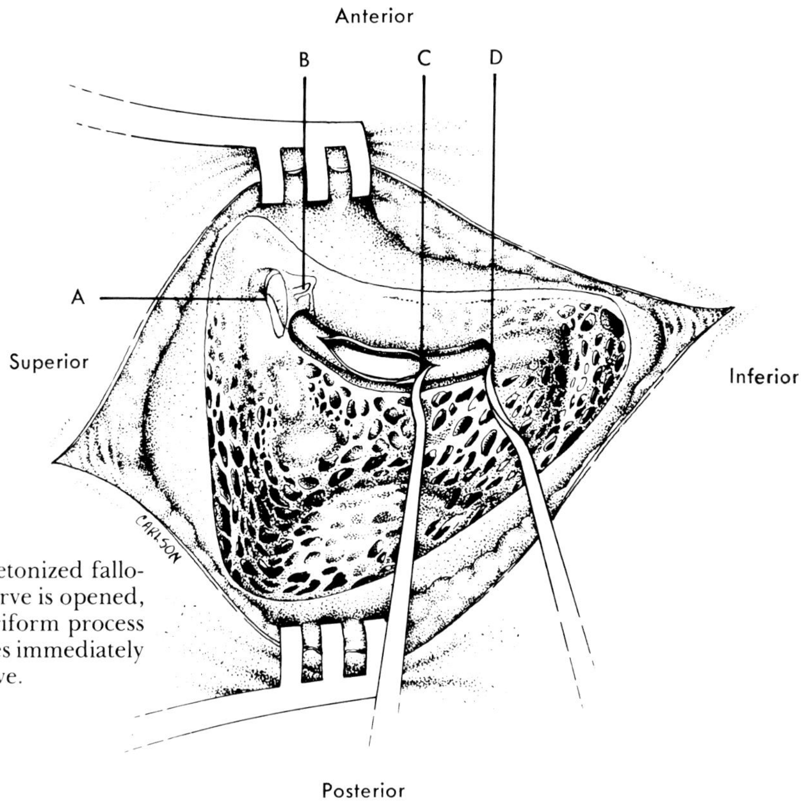

Fig. 34-7. Right ear: thinned bone of skeletonized fallopian canal is removed, *D,* and sheath of nerve is opened, using fine cataract knife, *C,* from cochleariform process to stylomastoid foramen. *A,* Incus. *B,* Stapes immediately inferior to horizontal course of facial nerve.

After the surgeon has outlined the facial nerve, the bone of the fallopian canal is then thinned down to eggshell consistency with a diamond drill. The facial nerve is thinned over its posterior 180 degrees in its vertical portion and over its lateral aspect at the external genu and horizontal and labyrinthine portions. The thinned bone is then removed from the facial nerve with a fine dental excavator in the vertical portion and a small sickle knife in the horizontal portion through the facial recess beneath the long process of the incus (Fig. 34-7).

After the bony fallopian canal has been unroofed and the facial nerve exposed, the sheath of the nerve is incised with a fine cataract knife. The sheath is incised parallel to the long axis of the nerve throughout the course of exposure to avoid cutting any of the nerve fibers. Upon completion of the decompression, the wound is closed without drainage with 3-0 Dexon or chromic catgut suture subcutaneously. Steri-Strips are used to approximate the skin edges, and a sterile mastoid dressing is applied.

MIDDLE CRANIAL FOSSA APPROACH

The middle cranial fossa approach to the facial nerve is indicated for exposure of the facial nerve in its labyrinthine course and within the internal auditory canal[8-10] (Fig. 34-8). It is used when the patient has serviceable hearing and intact vestibular function. This approach is most frequently used in conjunction with the transmastoid approach in order to perform a total facial nerve decompression (Fig. 34-9).

With the patient in the supine position and under general anesthesia, the head is turned to the uninvolved side and shaved to the midline. A standard preparation and draping is performed using povidone-iodine (Betadine) soap and solution. The line of incision is initially injected with 1% lidocaine (Xylocaine) with epinephrine 1:100,000. An incision is then made in the hairline just anterior to the ear above the level of the zygomatic arch (to avoid fibers of the facial nerve going to the frontalis muscle) and is carried superiorly and posteriorly in a gentle curve to approximately 4 cm above the helix. The temporalis muscle is then incised down to the periosteum of the calvaria parallel to the direction of its fibers. The attachment of the temporalis muscle and fascia to the zygomatic arch is then incised parallel to the arch to gain additional exposure. The superficial temporal artery is usually divided with this maneuver, and hemostasis is obtained with co-

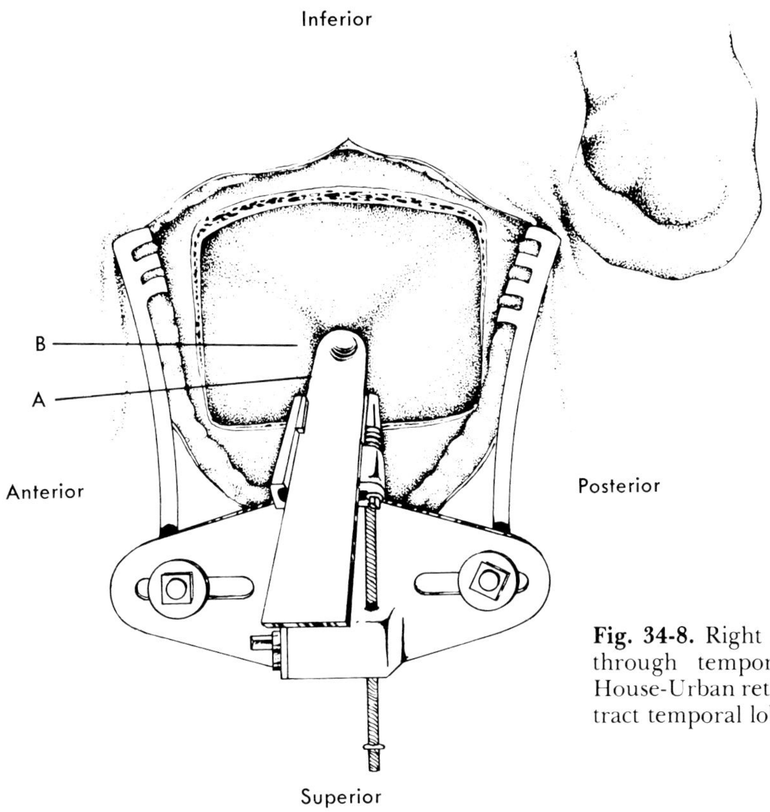

Fig. 34-8. Right middle fossa is entered through temporal craniectomy, using House-Urban retractor, *A*, to medially retract temporal lobe, *B*, extradurally.

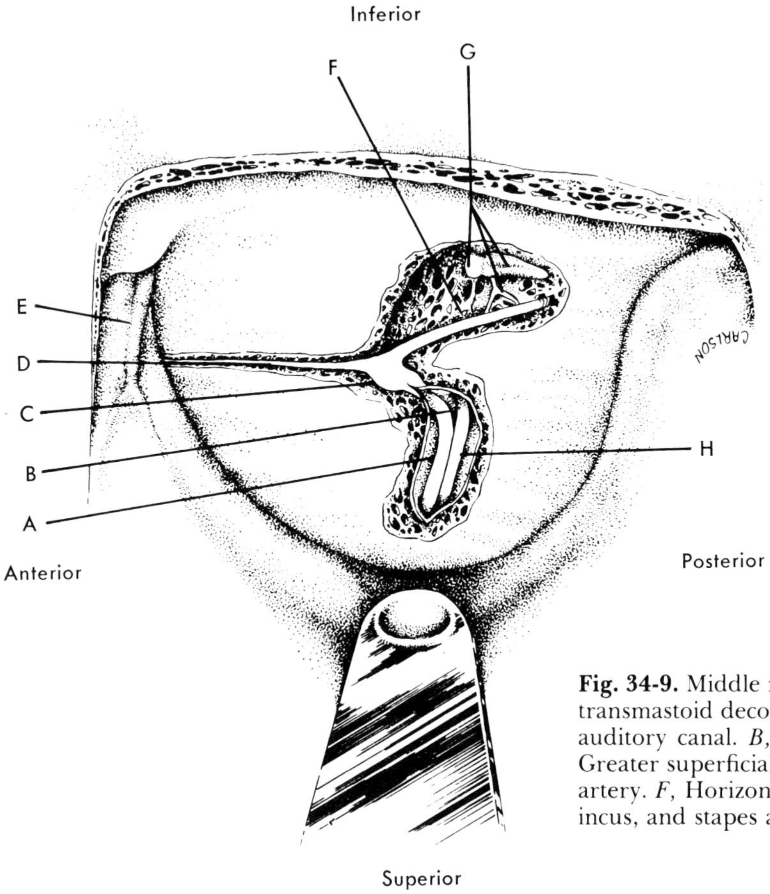

Fig. 34-9. Middle fossa decompression is combined with transmastoid decompression. *A,* Facial nerve in internal auditory canal. *B,* Bill bar. *C,* Geniculate ganglion. *D,* Greater superficial petrosal nerve. *E,* Middle meningeal artery. *F,* Horizontal course of facial nerve. *G,* Malleus, incus, and stapes as seen from above.

agulation or suture. The muscle and periosteum are then elevated, and the exposure is maintained with a self-retaining retractor positioned beneath the muscle. A rectangular temporal bone flap is then fashioned, with the base of the flap approximating the floor of the middle cranial fossa. Its anterior-posterior dimensions should be two thirds in front of the external auditory canal and one third behind this point. It is important that the temporal bone flap is fashioned with parallel sides to facilitate placement of the House-Urban retractor, which is used to elevate the temporal lobe and to maintain exposure during the procedure.

The bone flap is carefully elevated away from the dura, and any bleeding from the branches of the middle meningeal artery is controlled with bipolar coagulation. Bone wax is used to stop any bleeding from the diploic bone of the skull. The House-Urban retractor is then inserted between the edges of the craniectomy, and the blade is placed between the dura and the bone of the middle fossa after this bone has been carefully elevated. The dura may be very thin and may adhere to the bone floor in elderly patients. An opening in the dura may result in a profuse leakage of cerebrospinal fluid. If an opening occurs, the defect is sutured with silk, and this area is protected with a Cottonoid pledget.

After elevating the dura, the surgeon identifies the middle meningeal artery emerging from the foramen spinosum. This artery is the basic landmark for middle fossa surgery. Just medial to the artery is the thin bony roof of the eustachian tube, and lateral is the roof of the temporomandibular joint. Once the surgeon has identified the middle meningeal artery, the dissection is carried posteriorly where the arcuate eminence and ridge of the petrous pyramid are identified. After the dome of the arcuate eminence has been identified, the retractor blade is advanced to the ridge of bone corresponding to the superior petrosal sinus, and the dura is elevated in a posterior-to-anterior direction. This technique is important since the geniculate ganglion may be dehiscent without a bony covering in 5% of patients and may be injured during this maneuver.[8]

With the dura now retracted, the greater superficial petrosal nerve is identified and followed posteriorly by removing its bony covering using a diamond bur with continuous suction-irrigation. The geniculate ganglion is then identified. The labyrinthine portion of the facial nerve is exposed as it runs medially to the fundus or lateral extent of the internal auditory canal. The labyrinthine portion also has a slight posterior direction due to the presence of the basal turn of the cochlea. The surgeon continues the dissection by carefully uncovering the thick bony roof of the internal auditory canal, exposing the dural covering.

After the dura has been exposed, the surgeon locates a triangular strut of bone (Bill bar) at the fundus of the canal. This vertical crest of bone separates the facial nerve anteriorly from the superior vestibular nerve posteriorly in the internal auditory canal. Once the landmarks have been identified, the dura is opened posteriorly over the superior vestibular nerve to allow for an anterior-based dural flap to protect the facial nerve. The wound is inspected for complete hemostasis after the completion of the middle fossa decompression. A small plug of temporalis muscle and fascia is placed over the internal auditory canal to prevent cerebrospinal fluid leakage. The retractor is removed and the temporal lobe allowed to reexpand to its normal location. The bone flap is replaced, and the temporalis muscle and fascia are then approximated. The galea and skin are closed with interrupted nonabsorbable suture. Drainage is not used. A sterile dressing is applied and the patient is observed in the intensive care unit until the afternoon of the first postoperative day.

TOTAL FACIAL NERVE DECOMPRESSION

Combined transmastoid–middle cranial fossa approach

The facial nerve may be exposed and decompressed throughout its entire intratemporal course in the fallopian canal from the porus acusticus in the internal auditory canal to its point of exit at the stylomastoid foramen. A total facial nerve decompression entails a combination of the transmastoid and middle cranial fossa approaches if serviceable hearing and vestibular function are to be preserved[16] (Fig. 34-10).

A transmastoid decompression is performed with the patient under general anesthesia. A small opening is made in the tegmen of the epitympanum above the malleus and incus and just lateral to the geniculate ganglion. This small opening serves as a reliable and readily identifiable landmark in the middle fossa. A separate incision is then made for the middle fossa decompression and the procedure carried out as previously described. Upon completion of the total facial nerve decompression a small piece of bone is placed over the opening to the epitympanum from above to prevent adhesions between the dura and ossicular chain, which could result in a conductive-type hearing loss. The wounds are each closed in layers and a sterile dressing applied. The patient is observed overnight in the intensive care unit.

Translabyrinthine approach

A total facial nerve decompression can be performed through the postauricular translabyrinthine approach. This approach allows for complete exposure of the facial nerve from the porus acusticus in the internal auditory canal to the stylomastoid foramen as it exits the mastoid. This procedure is used when total decompression of the facial nerve is indicated in a patient who does not have serviceable hearing or vestibular function.

With the patient in a supine position under general anesthesia the postauricular and temporal areas are prepared and draped in a sterile field. A postauricular incision is made approximately 2 cm posterior to the postauricular fold, extending from 1 cm above the superior level of the helix to 2 cm posterior to the mastoid tip. This incision is carried down to the periosteum of the mastoid, which is elevated along with the soft tissues up to the external auditory canal. A complete wide mastoidectomy is performed, and the mastoidectomy is extended above the external auditory canal into the epitympanum, exposing the malleus and incus from behind. The facial nerve is then skeletonized in its vertical course to its exit from the mastoid at the stylomastoid foramen. The external genu of the facial nerve is identified, and a thin layer of bone is left covering the genu for protection during the labyrinthectomy. The sigmoid sinus and superior petrosal sinus are carefully skeletonized, leaving a thin layer of bone over them.

A complete labyrinthectomy is then performed by fenestrating the posterior, horizontal, and superior semicircular canals, followed by a complete exenteration of the labyrinth until the vestibule of the inner ear is identified (Fig. 34-11). The internal auditory canal is then skeletonized in its posterior 180 degrees. The fibers of the superior vestibular nerve are identified as they enter the vestibule, and bony removal is carried out along the superior vestibular nerve to the internal auditory canal. The facial nerve is then identified as it enters the internal canal by removing bone superior to the superior

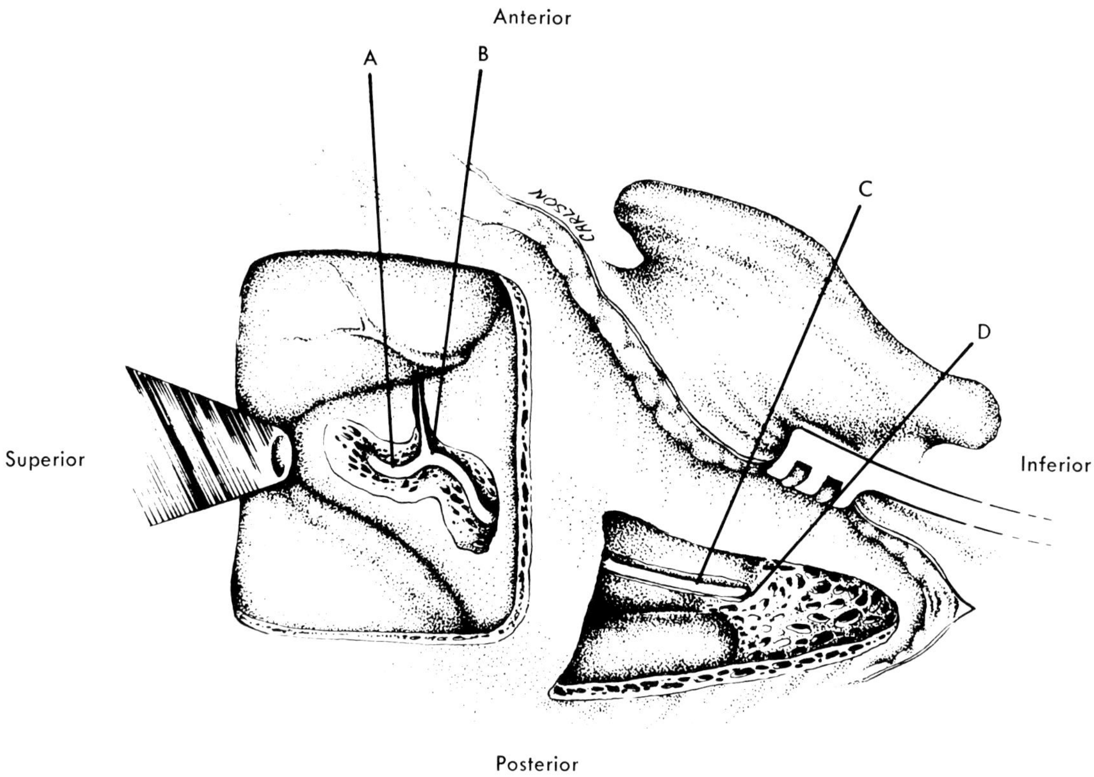

Fig. 34-10. Total facial nerve decompression by combined transmastoid–middle fossa approach has been completed with preservation of audiovestibular function. *A,* Facial nerve in internal auditory canal. *B,* Geniculate ganglion. *C,* Vertical course of facial nerve in mastoid. *D,* Facial nerve exiting mastoid at stylomastoid foramen.

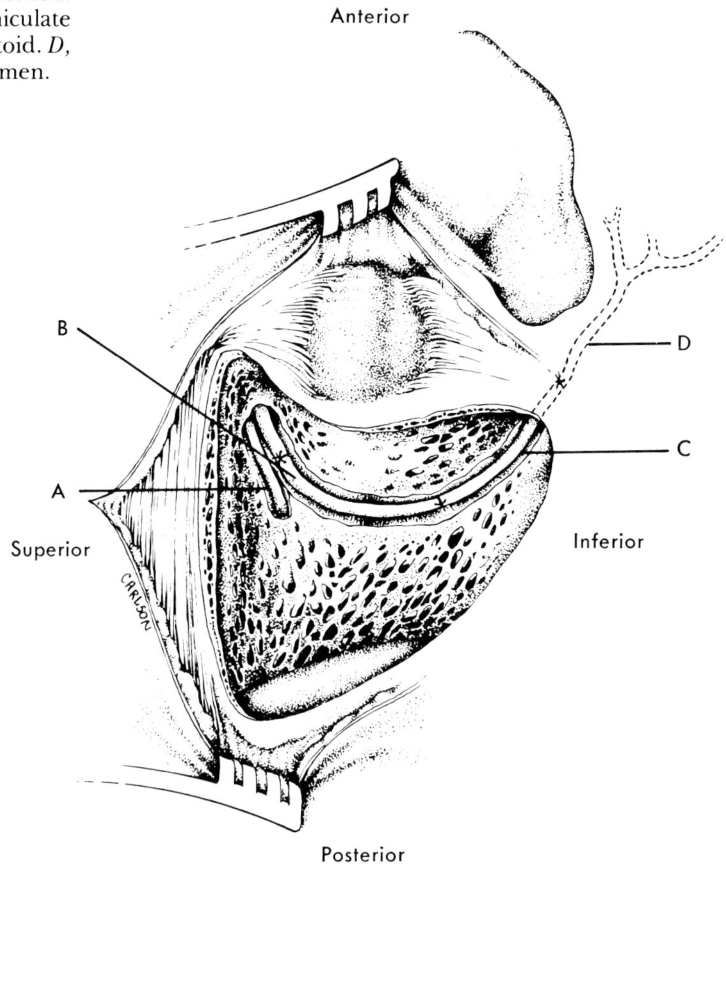

Fig. 34-11. Right labyrinthectomy has been performed, and facial nerve is exposed throughout its entire intratemporal course to internal auditory canal, *A. B,* Graft of facial nerve within mastoid. Facial nerve can be grafted from its vertical course in mastoid, *C,* to its extratemporal course, *D.*

vestibular nerve and identifying a vertical crest of bone (Bill bar) that lies between the facial nerve and the superior vestibular nerve at the fundus of the internal auditory canal.

The entire course of the facial nerve is then exposed from the porus acusticus to the stylomastoid foramen by use of a diamond stone bur and continuous suction irrigation. The incus and malleus head are removed to facilitate exposure of the horizontal course. If exposure and access are limited, bone may be removed from the sigmoid sinus and posterior fossa dura. The exposure can be maintained by using the Leyla retractor to keep the sigmoid sinus compressed during the remainder of the procedure. When the nerve has been totally exposed, the sheath of the nerve is then incised throughout its entire course. A vestibular nerve section may be performed during the procedure to allow for examination of the facial nerve within the internal canal.

When the procedure has been completed and hemostatis obtained, the epitympanum is sealed with a plug of temporalis muscle, and temporalis fascia and a muscle plug are used to cover the opening to the internal auditory canal to prevent cerebrospinal fluid leakage. The wound is closed in layers, and a sterile mastoid dressing is applied. The patient is observed in the intensive care unit until the morning of the first postoperative day.

Retrolabyrinthine approach

The retrolabyrinthine approach may be used to gain access to the facial nerve in the posterior fossa as it exits the brain stem to the internal auditory canal. Hearing and balance function can be preserved. The procedure is performed under general anesthesia in a supine position with the head turned so that the involved side is up. A postauricular incision is made, and the soft tissues and periosteum are elevated from the mastoid. A wide complete mastoidectomy is performed, and bone over the sigmoid sinus and the bone immediately posterior to the sinus are removed. The bone covering the posterior fossa dura is removed down to the level of the posterior semicircular canal. The middle fossa plate superiorly and the jugular bulb inferiorly are skeletonized to serve as landmarks for the limits of the dissection. When the bone removal is completed, the dura is incised anterior to the sigmoid sinus but posterior to the endolymphatic sac in order to preserve its function.

As cerebrospinal fluid is released from the posterior fossa, the cerebellum will recede posteriorly, allowing for visualization of the exiting cranial nerve roots. The seventh and eighth cranial nerves can be visualized along with the brain stem and adjacent blood vessels. Anterior to the seventh and eighth cranial nerves lies the trigeminal nerve, and the ninth and tenth cranial nerves can be seen as they travel to the jugular foramen.

Prior to wound closure, bleeding is controlled. The dura is closed with silk suture, and a temporalis muscle plug is then placed over the surgical defect to prevent cerebrospinal fluid leakage. The remainder of the wound is closed in layers, without drainage, and a sterile mastoid dressing is applied. The patient is observed overnight in the intensive care unit; his usual postoperative stay is approximately 5 days.

Facial nerve grafting

When the continuity of the facial nerve has been disrupted by either trauma or tumor removal, an autogenous nerve graft may be used to bridge the gap. Grafting is the primary means by which emotional expression can be restored; however, complete restoration of function is not usually attainable.[4] The factors responsible are proliferation of connective tissue between the anastomotic surfaces of the nerve ends and nondirected growth of the regenerating fibers.[13] Mass movement of the reinnervated facial muscles is usually the result of the haphazard regeneration of the nerve fibers.

Precise approximation of the nerve ends by an atraumatic technique is very important. This is accomplished by using the operating microscope and avoiding tension at the anastomotic site. When an end-to-end anastomosis cannot be accomplished without tension, a free graft should be used. The graft should be 3 mm longer on each side of the gap in order to avoid tension.[7] Minimal suturing will decrease the amount of trauma and subsequent connective tissue proliferation. Millesi has shown that the source of connective tissue ingrowth is the epineural layer of the nerve trunks.[15] Circumferential resection of this layer at the anastomotic site may avoid this source of connective tissue ingrowth.

The great auricular nerve is the most common nerve used in facial nerve grafting. Other suitable nerves are the sural nerve and the lateral femoral cutaneous nerve. The great auricular nerve has the advantages of proximity to the operative site and of suitable length and diameter for grafting the facial nerve. It can be located along a line perpendicular to the midpoint of the distance between the mastoid tip and the angle of the mandible.

Trauma and surgical lesions are the most common causes of repair of the horizontal or vertical course of the facial nerve. It is usually possible to use the fallopian canal as the graft bed, and small sutures are used to approximate the graft.[17] Because of the natural self-adherence between cut nerve surfaces, the suturing may be avoided within the mastoid and middle ear portions of the facial nerve. The grafts can be secured by thrombin glue made from the patient's plasma and combined with topical thrombin at the anastomotic site. Gelfoam saturated in topical thrombin may also be used to secure the anastomosis. When the anastomosis will be subject to movement from surrounding muscles in extratemporal areas or from pulsations from the cerebrospinal fluid, very fine monofilament suture should be used to maintain the anastomosis.

It may be possible to reroute the nerve through the middle ear to obtain a direct end-to-end anastomosis. However, due to the potential loss of blood supply most surgeons prefer to graft the nerve rather than to reroute it. If a large segment has been destroyed in the middle ear and labyrinthine portions, the nerve can be directly anastomosed from the internal auditory canal to the vertical course with little tension by using the translabyrinthine approach if the hearing is not serviceable. If the hearing is serviceable, a combined transmastoid–middle cranial fossa approach may be used and the geniculate ganglion bypassed in performing a direct end-to-end anastomosis of the labyrinthine and horizontal portions of the facial nerve.[6] If an intratemporal graft or end-to-end anastomosis cannot be accomplished, then one of many extratemporal reconstructive procedures will be required.

COMPLICATIONS OF SURGERY

Due to the very compact anatomy of the temporal bone and the course of the facial nerve, several structures are at risk during temporal bone surgery. Injury to the sigmoid sinus may result in profuse venous bleeding. The sinus may lie superficial to the mastoid cortex or deep to it if the mastoid is well pneumatized. The sinus may also lie far anteriorly, almost adjacent to the posterior wall of the external auditory canal. If the sigmoid sinus is injured and bleeding occurs, extraluminal packing with Surgicel will usually control the hemorrhage. If this bleeding is not controlled, proximal and distal extradural packing of the sigmoid sinus may be necessary.

Hearing loss and disturbances of balance function may also occur during the course of facial nerve surgery. The auditory ossicles are in close proximity to the horizontal or tympanic course of the facial nerve. They may be dislocated or traumatized when opening the facial recess or in decompression of the horizontal portion of the facial nerve. If the incudostapedial joint is intact and the drill contacts the ossicular chain, vibrations transmitted to the cochlea may result in an irreversible sensorineural hearing loss. Any invasion into the perilymphatic space through either the vestibule or the semicircular canals may result not only in vestibular dysfunction but also in sensorineural hearing loss. This damage may occur from instruments or from removal of diseased tissue adjacent to or involving the facial nerve.

The jugular bulb may be encountered, particularly when working medial to the vertical course of the facial nerve. Occasionally the jugular bulb may have a high placement adjacent to the inferior crus of the posterior semicircular canal or even directly inferior to the internal auditory canal. Damage to this structure can result in profuse bleeding. Control of hemorrhage can be obtained by extraluminal packing. If necessary, the sigmoid sinus can be packed extradurally for proximal control, and the internal jugular vein can be ligated high in the neck for distal control. This ligation will prevent any embolization of packing or thrombus from the jugular bulb.

The dura of both the middle fossa and the posterior fossa may be exposed during any type of temporal bone surgery. An injury or tear of the dura can result in a cerebrospinal fluid leak or a herniation of part of the temporal lobe or of the cerebellum. Cerebrospinal fluid leakage can usually be controlled by packing with fascia and muscle.

Bleeding can also occur as a complication of middle fossa surgery, resulting in a subdural or epidural hematoma. Retraction of the temporal lobe can produce a postoperative hemiparesis. If the physician is operating over the dominant hemisphere, an expressive aphasia or dysphasia can occur.

Infection can occur in any type of surgery during the postoperative period. However, when the subarachnoid space has been entered or the dura of the middle or posterior fossa surgically traumatized, meningitis can develop during the first postoperative week. The patient is carefully observed, with frequent monitoring of temperature during this postsurgical period.

SUMMARY

Modern techniques of neuro-otologic surgery enable the otologist to surgically expose the facial nerve throughout its entire course without further trauma to the nerve itself. Auditory and vestibular function can be preserved, and the production of a mastoid cavity can be avoided. Each procedure described has its specific indications, depending on the site of the pathology and the status of the auditory and vestibular function.

The facial nerve travels through a longer bony canal than any other motor nerve. In 90% of patients the abnormality is located in the intratemporal course of the nerve and requires detailed analysis and careful otologic surgical technique.

REFERENCES

1. Alford, B. R., Sessions, R. R., and Weber, S. C.: Indications for surgical decompression of the facial nerve, Laryngoscope **81:**620-635, 1971.
2. Alford, B. R. Jerger, J. F., Coats, A. C. et al.: Neurophysiology of facial nerve testing, Arch. Otolaryngol. **97:**214-219, 1973.
3. Cawthorne, T.: Intratemporal facial palsy, Arch. Otolaryngol. **90:**789-799, 1969.
4. Conley, J.: Facial nerve grafting, Arch. Otolaryngol. **73:**322-327, 1961.
5. Crabtree, J. A.: Herpes zoster oticus, Laryngoscope **78:**1853-1878, 1968.
6. Fisch, U.: Operations of the facial nerve in its labyrinthine and meatal course. In Miehlke, A. editor: Surgery of the facial nerve, Philadelphia, 1973, W. B. Saunders Company.
7. Fisch, U.: Facial nerve grafting, Otolaryngol. Clin. North Am. **7:**517-529, 1974.
8. Glasscock, M. E.: Middle fossa approach to the temporal bone. An otologic frontier, Arch. Otolaryngol. **90:**41-53, 1969.
9. House, W. F.: Surgical exposure of the internal auditory canal and its contents through the middle cranial fossa, Laryngoscope **71:**1363-1385, 1961.
10. House, W. F., and Crabtree, J. A.: Surgical exposure of the petrous portion of seventh nerve, Arch. Otolaryngol. **81:**506-507, 1965.
11. Jongkees, L. B. W.: Tests for facial nerve function, Arch. Otolaryngol. **89:**127-130, 1969.
12. Lewis, M. D., Jr.: A variation in technique of facial nerve decompression, Laryngoscope **66:**1451-1463, 1956.
13. McCabe, B. F.: Facial nerve grafting, Plast. Reconstr. Surg. **45:**70-75, 1970.
14. McHugh, H. E.: Surgical treatment of facial paralysis and traumatic conductive deafness in fractures of the temporal bone, Ann. Otolaryngol. Chir. Cervicofac. **68:**855-899, 1959.
15. Millesi, H., et al. as cited in Fisch.[7]
16. Pulec, J. L.: Total decompression of the facial nerve, Laryngoscope **76:**1015-1028, 1966.
17. Pulec, J. L.: Facial nerve grafting, Laryngoscope **79:**1562-1583, 1969.
18. Pulec, J. L.: Facial nerve tumors, Ann. Otol. Rhinol. Laryingol. **78:**962, 1969.
19. Shambaugh, G. E., and Clemis, J. D.: Facial nerve paralysis. In Paparella, M. M., and Shumrick, D. A., editors: Otolaryngology, vol. 2, Philadelphia, 1973, W. B. Saunders Company.

SUGGESTED READINGS

Ballance, C., and Duel, A. B.: The operative treatment of facial palsy by introduction of nerve grafts into the fallopian canal and by other intratemporal methods, Arch. Otolaryngol. **15:**1-70, 1932.

Bunnell, S.: Suture of facial nerve within the temporal bone, with report of first successful case, Surg. Gynecol. Obstet. **45:**7, 1927.

Dott, N.: Facial nerve reconstruction by graft bypassing the petrous bone, Arch. Otolaryngol. **78:**426, 1963.

Ducker, T. B., Kempe, L. G., and Hayes, G. J.: The metabolic background for peripheral nerve surgery, J. Neurosurg. **30:**270-280, 1969.

Rosenberg, J. J., and Alford, B. R.: Experimentally controlled facial nerve injuries, Arch. Otolaryngol. **84:**337-342, 1966.

Chapter 35

Palpebral magnets for paretic lagophthalmos

Wolfgang D. Mühlbauer

In the paralyzed eyelid, sphincter function may be restored by implanting two small permanent magnetic rods near the upper and lower eyelid margin[1-5] (Fig. 35-1). These not only achieve eye closure but also act as antagonists to the intact levator muscles, thus mimicing near-normal lid function.

Modern permanent magnets are characterized by a high-energy product and coercivity that exert a maximum of attractive force with a minimum of volume and weight. Platinum-cobalt (Pt Co) was found to be the most suitable permanent magnetic material for eyelid surgery. The magnets* are manufactured as slightly curved rods with radii of 15 to 17 mm, contoured to the eyelid margin. They vary from 8 to 15 mm in length and weigh between 50 and 250 mg (Fig. 35-2). The north pole faces are marked, and the rods are perforated for better suture fixation to the tarsus. As platinum-cobalt is biologically inert, the magnets need not be coated before implantation.

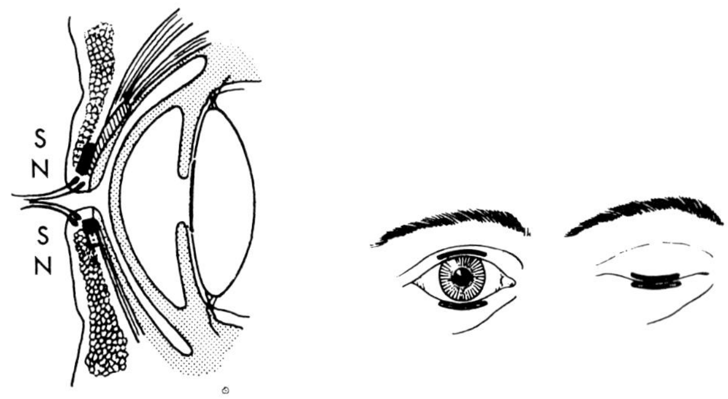

Fig. 35-1. Topography of palpebral magnets. (From Mühlbauer, W. D., Segeth, H., and Viessmann, A.: Chir. Plast. **1**:295-304, 1973.)

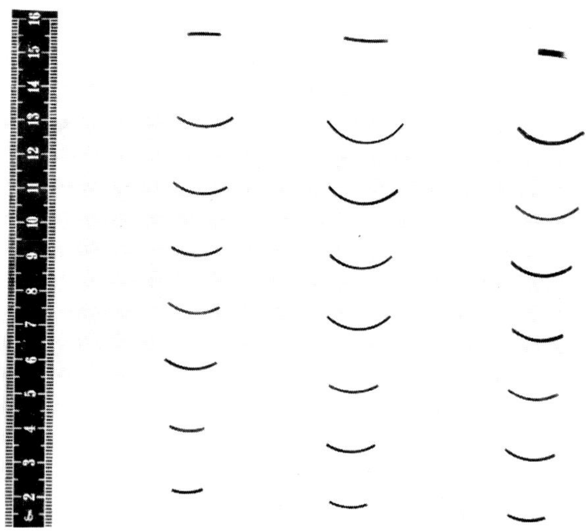

Fig. 35-2. Palpebral magnets with centimeter scale for comparison of size. (From Mühlbauer, W. D., Segeth, H., and Viessmann, A.: Chir. Plast. **1**:295-304, 1973.)

DETERMINATION OF ATTRACTIVE FORCE

The attractive force of a double magnet system is a function of the air gap between the pole faces. As the air gap increases, the attractive force decreases by the square of the distance. In the open eye position with lid angles of 45 to 60 degrees, very little magnetic force is exerted (Fig. 35-3).

When the patient tries to close the paralyzed eyelids, the levator muscles relax, and the upper eyelid comes down a few millimeters, thus decreasing the lid angle to approximately 30 degrees. This

*Magnet-service F. Henning, 8035 Gauting b. Munchen Postfach 237, Ammersee Strasse 28⅓ Ger.

increases the attractive force of the magnets enough to take over and complete eyelid closure (Fig. 35-4). When the eyelids are closed, 1,600 to 2,000 milliponds (mp) are sufficient to close the eye securely and still permit the intact levators to open the eye physiologically. When the levator muscles are chosen correctly, the magnetic sphincter thus becomes a true antagonist to them.

Clinically, a pair of palpebral magnets, taken from a set of standard sizes, is taped to the upper and lower eyelid approximately 2 mm away from the margin (Fig. 35-5). Lid function is observed for some time at various positions. If the magnets differ in size, the larger one should be used for the upper eyelid so as not to compound an existing lower eyelid ectropion. The standard sizes may be shortened for additional variation of the attractive force.

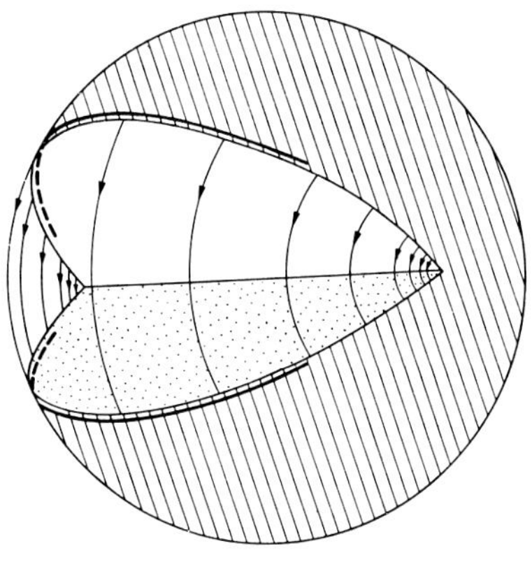

Fig. 35-3. Eyelid opening angle as parameter of action of palpebral magnets. (From Mühlbauer, W. D., Segeth, H., and Viessmann, A.: Chir. Plast. **1**:295-304, 1973.)

An alternative approach is to implant magnetically saturated magnets from a standard set and demagnetize them selectively in situ with a degaussing device (Fig. 35-8). Selective demagnetization in situ is an elegant way to gradually decrease the attractive force, where progressive reinnervation of the seventh nerve takes place. Adding magnetism to the prefabricated rods would be of equal interest,

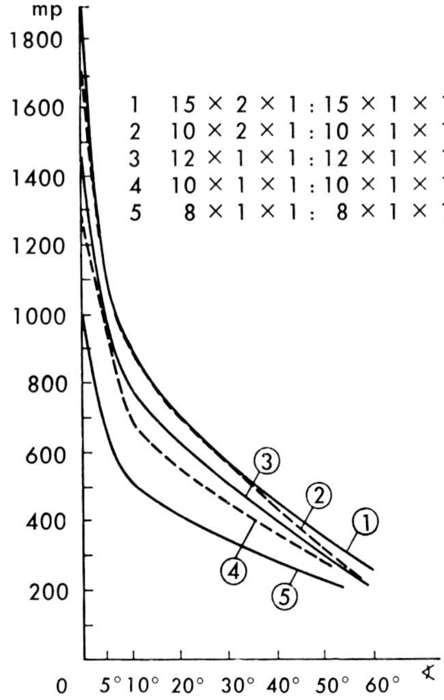

Fig. 35-4. Range of action of two palpebral magnets. Attractive force, P, in millipонds (mp) as function of lid angle from zero to sixty degrees. Lines *1* to *5* represent measurements of double magnet systems of various dimensions ($Sr \cdot O \cdot 6 \cdot Fe_2O_3$). (From Mühlbauer, W. D., Segeth, H., and Viessmann, A.: Chir. Plast. **1**:295-304, 1973.)

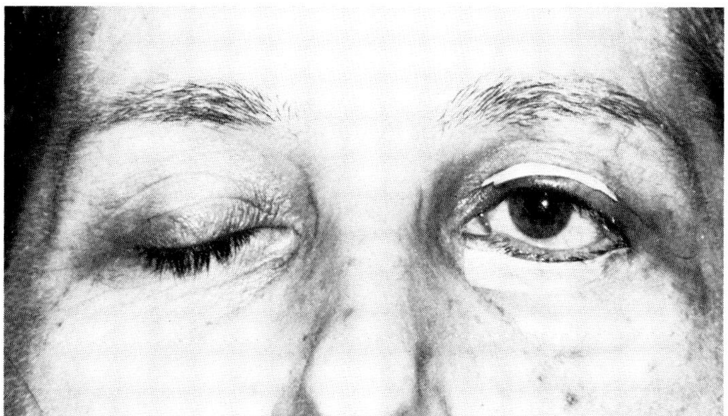

Fig. 35-5. Empirical determination of necessary attractive force with magnets taped to lids.

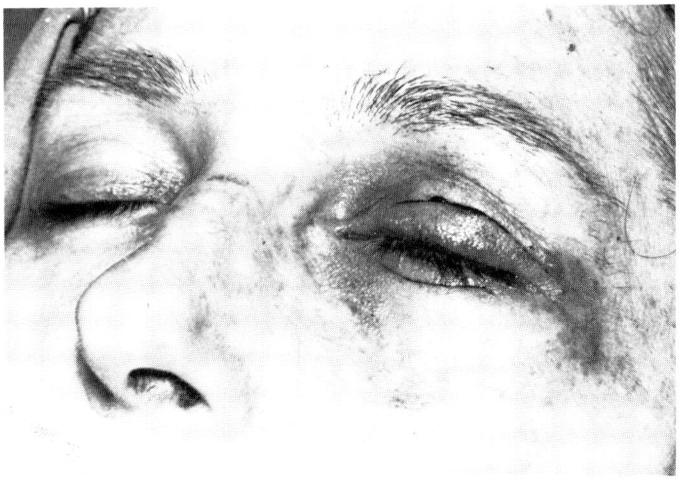

Fig. 35-6. Incisions in upper and lower eyelid with palpebral magnets already implanted.

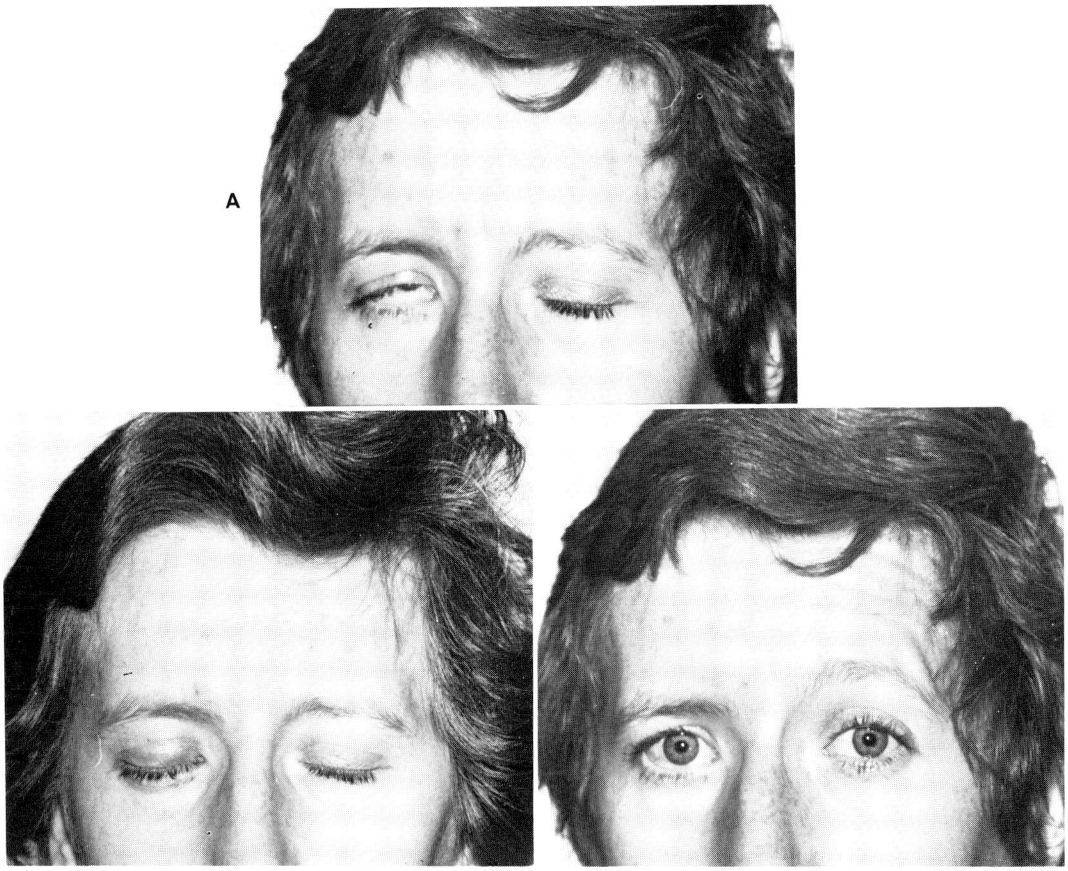

A

B

C

Fig. 35-7. Restoration of eyelid function in facial palsy with palpebral magnets. **A,** Before, and **B** and **C,** 3 months after implantation.

but no handy and portable device has been developed.

More sophisticated methods to determine the necessary attractive force are restricted to the laboratory.

OPERATIVE TECHNIQUE

With the patient under local anesthesia, this procedure can be easily performed. Incisions through the skin and orbicularis are made in the upper eyelid fold and 3 to 4 mm from the lower lid margin down to the tarsal plate (Fig. 35-6). A small pocket is dissected between tarsus and orbicularis muscle fibers as close to the lid margin as possible. The magnets are then secured to the tarsus with three or four permanent sutures through the prefabricated holes. Great care must be taken that alternating (north-south) poles face and attract each other because similar poles will repel. The orbicularis fibers and skin are then repaired. No dressing should be applied.

RESULTS

Since 1972, 114 patients with unilateral lagophthalmos and three patients with bilateral lagophthalmos were treated with this procedure (Table 13). Roughly two thirds of the cases were operated on within days or weeks of the onset of paralysis. The rest had long-standing irreversible facial palsies with various inadequate attempts at correction of the lagophthalmos. In these late cases, additional procedures were frequently necessary to correct a pronounced lower lid ectropion at the same time. Medial or lateral tarsorrhaphies, silicone plates, or small silicone tubes in which the lower lid magnet was incorporated for static suspension of the lower eyelid were performed.

In 74 cases a good result was obtained with freedom of symptoms and restoration of lid function to near normal. The shape, height, and width of the palpebral fissure remained undisturbed and corresponded favorably to the normal side (Fig. 35-7).

Table 13. Palpebral magnets for paretic lagophthalmos

Results (1972-1976)	*Cases*	*Percent*
Good	74	61.7
Satisfactory	27	22.5
Not improved	4	3.3
Extrusions	15	12.5
TOTALS	120	100

Twenty-seven cases were rated satisfactory with a residual lagophthalmos of 1 to 1.5 mm as a result of slightly underestimating the necessary magnetic force. Yet the cornea was covered and fully protected during sleep so that no gross irritation was present.

In four cases no improvement was seen due to marked spasticity and retraction of the levator muscles after long-standing disease.

In 15 patients one or both magnets were extruded through the skin, but the globe was never injured. Two extrusions were due to infection. Gradual erosion and perforation of the lateral end of the magnets resulted from insufficient soft tissue cover, loosening of the anchoring stitches, or sharp edges of the early models.

In all cases the magnets were replaced either immediately or some weeks later. All healed with satisfactory or good results.

DISCUSSION

Palpebral magnets are useful in the majority of patients to restore dynamic function to paretic eyelids to protect the vulnerable cornea. The tiny foreign bodies are well tolerated and practically invisible. The natural shape and size of the palpebral fissure remain undisturbed. No fading of the magnetic energy is to be expected in these high-quality permanent magnets. Although the blinking reflex is a bit slow, the voluntary eyelid movements are near normal. Best results are obtained in patients who are operated on within days or weeks of the onset of paralysis. It seems important to restore the missing antagonist to the levator early in the course.

In many long-standing palsies one observes levator retraction or spasticity with a sort of paradoxical motion when the patient tries to close his eyes. In these cases it may take weeks after implantation of the magnets before lid functions return to normal. I found it helpful to tell these patients to look downward when trying to close the eyes to encourage relaxation and stretch of the levators and possibly the superior rectus muscle.

In some patients a partial or total levator recession is necessary. Great care must be taken to test and select the correct pair of magnets preoperatively so as to accurately restore the delicate balance of power between the intact levators and the magnetic sphincter. In situ decrease of the magnetic force is possible with a degaussing device. One should not attempt to obtain a "click" closure mech-

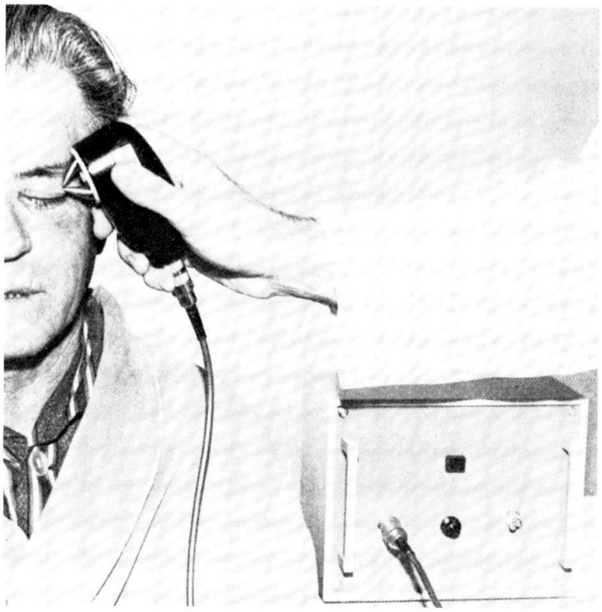

Fig. 35-8. Demagnetization in situ in bilateral facial palsy with special device.

anism. The result might be quite impressive, but the necessary antagonistic force is not physiologically strong, resulting in late pain and difficulty in opening the eye in the morning. Too much pressure on the lid margins was the major cause of extrusion of the magnets.

A pronounced lower lid ectropion requires simultaneous correction with an appropriate procedure.

The palpebral magnets provide excellent temporary palliation in reversible facial palsy and function well as permanent palliation in irreversible palsies. They may also be used as an adjunct to other operative procedures to augment an otherwise incomplete correction of paretic lagophthalmos. Marked atrophy of the lid structures and poor skin coverage is the only contraindication.

SUMMARY

A method has been presented to restore dynamic eyelid function in facial palsy with the implantation of two permanent magnets near the upper and lower eyelid margin. The attractive force characteristics of the double magnet system closely simulate the action of the paralyzed orbicularis sphincter. Normal lid opening is accomplished by the intact levators. The width and contour of the palpebral fissure remain undisturbed and are comparable to those of the normal side. The magnetic material used is characterized by a high-energy product and coercivity, which permit minimal volume and weight. The magnets are biologically well tolerated without coating.

Clinical experiences on 114 patients with unilateral and three patients with bilateral paretic lagophthalmos due to complete facial palsy have been reported. In the majority of cases near-normal lid functions could be restored with full protection of the eye. In 15 patients one or two magnets were extruded usually due to technical error. Palpebral magnets are indicated as temporary palliation in reversible palsy, as permanent palliation in irreversible facial palsy, and as adjuncts to other procedures to augment an incomplete correction of the lagophthalmos.

REFERENCES

1. Hinzpeter, E. N., and Riehn, E.: Preliminary experience with lid magnets for paralytic lagophthalmos, Trans. Ophthalmol. Soc. U.K. **96:**73-78, 1976.
2. Momma W. G., and Biermann, B.: Eine einfache Methode, die Lidfunktion bei Fazialisparese mit Permanentmagneten wiederherzustellen, Klin. Monatsbl. Augenheilkd. **169:**529-533, 1976.
3. Mühlbauer, W. D.: Palpebral magnets in facial palsy. Marchac, D., and Hueston, J., editors: In transactions of the sixth International Congress of Plastic and Reconstructive Surgery, Paris, 1976 Masson, p. 333.
4. Mühlbauer, W. D., Segeth H., and Viessmann, A.: Restoration of lid function in facial palsy with permanent magnets, Chir. Plast., **1:**295-304, 1973.
5. Mühlbauer, W. D., Segeth H., and Viessmann, A.: Wiederherstellung eines funktionellen Lidschlusses bei Fazialisparese durch Implantation von Dauermagneten. In Höhler, H., editor: Plastische und Wiederherstellungschirurgie aus Klinik und Forschung, Stuttgart, 1975, Schattauer.

Chapter 36

Temporalis muscle transposition technique for late permanent facial paralysis

Leonard R. Rubin

Our attempts to find the substitute for a paralyzed facial motor apparatus have fallen short of their mark. This symposium has demonstrated that in most cases nerve suturing immediately after seventh nerve disruption can result in a good return of function—well almost. The result will depend on the location of the nerve suturing. If nerve severence occurs in the cranium after removal of an acoustic nerve neuroma, the chances of nerve regeneration into the distal segments after resuturing is about 50% of normal and the results can be seen only after 2 years.[5] However, if the seventh nerve trunk is sutured as it emerges from the temporal canal, the expected result can be considered to be good, with return of muscle function expected within several months. In a similar fashion, suturing distal branches of the seventh nerve in the parotid gland or the distal portion will usually result in an excellent facial movement. However, nerve grafting in the cranium temporal canal and even in the parotid is far less certain and in the best of circumstances seems to give but a limited result. A similar end result seems to occur with nerve transfers such as the twelfth and eleventh nerve sutured to the distal portion of the severed seventh nerve. All of this, despite the magnificent advances in nerve grafting and suturing as demonstrated by Dr. Millesi,[7] why?

There are at least two factors present in all nerve grafting. The most important is the suture junction. Fibroblasts and scar formation across the junction set up a barrier, limiting axon penetration to the distal end. Second, the moment nerve impulses to a facial muscle are interrupted, atrophy commences. Thereafter it is a race between fibrosis and regeneration of the muscle, which can recover completely only after the nerve impulse arrives through the scar barrier to its muscle destination.[11] Whereas research definitely shows that the degenerating facial muscle can survive longer than other muscles, there is little doubt but that regeneration is not total and that functional return is most varied.[11] An authority of cross-face grafting in facial paralysis is Dr. Hugo Fisch. In a recent article[2] he stated that the results in cross-face grafting are at best uncertain. He set a standard of 18 months as the time limit after which return of facial muscle function with the nerve grafting is indeed poor. It has been our policy to substitute the temporalis muscle as a new motor apparatus when the time has exceeded 18 months from the initial injury. Temporalis muscle supplied by the fifth cranial nerve is rarely paretic and makes an excellent facial contracting motor apparatus. Whereas this method has limitations such as the need to develop synchronized facial movements by relearning how to smile evenly on both sides, the consistency of obtaining immediate facial movements such as smiling and closing the eyelids on the affected side makes this operation a most desirable one.

The technique of transposing the temporalis muscle is not complicated. However, the expected good result can only be obtained by the most constant attention to detailed technique.

In 1933, Gillies transplanted the anterior portion of a temporalis muscle to activate the corners of the mouth and nasolabial folds.[4] Fascia lata was used as tendon for the length needed beyond the ends of the muscle. In 1938, Sheehan[10] included the eyelid in a similar fashion. Anderson[1] modified Gillies technique by employing temporalis fascia instead of the fascia lata to activate eyelids. In 1952

McLaughlin[6] detached the coronoid process of the mandible, leaving the bone attached to the temporalis tendon. A sling of fascia lata was placed around the lips to simulate an orbicularis oris and was then inserted into a hole in the coronoid process, which in turn was elevated by the entire temporalis muscle.

The most commonly used procedure by plastic surgeons has been a static sling of fascia lata[3] threaded around the mouth and fastened to the zygomatic arch to give support to the lips and the nasolabial fold. The anterior portion of the masseter muscle has also been used to give tone to the upper lips. Unfortunately, the line of contraction is poor (Fig. 36-1).

In 1966[8] I presented a paper to the Third International Congress in Rome describing bilateral temporalis muscle transplantation with temporal fascia added as tendons to activate the eyelids, cheeks, upper lips, and nasolabial folds. In this one-stage procedure almost all the muscle is used. The operation is still being used as described in 1966 with very little change. Animation of the face can be accomplished in a one-stage procedure in about 3 hours of operating time.

ANATOMY OF THE TEMPORALIS MUSCLE

The temporalis muscle is a fan-shaped, thick, broad muscle that occupies the temporal fossa on the external surface of the skull's temporal bone. It is covered with a dense, firm fascia. The muscle fibers are attached to the periosteum of the temporal fascia, converge to pass under the zygomatic arch, and are finally inserted into the anterior border of the coronoid process. The muscle is covered by a dense fascia continuous with the deep fascia rising from the neck. The fascia envelops the mandible, the facial muscles, and the zygomatic arch. At the superior border of the latter it fuses to form the thick sheet covering the muscle up to the superior temporal line, where it merges into the galea of the scalp.

The function of the temporalis muscle is to assist in elevating the mandible by contracting its fibers. It also aids in protrusion and retraction of the mandible. The temporalis muscle nerve supply is derived from the temporal branch of the motor division of the fifth cranial nerve. The anatomic division of the temporal nerve is fortuitous in that it splits into three separate branches, innervating the anterior, mid, and posterior aspects of the muscle. The nerve is found in the mid level of the zygomatic arch, where it divides into its three branches, each penetrating the muscle at about the junction of its lower one third and upper two thirds. Thus the muscle can be freed from the temporal bone down to the upper level of the zygomatic arch without injuring the nerve supply.

The technique of the temporal muscle transfer in facial paralysis is possible because of the attachment of the upper one half of the muscle to the temporal bone above the level of the zygomatic arch. When the superior part of the muscle is freed from the bone and draped over the zygomatic arch, the lower one half has sufficient attachment to the temporal bone to contract and serve as a motor apparatus to raise the lips and corner of the mouth and to activate the eyelids. In most cases the length of the draped muscle is insufficient to reach the nasolabial fold and the lips. The temporal fascia can then act as tendons to reach and be inserted into the upper lip, corner of the mouth, lower lip, and the eyelids.

Before starting the operation the surgeon must examine the patient's smile on the normal side. I have described three types of smiles produced by the dominant muscles of the lips and the corners of the mouth.[1] The surgeon can locate, on the normal side, the exact position of major muscle pull and plan to place the temporalis muscle and its facial tendons into the exact mirror image on the affected side. These points of attachment must be predetermined prior to the operation.[9]

TECHNIQUE FOR TEMPORALIS TRANSPOSITION PROCEDURE (Fig. 36-1)

Fig. 36-1, A. The temporalis scalp region of the affected side is prepared by cutting the hair close to the scalp. The scalp is not shaved. After careful and thorough scrubbing with povidone-iodine (Betadine) soap and solution, a line is marked out corresponding to *ab*. An incision is made through the scalp from the level of the upper margin of the zygomatic arch, *ZY*, to the superior temporal line. The superior temporal line denotes limits of the superior border of the temporal muscle. In an elderly person, the incision is usually made in the preauricular area similar to the incision for a facelift. Redundant skin can then be removed.

Drapes are sutured to the scalp with 3-0 black silk to ensure hair coverage. An incision is made through the scalp skin to the depth of the deep fascia. The exposed fascia resembles a thick white-gray film.

Tunnels are dissected through the cheek from the lower border of the incision and superficial to the zygomatic arch down to the nasolabial fold, the upper lip, corner of the mouth, and portions of the lower lip (see shaded areas, Fig. 36-1, *A*). An incision is made in the skin just lateral to the outer canthus in the lines of the face, *C*. Horizontal incisions, no longer than 3mm, are made through the skin in the mid area of the upper and lower eyelids just above and below the eyelashes, *E* and *D*. Another incision is made medial to the inner canthus to expose the medial inner canthal ligaments, *F*. An incision is made in the nasolabial fold *G* and *I*, to match the shape and location of the normal nasolabial fold. This incision runs from 1 cm below the ala–nasolabial fold junction to the level of the corner of the mouth. The incision in this area goes into the deep tissue and will allow the scissors to exit, making the tunnel from the zygomatic arch. An incision, *J*, is made in the cheek along the facial lines. It measures about 1 cm in length. A vertical incision, *K*, is made in the lower lip about 2 cm medial to the corner of the mouth and just below the vermilion tissue. It is no more than 1 cm long.

Fig. 36-1, B. In the operation performed, good exposure of the fascia and the muscle can be obtained by using broad retractors to hold back the scalp. Fig. 36-1, *B*, shows a flap of deep temporal fascia to be lifted off the muscle as a sheet. A first

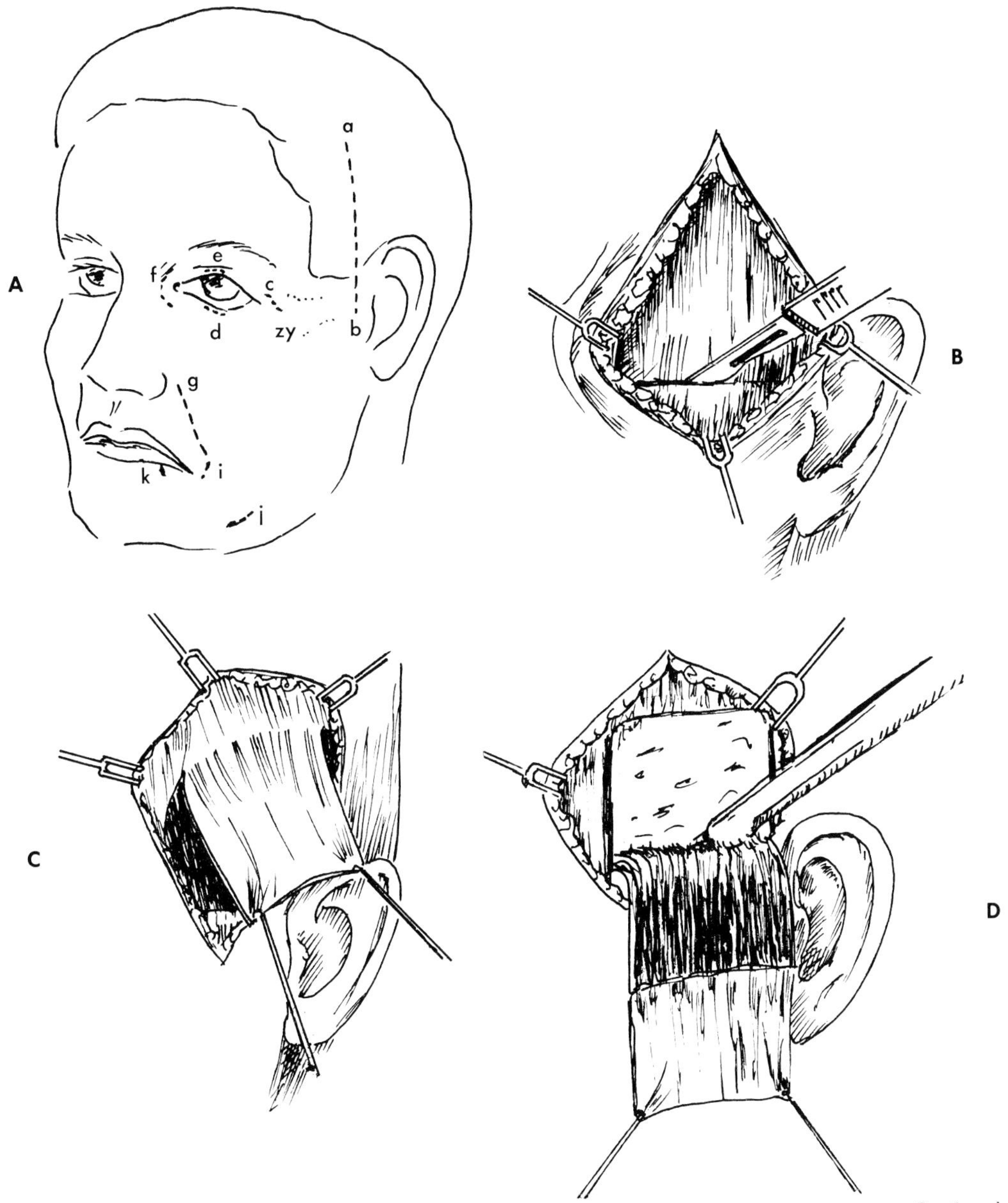

Continued.

Fig. 36-1. Technique for temporalis transposition procedure.

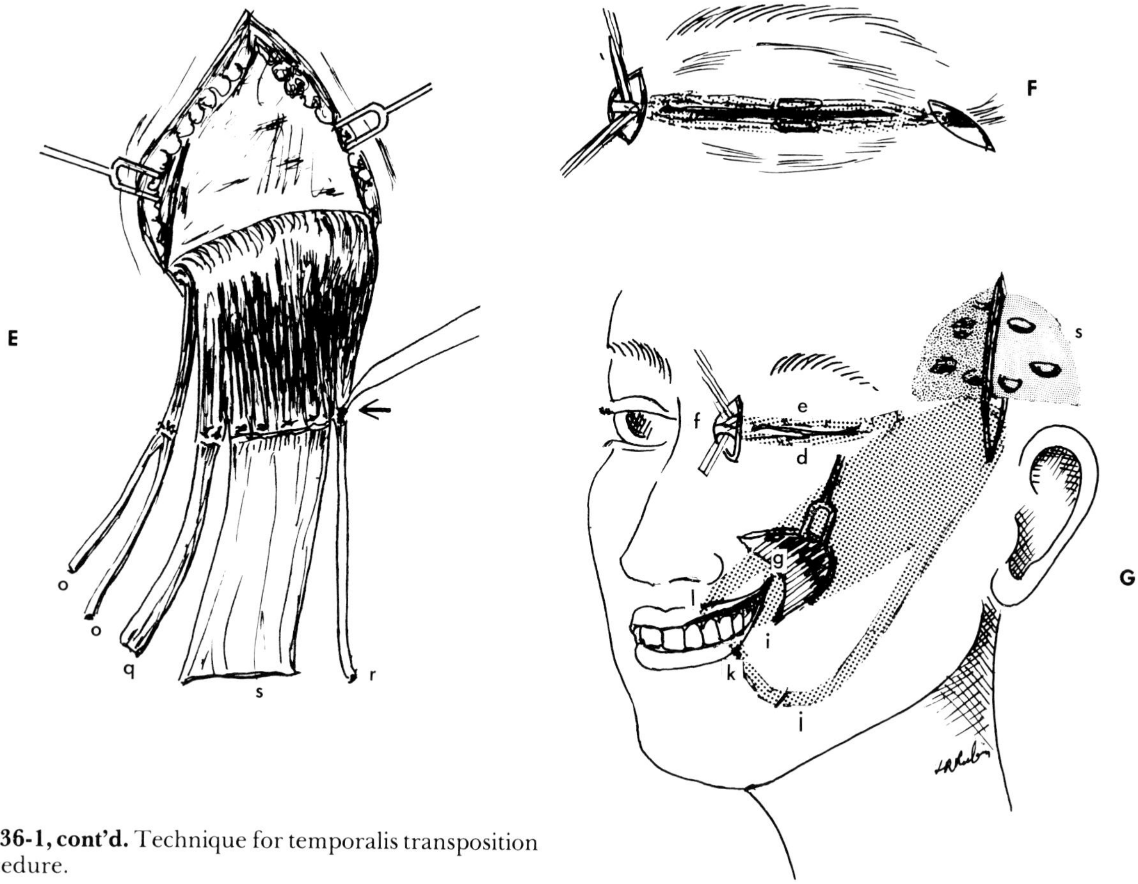

Fig. 36-1, cont'd. Technique for temporalis transposition procedure.

incision is made horizontally at the level of the zygomatic arch.

Fig. 36-1, C. Two vertical incisions are then made through the fascia anteriorally and posteriorly, creating a superiorly based flap (Fig. 36-1, *C*). The anterior vertical incision is level with the outer canthus of the eye, and the posterior incision is made behind the helix of the ear. The fascia is lifted off the muscle by blunt dissection almost to the height of the superior temporal line, where it is left attached to the underlying muscle. A horizontal incision is cut above the temporal line through the fascia to the bone joining each vertical incision, thus creating a rectangular flap of muscle and fascia.

Fig. 36-1, D. The muscle is stripped downward off the temporal bone (Fig. 36-1, *D*) with a blunt instrument. The muscle flap is the same size as the overlying fascial flap. The stripping is carried downward to the level of the upper border of the zygomatic arch with the assistant, using fine hooks, gently holding the attached fascia. It is most important not to strip the muscle below the level of the zygomatic arch since the nerve entering the muscle is located halfway down the width of the zygomatic arch and is subject to injury.

Fig. 36-1, E. After the muscle is draped over the arch, it becomes obvious that it cannot reach the lips or the inner canthi of the eyelids (Fig. 36-1, *E*). The fascia now takes the role of tendons. On the medial side, two narrow strips of fascia are cut, each 4 mm wide. They will serve as tendons for the eyelids *o*. The motor muscle for these fascial strips to the eyelids is now cut from the medial aspect of the temporalis muscle flap and is no more than 8 mm wide. The fascia attachment is reinforced with white 4-0 Mersilene mattress sutures. The remaining fascia is now divided into three parts: *q*, a strip medially, about 5 mm wide which activates the upper lip and substitutes for the levator superior portion of the quadratus labii superior muscle (this strip is used if the patient has demonstrated a dominant canine smile); a 5 mm wide strip farthest laterally to serve as a long tendon to thread through the cheek and fasten to the lower lip; and *r*, the remaining intervening fascia, about 4 cm wide, used to activate the nasolabial fold, lateral portions of the upper lip, and the angle of the mouth.

The junctions of each facial strip to the muscle must be reinforced with many white 4-0 Mersilene mattress sutures.

Many sutures are used to ensure a firm union (Fig. 36-1, *E*). The strips should be tested by pulling them taut. There should be no separation of fascia from muscle. These junctions must withstand firm stretching when they are inserted into their new position.

Fig. 36-1, F. Strips of the fascia, acting as tendons, are tested for proper length to the desired areas. Note the two tendons for the eyelids (Fig. 36-1, *F*). They must be long enough to fasten to the inner canthus.

Fig. 36-1, G. The strip to the lower lip (Fig. 36-1, *G*) is too short to reach its destination, requiring additional length by suturing an extra piece to the end. Care must be made to ensure that the suturing is beyond the cheek incision, *J*, where the tendon turns upward toward the lip. This point, *J*, acts as a pulley, and should the lengthening strips be sutured proximal to the pulley, it could be snagged when the muscle is contracted.

The tendons have been threaded through the tunnels. The tendons to the eyelids must be very close to the lid margins. A suture of 5-0 Mersilene is usually placed in the soft tissue around the tendons to keep them close to the margins and to keep them from slipping down the lids, *ed*. This could produce an ectropion when the tendons are tightened. The strips are threaded under and around the medial canthus and intertwined after being pulled *taut, f*. They are sutured into the inner canthus with 4-0 white Mersilene. The sketch shows the strips coming through the medial incision after being threaded under the medial inner canthal ligaments, *f*.

The medial strip to the upper lip will be fastened to the mirror position of the levator superior on the normal side, *l*. The wide strip is attached to the lip laterally, to the corner of the mouth, and to the lateral portion of the lower lip. It is sutured to the deep fascia, remaining muscle, or dermis if need be with 4-0 white Mersilene mattress sutures. *The suturing is done under tension;* two dull rakes are used to pull the cheek upward, while the pull on the tendons will be downward, stretching the muscle as much as possible.

The tendon to the lower lip is pulled upward around the pulley in the cheek and then sutured to the lower lip, which is held in a neutral position, *k*. This tendon will act as a restraining force to exert counterpull to the upward force at the mouth angle. The temporalis muscle can be seen in Fig. 36-1, *G*, as a bulge above the level zygomatic arch. This bulge is unavoidable and makes the face somewhat asymmetric in the region of the zygomatic arch. The sketch also shows a silicone, shaped block being inserted above the muscle to fill the temporal fossa, previously occupied by the temporalis muscle, *s*.

The tendons have been pulled taut and sutured under tension to the inner canthi, the upper lip, angle of the mouth, and lower lip. All face skin wounds have now been closed with 4-0 Dexon for the deep tissue and 5-0 nylon pull-out subcuticular stitches for the superficial skin. The defect in the temporal fossa created by turning the muscle downward is filled with a soft, silicone block carved at the table. Holes are made in the block to allow scar tissue invasion for fixation.

The final closure of the scalp is made with 3-0 interlocking continuous black silk sutures. Fig. 36-1, *G*, shows a suction tube being placed deep in the face and the scalp pocket to evacuate any residual hematoma. The tube is removed in 24 to 48 hours. A tight pressure dressing is placed over the entire cheek to help close the space created by the extensive undermining.

When skin closure is completed on the paralyzed side, attention is shifted to the normal side. Weakening of the dominant muscle is needed to equalize the disproportionate contracting force of the normal side as compared to the weak temporalis contractions. Once the surgeon has predetermined which muscles are dominant, a curving incision is made in the mouth mucosa above the orbicularis on the normal side, exposing the quadratus levator superior and the zygomatic major muscles. A 0.5 cm strip is excised from each muscle just as it reaches the orbicularis oris. The muscle will contract and separate immediately. A similar incision is made in the mucosa of the lower lip, exposing the quadratus labii inferior and the triangularis, the major depressors of the lower lip and corner of the mouth. A 0.5 cm strip is removed from each of these muscles. There is little fear of paralysis. Marked weakening only creates a more pleasant balance. As time goes on, muscle reattachment occurs, and the contracting forces on the normal side start approaching their original contractions. However, if moderate excisions are made, the lessened contracting force is beneficial. The mucosal wounds are sutured with 4-0 Dexon sutures, which need no removal.

The sagging of the eyebrow is corrected by removing a crescent of skin above the brow. The amount of skin to be taken can be determined by pulling the brow upward to the best level to correspond to the normal eyebrow shape. It is advisable to overcorrect the brow height. The shape of the skin patch removed seems best suited when cut as shown in Fig. 36-1. The incision is made just at the brow line, and the final closure with a pull-out of 4-0 nylon subcuticular sutures leaves but a minimal scar.

POSTOPERATIVE COURSE

The immediate postoperative course creates an extremely edematous face. The eyelids are shut tightly. All the teeth are exposed in an extreme grimace. The nasolabial fold and the corner of the mouth are pulled upward and backward. The soft pressure dressings are removed by the fourth day. Several more days will elapse before the eyelids start functioning. Levator function will slowly open the upper lids. The corner of the mouth and the nasolabial fold will return to a normal position covering the teeth within approximately 10 days.

Muscle movements become apparent within 24 to 48 hours after surgery and continue to function with greater efficiency as the patient, clenching his teeth, stimulates the temporalis contractions. The full muscle function may take about 1 year to be completed. Edema of the face persists for months. During this time the patient must observe himself in front of a mirror and practice exposing his teeth in an expression of happiness or pleasure that can now be called a smile. This can always be accomplished by clenching the teeth tightly on the affected side. After the edema subsides, the muscle contracts the upper lip and the nasolabial fold to a greater degree, since the edema of the facial tissue is no longer a restricting force. The greater the overcorrection of the smile at the time of surgery by stretching the temporalis muscle, the greater will be the excursion when the patient clenches his teeth.

A number of our patients have in time been able to control movements of eyes and mouth independently. It is our feeling that some of this independent action may take place because of changes in the brain or that the three branches of the nerve to the temporalis muscle may be sufficient to cause the different portions of the muscle to move independently.

PITFALLS TO BE AVOIDED

1. The possibility of a weak or underdeveloped temporalis muscle exists. Testing must be done in advance to ensure the temporalis function. If the fifth nerve is injured, the operation obviously cannot be performed. If the muscle is weak, the patient can strengthen it by active exercise such as clenching his teeth continuously or chewing gum. Several months of exercise prior to the surgery may be needed to obtain the increased strength.

2. The temporalis fascia, acting as tendons, must be carefully sutured to the muscle to reinforce the junctions, since the fascia and the muscle must be pulled taut in extreme tension.

3. The tendons threading through the eyelids must be at the lid margins. Failure can cause ectropion as the tendons slip beyond the margins to evert the eyelids. I have found that a 4-0 Dexon suture may often act as a tunnel check in the mid-eyelid incision area to help hold the marginal position.

4. Facial configuration must be carefully planned before surgery. Proper placement of the nasolabial fold incision can create a pleasant, normal result. By predetermining the optimal direction of the pull, the muscle and its fascia can be placed in the mirror position of the normal side to develop a pleasant smile when all muscles contract simultaneously.

The temporalis transplantation procedure has one definite limitation. It does not provide for a coordinated, synchronized, balanced face during speech. However, a solution is in sight. Our recent work with dogs has confirmed the principle of neural neurotization. The implantation of a free nerve graft into a denervated muscle will stimulate nerve end–axon sprouting and reanastomosis with the neuromuscular junction. A sural nerve anastomosed with buccal fascicles of the opposite normal side can be threaded across the face and inserted into the belly of the temporalis muscle, which has been transplanted to activate the face. This may be done only after the functioning temporalis muscle has had its fifth nerve motor function cut at least 2 weeks prior to the implantation. Whereas the possibility exists of doing a direct nerve anastomosis to the end of the fifth nerve as it enters the temporalis, the logistics of suturing under microscope make it a most difficult approach.

SUMMARY

I have described a comparatively simple procedure in which the temporalis muscle and its overlying thick fascia, acting as tendons, are used to provide a dynamic motor force that activates the paralyzed upper portions of the face, including the eyelids. The temporalis muscle is innervated by the fifth cranial nerve, which is rarely paretic. The temporal muscle transplantation has been a satisfactory motor apparatus for facial paralysis (Figs. 36-2 to 36-6). Many static procedures using fascia lata have been described in textbooks. I feel that these should not be used under any circumstances since the re-

Text continued on p. 300.

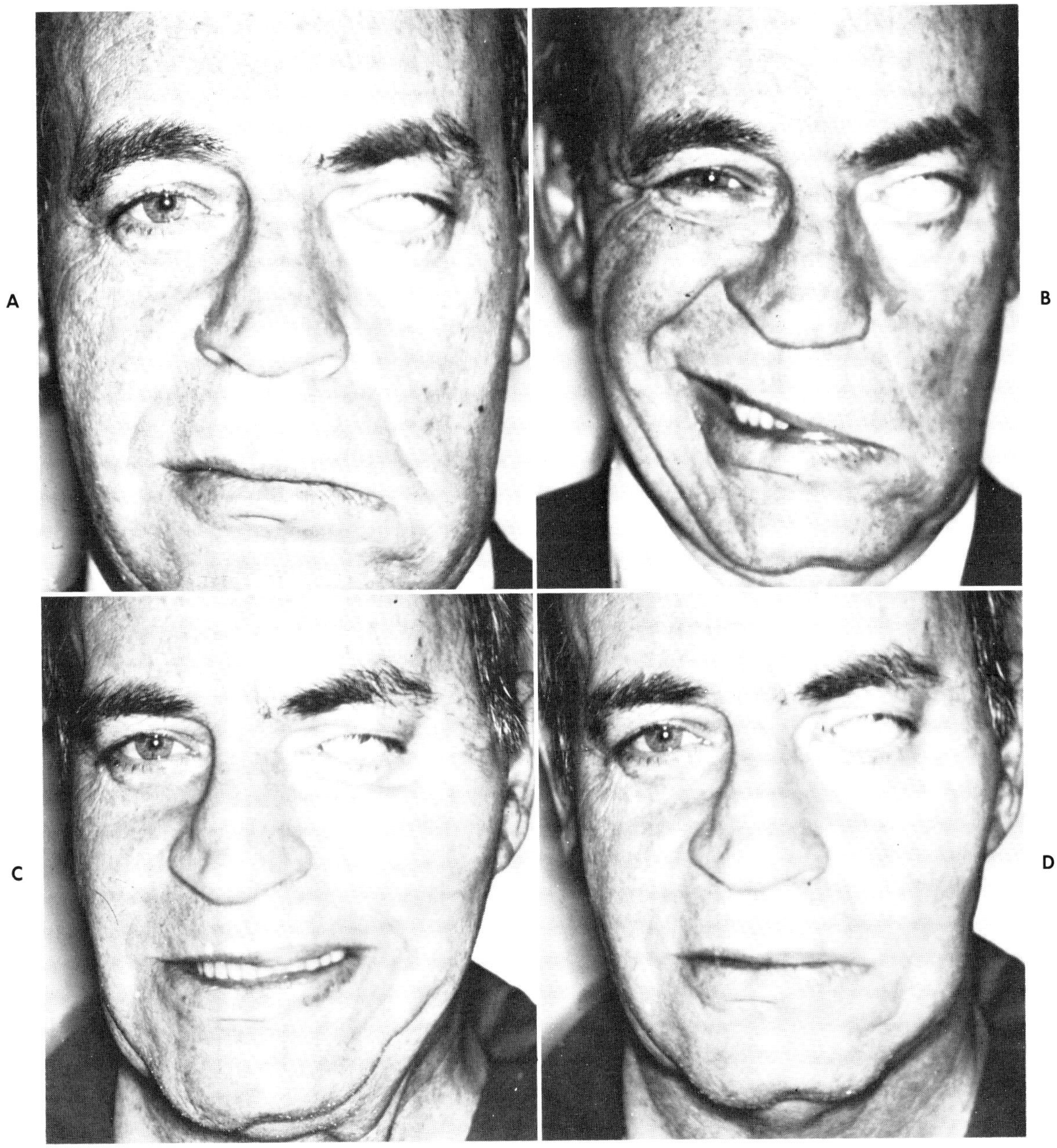

Fig. 36-2. Patient is a 51-year-old man who had an acoustic nerve neuroma removed 25 years previously with resultant complete left side facial paralysis. Nerve studies showed no activity. **A,** Preoperative view with patient in repose. Clouded eyeball was unrelated to paralysis. **B,** Preoperative view of patient trying to smile and close left eyelid. **C,** Postoperative view 1 year after temporalis muscle transposition. Eyelids contract, and patient smiles when he tenses left jaw. By practice in front of mirror, he has been able to correlate and balance his smile. **D,** Patient in repose. (From Rubin, L.: Reanimation of the paralyzed face, St. Louis, 1977, The C. V. Mosby Co.)

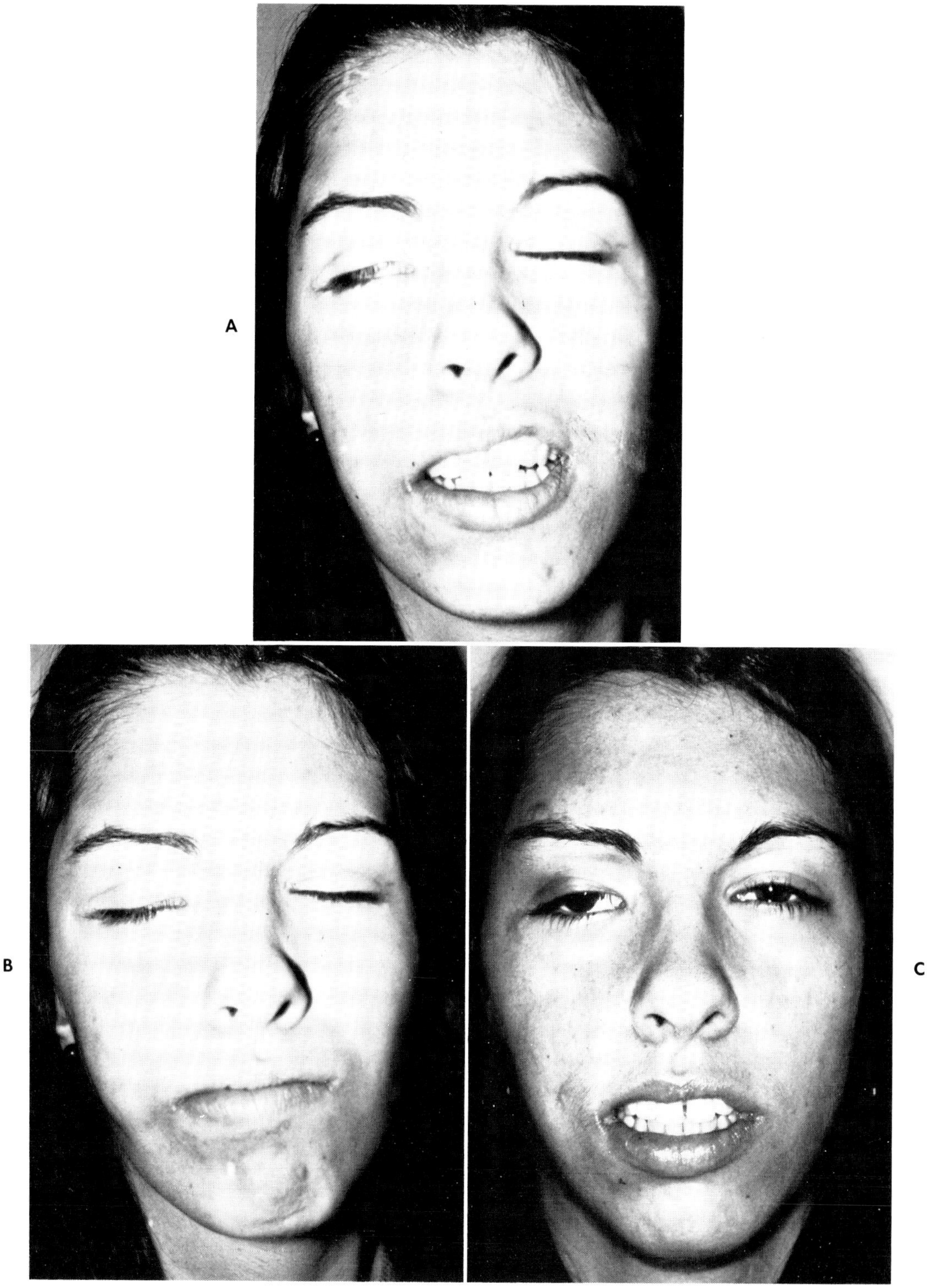

Fig. 36-3. An 18-year-old woman who suffered severe cerebral damage following a fractured skull. She had been unconscious for several weeks and was left with permanent facial paralysis as well as partial hemiplegia. Accident had occurred 18 months prior to photographs. Eight months previously, patient had a partial masseter muscle implant to corner of mouth and a fascia lata sling from mouth to temporalis muscle by another surgeon. Electronic testing just prior to present operation showed complete absence of facial nerve function on paralyzed face. **A,** Preoperative view of patient trying to smile and close right eyelid. **B,** Patient with face in repose. Note thick pad in right cheek lateral to mouth corner. This is masseter muscle attachment to mouth corner done 8 months previously. **C,** Postoperative view after temporalis muscle transplant to cheeks, lips, and eyelids. Patient also had weakening of levator superior muscle on normal side. Patient is now able to close eyelids. (From Rubin, L.: Reanimation of the paràlyzed face, St. Louis, 1977, The C. V. Mosby Co.)

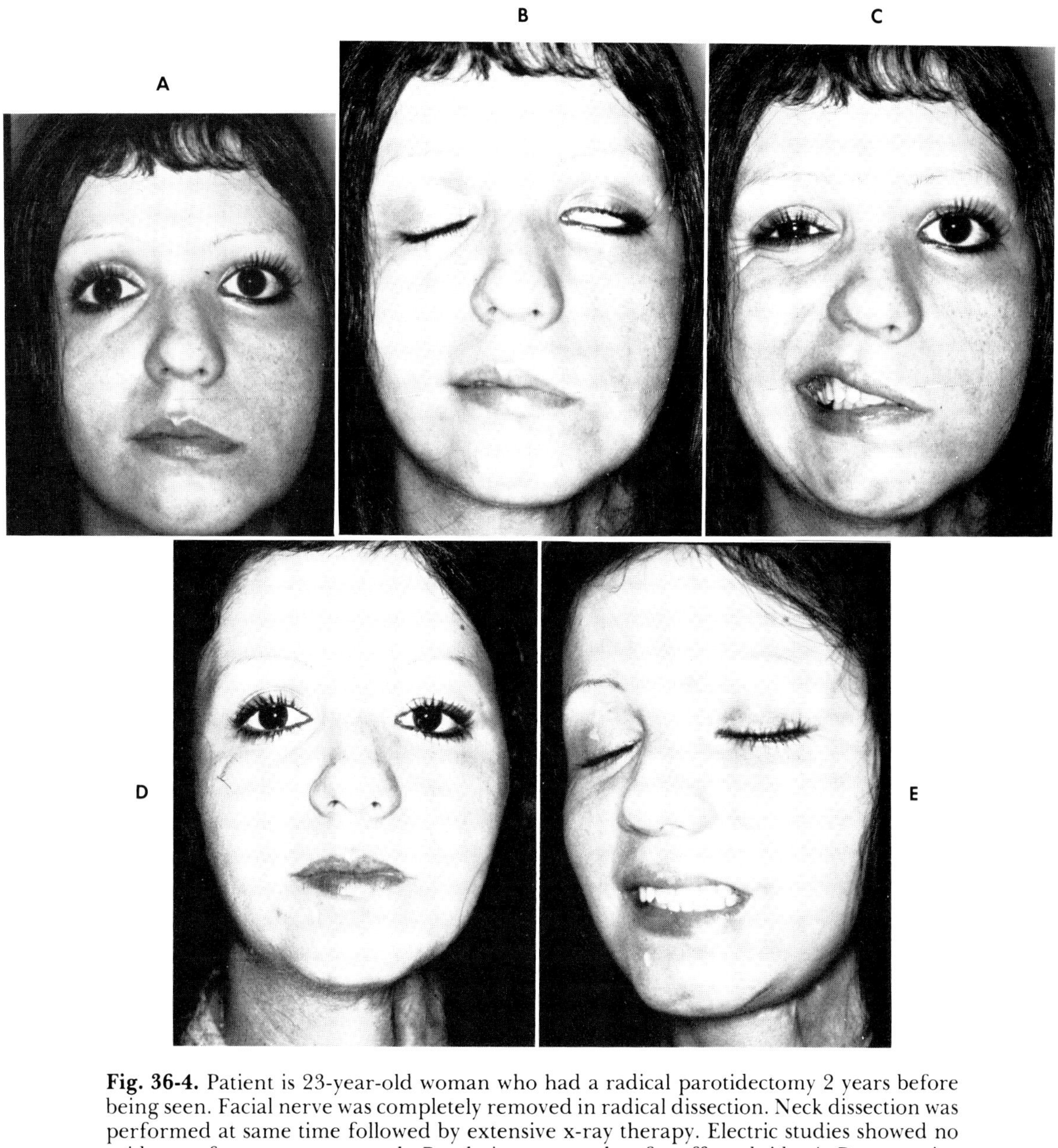

Fig. 36-4. Patient is 23-year-old woman who had a radical parotidectomy 2 years before being seen. Facial nerve was completely removed in radical dissection. Neck dissection was performed at same time followed by extensive x-ray therapy. Electric studies showed no evidence of any nerve regrowth. Paralysis was complete for affected side. **A,** Preoperative view in repose. **B,** Patient trying to close left eye. **C,** Patient trying to smile. **D,** Postoperative view of patient in repose 1 year after surgery. **E,** Postoperative view, showing patient smiling and closing eyelids. Repeat electronic studies showed no facial nerve recovery on affected side. (From Rubin, L.: Reanimation of the paralyzed face, St. Louis, 1977, The C. V. Mosby Co.)

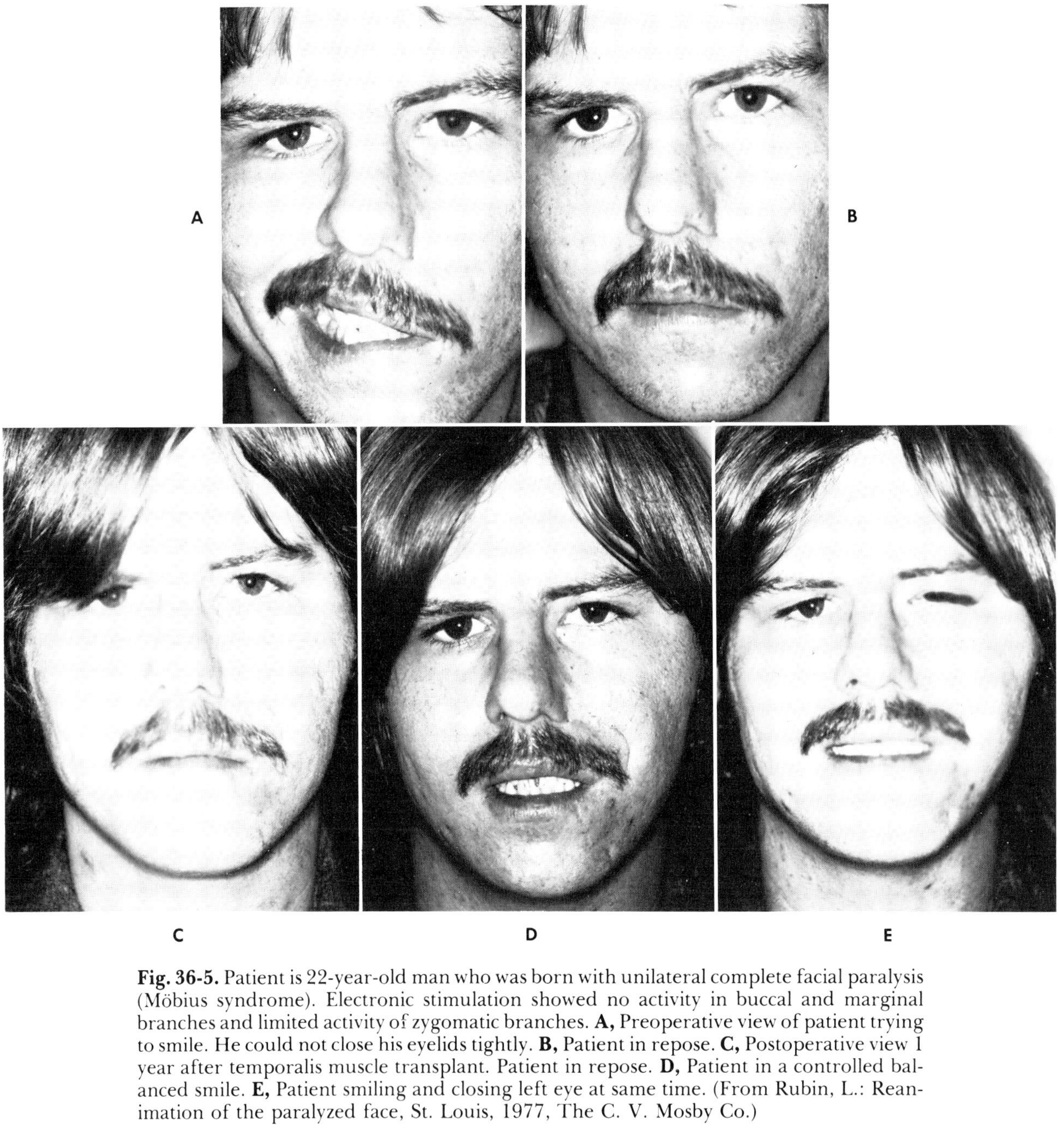

Fig. 36-5. Patient is 22-year-old man who was born with unilateral complete facial paralysis (Möbius syndrome). Electronic stimulation showed no activity in buccal and marginal branches and limited activity of zygomatic branches. **A,** Preoperative view of patient trying to smile. He could not close his eyelids tightly. **B,** Patient in repose. **C,** Postoperative view 1 year after temporalis muscle transplant. Patient in repose. **D,** Patient in a controlled balanced smile. **E,** Patient smiling and closing left eye at same time. (From Rubin, L.: Reanimation of the paralyzed face, St. Louis, 1977, The C. V. Mosby Co.)

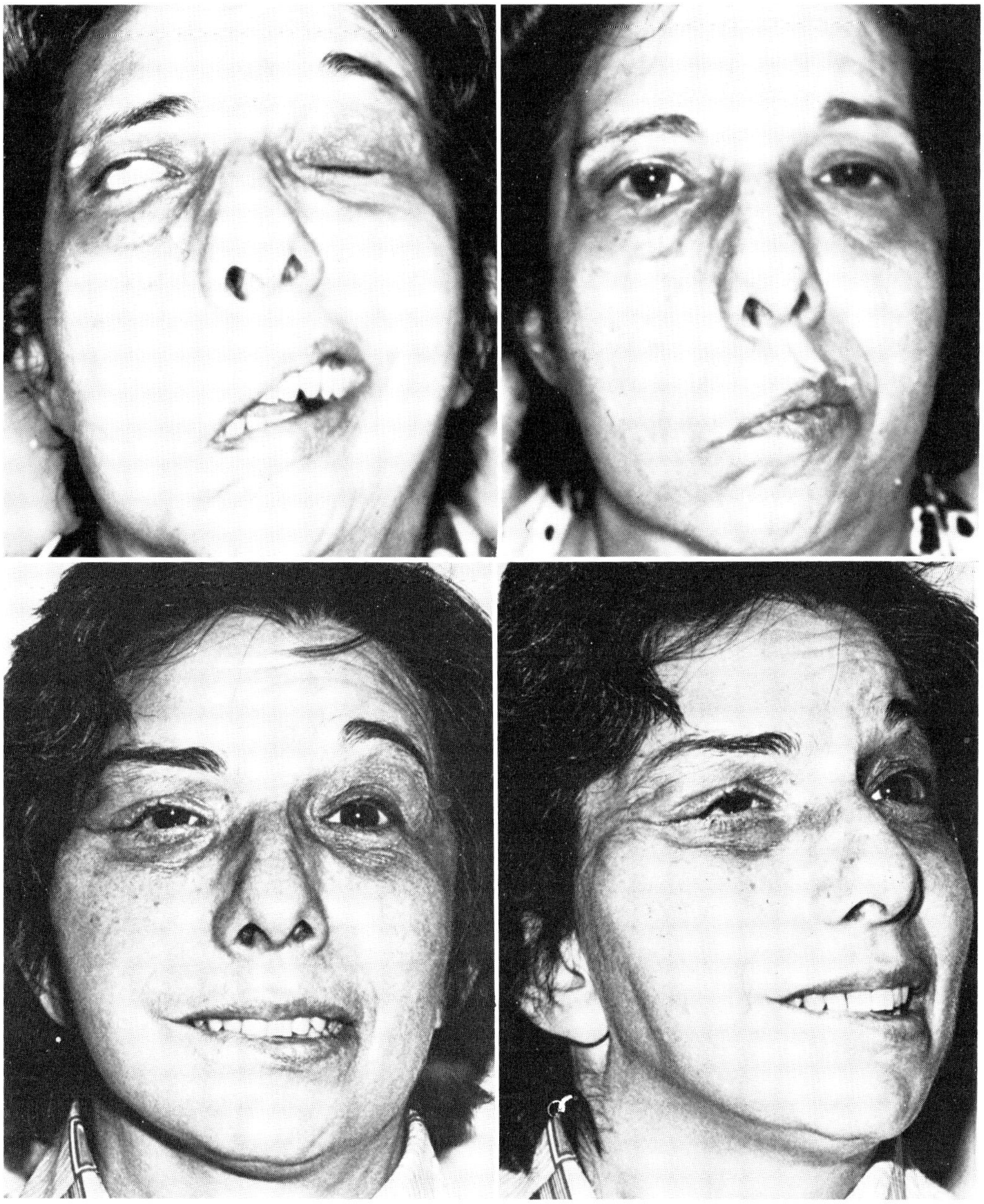

A B

C D

Fig. 36-6. A 56-year-old woman who had acoustic nerve tumor removed approximately 3 years prior to temporal muscle transposition. Electronic studies showed muscle degeneration and no nerve regeneration prior to temporalis muscle operation. **A,** Patient attempting to smile and close eyes. **B,** Patient in repose. **C** and **D,** Patient has had temporalis muscle transplantation and removal of about 1 cm of levator superior and zygomatic major muscles on normal side. (From Rubin, L.: Reanimation of the paralyzed face, St. Louis, 1977, The C. V. Mosby Co.)

sults leave a face fixed and immobile instead of giving it a dynamic, moving expression.

The temporalis muscle transposition has one great limitation. The face cannot be synchronized during speech. New techniques of nerve grafting have brightened the picture for a solution to this problem.

REFERENCES

1. Anderson, J. G.: Surgical treatment of lagophthalmos in leprosy by the Gillies temporalis transfer, Br. J. Plast. Surg. **14:**339, 1961.
2. Fisch, U.: Cross-face grafting in facial paralysis, Arch. Otolaryngol. **102:**453-457, 1976.
3. Freeman, B.: Facial paralysis. In Converse, J. M., editor: Reconstructive Plastic Surgery, Philadelphia, 1964, W. B. Saunders Company.
4. Gillies, H. D.: Facial paralysis procedures, Proc. R. Soc. Med. **27:**1372, 1933.
5. Malis, L.: Nerve grafting by microscope in the cranium. In Rubin, L. R., editor: Reanimation of the paralyzed face, St. Louis, 1977, The C. V. Mosby Co.
6. McLaughlin, C. R.: Surgical support in permanent facial paralysis, Plast. Reconstr. Surg. **11:**302, 1953.
7. Millesi, H.: The technique of free nerve grafting in the face. In Rubin, L. R., editor: Reanimation of the paralyzed face, St. Louis, 1977, The C. V. Mosby Co.
8. Rubin, L. R., Bromberg, B. E., and Walden, R. H.: Congenital bilateral facial paralysis Möbius syndrome. Surgical animation of the face. In Transactions of the Fourth International Congress of Plastic and Reconstructive Surgery, Amsterdam, 1969, Excerpta Medica Foundation, pp. 740-745.
9. Rubin, L. R.: The anatomy of a smile—its importance in the treatment of facial paralysis, Plast. Reconstr. Surg. **55**(4):384-387, 1974.
10. Sheean, J. F.: Manual of reparative plastic surgery, New York, 1938, Macmillan Publishing Co.
11. Sher, J. H.: The pathophysiology of degeneration in the facial neuromuscular motor unit. In Rubin, L. R., editor: Reanimation of the paralyzed face, St. Louis, 1977, The C. V. Mosby Co.

Chapter 37

Free muscle grafts

Timothy A. Miller
Ervin S. Wheeler

With the exception of skeletal muscle, autogenous grafts of virtually every type of tissue are routinely employed in reconstructive surgery. The principal consideration in almost all tissue transfers is the establishment of an adequate blood supply to maintain graft viability. Grafts of skeletal muscle, however, have the *additional* requisites of neural innervation and mechanical tension. The singular loss of any one of these three requirements will result in eventual complete atrophy and fibrous replacement.

INNERVATION

It is well known that muscle atrophy and fibrous replacement even in situ are the inevitable consequences of motor nerve severance. The evolution of this process following denervation has been presented in great detail by Gutmann.[10] The fact that nerve has a profound trophic influence on muscle has also been well documented. Innervation is indispensable for synthesis of new acetylcholinesterase by the motor end-plate.[7] It has also been shown that innervation controls the muscle fiber type. For example, experimental denervation substantially retards the rate of contraction of fast (white) muscle,[5] and slow (red) muscle exhibits a shortened contraction time.[1] In cross-innervation studies, where the nerve to a fast muscle is implanted into a slow muscle, the former will develop a slow contractile response and the latter a fast response.[4] From these and numerous other studies, it has been shown that the nerve determines the metabolic profile of any given muscle. This principle has been utilized in documenting the reinnervation of a denervated muscle. Karpati and Engel[17] demonstrated "type grouping" of muscle fibers in reinnervated muscles. Most mammalian muscle fibers demonstrate a mosaic pattern histochemically. The appearance of clusters or groups of muscle fibers of the same type indicates that axonal regeneration with collateral branching has reinnervated groups of muscle fibers and induced a single fiber type in that area within the muscle.

Studitsky and associates[24] have noted the importance of motor nerve influence in studies on the regenerative capacity of skeletal muscle. They found that when minced muscle tissue in young rats is reimplanted in its original location it undergoes a myoblastic proliferation phase. If nerve is implanted, muscle fibrils eventually develop, motor end-plates are formed within them, and the muscle is reconstituted. If the nerve is absent, however, the myoblasts degenerate, and muscle tissue does not regenerate.

MECHANICAL TENSION

Muscle must also be maintained under tension. Skeletal muscle fibers atrophy and undergo biochemical changes following tenotomy despite intact neural and vascular supply.[16] It has been shown experimentally that mechanical tension plays a vital role in the regeneration of striated muscle. In the absence of tension, differentiation of the myogenous elements is inhibited, and the fibers do not reach maturity.[33] Studitsky and associates[24] demonstrated that minced muscle placed in the bed of the extirpated gastrocnemius in the rat will regenerate if the distal tendon is intact. However, when the foot is amputated and the tendon has no point of attachment to develop tension, the muscle fibers lack orientation and do not mature.

Research reported in this chapter was partially supported by VA Fund #5733.

BLOOD SUPPLY

If any transplanted tissue is to survive, adequate blood flow to the graft must be provided to maintain metabolic integrity. Several studies have shown that muscle is exquisitely sensitive to anoxia and deteriorates rapidly. In extensive experimental efforts directed toward muscle grafting, there have been frequent reports that death of the grafts was ischemic in etiology.[3,15,22]

HISTORY OF EXPERIMENTAL FREE MUSCLE GRAFTS

It seems generally agreed that Zielonko[35] in 1874 was the first to attempt to graft muscle. In experiments on the frog he observed that the graft was completely replaced by fibrous tissue, an observation that was to be repeated by numerous investigators in a variety of experimental circumstances over the subsequent 100 years. Shortly thereafter, however, Gluck[9] reported that he had been successful; moreover, he claimed that he had grafted muscle from a rabbit to a chicken! The controversy began. In a vain attempt to repeat Gluck's achievement, Magnus[19] in 1890 performed autografts of the quadriceps muscle in the rabbit, but all resulted in fibrous scar. In 1893 Volkmann[30] stated firmly that free muscle grafts could simply not be performed. Noting avascular necrosis in these grafts, he pointed out the early occurrence of this process in the transfer of a muscle graft.

In an attempt to devise a novel and successful method of muscle transplanting, Hildebrandt[15] performed grafts that still had intact nerves attached to them. The grafts failed, and again it was noted that without blood supply the muscle deteriorated rapidly, usually within hours.

During a time when great success was achieved in clinical work on autogenous skin grafts, virtually no progress was achieved with muscle grafts. Clinical attempts at free muscle grafts in human beings were made by Eden in 1919 and by Peer and Walker in 1951.[21] Even though Peer placed the muscle grafts in proximity to other muscles and established a blood supply by the fourth day, he eventually concluded that fibrous replacement was the inevitable consequence of free muscle grafting.

If it is possible to define a modern era in a field such as skeletal muscle transplantation, the work of Studitsky and his colleagues[24-26,33] in Russia clearly leads the way. In 1960, Studitsky and Bosova[26] performed what was probably the first successful muscle graft when they transferred the middle third of the gastrocnemius muscle in the rat. Studitsky believed that the grafting process stimulated a myoblastic response within the traumatized muscle. Although he was successful in autografting portions of a muscle, his attempts at homografting muscle segments were, not suprisingly, distinct failures. However, while carrying out these unsuccessful attempts, several interesting observations were made at a time when it was not widely appreciated that muscle possessed regenerative potential. During the healing process following homograft failure, Studitsky noted that the process apparently involved muscle regeneration. This regenerative capacity was confirmed by subsequent studies. In 1964 he reported grafting a muscle after mincing it into a semiliquid porridge-like state. During these experiments the requisites of tension and nerve innervation needed in muscle grafting were reinforced. He observed that the minced muscle actually regenerated into a newly formed muscle belly. In order to enable the process to take place, however, the nerve and tendon in the orthotopic site must be present; if either were absent, muscle regeneration would not occur. In 1965, Zhenevskaya and Studitsky successfully grafted whole muscle bellies in rats. In this and previous work they introduced the concept of preoperative denervation, holding the belief that denervation was a form of stimulus or inducement toward a "plastic state" within the muscle. Mincing, denervation, and tenotomy all resulted in a similar dedifferentiation response eventually followed by the regenerative process: "enlargement and division of nucleoli, amitotic division of nuclei, the growth of sacroplasma masses with corresponding accumulation of nuclei, the formation of myofibrils, and, in case of mechanical trauma, the development of myoblasts with multiplication of them by means of mitotic divisions."[25]

FREE MUSCLE GRAFTS IN CLINICAL SITUATIONS

In 1971 Thompson[27] was the first to report successful free muscle grafts in human beings, principally in reanimation of the face following seventh nerve palsy. He also presented experimental evidence in dogs to substantiate his clinical studies.[27,28] A number of other reports from Thompson followed, causing a mild controversy that still persists. Prior to 1971 the vast majority of clinical surgeons were not aware of the research in Russia and were influenced chiefly by the pessimistic viewpoint of Peer as well as more recent unsuccessful attempts to graft muscle in dogs reported by Roy in 1966.[23] After Thompson's initial clinical success, free muscle grafts were attempted unsuccessfully,[18,31] and it was several years before news of effective free muscle grafting in clinical situations appeared from other surgeons.[8,11-14] Why it was and has been so difficult to reproduce successful muscle grafts in the usual clinical instance is not entirely clear. However, it has become increasingly apparent that if muscle grafting is a potential reconstructive method, it certainly is not easily accomplished clinically. Indeed, a great deal remains to be learned about this technique.

As recently as 1976, in a carefully designed study, Watson[31] again encountered failure with free muscle grafts in dogs. He pointed out that while Thompson's "patients appeared to have been clinically improved, the evidence of functioning graft survival did not seem convincing in many cases." It was also noted when reviewing Thompson's experimental evidence that in five out of eight dogs less than 50% of the muscle bulk survived. Watson's study took into account the highly important concepts of preoperative denervation, transplantation of entire muscle bellies, preservation of physiologic tension, and removal of fascia. Positioning the graft at right angles to the recipient, Watson employed histology, histochemistry, and contraction studies to evaluate the results, but all to no avail. He was completely unsuccessful. Although he suggested that this could be due to excessive muscle size utilized in his study, his investigation seemed to underline the fact that there are a number of variables involved in free muscle grafts and that they cannot be routinely performed at this time. Perhaps one of the principal difficulties is that many of the concepts regarding muscle and muscle grafting are open to question. Thompson attributed his success with free muscle grafts in spite of so many previously negative experiments by others to two innovative concepts: (1) transplantation of an entire muscle belly, thereby including only undamaged muscle cells, and (2) preoperative denervation (to render the transplanted muscle more suitable metabolically for the initial anoxic period associated with grafting).[27-29] Neither of these concepts, however, is entirely supported by experimental or clinical evidence.

In considering the necessity of transplanting an entire undamaged muscle, several contradictions seem appropriate to mention. Perhaps one of the most successful examples of clinical muscle grafts is the Abbe lip flap, a reconstructive method that has also been modified and used successfully as a free composite from lower lip to upper lip graft.[32] The design of the flap certainly divides the majority if not all of the muscle cells within the orbicularis oris muscle, yet the technique is quite effective. Moreover, it would seem that the successful mincing of experimental muscle grafts would argue against this theory. With respect to the concept of denervation, preoperative denervation is known to substantially alter the metabolic activity of a muscle. Nevertheless, human muscle is a mosaic mixture of fast and slow muscle types; while denervation may change the metabolism of aerobic (slow) muscle and make it more suitable to endure an anoxic period associated with grafting, it is likely to have a potentially unfavorable effect on the anaerobic (fast) fibers within the same muscle. It is certainly more reasonable to argue that preoperative denervation increases the capillary circulation within the involved muscle and initiates the "plastic state" associated with muscle regeneration. Indeed, prior denervation may increase the number of functional muscle fibers in a free transplant. Recent evidence suggests that denervation acts as a stimulus to dormant cells adjacent to the mature muscle fibers (satellite cells) to develop a myogenic potential. It is theorized that prior denervation stimulates these myoblasts, which are thought to be a more undifferentiated cell that is better able to withstand the relative anoxia of free grafting.[2]

Despite these theoretic questions, the substantial contribution and success with difficult problems reported by Thompson in clinical reanimation remain. This work has recently been reaffirmed by reports from Hakelius and Freilinger[8,13,14] who have utilized and documented survival of transplanted muscle. Hakelius has presented convincing evidence of muscle graft survival in a group of 23 patients with varying degrees of facial palsy. Utilizing the techniques described by Thompson, he noted generally satisfactory results, particularly in the reconstruction of lagophthalmos, and he concluded that muscle grafting was superior to any other reconstructive method.

MUSCULAR NEUROTIZATION

In the technique of muscle grafting the graft is sutured over the normal orbicularis oculi muscle (in the case of lagophthalmos) from which it will obtain its neural innervation: the process of muscular neurotization. Can a denervated muscle such as a graft obtain its neural innervation from an adjacent normally innervated muscle? It is on this process that the success or failure of a free muscle graft depends. The phenomenon was first noted by Erlacher[6] in 1915 but was not formally investigated until the recent surge of interest in muscle grafting. Certainly the success reported in free muscle grafts strongly argues for the existence of this phenomenon. In a study recently concluded in our laboratory a model was developed in the forelimb of a rabbit to study reinnervation at a muscular level[20] (Fig. 37-1). We found that a denervated muscle can become reinnervated following removal of fascia and surgical approximation to an adjacent normal muscle. In this investigation, muscle tension of the denervated muscle was not altered, and the blood supply was essentially undisturbed. A number of parameters were used to ascertain whether reinnervation had occurred; unexpectedly this was a diffi-

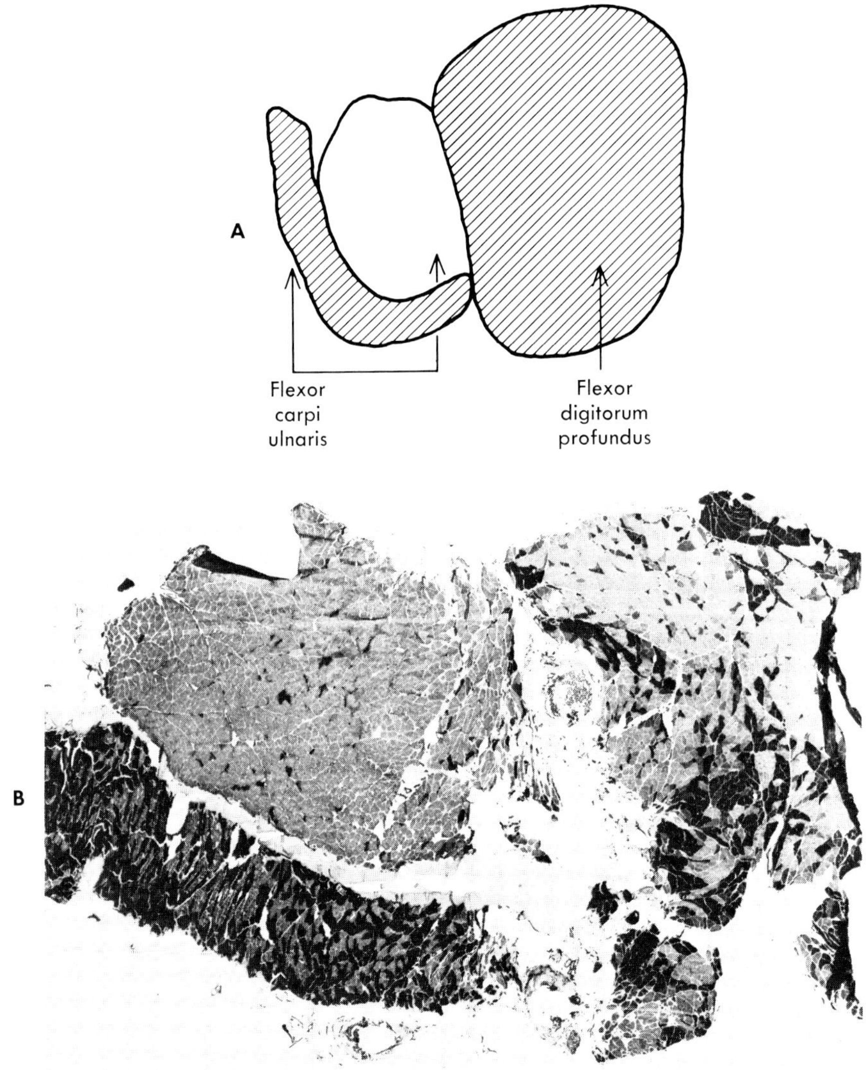

Fig. 37-1. A, Cross-section diagram of normal relationships of forearm muscle in rabbit. Flexor carpi ulnaris (FCU) is innervated by ulnar nerve and is smaller than flexor digitorum profundus (FDP), which is innervated by median nerve. Note that FCU has two muscle heads. Broad flat lateral component stains darkly for anaerobic enzymes (e.g., ATPase) and is therefore characterized as fast. Other portion of FCU is essentially slow, and light staining indicates low content of anaerobic enzymes. Active FDP is dark staining. **B,** ATPase stain of cross section of forearm musculature of rabbit where the median nerve has been sectioned, and denervated FDP (far right) was sutured to normally innervated FCU 1 year previously. These staining characteristics of FCU are normal. Previously denervated FDP (which should stain darkly) is now predominantly lightly stained, indicative of reinnervation from adjacent slow portion of FCU.

cult task. It was determined, however, that histochemistry offered the best evidence of whether nerve regrowth had occurred. In this model a predominantly fast muscle was approximated to a predominantly slow one. It was found that the denervated muscle assumed the general metabolic pattern (fast changed to slow or vice versa) of the innervated muscle. Histologically, type grouping of muscle fibers indicative of reinnervation was seen within the previously denervated muscle (Fig. 37-1). The general histochemical pattern of the muscles that had been left in situ was similar to that noted in successful experimental muscle grafts in cats as recently reported by Hakelius. It is important to emphasize that in our study the amount of atrophy within the denervated muscle was substantial. We observed that frequently only 30% of the original denervated muscle volume was present, a disturbing fact considering that the denervation and muscle approximation were performed simultaneously. It was the purpose of this study to focus on the reinnervation process at the muscular level. The variables of mechanical tension and blood supply were unchanged as best we could determine. Even though there was definite evidence of reinnervation, the substantial amount of atrophy seen suggests that the amount of functioning muscle mass resulting when free grafts of muscle are performed would have to be rather small. However, the functional clinical consequences of this loss in muscle volume have yet to be determined.

We found it surprisingly difficult to *prove* that a free muscle graft is alive and well in its new location. For example, a biopsy showing viable muscle does not necessarily prove that the muscle is indeed the one that was grafted. In addition, there are a number of pitfalls associated with the use of conventional electromyographic techniques, which were extensively employed to prove success in free muscle grafting. Perhaps the greatest problems are those involving volume conduction from adjacent normal muscles. One cannot be entirely sure where the electrode probe is located, and this is particularly important in evaluating relatively small muscles that have been surgically approximated side to side. In this regard, however, when reporting their success with free muscle grafts, Hakelius and Stalberg[14] not only employed conventional electromyography but also single fiber electromyography. Review of their data seems clearly to establish the fact that the grafts have developed a blood supply and neural innervation. From a clinical standpoint, in our experience, single fiber electromyography is a highly reliable tool for the documentation of muscle graft survival.

SUMMARY

Although there has been some controversy regarding free muscle grafts, on the basis of recent experimental and clinical experience it seems certain that under very specific circumstances skeletal muscle can be transferred as a free graft in a variety of animals and in humans. To survive and to function, a muscle graft requires tension and innervation as well as a new vascular supply. The requisite of tension can be satisfied by proper surgical technique. The speed of neovascularization limits the size of the graft. In the early period after transfer the central area of the graft is most vulnerable to anoxic necrosis because the supply of oxygen and nutrients is limited by the distance of diffusion. However, prior denervation stimulates increased capillary vascularity in the graft and increases the chance of vascular anastomoses returning blood flow to the graft. Moreover, prior denervation produces a myoblastic response in dormant satellite cells, thus providing improved conditions for graft regeneration. Current evidence suggests that the original muscle fibers rapidly degenerate and that the more resilient myoblasts ultimately reconstitute the functional fiber units. In order that the graft function, it must obtain innervation from adjacent normally innervated muscle. The process of muscular neurotization does occur. To what extent axonal ingrowth from adjacent muscle will proceed is not fully understood. Further experimental work is necessary to explore the numerous parameters and variables involved in muscle grafting and to corroborate the theoretic physiologic mechanisms before the general use of free muscle grafts in clinical surgery can be recommended.

REFERENCES

1. Buller, A. J., and Lewis, D. M.: Factors effecting the differentiation of mammalian fast and slow muscle fibers. In Gutman, E. and Hink, P. editors: The effect of use and disuse of neuromuscular functions, Prague, 1963, Academia, Publishing House of the Czechoslovak Academy of Science, p. 149.
2. Carlson, B. M.: A qualitative study of muscle fiber survival and regeneration in normal, predenervated, and marcaine-treated free muscle grafts in the rat, Exp. Neurol. **52**:421, 1976.
3. Clark, W. E. L.: An experimental study of the regeneration of mammalian striped muscle, J. Anat. **80**:24, 1946.
4. Close, R.: Effects of cross-union of motor nerves to fast and slow muscles, Nature **206**:831, 1965.
5. Eccles, J. C., Eccles, R. M., and Kozak, W.: Further investigations on the influence of motor neurons on the speed of muscle contraction, J. Physiol. (Lond.) **163**:324, 1962.
6. Erlacher, P.: Direct and muscular neurotization of paralyzed muscles: experimental research, Am. J. Orthop. Surg. **13**:22, 1915.

7. Filogamo, G., and Gabella, G.: Cholinesterase behavior in the denervated and reinnervated muscles, Acta Anat. (Basel) **63:**199, 1966.
8. Frielinger, G., Holle, H., and Mancoli, B.: Free muscle transplants for anal sphincter reconstruction in pigs, Chir. Plast. **2:**133, 1974.
9. Gluck, T.: Ueber Muskei-und Schenplastik, Langenbecks, Arch. Klin. Chir. **26:**61, 1881.
10. Gutman, E.: The denervated muscle, Prague, 1962, Academia, Publishing House of the Czechoslovak Academy of Science.
11. Hakelius, L.: Transplantation of free autogenous muscle in the treatment of facial paralysis, Scand. J. Plast. Reconstr. Surg. **8:**220, 1974.
12. Hakelius, L.: Free autogenous muscle transplantation in two cases of total anal incontinence, Acta Chir. Scand. **141:**69, 1975.
13. Hakelius, L., Nystron, B., and Stalberg, E.: Histochemical neurophysiological studies of autotransplanted cat muscle, Scand. J. Plast. Reconstr. Surg. **9:**15, 1975.
14. Hakelius, L., and Stalberg, E.: Electromyographical studies of free autogenous muscle transplantation in man, Scand. J. Plast. Reconstr. Surg. **8:**211, 1974.
15. Hildebrandt: Ueber eine neus Methods der mustrel Transplantation, Arch. Klin. Chir. **78:**75, 1906.
16. Humoller, F. L., Griswald, B., and McIntire, A. R.: Biochemical and metabolic changes in skeletal muscle following denervation and tenotomy, Am. J. Physiol. **161:**406, 1950.
17. Karpati, G., and Engel, W. K.: The gripping in skeletal muscle after experimental reinnervation, Neurology (Minneap.) **18:**447, 1968.
18. Lavine, D., and Cochran, T.: The failure to survive of autogenous free grafts of whole gracilis muscles in dogs, Plast. Reconstr. Surg. **58:**221, 1976.
19. Magnus, R.: Ueber Muskeltransplantation, Munchen Med. Wochenschr. **37:**515, 1890.
20. Miller, T., Korn, H., Wheeler, E., and Eldridge, L.: Can one muscle reinnervate another? A laboratory study of muscular neurotization, Plast. Reconstr. Surg. **61:**50-57, 1978.
21. Peer, L. A., and Walker, J. C.: The behavior of autogenous human tissue grafts, Plast. Reconstr. Surg. **7:**73, 1951.
22. Peer, L. A.: Transplantation of tissue, Baltimore, 1955, The Williams & Wilkins Company.
23. Roy, P. R.: Behavior-free autogenous muscle graft in skeletal muscle of dogs, J. Exp. Med. Sci. **9:**78, 1966.
24. Studitsky, A. N.: Dynamics of the development of myogenic tissue under conditions of explanation and transplantation. In Rose, G. G., editor: Cinemicrography in cell biopsy, New York, 1963, Academic Press, p. 171.
25. Studitsky, A. N.: Free auto- and homographs of muscle tissue in experiments on animals, Ann. N.Y. Acad. Sci. **120:**789, 1964.
26. Studitsky, A. N., and Bosova, N. N.: Development of atrophic muscular tissue transplanted to supply a defect of mechanically injured muscles, Arch. Anatomii, Gistologii i Embryologii **39:**18, 1960.
27. Thompson, N.: Autogenous free grafts of skeletal muscle. A preliminary experimental and clinical study, Plast. Reconstr. Surg. **48:**11, 1971.
28. Thompson, N.: Investigation of autogenous skeletal muscle free grafts in the dog, Transplantation **12:**353, 1971.
29. Thompson, N.: Treatment of facial paralysis by free skeletal muscle grafts. In Transactions of the Fifth International Congress of Plastic and Reconstructive Surgery, London, 1971, Butterworth, p. 66.
30. Volkmann, R.: Uber die regeneration des quergestreiften muskelgewebes beim menshen ung saugethier, Zigler's Beitr. Pathol. Anat. **12:**233, 1893.
31. Watson, A., and Muir, A.: Failure of free muscle grafts in dogs, Br. J. Plast. Surg. **29:**27, 1976.
32. Walker, J. C., Jr., and Sawhney, O. P.: Free composite lip grafts, Plast. Reconstr. Surg. **50:**142, 1972.
33. Zhenevskaya, R. P.: Experimental histologic investigation of striated muscle tissue, Rev. Can. Biol. **21:**457, 1962.
34. Zhenevskaya, R. P., Rumyantseva, O. N., Novosylova, I. L., and Proshlyahova, E. V.: Regeneration process in the transplant of intact muscle of young rats, Zh. Obshch. Biol. **26:**569, 1965.
35. Zielonko, J.: Ueber die Entwicklung und Proliferation von Epithelien und Endothelien, Arch. Mikroscop. Anat. **10:**351, 1874.

Chapter 38

Ancillary techniques for the amelioration of facial palsy

Bromley S. Freeman

A review of 100 patients who were referred for treatment of facial paralysis and were followed-up from 5 to 30 years forcefully confirms the fact that multiple procedures were necessary after most primary reconstructions. The attempt to restore the delicate orchestral balance of multiple fine muscular interplay by gross transfer of two or even three slow-moving muscles or large fascial slings can be frustrating. Despite multiple modifications of these techniques, at the time of the initial surgical procedure compensatory techniques must be used and constantly tuned over the years. The operations used during the past 30 years for reconstruction of the paralyzed face have included nerve transfers, nerve grafts, masseter and temporalis muscle transfers, as well as suspension and sphincteric reconstruction using fascia, Marlex mesh, and dermis. Auxiliary techniques include release of the pull of overactive contralateral muscles and aesthetic aids such as face-lift, brow-lift, and the creation of nasolabial folds. Dynamic, supportive, gravitational, and reconstructive lid and lip procedures have been added. The type and number of procedures used for each patient are abstracted in Tables 14 and 15.

Invariably patients required one or more accessory procedures as listed in the outline below. Some operations, although considered primary reconstructions, have been added occasionally to modify the results of the initial operation over the years. All of the original methods have been refined and modified (Fig. 38-1).

The following are nonneural operative procedures used for the amelioration of facial paralysis:

A. Dynamic
  1. Muscle transfer
    a. Temporalis
    b. Masseter
    c. Digastric
    d. Sternocleidomastoid
    e. Muscle grafts (free)
  2. Alloplastic motors
    a. Metal spring (upper lid)
    b. Silastic bands on lip and lid
    c. Lid weights
B. Static
  1. Suspension materials
    a. Fascia
    b. Dermis
    c. Silastic rubber
  2. Stabilization materials
    a. Dermal flaps
    b. Marlex
    c. Bone fixation
C. Sphincteric reconstruction
  1. Orbital
    a. Canthoplasties
    b. Bucco-oral reconstruction
    c. Septoplasty
D. Control of antagonist muscles
  1. Neurectomy (temporary chemical or permanent surgical)
  2. Myectomy
E. Rhytidoplasties
  1. Modified cheek plastic surgery
  2. Blepharoplasty
  3. Nasolabial excision
  4. Supraorbital excision and brow-lift
  5. Temporal lift
  6. Labial and mucosal excisions

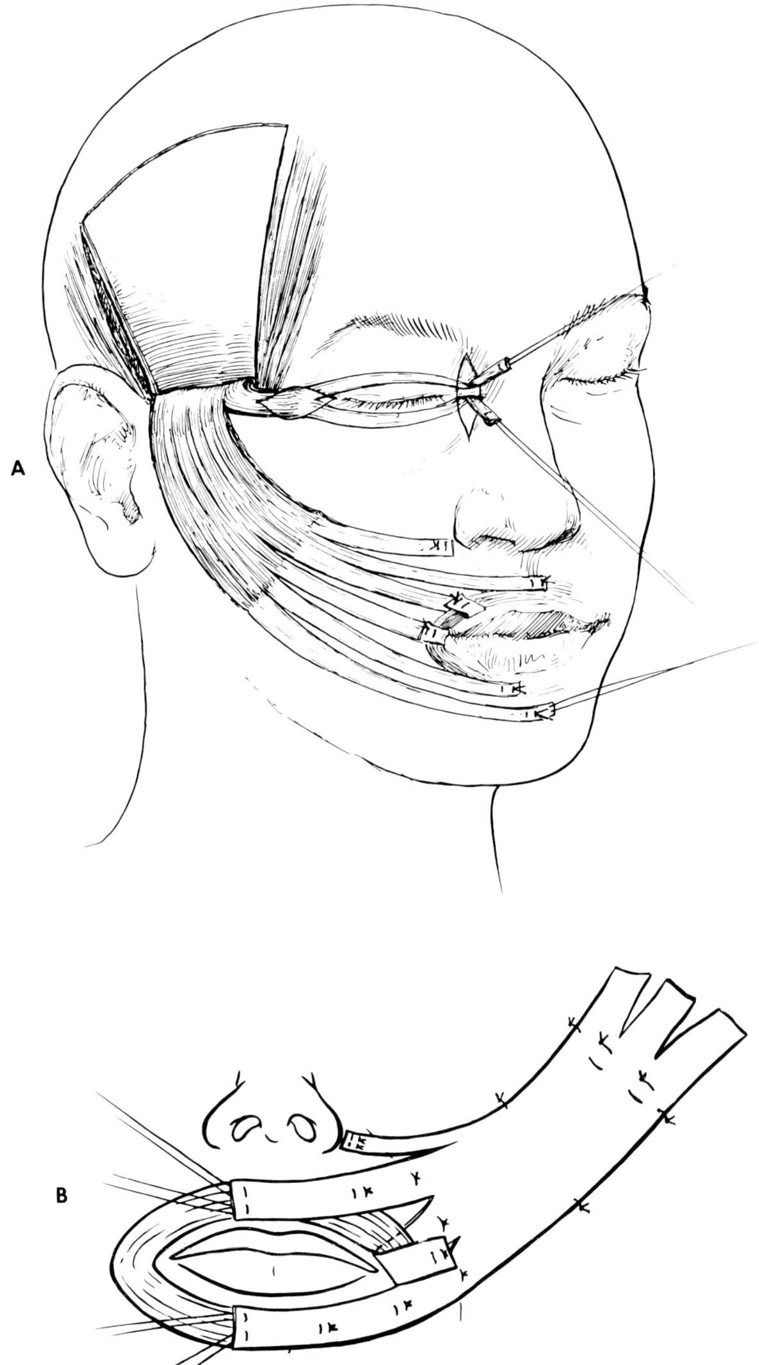

Fig. 38-1. A, Modification of subtotal temporalis muscle transfer for control of sphincters around eye, nose, and mouth. Multiple aponeurotic bands permit some variation in response as well as connect to opposite side, thus combining suspension, dynamism, and reconstruction of sphincter with attempt to simulate facial muscle insertions. Modification has been in use for past 10 years and is superior to gross attachments to orbicularis oris previously used or to combination of masseter and temporalis, also used. **B,** Classic suspension operation using either fascia or Marlex mesh and presently modified by swinging posterior inferior leaf around back of ear and attaching to both concha and mastoid periosteum. (From Converse, J. M., editor: Reconstructive plastic surgery, ed. 2, Philadelphia, 1977, W. B. Saunders Company, vol. 3, pp. 1774-1867.)

After a muscle transplant to the paralyzed side has contributed support and action, selective myectomy or weakening of the muscles on the nonparalyzed side provides better balanced facial expression. Myotomy or the neutralization of antagonistic muscles by neurotomy of the marginal mandibular and temporal branches of the facial nerve or both are usually combined with suspension by fascia or mesh, skin excision, and a modified face-lift, allowing elliptic excision of supraorbital, infralabial, and nasolabial sag. Although those muscles most frequently causing distortion during speech, emotion, and associated actions are the quadratus labii superioris, the depressor labii inferioris, and the zygomaticus, a study of the muscle groups responsible for the distortion permits these to be isolated and sectioned and varying amounts of muscle tissue to be resected. This procedure is of special value in the residual partial palsies after poliomyelitis, after nerve grafting or anastomoses, or in segmental paralyses not amenable to surgical neurorrhaphy or grafting. Dampening the contralateral, often overactive, muscle power in some measure restores

Table 14. Primary procedures for amelioration of facial palsy in 69 adults aged 16 to 75 (average number of operations: 2; average number of procedures per operation: 3)*

Procedure	*No.*
Total suspension	
Fascia	22
Mesh (includes 8 with nerve transfer also)	12†
Dermis	2
TOTAL	36
Nerve transfers	
Eleventh	7
Twelfth	9
TOTAL	16
Muscle transfers	
Temporalis	15
Masseter	2
TOTAL	17

*From Freeman, B. S.: Longterm results following varying techniques for facial palsy. In Marchac, D., editor: Transactions of the Sixth International Congress of Plastic and Reconstructive Surgery, Paris, 1976, Masson, A. S.

Table 15. Primary procedures for amelioration of facial palsy in 31 children aged 2 to 15 (average number of operations: 3; average number of procedures per operation:2)*

Procedure	*No.*
Masseter transfer	6
Temporalis transfer	12
Combined nerve transfer	1

*From Freeman, B. S.: Longterm results following varying techniques for facial palsy. In Marchac, D., editor: Transactions of the Sixth International Congress of Plastic and Reconstructive Surgery, Paris, 1976, Masson, A. S.

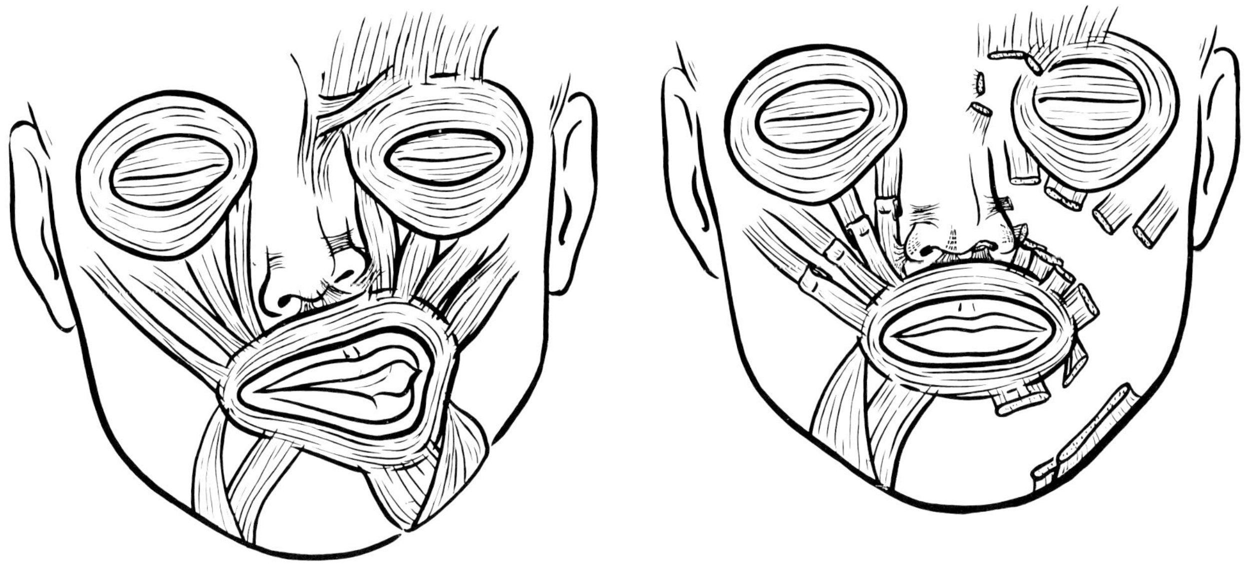

Fig. 38-2. Resection of antagonist (modified considerably from Niklison but retaining no-longer-used "tacking" of lax or flaccid muscles). Resection of all facial muscles is never done, but selection is made individually and when necessary can be repeated. (From Converse, J. M., editor: Reconstructive plastic surgery, ed. 2, Philadelphia, 1977, W. B. Saunders Company, vol. 3, pp. 1774-1867.)

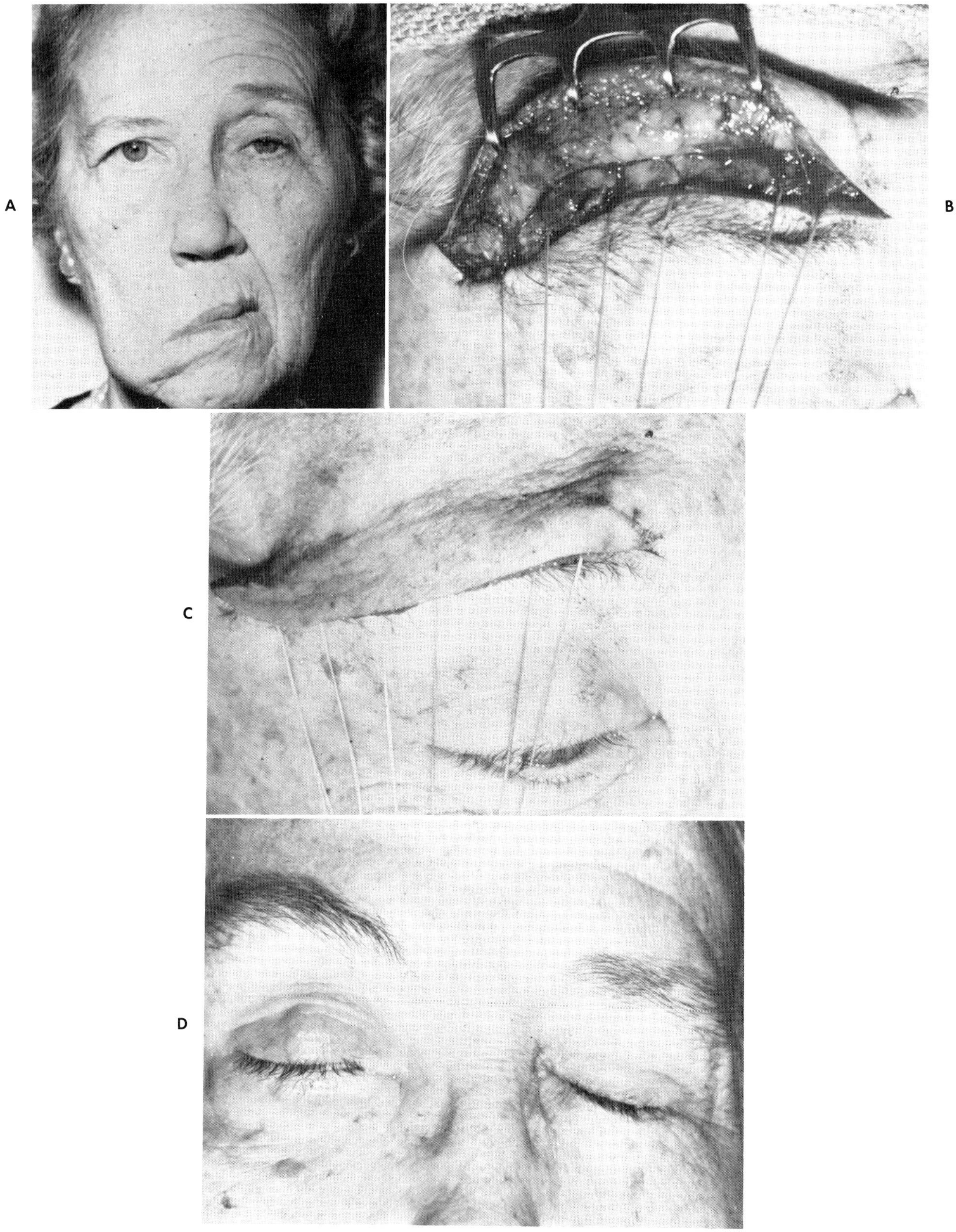

Fig. 38-3. Multiple accessory procedures used to rehabilitate neglected facial paralysis. **A,** Unreconstructed. **B,** After fascial suspension and reconstruction of periorbital and perioral sphincters, attaching dermis of brow to selected position on galea. **C,** Overlap of frontal skin removed. **D,** Several years after surgery, eyes closed.

E

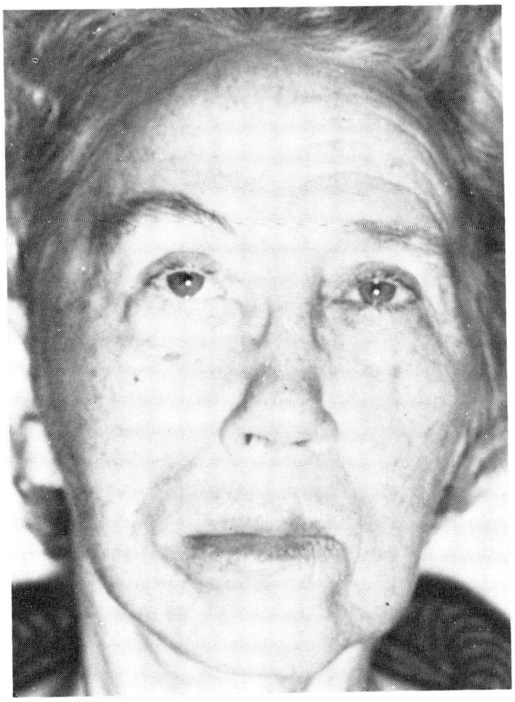

F

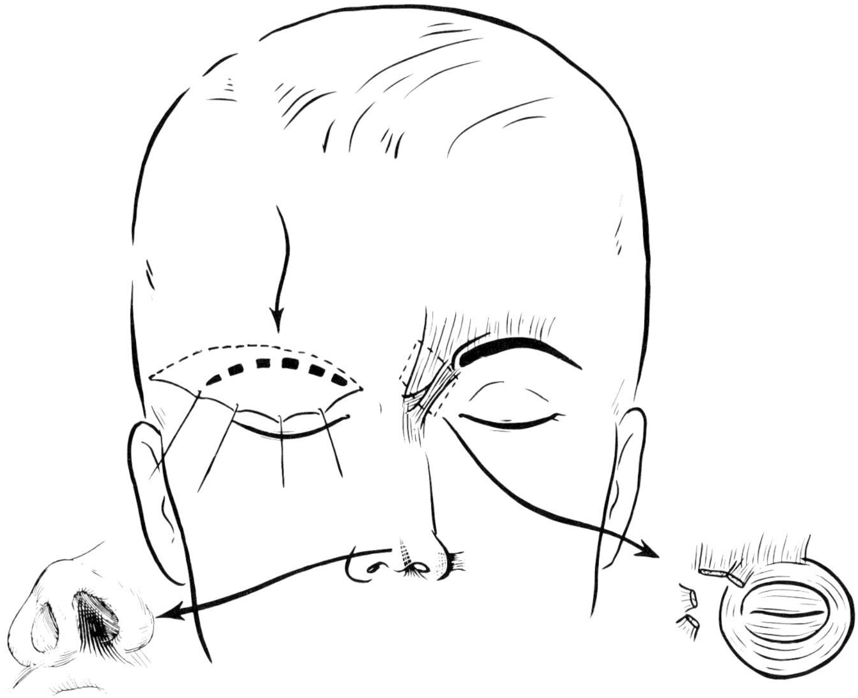

Fig. 38-3, cont'd. E, Eyes opened and relaxed. **F,** Diagram of brow-lift combined with opposite corrugator resection and anterior, septal unopposed pull. (From Converse, J. M., editor: Reconstructive plastic surgery, ed. 2, Philadelphia, 1977, W. B. Saunders Company, vol. 3, pp. 1774-1867.)

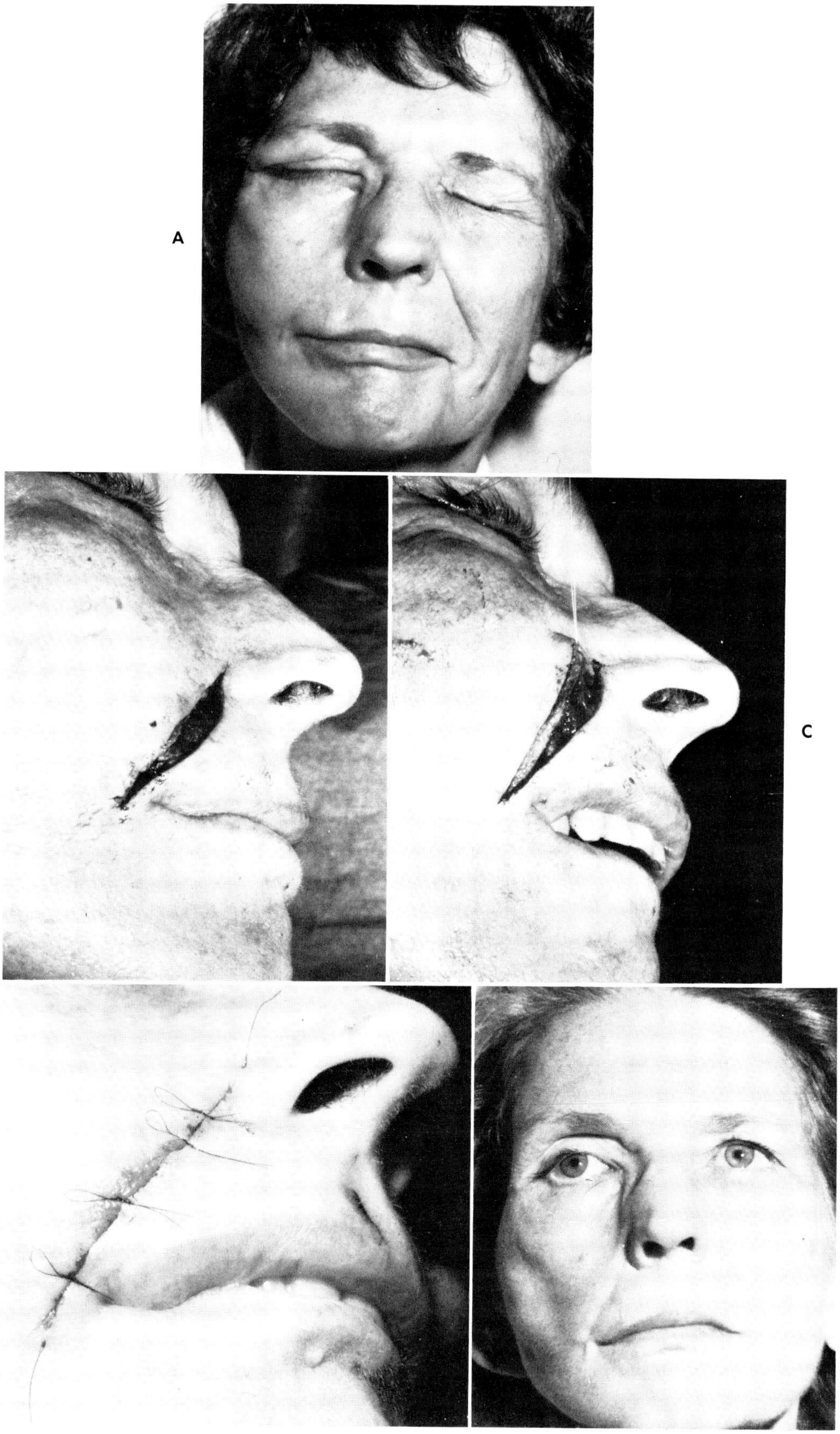

Fig. 38-4. Creation of nasolabial fold. **A,** Patient after total temporalis muscle transfers and face-lifts with absence of right nasolabial fold. **B,** Creation of deepithelialized fat. **C,** Swinging, superior end of deepithelialized flap prior to freeing and attachment to malar fascia (see text). **D,** Dermis-to-dermis closure. **E,** Controlled face, with nasolabial folds, 5 years later. (From Converse, J. M., editor: Reconstructive plastic surgery, ed. 2, Philadelphia, 1977, W. B. Saunders Company, vol. 3, pp. 1774-1867.)

functional balance and symmetry in repose, voluntary activity, and spontaneous emotional action. When myectomy or neurectomy is carried out at the same time as the primary supportive or dynamic reconstruction, there is less strain on new insertions (which require at least 5 weeks to heal). In children, although the residual deformity is diminished by baby fat and the persistence of a certain amount of tissue tone, *antagonist muscle resection* was the most frequent secondary procedure advocated when the face lengthened and the skin and subcutaneous layer thinned (Fig. 38-2).

In adults modification of the contralateral muscles, usually combined with the primary procedure and *balanced cosmetic procedures,* especially brow-lifts and face-lifts, was the most common secondary operation recommended after neural, muscular, or suspensory repair. These multiple aesthetic improvements were necessary because of progressive facial imbalance and its accentuation by age. Except for those patients who had had a nerve crossing or a massive temporalis muscle transfer, all "aged" more rapidly on the paralyzed side. The brow-lift used is that popularized by Castarnares but modified to permit attachment of a deepithelialized flap from the inferior border to the galea or pericranium (Fig. 38-3).

Flattening of the nasolabial fold can be restored by muscle transfer or suspension, but not infrequently a dermal flap reconstruction was used. Formation of the nasolabial fold is preferred to the simple excision of the stretched nasolabial skin. Based on the new nasolabial crease line the thin flap is formed by the "deepithelialized" excess of the stretched skin of the upper lip and cheek. After the "deepithelialized" skin is freed from the underlying subcutaneous tissue and muscle and tailored, the flap swung through a dissected pocket is attached by permanent sutures to the periosteum of the malar bones. A right-angle malar-labial–to–nasolabial attachment of dermis to dermis fashions the new skin fold. Again the perioral area must be splinted for 5 weeks until it is healed, as the opposing muscle pull can loosen the attachment. This procedure is most gratifying to the patient, especially after a face-lift has flattened the nasolabial fold (Fig. 38-4).

Muscle transposition, masseter, or temporalis, maintains support and does not require buccal hernia repair. The segment of broad muscle acts as the buccinator, and sphincter control varies from good to fair. *Mechanical control of the sphincteric weakness* is most important and is immediately regained in muscle transfers and aided in static suspension by

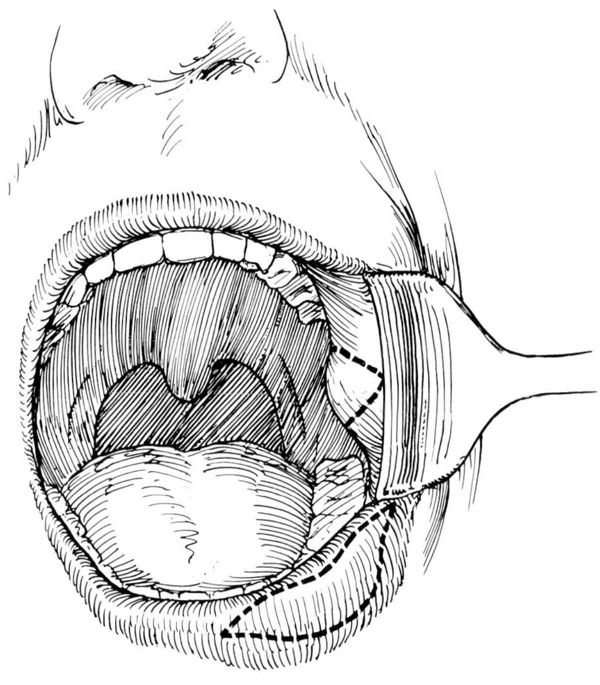

Fig. 38-5. Excision of mucosal and vermilion excess for reduction of protrusion of buccal and labial mucosa in untreated patients. (From Converse, J. M., editor: Reconstructive plastic surgery, ed. 2, Philadelphia, 1977, W. B. Saunders Company, vol. 3, pp. 1774-1867.)

substitution or reinforcement of the defect by a broad sheet of fascia, dermis, or mesh. This may be followed later by buccal and labial mucosal protrusion. Patterned mucosal and vermilion excision will correct this (Fig. 38-5).

The earlier muscle transplants not attached to the ala allowed nasal septal deviation with occasional nares blockage and distortion but only after many years. The adjustment was by septoplasty, and resection of the spastic contralateral muscles (Fig. 38-3, *F*). Muscle transfer (or even the fascial or mesh suspension slip) attached to the ala seems to prevent a septal twist.

COMPLICATIONS

Complications were not too frequent and were those incident to the surgical technique and the age and cooperativeness of the patient. In the very early patients in whom narrow fascial strips were used the bands showed through thinned skin; after 2 or 3 years, some large-band, fascial suspensions in use during the past 20 years slackened and required considerable adjustment. Marlex mesh suspension showed no evidence of contracture, but several required elevation and reattachment of the posterior

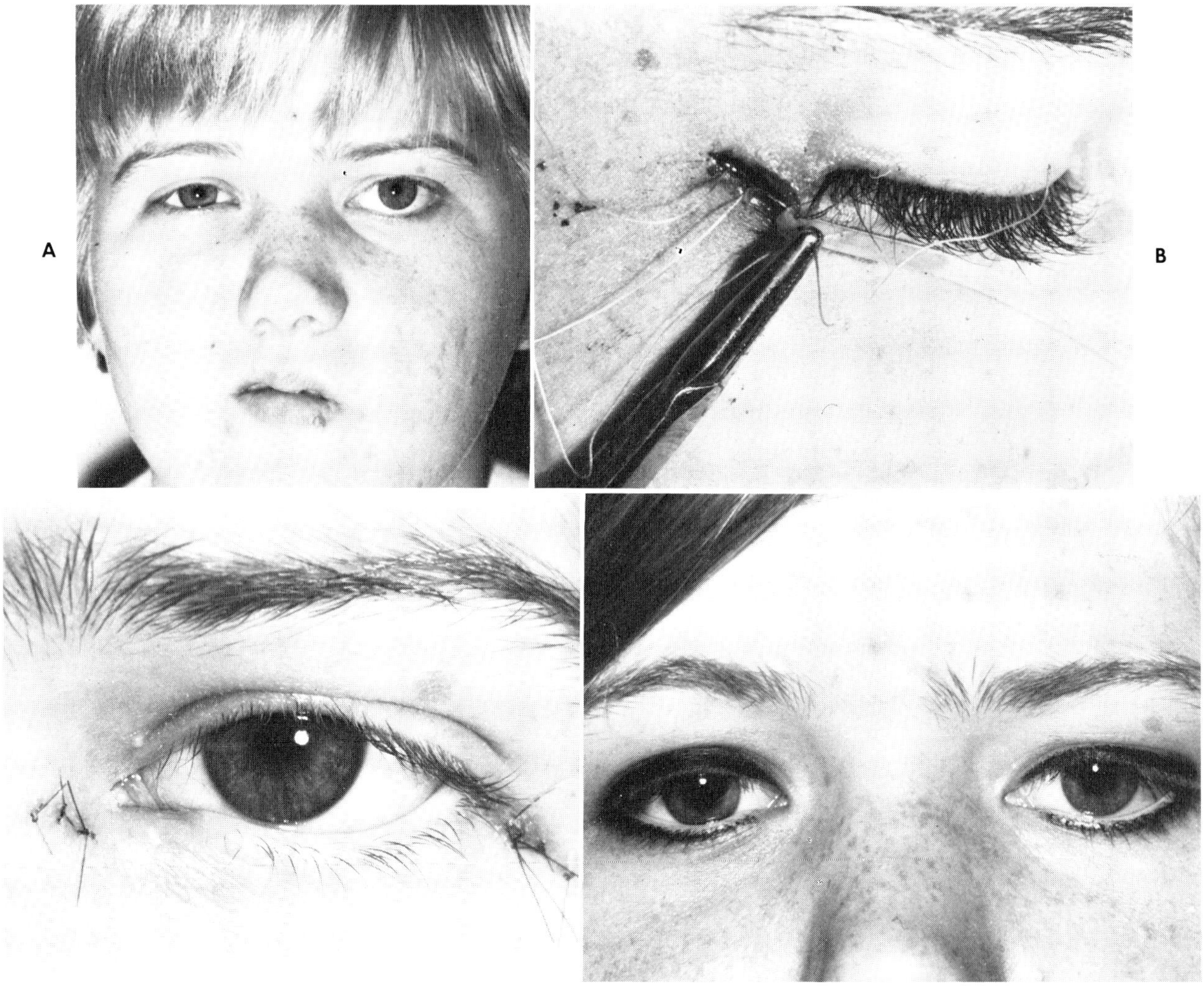

Fig. 38-6. Suspensory Silastic band secured to orbital rim. **A,** Four years after muscle suspension with loss of control of lower lid. **B,** Insertion of Silastic into lower lid just below margin and secured to drill holes in bone with small medial and lateral incisions. **C,** Closure of incisions. **D,** Static suspension of lid still present some 2 years later. (From Converse, J. M., editor: Reconstructive plastic surgery, ed. 2, Philadelphia, 1977, W. B. Saunders Company, vol. 3, pp. 1774-1867.)

leafs to the mastoid and temporal areas because of slackening. In several, however, tension, prominent teeth, and an associated anesthesia of buccal mucosa caused exposure of the mesh. Segmental removal of the mesh and closure of the mucosal defect allowed healing with the residual scar maintaining the buccinator pillow and sphincter continuity. The best results were obtained by staged insertion of the anterior attachment and later elevation and posterior fixation to the mastoid, concha, and temporal regions. Silastic sphincters for lids eventually broke. Suspensions of the lower lid were of much value when fixed to bone (Fig. 38-6).

RESULTS

At rest the majority of the cases looked good. In purposeful activity all of the transferred muscles worked well if further adjustments, such as taking up slack and releasing adhesions, had been carried out. During unguarded, emotional speech, most patients had some form of sphincteric distortion, which could be noted by the trained observer. Patients who practiced in front of a mirror were stilted or affected in their speech yet controlled their grimaces readily. All who had the patience to practice eating, speaking, and showing controlled emotion in front of the mirror improved after months of

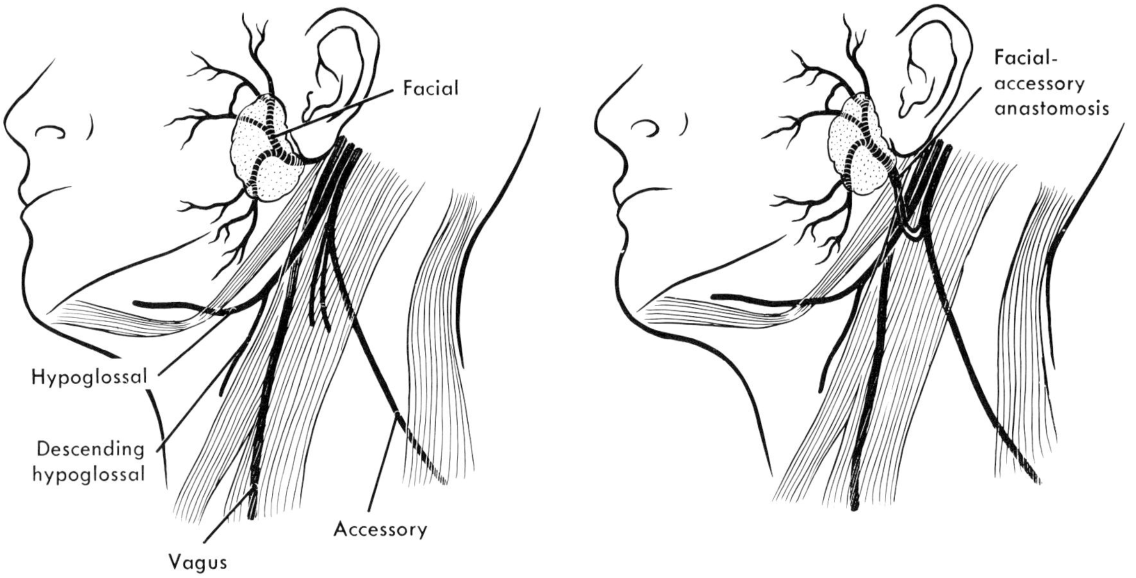

Fig. 38-7. Facial nerve crossover to restore tone. Use of sternocleidomastoid branches of spinal accessory nerve to restore tone without denervation of trapezius. As noted in text, multiple cranial nerves have been used, and although end results of hypoglossal crossover are good, patients had some dysarthria. Patients with this modification of spinal accessory nerve anastomosis have relatively little true motion, and now it would seem that transfer of masseter branch of fifth cranial nerve may become popular (Spira, 1977). (From Converse, J. M., editor: Reconstructive plastic surgery, ed. 2, Philadelphia, 1977, W. B. Saunders Company, vol. 3, pp. 1774-1867.)

assiduous training. It is sad to say that many, after their deformities had been accepted by their friends, desisted in their training efforts after a year or so unless stimulated by continued medical observation.

EXPECTATIONS

All nerve grafts, whether bypass, crossover, or in continuity, are potentially subject to the same mass reflex or irregular response prevalent after facial anastomosis to the fifth, tenth, eleventh, or twelfth nerve (Fig. 38-7). In our hands a degree of this complication has been found even after direct funicular suturing! The approach of greatest promise would seem to be that of Dott in his use of an immediate nerve rerouting from the brain stem through a nerve graft with later secondary reanastomosis to the facial trunk. This, a true bypass, should give a close approximation of the normal in this era of the operating microscope. But, even here the discriminating surgeon may find ancillary procedures necessary! I would anticipate the cross-face nerve grafts of Smith and Anderl to require some amelioration of these irregular responses. Patients operated upon soon after the diagnosis was established had less edema and were rehabilitated earlier, that is, back to work or to normal social customs. Penalties for the delay of surgical, mechanical aid include the development of faulty facial and sphincteric habits, dependent cheek edema becoming organized, with fibrosis of the paralyzed muscle inhibiting the return of tone after neural anastomosis and frequently progressive social seclusion.

DISCUSSION

The interesting, if delayed, results after segmental cross-face-nerve grafts, muscle grafts, and combined neural and muscular grafts may be ushering us into a new era of repair, but caution must be used in attributing the total results to the muscle neurotization or the nerve reanastomosis. The reported good results in cross-face-nerve and muscle grafts undoubtedly have been aided by the modification or dampening of the nonparalyzed side by either severance of multiple small branches of the normal nerve used to innervate the cross-face-nerve grafts or the wide dissection necessary to revascularize and neurotize the free muscle grafts. In the former, during the considerable period of delay, as long as 2 years, many of the complications of untreated paralysis can occur, especially in the elderly. Sphincteric control by shortening, fascial suspension, and myectomy may seem crude and old-fashioned, but it offers immediate support, can be carried out rapidly and early, and can and should be combined with cross-face-nerve grafts.

INDICATIONS

The selection of procedures to be utilized for the individual patient with facial paralysis should be based on an exacting analysis of the deformity, knowledge of the usual results of specific procedures in the individual surgeon's hands and of the requirements, capabilities, and physical condition of the patient. Factors include the degree, extent, and longevity of the paralysis, and the age, life expectancy, and overall prognosis of the patient, as well as his occupation, emotional balance, and social activities. Procedures gauged as to their efficiency are modified and suited to the individual.

Facial gymnastics, precisely outlined by the surgeon and encouraged by relatives and friends, are of great importance. However, after being accepted by their friends, the majority of the adult patients desisted in their training efforts after a year or so. Most children practiced through adolescence. For adults we have advocated crossover facial nerve anastomosis to branches of the opposite facial nerve, to the masseter branch of the fifth nerve, or to the sternocleidomastoid branch of the eleventh nerve, temporalis transfer, hemi–face-lift and brow-lift, selective antagonist myectomies, and reconstruction of the nasolabial fold.

In children the combination of a massive temporalis muscle transfer, selective antagonist myectomy, canthoplasty if required, and a temporary upper lid weight has proved of lasting value. With the advent of microsurgery, neural techniques will be used more frequently.

If the paralysis is thought to be temporary, we use the following procedures: hemi–face-lift, massive fascial or mesh suspension, reconstruction of nasolabial fold, lid adjustment, and elevation of brow.

However, in the aged patient of feeble constitution or in those with a poor prognosis, local anesthesia can be used to perform a hemi–face-lift with brow-lift, mesh suspension, and transfer of the sternocleidomastoid branch of the eleventh nerve to the facial nerve stump. A lid weight and canthoplasty or construction of a Silastic sphincter protects the eye.

SUMMARY

A retrospective study of 100 patients with unilateral palsy of the facial nerve followed-up from 5 to 30 years has shown that few operative procedures for facial paralysis are immune from complications or gradual deterioration of the initial result. Even most patients with successful reanastomosis or rerouting of the seventh nerve require further surgery. Expectations are sufficiently good, contrasted against the alternative, progressive deterioration after paralysis, to warrant early and repeated auxiliary measures; after the preliminary delay in order to allow for a positive and accurate diagnosis a total approach should be considered. Repeated review of the individual is essential as all patients require repeated ancillary surgical aid if followed-up over a sufficiently long period. In few conditions is the continued physician's interest as important as in facial palsy.

In addition to a clinical assessment of spasticity, overflow activity, and volitional control in the muscles, as well as neural and electromyelographic evaluation, any presentation of the results of the amelioration of facial paralysis requires preoperative and postoperative motion study records. Their absence might conceivably lead to a doubt of the validity of the observations. Indeed, audio recordings would help evaluate speech improvement or at least establish a baseline.

SUGGESTED READINGS

Dott, N. M.: Facial paralysis—Restitution by extrapetrous nerve graft, Proc. R. Soc. Med. Lond. **51:**900, 1958.

Freeman, B. S.: An immediate combined approach for rehabilitation of the patient with facial paralysis, Plast. Reconstr. Surg. **37:**341, 1966.

Freeman, B. S.: Silastic rod sling to elevate the paralyzed lower lid, Plast. Reconstr. Surg. **44:**401, 1969.

Freeman, B. S.: Techniques for sphincteric control in facial paralysis. In Conley, J., editor: Plastic and reconstructive surgery of the face and neck, vol 2, Stuttgart, 1972, Thieme. p. 103.

Freeman, B. S.: Late reconstruction of the lax oral sphincter in facial paralysis, Plast. Reconstr. Surg. **51:**144, 1973.

Freeman, B. S.: Longterm results following varying techniques for facial palsy. In Marchac, D., editor: Transactions of the Sixth International Congress of Plastic and Reconstructive Surgery, Paris, 1976, Masson.

Freeman, B. S.: Facial paralysis. In Converse, J. M., editor: Reconstructive plastic surgery, Philadelphia, 1977, W. B. Saunders Company.

Spira, M.: Another method of treatment for facial paralysis: a preliminary report. Presented at the American Association of Plastic Surgery meeting, Chicago, May 1977.

Panel discussion on paralysis of the facial nerve

LEONARD RUBIN, Moderator
HANS ANDERL
MARGARET E. BRAND
JOHN J. CONLEY
BROMLEY S. FREEMAN
MELTON J. HORWITZ
TIMOTHY A. MILLER

Question: At what point are the facial muscles atrophied beyond the possibility of reinnervation?

Anderl: This is not a simple question. Certainly it is age related, as the younger the patient, the longer the expected period of viability. Just before attending this symposium I operated on a 35-year-old man 8 months after removal of a frontocerebellar tumor. He had no muscle activity on EMG in the orbital region, and biopsy showed extensive fibrosis. This contradicts the commonly held opinion that one can wait 1½ to 2 years. I prefer to do the procedure within 6 months, and if we are certain that there will be no nerve recovery, we will do the first stage sooner. You then have another 4 months before you commit the distal end.

Conley: One can evaluate muscle function clinically by looking for residual motion or by EMG evaluation. The facial nerve may have as many as 12 or 13 different connections with other nerves in the area, and by collateral budding the muscles may continue to get some stimuli so that they can be preserved for 1 or 2 years. This mechanism becomes less operative as the patient ages. There may also be segmental differences among the facial thirds. I have examined facial muscles and nerves under the electron microscope up to 50 years after injury and found some muscle fiber, axons, and neurilemmal sheaths. Certainly there were only a few, but nevertheless there were always some present. The facial nerve will grow through barbed wire and concrete if there is a functional muscle to receive it.

Question: Dr. Freeman, would you give us your indications for selecting temporalis versus masseter versus fascia and Marlex?

Freeman: If a neural transplant is not available, then I prefer a temporalis transplant plus a contralateral myectomy. I have used temporary fascial slings, either freeze-dried or autogenous, for support in debilitated patients even 5 or 6 days after craniotomy. I use the masseter mostly for Möbius syndrome, but basically the temporalis is by far the best motor.

Rubin: I agree. The masseter at best pulls directly posteriorly, which is really less satisfactory than the upward pull of the temporalis.

Question: Would Dr. Millesi and Dr. Conley discuss the technical details of direct nerve implantation into muscle?

Millesi: We try to lay the nerve into the muscle as close as possible to the hilum. The muscle is split and the nerve inserted close to the motor end-plates. No sutures are used.

Conley: I just make a small hole in the muscle and plug the nerve in. This technique is not as successful as nerve anastomoses. I've said before that you only have to get the nerve ends in reasonable proximity. They'll come together like a teenage boy and girl in the springtime.

Question: Dr. Brand, when would you decide to use a temporalis muscle transfer for lagophthalmos as opposed to the other available procedures?

Brand, M.: The patient who is obviously beyond recovery of his orbicular function and whose frequent attempts at blinking are evidenced by repeated Bell phenomenon is an excellent prospect for transfer. I have seen some patients who make no attempt to blink and seem to have no urge to do so. Muscle transfers in these patients can be performed perfectly well but will not be used without the subconscious stimulus to protect the eye. For the latter group, Dr. Mühlbauer's lid magnets seem to be an exciting alternative, and I can't wait to try it.

Question: When would you begin reconstruction of a child with congenital palsy?

Rubin: My only experience with transfers in young children has been disastrous. I believe one must wait until there is motivation and cooperation in using the new muscle. I prefer to wait until age 12 or so.

Millesi: We have operated on children as young as 5 or 6, but they must be strongly motivated.

Freeman: I would confirm the importance of patient motivation. I have done the procedures on a 2 year old who is now 10 and using it fairly well. Those patients who had the patience to practice extensively in front of a mirror improved after many months. Their expressions were less stilted, and they grimaced less. If, however, they relaxed their training efforts, the skill was soon lost.

Conley: Congenital seventh nerve palsy can mean anything from a birth injury, to nondevelopment of the nerve, muscle, or both, to an early viral infection. Treatment will depend on the cause. Laminagrams will demonstrate the presence of the fallopian canal, and if it is absent you can assume that there is no nerve, and therefore facial nerve rehabilitation is useless. Similarly electric stimulation will tell you whether there is any functional muscle. I do agree that muscle transfers in children do not work well.

Question: Dr. Miller, do you think there is an actual indication for free muscle grafting in the face?

Miller: Quite frankly, on the basis of Dr. Thompson's work, I'd have to say "no." However, the reports of Hakelius from Sweden are most encouraging. Certainly it seems successful in rats and lower animals. However, I don't believe that the muscle survives as a graft but rather that just its periphery becomes neurotized, and the rest fibroses and becomes a passive sling. I'm not sure that it is a procedure that is certain enough to justify its use today.

Millesi: We also have done some cases as Thompson described, with little certainty that they functioned any better than a fibrous sling. We have had success, however, by interposing a long nerve graft to a functioning muscle, and after this is healed we transfer the muscle with its new lengthened nerve supply intact. This is too new to really comment on its efficacy.

Question: Dr. Mühlbauer, how available are your magnets?

Mühlbauer: They are commercially available from the firm that produces them in Munich (see p. 284). Hopefully, they will be distributed here in the United States for between \$10 and \$20 per magnet.

Index